Handbook of Geriatric Medicine

Handbook of Geriatric Medicine

Edited by Mason Button

hayle
medical

New York

Hayle Medical,
750 Third Avenue, 9th Floor,
New York, NY 10017, USA

Visit us on the World Wide Web at:
www.haylemedical.com

ISBN: 978-1-63241-549-3

Printed in China.

Cataloging-in-Publication Data

Handbook of geriatric medicine / edited by Mason Button.
p. cm.
Includes bibliographical references and index.
ISBN 978-1-63241-549-3
1. Geriatrics. 2. Aging. 3. Gerontology. 4. Older people--Diseases.
5. Older people--Health and hygiene. I. Button, Mason.
RC952 .H36 2019
618.97--dc23

Table of Contents

Preface

This book has been an outcome of determined endeavour from a group of educationists in the field. The primary objective was to involve a broad spectrum of professionals from diverse cultural background involved in the field for developing new researches. The book not only targets students but also scholars pursuing higher research for further enhancement of the theoretical and practical applications of the subject.

Geriatric medicine is aimed at the promotion of health in older adults. There is no particular age at which patients are placed under the care of a geriatrician. It depends on the patient's needs. Owing to a physiologic decline in organs, older adults develop certain diseases and complications from even minor problems. Sometimes, even multiple problems can compound, often leading to polypharmacy. This can lead to adverse drug reactions and drug interactions. Geriatric medicine can have several specializations, depending on the care provided to the elderly. Some of such specializations are geriatric nephrology, geriatric dentistry, geriatric rheumatology, geriatric urology, etc. This book provides comprehensive insights into the field of geriatric medicine. It presents researches and studies performed by experts across the globe. It will help the readers in keeping pace with the rapid changes in this field.

It was an honour to edit such a profound book and also a challenging task to compile and examine all the relevant data for accuracy and originality. I wish to acknowledge the efforts of the contributors for submitting such brilliant and diverse chapters in the field and for endlessly working for the completion of the book. Last, but not the least; I thank my family for being a constant source of support in all my research endeavours.

Editor

1

Preliminary evidence for an increased likelihood of a stable trajectory in mild cognitive impairment in individuals with higher motivational abilities

Myriam V. Thoma[1,2,13*], Simon Forstmeier[1,3], Roger Schmid[4], Oliver Kellner[5,6], Franziskos Xepapadakos[7], Ursula Schreiter Gasser[8], Andreas Blessing[9], Axel Ropohl[10,11], Gabriela Bieri-Brüning[12], Dries Debeer[1] and Andreas Maercker[1,2]

Abstract

Background: Motivational abilities (MA), that describe skills in relation to goal-oriented behavior, have recently been found to be associated with neuropathological aging. Here we examine the impact of MA on the long-term course of mild cognitive impairment (MCI).

Methods: We followed-up $N = 64$ individuals diagnosed with MCI ($M_{age} = 73$ years, 44% female) for 3 years. MA were assessed by long-term informants of the participants using two scales: motivation and decision regulation [Volitional Components Questionnaires, VCQ, (Kuhl and Fuhrmann, Decomposing self-regulation and self-control: the volitional components inventory, 1998)]. Cognitive abilities were assessed with the Mini Mental State Examination (J Psychiatr Res 12:189-98, 1975). Survival analyses and multilevel modeling (MLM) were applied to determine the predicting effect of informant-rated MA at baseline on the likelihood of MCI stability and on the trajectory of cognitive abilities.

Results: Fifty percent ($n = 32$) of the MCI participants remained stable, while 32.8% ($n = 21$) and 17.2% ($n = 11$) converted to Alzheimer's disease (AD) or dropped-out, respectively. Survival analyses revealed that MCI cases with higher-rated MA at baseline were more likely to exert a stable course in MCI over 3 years ($p = 0.036$) when controlling for demographic characteristics and executive function. MLM analyses indicated that higher informant-rated MA at baseline were significantly related to higher cognitive abilities, even when controlling for MCI subtype ($p = 0.030$).

Conclusions: This study provides preliminary longitudinal evidence for a lower risk of conversion to AD and higher cognitive abilities by higher rated MA at an early stage of MCI.

Keywords: Mild cognitive impairment, Stability, Informant-rated motivational abilities

* Correspondence: m.thoma@psychologie.uzh.ch
[1]University of Zurich, Binzmuehlestr, 14, 8050 Zurich, Switzerland
[2]University Research Priority Program "Dynamics of Healthy Aging", University of Zurich, Zurich, Switzerland
Full list of author information is available at the end of the article

Background

Mild cognitive impairment (MCI) is defined as an objectified decline of cognitive abilities in an individual over time in at least one cognitive domain, while independence with regard to functional abilities prevails and dementia criteria are not met [1]. Alzheimer's disease (AD) dementia is a slowly progressive neurodegenerative disorder including a gradual cognitive decline in more than one cognitive domain, most common is the amnestic syndrome, and in functional abilities of daily living [2]. AD differs from other dementia by the 'cause' of the dementia, i.e., the underlying pathophysiological changes within the brain. On a biochemical level, the accumulation of the amyloid-beta peptide (A*B*) in the brain has been identified as a crucial element in the pathology of AD [3].

While in many AD cases, MCI can be identified as a prodromal syndrome, not all MCI cases progress to AD or other types of dementia [4]; rather, some cases remain stable or even revert to previous cognitive performances (e.g., [5]). However, an increased understanding of why individuals differ in their stability or progression of MCI, i.e., what factors predict favorable courses, rather than a further decrease in cognitive abilities and thus conversion to dementia, would provide crucial indications about how preventive measures and therapeutic interventions could best be applied.

This study has been conducted to understand the predictive role of motivational abilities on the course of MCI. Given the strong link to current brain and cognitive reserve models, we start with describing these models in more detail. In a next step, we provide an extensive definition of motivational abilities, as those build the basis for the motivational reserve (MR) model. Due to its relatively new emergence into the scientific literature, we further describe the MR model and the rationale behind its supposedly protective effect against cognitive decline. For this, we provide an overview over previous studies conducted with cognitively intact and cognitively impaired older adults. Finally, we present our main research question.

Brain and cognitive reserve and resilience

Dementia progression is characterized by a substantial interindividual heterogeneity that cannot be sufficiently explained with disease characteristics [6]. Contextual factors, including social aspects, psychological and physical factors have to be taken into account when aiming to predict progression of dementia [6]. Previous research indicates that living a physically, socially and intellectually stimulating and active life may have a protective impact on the pathophysiological process of MCI and AD (for an overview see [7]). This phenomenon became known as the so-called brain or cognitive reserve [8–10]. The cognitive reserve model builds upon the epidemiological observation that despite the presence of AD neuropathology, some older individuals do not show clinical signs of cognitive impairment (e.g. [11]). Within a new framework proposed by Arenaza-Urquijo and Vemuri [12] this phenomenon that has been described as 'resilience'to AD, i.e., normal cognitive functioning despite underlying substantial AD pathologies (versus 'resistance'i.e., normal cognitive functioning without/low underlying substantial AD pathologies). According to the cognitive reserve model, the available reserve within the brain (of hereditary or acquired origin, or both) can tolerate or absorb neurodegenerative processes before the underlying pathophysiological process becomes clinically manifested [13]. The higher the reserve within the brain, the more neuropathology is required in order to interfere with cognition and functional abilities [14].

While the brain and cognitive reserve models are crucial in the understanding of interindividual differences in the susceptibility for developing clinically relevant AD pathology [14], the current models lack to acknowlegde factors that influence the "whys" an individual initiates and carry out those activites in the first place. This question relates to motivational abilities, that lie at the bottom of such behavior [15].

Motivational abilities

Motivational abilities are crucial for the understanding of the trajectory of an individual's personal and professional life as they are skills necessary to pursue goals. The way an individual pursues a particular goal, changes as a function of age. Several motivational theories exist that focus on variabilities in goal management over the life-course, such as the dual-process framework [16], the model of selection, optimization and compensation [17] or the life-span theory of control [18].

In general, two different stages can be differentiated in the pursuit of goals: the stage of selecting a particular goal (=goal-setting phase) and the stage of goal-striving [19]. For the goal-setting phase, aspects of control and expectancy are needed. A prominent concept related to this is the self-efficacy concept by Bandura [20] which describes the strength of belief one has in his or her own capabilities to deal with life's challenges. For the goal-striving phase, aspects of volition and self-regulation are of importance, such as motivation, decision and activation regulation. Motivation regulation refers to the ability to keep oneself motivated when difficulties arise [21]. Decision regulation describes the ability to make self-congruent decisions [21]. Activation regulation finally is essential to initiate activities planned to reach a set goal [22]. These regulation processes are illustrated by the following hypothetical example: decision regulation processes are required when an individual makes the decision to register for an exam which is mandatory to graduate from college (=

self-congruent goal). The repeated process to activate oneself to study for this exam, rather than spending time with friends, requires activation regulation processes. To keep up with the study plan despite adverse circumstances, such as also having to work night shifts, requires motivation regulation. Finally, the belief that one can achieve the set goal despite a potentially unfavorable environment involves self-efficacy. Together, motivational abilities are involved in the phases of setting and striving a particular goal and are of thus integral part of goal-directed human behavior.

Possible mechanisms underlying the association between motivational reserve and cognitive trajectories

It follows that motivational aspects are intrinsically connected to activities and behaviors traditionally associated with cognitive reserve. This notion is supported by previous empirical work in varying areas. Objective career success has been found to be meaningfully related to motivation [23]. Self-motivation, expected benefits, intention to exercise are all relevant aspects in explaining "why" an individual engages in physical activity [24]. It becomes obvious that motivation ('will') and cognition ('skill') are both crucial factors for achievements by self-regulated learning [25]. Given this close link between the psychological entities of motivation and cognition [26] "cognitive" activities or behaviors may not be examined in isolation of motivational abilities that lie at the bottom of such behavior. Given the intrinsic connection between motivation and cognition, our research group expanded existing reserve models with motivation-related aspects (motivational reserve [MR], [27]).

The basic assumption of the MR model is that motivational abilities of an individual exert a protective influence against neuropathological damage. The assumed underlying mechanism is believed to work in analogy to the brain or cognitive reserve concepts [8–10, 28]. With regard to possible mechanisms, current understanding is that an adequate stimulation of the brain through particular experiences, training or exercise of certain abilities, such as within the context of education, occupation or leisure activities throughout the lifespan is a prerequisite to increase cognitive reserve [14]. The suggested underlying neural basis discussed hereby are the enhancement of the interconnectivity of various brain networks in form of higher efficiency and capacity and compensatory mechanisms [14, 29]. The increased use of brain areas specifically related to motivational abilities is assumed to promote synapse formation and neuronal growth, which then lead to higher efficiency within the brain, that in turn allows the compensation of impaired neuronal networks [30, 31]. For instance, self-efficacy has been found to predict performances in a memory task after 6 years in a sample of older adults [32]. Or internal locus of control, which describes the confidence that one's action lead to a particular outcome, a construct with strong similarities to self-efficacy [33], were found to be related to the volume of the hippocampus in older adults [34]. A potentially indirect mechanism may also be assumed by which motivation influences the experience of stress, and promotes emotional health or cognition [30, 31].

Previous research on the association between midlife motivational abilities and cognitive decline

Previous research efforts provided first evidence of a meaningful association between higher motivational abilities and decreased cognitive decline. In a cross-sectional study with non-demented individuals of 60-years of age and older, it was examined whether midlife motivational abilities, that were estimated on the basis of participant's professional history, were related to cognitive status, well-being and the risk to develop MCI [30]. For this, the *Occupational Information Network* (O*Net; [35, 36]) was used to code all occupations a participant had in his / her professional life. For each profession, motivational abilities necessary to conduct the job were rated by two individual raters (for an extensive description of the exact method, see [30]). It was found that motivation-related occupational abilities were related to the risk of MCI, as well as cognitive status and well-being [30]. This was found even when factors were controlled that are generally related to cognitive reserve concepts, such as education and cognitive ability. In a next step, our research group took this question one step further and examined the same research question in the context of a prospective study with a larger (over 2000 older adults) and older (age of 75-years or older), non-demented sample [31]. It was found that high motivation-related occupational abilities were related to reduced risk (– 35%) to develop MCI and AD (in ApoE epsilon4 carriers only, [31]). These studies provided initial support that motivational abilities are associated in a meaningful way with the risk for the development of cognitive decline.

Predictive effect of current motivational abilities on cognitive decline

It remains unclear whether motivational abilities can be used to predict the course of existing cognitive decline. It is assumed that individuals with higher motivational abilities may exert a more stable course as compared to individuals with lower motivational abilities due to their higher reserve.

Palmer and colleagues showed that motivational abilities may still exert a protective influence in the context of existing cognitive decline [37]. This study was centered around the syndrome apathy, which includes a lack of motivation in its set of criteria [38]. The authors reported significant increases in the risk for conversion from MCI to AD in apathetic patients [37].

Goals of the present study

In previous studies, a retrospective estimate of motivational abilities has been used to examine the potentially protective effect of motivational abilities on cognitive decline [30]. This retrospective estimate was created by rating midlife motivational abilities on the basis of a participant's occupational history (O*Net; [35, 36]). While this method showed to be a valuable approach to estimate midlife motivational abilities, they are nonetheless indirect measures. In the presence of a lack of assessment of motivational abilities in midlife, which would have been the optimal measure for the use as predictor, what are acceptable alternatives? Retrospective assessments suffer from recall biases (e.g. [39]). What is more, given the reduced abilities of accurate self-judgements in individuals with cognitive decline [40] current self-reports of one's abilities may be less accurate. We therefore chose informant-rated motivational abilities as predictors for this study to examine whether they can be used to predict the long-term course of MCI.

Therefore, we aimed to examine the hypothetically protective influence of current motivational abilities that were rated by informants of the participants, on the stability of MCI. In this study, we focused on the motivational abilities 'decision regulation' (= to decide to do a specific task) and 'motivation regulation' (= to stay with the task). These two motivational abilities were chosen as, in contrast to the rather robust self-efficacy 'belief', they are modifiable and thus well applicable for potentially future intervention. From a content-related as well as methodological perspective, decision and motivation regulation belong together and should as such be assessed in combination, without the additional assessment of other motivation-related constructs (e.g. activation regulation). We hypothesized that individuals with higher-rated motivational abilities would exhibit an increased likelihood for stability of MCI, as compared to MCI individuals with lower informant-rated motivational abilities, when followed-up for a period of 3 years.

Methods

The data presented here have been sampled in the context of the longitudinal study "Motivational Reserve as a Protective Factor in Mild Alzheimer's Dementia and Mild Cognitive Impairment" (MoReA, [41]).

Study participants

For recruitment and diagnostic purposes, we cooperated with several different German-speaking Swiss and Austrian memory clinics and specialized institutions for cognitive impairment and dementia. Diagnostic assessments were conducted by neuropsychologists and medical doctors at the respective institutions, independently, and before the partaking of the participants in the current study. In each of the cooperating memory clinics, diagnoses for participants were made in consensus in an interdisciplinary team, after an extensive psychiatric, neurological, clinical and neuropsychological assessment (see detailed diagnostic assessment below). Inclusion criteria for study participation were as follows: willingness to partake in the longitudinal study, minimum age of 60 years, and the clinical diagnoses of MCI and mild AD. For this study, only individuals diagnosed with MCI were included. Exclusion criteria applied in the MoReA-study were the diagnosis of a pure vascular dementia or diagnoses of Parkinson's, Creutzfeld-Jakob's or Pick's disease, as well as traumatic injuries to or previous surgeries of the brain, as well as neurological diseases or syndromes such as epilepsy, post-encephalitic or post-concussional syndromes. Further exclusion criteria were chronic diseases (such as HIV, metabolic or hematologic disorders), severe organ failure, history of malignant diseases or current psychiatric disorders other than mild AD. Potential participants and their informal caregivers were informed about the study by the clinical experts at the specialized clinics and institutions. In case of expressed interest by the patients to partake in the study, participants had to complete a written informed consent at the respective clinic allowing the project researchers to contact them. Contact details, diagnostic information and neuropsychological data were provided to the researchers. Together, the memory clinics referred $n = 133$ individuals to the study center (= baseline participation rate). Almost 30% ($n = 22$) refused at that stage to participate in the study. Reasons for non-participation were excessive demands after learning about the diagnosis, or the informants had no time to take part in the study.

Informants

In order to be able to participate in the study, patients were required to be accompanied by an informant, i.e., a reliable source of information. Those informants were predominantly partners of the participants (70%), children (17%), or other relatives and friends of the patients (13%). Most of the informants see the patients on a daily or almost daily basis (73.6%) or several times per week (5.7%). On average, informants know the patients since 46 years (SD = 14.02), with a range of 6 to 70 years. Written informed consent was obtained from all informants.

Procedure

Baseline assessment (time 1, t1)

A first appointment was arranged with the patients and their informants, during which in-depth information with regard to content and procedure of the study was provided by the researchers. In the case of persisting interest, the patients and their informants both provided written informed consent. During the remaining time of this first appointment, data collection started, separately for the patient and the informant, in two different rooms. Neuropsychological, psychiatric, motivational, cognitive and socio-demographic information were assessed during the second part of the first meeting and completed on a second meeting, an approximately 2.5 h appointment conducted within the next week.

Follow-ups (t2, t3, t4)

Clinical, neuropsychological and cognitive data were re-assessed during meetings of approximately 1.5–2 h, separated by 12-month intervals. Data sampling was executed in a similar fashion as on the baseline assessment (i.e., separately for the patient and the informal caregiver). The informal caregiver was interviewed once per follow-up. All patient interviews over the course of the 3 years were conducted by the same interviewer. This research assistant has also been the constant contact person for the patients and informal caregivers. The interviewer for the informal caregivers varied. For the assessment at t1, as well as for all follow-ups, participants were reimbursed with 50 Swiss Francs. The ethics committees of the Zurich cantonal medical authority approved the research protocol.

Diagnostic assessment of MCI and AD

An extensive battery of diagnostic instruments for MCI and AD has been used in the MoReA study (for a complete overview see, [41]). In the following, we list those instruments that have been applied in the present analyses.

Taking into account the international consensus criteria [42], MCI was operationalized in the current study as following: a) not meeting the DSM-IV criteria for dementia (Mini Mental State Examination, MMSE, score of 24 points or higher, [43]), b) cognitive decline reported by the patient and / or informant, and / or quantifiable deteriorating cognitive abilities over time, c) no impairment in basic activities of daily living and only minimal impairment in complex instrumental functions (Clinical Dementia Rating Scale, CDR, required score of 0.5 points, [44]) and d) impairment (at least mildly) in one or more of the subsequent domains: memory, executive function, attention, language and praxis. The criterion for cognitive decline was > 1.5 standard deviation impairment compared to age and education corrected norm scores.

The diagnostic criteria given by the *Diagnostic and Statistical Manual of Mental Disorders* (DSM-IV-TR, American Psychiatric Association, [45]) and those of the *National Institute of Neurological and Communicative Disorders and Stroke-Alzheimer's Disease and Related Disorders Association* (NINCDS-ADRDA, [2]) were used for the diagnosis of probable AD. The NINCDS-ADRDA criteria require a history of cognitive decline and evidence of impairment in memory and at least one other cognitive domain. Possible AD cases (in NINCDS-ADRDA terminology) were also included, i.e., persons who met these criteria and also had another condition thought to be contributing to cognitive impairment. Diagnostic criteria for AD involved an insidious onset and observable progression or quantifiable worsening of cognitive impairment (in memory and at least in one other cognitive domain) and meaningful functional impairment. Mild AD cases were selected on the basis of a CDR score of 1 [46] and MMSE score between 18 and 28 points (DSM-IV-TR, American Psychiatric Association, [45]).

For the assessment of cognitive function, we applied the *Consortium to Establish a Registry for Alzheimer's Disease – Neuropsychological Assessment* NINCDS-ADRDA, (CERAD-NP, [44]). The CERAD-NP consists of the MMSE [43] and an additional 13 measures related to cognitive functioning (for a complete overview see, [41]). To diagnose and determine the severity of AD, we applied the widely used, semi-structured CDR interview [44].

Classification of participants into subgroups

The participants that were diagnosed with MCI at both t1 and all follow-ups until t4 (i.e., those participants that remained stable with regard to their cognitive decline throughout the observation period of 3 years), were classified into the subgroup *'MCI stability'*. Those participants that converted to (any degree of severity of) AD by the assessment at t4, were classified into the group *'MCI conversion'*.

Psychometric assessment of motivational abilities – main predictor

We further assessed a composite measure of patients' motivational abilities at baseline (= current motivational abilities) through informant-ratings of two different scales for motivation and decision regulation. Two scales of the *Volitional Components Questionnaires* (VCQ) [21] were applied to measure 'motivation regulation' (e.g., "I can usually motivate myself quite well if my determination to persevere weakens"; Cronbach's alpha = .87) and 'decision regulation' (e.g., "When I think about doing or not doing something, I usually arrive at a decision quickly"; Cronbach's alpha = .69).

The original scales are all constructed as self-report measures. To receive informant-rated measures, we reformulated the original items in such a way that the item can be applied as informant-rated measures (e.g., original item "I can usually handle whatever comes my way"; re-formulated item "He/she can usually handle whatever comes his / her way"). There is a small to moderate correlation between informant and self-rated motivational abilities [41].

To summarize, a composite measure including two scales, which were z-transformed beforehand, was created for the assessment of the current informant-rated motivational abilities of the participants.

Additional variables

General information, including living situation, family status, education, former occupation and health, were assessed with self-reports. For an extensive description of former occupation of the sample and how it was assessed, we refer to Forstmeier and Maercker [41]. Rather than a measure for physical health in general, we assessed risk factors with regard to cardiovascular health, as those have previously been found to meaningfully increase risk for AD (e.g. [47]). We assessed following factors to calculate a proxy for cardiovascular risk: diagnosis of diabetes mellitus, diagnosis of elevated cholesterol and high blood pressure. Out of these variables we calculated a composite measure for cardiovascular risk.

To control for depression, we applied the German version of the *Geriatric Depression Scale* (GDS, [48, 49]). The Cronbach's alpha of 0.91 indicates a high internal consistency [48]. As protective factor, we included education (numbers of years of education) as a proxy for cognitive reserve. To control for the effect of higher or lower executive functions on MCI stability or conversion or the trajectory of cognitive abilities, we included the Stroop-Color Word test [50].

Statistical analyses

All statistical analyses were performed using SPSS for Mac OSX (22.0) software packages (IBM, Chicago, IL, USA). Descriptive analyses were used for the calculation of mean (M) and standard deviation (SD). To assess potential demographic differences between groups, t-tests, and chi-square tests were applied. Bivariate correlations were performed to identify relationships between variables of interest. Little's missing completely at random (MCAR) test was conducted to test whether data was missing in a random way [51]. All data was found to be MCAR. Multiple imputation was used to address missing data. The incomplete variables were imputed variable by variable: a filled-in variable is then used as a predictor in subsequent steps. SPSS automatically used the monotone method (multiple imputation algorithms). SPSS applies sequential regression imputation, i.e., linear and logistic regression for continuous variables and categorical variables, respectively. Diagnoses of drop-outs were not imputed. The variables age, sex, MCI subtype, education (years) had no missing values. The variables 'motivational abilities', 'children', and 'cardiovascular risk factors' had 1.89, 15.09, and 24.53% missing values, respectively. Analyses of whether conclusions depend on the imputed variable revealed only minimal differences between the imputed and non-imputed data set with no change in the conclusions.

The analytic method of survival analysis using logistic regression has been chosen to predict which patients are most likely to stay stable, i.e., keep MCI diagnosis within the observation period of 3 years [52]. Hosmer and Lemeshow test results were used to test whether the models were a good fit for the data. An odds ratio (OR) lower than 1 is indicative of an increased risk for conversion, while an OR higher than 1 indicates a reduced risk for conversion. Given the limited power due to the relative low number of observations and the data reduction due to dichotomizing into 'MCI stability' and 'MCI conversion', we added additional calculations with multilevel modeling [53]. Multilevel modeling was used to test whether the trajectory in cognitive abilities, as measured with the MMSE, can be predicted by informant-rated motivational abilities. Our sample size for multilevel modeling is sufficient for an accurate estimation [54, 55]. Multilevel modeling was conducted with a non-imputed data set. As a measure of fit, the Akaike information criterion (AIC) was applied. Smaller values in the AIC are indicative of a better fit of a model [53]. For the calculation of R^2 for multilevel modeling, we used calculations provided by Xu [56]. Data sets for the survival analyses as well as for the multilevel model were vertically arranged, resulting in number of observations rather than number of patients.

All reported results were considered to be significant at the $p \leq 0.05$ level and were considered a trend at the $p \leq 0.1$ level.

Results

Sample characteristics

At t1, the study included $n = 64$ MCI participants. Sample characteristics at t1 are shown without the inclusion of participants that dropped-out from the study ($n = 11$) within the observation period of 3 years (for sample characteristics at t1, see Table 1). Drop-out was not related to sample characteristics (e.g. age, sex), cardiovascular risk, cognitive and motivational abilities or depression at t1. Reasons for drop-out from t1 to t2 ($n = 7$) were: lost interest ($n = 4$), death ($n = 2$), and severe somatic illness ($n = 1$). Reason for drop-out from t2 to t3 was death ($n = 1$). Reasons for drop-out from t3 to t4 were: severe somatic illness ($n = 1$), excessive demand of the testing situation ($n = 1$) and not reachable ($n = 1$).

Table 1 Sample characteristics at baseline of Mild Cognitive Impairment (MCI) cases, excluding drop-outs ($n = 53$), and comparison of basic characteristics between subgroups 'MCI Stability' ($n = 32$) and 'MCI Conversion' ($n = 21$) at last follow-up (t4)

Variables	MCI total ($n = 53$)	MCI stability ($n = 32$)	MCI conversion ($n = 21$)	t / χ^2-test	p	d / phi
Age (years), *M* (SD)	73.09 (7.12)	71.16 (7.61)	76.05 (5.19)	2.57 (*t*)	**0.013**	−0.75 (*d*)
Sex, female, *n* (%)	26 (49.1)	20 (62.5)	6 (28.6)	5.84 (χ^2)	**0.016**	−0.33 (phi)
Education (years), *M* (SD)	12.32 (2.52)	12.09 (2.37)	12.67 (2.75)	−0.95 (*t*)	0.346	−0.23 (*d*)
Living Situation, *n* (%)				1.79 (χ^2)	0.409	0.18 (phi)
- Alone	14 (26.4)	10 (31.3)	4 (19.0)			
- Partner	38 (71.7)	21 (65.6)	17 (81.0)			
- Family member	1 (1.9)	1 (3.1)	0			
Marital status, *n* (%)				1.54 (χ^2)	0.674	0.17 (phi)
- Single	3 (5.7)	2 (6.3)	1 (4.8)			
- Married	38 (71.7)	21 (65.6)	17 (81.0)			
- Divorced /separated	4 (7.5)	3 (9.4)	1 (4.8)			
- Widowed	8 (15.1)	6 (18.8)	2 (9.5)			
Children, *M* (SD)	2.36 (0.88)	2.00 (0.68)	2.89 (0.90)	3.77 (*t*)	**< 0.001**	−1.12 (*d*)
MMSE score, *M* (SD)	27.25 (2.04)	27.69 (2.22)	26.57 (1.54)	−1.79 (*t*)	*0.081*	0.57 (*d*)
CDR, *M* (SD)	0.42 (0.19)	0.39 (0.21)	0.45 (0.15)	−1.25 (*t*)	0.218	−0.33 (*d*)
GDS-S, *M* (SD)	2.93 (2.3)	3.34 (2.55)	2.30 (1.97)	1.58 (*t*)	0.121	0.46 (*d*)
MCI Subtype, *n* (%)				11.76 (χ^2)	**0.008**	0.47 (phi)
- Amnestic s-d	11 (20.8)	5 (15.6)	6 (28.6)			
- Amnestic, m-d	17 (32.1)	6 (18.8)	11 (52.4)			
- Non-amnestic, s-d	22 (41.5)	19 (59.4)	3 (14.3)			
- Non-amnestic, m-d	3 (5.7)	2 (6.3)	1 (4.8)			
Cardiovascular risk, *n* (%)						
- Diagn. diabetes mellitus	11 (20.8)	9 (28.1)	2 (9.5)	3.64 (χ^2)	0.162	0.28 (phi)
- Diagn. elevated cholesterol	15 (28.3)	12 (37.5)	3 (9.4)	2.63 (χ^2)	0.105	−0.25 (phi)
- Diagn. high blood pressure	22 (41.5)	16 (50)	6 (28.6)	1.21 (χ^2)	0.545	0.16 (phi)

CDR clinical dementia rating scale, *d* Cohen's d, *Diagn.* diagnosis, *GDS-S* geriatric depression scale – self-report, *M* mean, *MCI* mild cognitive impairment, *m-d* multi-domain, *MMSE* Mini-Mental State Examination, *n* number, *p* probability, *phi* Cohen's phi, *SD* standard deviation, *s-d* single-domain, *t* independent t-test, χ^2 chi-square test

The bold values indicate a statistically significant difference with a *p*-value less than 0.05

Clinical phenotypes of the $n = 53$ MCI patients at t1 were as follows: amnestic, single-domain ($n = 11$), amnestic, multi-domain ($n = 17$), non-amnestic, single-domain ($n = 22$), and non-amnestic, multi-domain ($n = 3$). From t1 to t4, 50% ($n = 32$) of the MCI participants remained stable (i.e., they kept their cognitive level), while 32.8% ($n = 21$) and 17.2% ($n = 11$) converted to AD or dropped-out, respectively (see Table 2). None of the MCI participants converted back to normal cognitive functioning within the observation period from t1 to t4.

Table 3 is a correlation matrix of variables used for the main analyses (see Table 3). It shows that higher age was significantly related to a higher number of children, to lower executive function and MCI amnestic subtype. Female sex was related to higher motivational abilities and lower education. Higher motivational abilities were related to fewer years of education (see Table 3).

Comparison of the subgroups of 'MCI stability' and 'MCI conversion'

In a next step, we compared the basic characteristics of the 'MCI stability' and 'MCI conversion' subgroups. We identified significant differences between these two subgroups with regard to age, sex, MCI subtype and number of children (Table 1). The participants in the 'MCI stability' subgroup were generally younger, of female sex, of non-amnestic MCI subtype and having fewer children. With regard to informant-rated motivational abilities, groups differed significantly with regard to the composite measure, as well as with regard to motivation and marginally with regard to decision regulation (Table 4). Over all these measures, informants rated the current motivational abilities of the participants in the 'MCI stability' group higher as compared to informants of the participants in the 'MCI conversion' group.

Table 2 Number of Mild Cognitive Impairment (MCI) and Alzheimer Disease (AD) cases and drop-outs at baseline and follow-ups in number (*n*) and percent (%) (*n* = 64)

	MCI	*Mild AD*	*Moderate AD*	*Severe AD*	*Drop-out*
Baseline (t1)	First Follow-up (t2)				
MCI (n = 64)	*44 (68.8%)*	13 (20.3%)	0 (0%)	0 (0%)	7 (10.9%)
First Follow-up (t2)	Second Follow-up (t3)				
MCI (n = 44)	38 (86.4%)	6 (13.6%)	0 (0%)	0 (0%)	0 (0%)
Mild AD (n = 13)	0 (%)	10 (76.9%)	2 (15.4%)	0 (0%)	1 (7.7%)
Second Follow-up (t3)	Third Follow-up (t4)				
MCI (n = 38)	32 (84.2%)	4 (10.5%)	1 (2.6%)	0 (%)	1 (2.6%)
Mild AD (n = 16)	0 (%)	11 (68.6%)	2 (12.5%)	1 (6.3%)	2 (12.5%)
Moderate AD (n = 2)	0 (%)	0 (%)	0 (%)	2 (100%)	0 (%)
Baseline (t1)	Third Follow-up (t4)				
MCI (n = 64)	32 (50%)	15 (23.4%)	3 (4.7%)	3 (4.7%)	11 (17.2%)

AD Alzheimer's disease, *MCI* mild cognitive impairment, *n* number, *t1* baseline, *t2* first follow-up, *t3* second follow-up, *t4* third follow-up

Prediction of MCI stability applying survival analyses using binary logistic regression

Survival analyses have been conducted using logistic regression to determine the predictive effect of informant-rated motivational abilities (= composite measure) at baseline (t1) on the likelihood of MCI stability (i.e., whether MCI participants remained stable with regard to their cognitive level over the course of 3 years). The differential predictive ability of the single components of the composite measure, i.e., motivation and decision regulation were also compared. Drop-outs were included in these analyses, resulting in $n = 138$ observations. Observations refer here to the information at each of the three follow-ups, of whether MCI patient remained stable or whether the individual converted to AD. As soon as the patient converted to AD, no more observations were added to this particular patient. This implies that if for example a MCI patient remained stable, we have three observations per patient. See also Table 3 for a correlation matrix of all included predictors (Table 3).

Model 1

The composite measure consisting of informant-rated motivation and decision regulation at baseline and the three follow-up measurement points, were the only predictors entered in the first model. Given that the model predicts the probability of MCI stability / conversion across time, the inclusion of the discrete measurement points was necessary. The results indicated that the predictors explained 53.1% (Nagelkerke R^2) of the variance. Higher informant-rated motivational abilities significantly predicted MCI stability (OR = 0.59; $p = 0.040$) (Table 5). A comparison between the predictive strength of the two motivational components of the composite measure indicated that while motivation regulation was

Table 3 Correlation matrix of all predictors included in survival analyses using binary logistic regression and multilevel model (*n* = 64)

	(1)	(2)	(3)	(4)	(5)	(6)	(7)
(1) Age							
(2) Sex (0 = male, 1 = female)	−0.20 (0.11)						
(3) Number of children	**0.29 (0.03)**	− 0.10 (0.47)					
(4) Motivational abilities [a]	− 0.09 (0.48)	**0.25 (0.05)**	0.04 (0.79)				
(5) Executive function [b]	**0.28 (0.03)**	−0.07 (0.58)	0.14 (0.31)	−0.004 (0.97)			
(6) Education (years)	0.02 (0.88)	**−0.33 (0.01)**	0.22 (0.11)	**−0.25 (0.05)**	− 0.23 (0.07) [d]		
(7) MCI subtype (0 = a; 1 = n-a.)	**− 0.30 (0.02)**	0.21 (0.10)	− 0.18 (0.18)	− 0.22 (0.09) [d]	− 0.22 (0.09) [d]	0.10 (0.46)	
(8) Cardiovascular risk [c]	0.24 (0.10)	0.05 (0.76)	−0.08 (0.64)	0.11 (0.48)	0.10 (0.50)	0.03 (0.84)	0.17 (0.27)

The bold values indicate a statistically significant correlation with a *p*-value less than 0.05
a amnestic, *MCI* mild cognitive impairment, *n-a.* non-amnestic
[a] Composite measure including informant-rated motivational abilities at baseline (t1)
[b] Interference score of the Stroop Color-Word Test
[c] Composite measure including the diagnosis of diabetes mellitus, elevated cholesterol and high blood pressure
[d] marginally significant
Values in brackets indicate *p*-values

Table 4 Informant-rated motivational abilities for all Mild Cognitive Impairment (MCI) cases at baseline ($n = 53$) and comparison of informant-rated motivational abilities between the subgroups 'MCI Stability' and 'MCI Conversion' as diagnosed at last follow-up (t4)

Motivational abilities [a]	MCI total ($n = 53$)	MCI stability ($n = 32$)	MCI conversion ($n = 21$)	*t*-test	*p*	*d*
Composite measure, min-max, *M* (SD)	2–14.5	3–14.5	2–11	2.31	**0.025**	0.665
	8.48 (2.88)	9.21 (2.93)	7.40 (2.50)			
Motivation regulation, min-max, *M* (SD)	2–15	2–15	2–11	2.23	**0.030**	0.654
	8.37 (3.24)	9.16 (3.53)	7.19 (2.38)			
Decision regulation, min-max, *M* (SD)	0–15	0–15	2–12	1.92	*0.061* [b]	0.545
	8.60 (3.10)	9.26 (3.10)	7.62 (2.91)			

d Cohen's *d*, *M* mean, *max* maximum, *min* minimum, *n* number, *SD* standard deviation, *t* independent t-test
[a] Composite measure including informant-rated motivational abilities at baseline (t1)
[b] marginally significant
The bold values indicate a statistically significant difference with a *p*-value less than 0.05

not found to be a meaningful predictor of MCI stability in this model (OR = 0.97; $p = 0.133$), decision regulation did significantly predict MCI stability (OR = 0.96; $p = 0.049$).

Model 2

In the second model, we added the control variables 'sex', 'age' and 'number of children'. Those were all statistically different between subgroups at t1. The results indicated that the predictors explained 63.3% (Nagelkerke R^2) of the variance. It was found that higher informant-rated motivational abilities marginally predicted MCI stability, when controlling for these control variables (OR = 0.52; $p = 0.052$). Neither 'age' (OR = 1.39; $p = 0.323$), nor 'sex' (OR = 0.59; $p = 0.376$), but 'number of children' (OR = 1.95; $p = 0.028$) were identified as significant predictors (Table 5). A higher number of children was thus associated with a decreased likelihood for MCI stability over 3 years. A comparison between the predictive strength of the informant-rated motivation and decision regulation showed a significant prediction of MCI stability with both components (motivation regulation: OR = 2.00; $p = 0.042$; decision regulation: OR = 1.95; $p = 0.040$).

Model 3

In the third model, we additionally included a measure for executive functions to test whether differences at baseline executive functions where meaningfully influencing MCI stability. The inclusion of a proxy for 'executive function', i.e., the interference score of the Stroop Color-Word Test, increased explained variance from 63.3 to 68.7% (R^2). 'Executive function' was not meaningfully associated with MCI stability (OR = 1.02; $p = 0.196$). Higher informant-rated motivational abilities significantly predicted MCI stability in this model (OR = 0.48; $p = 0.036$). Again, 'age' and 'sex' were not meaningfully predicting MCI stability, contrary again to 'number of children' (Table 5). While informant-rated motivational regulation did not predict MCI stability (OR = 0.97; $p = 0.276$), 'informant-rated decision regulation' did significantly (OR = 0.91; $p = 0.008$).

Model 4

The fourth model includes, besides the main predictor of 'informant-rated motivational abilities' and the demographic characteristics, the predictor (years of) 'education'. 'Education' was added to the predictors of *Model 2* and not to those of *Model 3*, as, given the rule of thumb of 15 observations per predictor, we are at the upper limit with 8 predictors per model and 138 available observations. 'Education' was included to test whether the predictive effect of 'informant-rated motivational abilities' is reduced when controlling for a proxy of cognitive reserve. The predictors explained a variance of 62.4% (R^2) in this model. 'Education' was not found to be meaningfully related to MCI stability (OR = 0.97; $p = 0.804$). Higher informant-rated motivational abilities marginally predicted MCI stability in this model (OR = 0.52; $p = 0.051$) (Table 5). Again, as in *Model 3*: while informant-rated motivational regulation did not predict MCI stability (OR = 0.97; $p = 0.258$), informant-rated decision regulation did (OR = 0.92; $p = 0.021$).

Model 5

The fifth model includes, besides the main predictor of 'informant-rated motivational abilities' and the demographic characteristics, the predictor 'MCI subtype'. We added 'MCI subtype' as predictor in addition to those included in *Model 2* (and not to *Model 3* or *Model 4*), due to a limited number of available observations. 'MCI subtype' was added as predictor as the clinical phenotype 'MCI amnestic' is commonly related to a higher conversion rate. Due to an unequal distribution of participants to the four MCI phenotypes, we combined the two amnestic and the two non-amnestic subtypes each into one group, resulting in a dichotomous MCI subtype variable (amnestic / non-amnestic). The inclusion of

Table 5 Survival analyses using binary logistic regression predicting likelihood of Mild Cognitive Impairment (MCI) stability (coded as 1) ($n = 64$)

Variable	*B*	SE	*P Value*	OR	95% CI
Model 1					
Follow-up 1	−1.24	0.66	**< 0.001**	0.289	0.153–0.546
Follow-up 2	−1.85	0.59	**< 0.001**	0.157	0.065–0.379
Follow-up 3	−1.78	0.56	**< 0.001**	0.168	0.064–0.436
Motivational abilities [a]	−0.53	0.36	**0.040**	0.587	0.353–0.976
Model 2					
Follow-up 1	−0.52	0.92	0.572	0.596	0.099–3.582
Follow-up 2	−1.85	1.05	*0.078* [c]	0.157	0.020–1.233
Follow-up 3	−0.76	1.01	0.454	0.468	0.064–3.413
Motivational abilities [a]	−0.65	0.33	*0.052* [c]	0.524	0.273–1.005
Age	0.33	0.33	0.323	1.389	0.725–2.661
Sex (0 = male, 1 = female)	−0.53	0.60	0.376	0.589	0.182–1.902
Children (number)	0.67	0.30	**0.028**	1.954	1.076–3.547
Model 3					
Follow-up 1	−1.07	1.02	0.294	0.345	0.047–2.519
Follow-up 2	−2.34	1.13	**0.038**	0.096	0.011–0.880
Follow-up 3	−1.27	1.10	0.247	0.280	0.032–2.414
Motivational abilities [a]	−0.74	0.35	**0.036**	0.477	0.239–0.952
Age	0.13	0.36	0.727	1.135	0.558–2.308
Sex (0 = male, 1 = female)	−0.54	0.60	0.372	0.584	0.179–1.902
Children (number)	0.73	0.32	**0.022**	2.082	1.109–3.908
Executive function [b]	0.02	0.01	0.196	1.016	0.992–1.042
Model 4					
Follow-up 1	−0.11	1.89	0.955	0.899	0.022–36.773
Follow-up 2	−1.46	1.91	0.446	0.233	0.005–9.854
Follow-up 3	−0.35	1.93	0.854	0.702	0.016–30.550
Motivational abilities [a]	−0.66	0.34	*0.051* [c]	0.515	0.264–1.003
Age	0.31	0.34	0.374	1.358	0.692–2.667
Sex (0 = male, 1 = female)	−0.58	0.64	0.360	0.559	0.161–1.940
Children (number)	0.70	0.32	**0.031**	2.003	1.066–3.763
Education (years)	−0.03	0.11	0.804	0.973	0.781–1.212
Model 5					
Follow-up 1	−0.07	0.96	0.940	0.930	0.141–6.120
Follow-up 2	−1.36	1.09	0.213	0.257	0.030–2.181
Follow-up 3	−0.17	1.07	0.876	0.845	0.103–6.941
Motivational abilities [a]	−0.63	0.33	*0.060* [c]	0.534	0.277–1.028
Age	0.16	0.38	0.684	1.169	0.551–2.479
Sex (0 = male, 1 = female)	−0.45	0.62	0.470	0.638	0.188–2.161
Children (number)	0.73	0.33	**0.024**	2.084	1.100–3.947
MCI amnestic (0 = amnestic, 1 = non-amnestic)	−1.47	0.62	**0.018**	0.230	0.068–0.773
Model 6					
Follow-up 1	−0.79	1.45	0.584	0.452	0.026–7.749
Follow-up 2	−1.35	1.64	0.408	0.258	0.010–6.381

Table 5 Survival analyses using binary logistic regression predicting likelihood of Mild Cognitive Impairment (MCI) stability (coded as 1) ($n = 64$) *(Continued)*

Variable	*B*	SE	*P Value*	OR	95% CI
Follow-up 3	−0.14	1.58	0.931	1.146	0.052–25.359
Motivational abilities [a]	−0.50	0.49	0.303	0.606	0.233–1.574
Age	0.78	0.52	0.135	2.181	0.784–6.064
Sex (0 = male, 1 = female)	−0.38	0.92	0.683	0.687	0.113–4.163
Children (number)	0.90	0.48	*0.060* [c]	2.455	0.963–6.255
Cardiovascular risk factors	−3.29	1.59	**0.038**	0.037	0.002–0.837

The bold values indicate a statistically significant correlation with a *p*-value less than 0.05
B coefficient, *CI* confidence interval, *MCI* mild cognitive impairment, *OR* odds ratio, *p* level of significance, *SE* standard error
[a] Composite measure including informant-rated motivational abilities at baseline (t1)
[b] Interference score of the Stroop Color-Word Test
[c] marginally significant

'MCI subtype' increased explained variance from 63.3 to 66.1% (R^2). The clinical phenotype 'MCI amnestic' was found to be associated with a decreased likelihood for MCI stability over 3 years (OR = 0.23; $p = 0.018$). The informant-rated motivational abilities marginally predicted MCI stability in this model (OR = 0.53; $p = 0.06$) (Table 5). While informant-rated motivational regulation did not predict MCI stability (OR = 0.97; $p = 0.296$), informant-rated decision regulation did (OR = 0.93; $p = 0.021$).

Model 6

We additionally calculated *Model 2* by adding a proxy for 'cardiovascular risk'. The predictors in this model explained 80% of the variance (R^2). The variable 'cardiovascular risk'was associated with a decreased likelihood for MCI stability over 3 years (OR = 0.04; $p = 0.038$). The informant-rated motivational abilities did not predict MCI stability in this model (OR = 0.61; $p = 0.303$) (Table 5), neither did the informant-rated motivational regulation (OR = 0.96; $p = 0.384$) nor the informant-rated decision regulation (OR = 0.96; $p = 0.249$).

Multilevel modeling

At first, we calculated whether the proportion in the variance of cognitive abilities, as measured with the MMSE, indicated the need for analyses with multilevel modeling. The intraclass correlation (ICC) was 43.90%, indicating that around 44% of the total MMSE variance resides between patients and around 56% within patient's repeated measures. The relatively large ICC indicates that data can be analyzed by multilevel modeling [53].

We found a significant between individual variance (Wald $Z = 4.22$, $p < 0.001$), indicating significant variation in the intercepts of MMSE (= random intercept; AIC = 1177). We also found a significant variation in the slope of MMSE between participants (= random slope; AIC = 1067; Wald $Z = 4.33$; $p < 0.001$). As of that, further analyses were conducted using the random intercept, random slope model. Additionally, we calculated the model with quadratic time to test for curvilinearity in the trajectory of MMSE. The effect was not significant ($p = 0.113$). Consequently, we calculated our models with linear time only.

In order to provide comparative analyses to the survival analyses models using logistic regression above, we calculated the multilevel models without interaction effects. Nonetheless, interaction effects of time with all predictors were calculated for all models (data not shown). The addition of interaction effects did not result in increasing the model fit as indicated by the model fit index AIC.

Model 1

In the first model, we were interested in the main effect of 'informant-rated motivational abilities' on the trajectory of cognitive abilities over a three-year observation period. As of that, we included only time and 'informant-rated motivational abilities' into the first model. We found a significant negative main effect of 'time' ($t = -3.08$; $p = 0.002$) and significant positive effect of 'informant-rated motivational abilities' ($t = 2.33$; $p = 0.023$) on the trajectory of cognitive abilities.

Model 2

In a second model, we added the demographic characteristics 'age' and 'sex'. Unlike the survival analyses, we did not add 'number of children' in these models, as current literature is not suggestive of a protective influence of having fewer children on the course of cognitive abilities. Again, we found a significant negative main effect of 'time' ($t = -3.08$; $p = 0.002$). In addition, we found a marginal positive effect of 'informant-rated motivational abilities' ($t = 1.95$; $p = 0.056$). The effect of the demographic characteristics 'age' ($t = -1.21$; $p = 0.231$) and 'sex' ($t = 1.54$; $p = 0.129$) were not significant.

Model 3

In the third model, we included a proxy for 'executive function'. We found a significant negative main effect of 'time' ($t = -3.28$; $p = 0.002$), a significant positive effect of 'informant-rated motivational abilities' ($t = 2.32$; $p = 0.023$), and a significant negative effect of the interference score of the Stroop Color-Word test ($t = -3.03$; $p = 0.004$), which can be translated into a significant positive effect of 'executive functions'. 'Age' ($t = -0.59$; $p = 0.558$) and 'sex' ($t = 1.64$; $p = 0.106$), were again not significant in this model.

Model 4

In the fourth model, we included a proxy for cognitive reserve, i.e., years of 'education'. We found a significant negative main effect of 'time' ($t = -3.28$; $p = 0.002$), a significant positive effect of 'informant-rated motivational abilities' ($t = 2.36$; $p = 0.022$), and a significant negative effect of the interference score of the Stroop Color-Word test ($t = -2.80$; $p = 0.007$), which, again, can be translated into a significant positive effect of 'executive functions'. 'Age' ($t = -0.59$; $p = 0.560$) and 'education' ($t = 0.40$; $p = 0.689$) were not significant, and 'sex' only marginally ($t = 1.68$; $p = 0.098$).

Model 5

In the final model, we additionally included 'MCI subtype'. We found a significant negative effect of 'time', a significant positive effect of 'informant-rated motivational abilities', a significant negative effect of the interference score of the Stroop Color-Word test, i.e., significant positive effect of 'executive functions'(see Table 6). The R^2 estimate for this final and best fitting model is 41.03.

Additional analyses

We also compared the predictive strength of informant-rated motivation and decision regulation in *Model 5*. We found that while 'motivation regulation' was not a meaningful predictor ($t = 0.92$; $p = 0.361$), 'decision regulation' had a significant positive effect on cognitive abilities in this model ($t = 3.03$; $p = 0.004$). Also, we added the predictor 'depression' to *Model 5* in order to control for influences of depressive mental states. 'Depression' predicted cognitive abilities significantly ($t = 2.10$; $p = 0.04$). Motivational abilities remained a significant predictor in this model ($t = 3.23$; $p = 0.002$). Finally, we added a proxy for health ('cardiovascular risk') to *Model 5* in order to control for the effect of health. While the measure for 'cardiovascular risk' did not significantly predict cognitive abilities ($t = 1.30$; $p = 0.201$), the inclusion of this somatic risk factor decreased the predictive ability of 'informant-rated motivational abilities' to a non-significant effect ($t = 1.15$; $p = 0.259$).

Figure 1 illustrates the differential trajectories of individuals with high and low decision regulation, as calculated with median split, over the four measurement time points with regard to their performances in the MMSE (Fig. 1).

Discussion

Here we aimed to examine the hypothesized protective influence of motivational abilities on the course of MCI. In the context of a longitudinal, prospective study, we compared the predictive effect of informant-rated

Table 6 Growth model parameter estimates of predictors for trajectories in cognitive abilities, as measured with the Mini Mental State Examination (MMSE) ($n = 64$)

Variable	MMSE					
	Fixed effects				Random effects	
	Estimate (s.e.)	*df*	*t*	*p*	Variance	Co-Variance
Intercept	26.11 (0.71)	63.73	26.80	**0.001**	1.26	−0.45 [a]
Time (years)	− 0.82 (0.25)	54.74	−3.29	**0.002**	2.96	−0.45 [a]
Motivational abilities [b]	0.56 (0.25)	60.90	2.23	**0.030**		
Age	−0.11 (0.23)	64.39	−0.49	0.623		
Sex (0 = male, 1 = female)	0.76 (0.48)	61.83	1.58	0.120		
Executive function [c]	− 0.62 (0.22)	60.85	−2.78	**0.007**		
Education (years)	0.08 (0.24)	62.15	0.32	0.751		
MCI subtype (0 = amnestic, 1 = non-amnestic)	0.16 (0.47)	62.92	0.35	0.731		
Residual					2.57	
AIC = 1047.86						

The bold values indicate a statistically significant correlation with a *p*-value less than 0.05

AIC Akaike information criterion, *df* degrees of freedom, *MMSE* Mini-Mental State Examination, *p* probability, *s.e.* standard error, *t* independent t-test

[a] Covariance of the Intercept and Time random effects

[b] Composite measure including informant-rated motivational abilities at baseline (t1)

[c] Interference score of the Stroop Color-Word Test

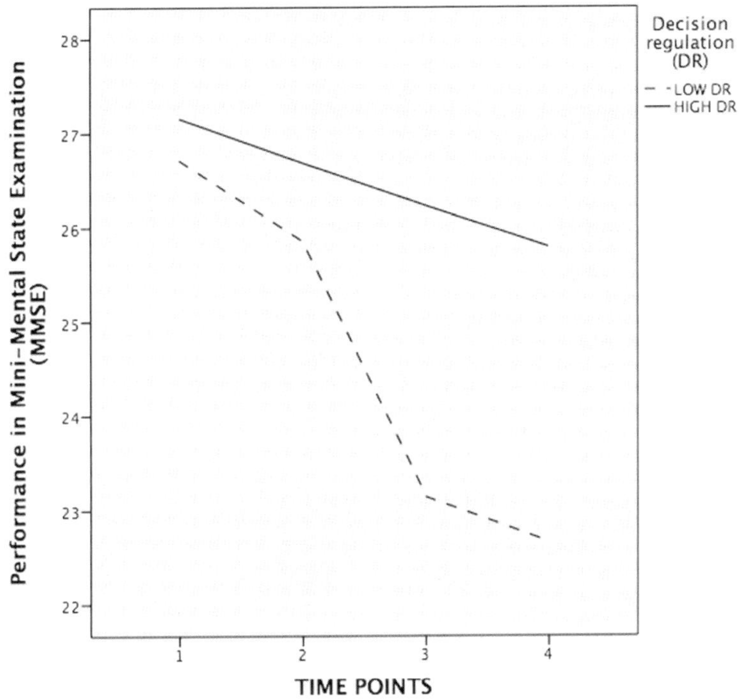

Fig. 1 Trajectories in performances in Mini-Mental State Examination (MMSE) over the four measurement time points for individuals with high and low informant-rated decision regulation, computed with median split

motivational abilities measured at baseline on the likelihood of MCI stability over a time period of 3 years. Our main finding was that informant-rated motivational abilities were meaningful predictors of MCI stability, even when controlling for demographic characteristics, executive functions at baseline or MCI subtype (i.e., amnestic vs. non-amnestic). The analyses conducted with logistic regression were partly supported by analyses using multilevel modeling. A comparison of the predictive strength of motivation versus decision regulation suggests that the potentially protective effect of motivational abilities may mainly be driven by the motivational ability 'decision regulation'. However, the control for the influence of cardiovascular risk at baseline resulted in the disappearance of a meaningful effect of motivational abilities. Given the relatively small sample size and the related low statistical power, in addition to the occasionally only marginally significant findings, our results may be considered as preliminary.

In our sample, we observed a conversion rate from MCI to AD of 32.8%. Given the relative short observation window of 3 years, this rate can be considered as comparatively high [4]. Previous studies have indicated that individuals who seek professional help due to their memory impairments [57], as well as individuals who complain about their memory loss [58], are at a higher risk for conversion. Given that we were recruiting our participants in specialized clinics and institutions, as well as by advertisements, we might have recruited individuals at a higher risk for conversion.

Our preliminary finding of a meaningful prediction of MCI stability by informant-rated motivational abilities corroborates previous cross-sectional [30] and prospective findings [31]. Given that in both previous studies, an indirect measure of motivational abilities (i.e., an estimate for motivational abilities that is based on the main occupation the individual had in midlife, by applying the O*NET, see description in [30, 31, 41, 59]) was used to predict MCI courses, we could extend those finding by showing that informant-rated motivational abilities can be used to predict MCI courses. We re-calculated all analyses with self-rated motivational abilities (data not shown). We found that self-rated motivational abilities are not effective in predicting the course of MCI stability. This corresponds to findings by Snow and colleagues, who concluded that self-reports of individuals with cognitive decline may be less accurate due to a diminished awareness [40].

On the basis of our analyses, it appears as if the motivational ability 'decision regulation' may be more closely related to MCI stability and cognitive abilities as compared to 'motivation regulation'. Decision regulation may be linked to the actual behavioral decision-making process. A recent longitudinal study with non-demented older adults (mean age of 83.5 years) found that poor decision-making reflected deteriorating cognitive abilities [60], rather than predicting cognitive decline. The authors concluded that their results "..suggest that even very subtle age-related changes in cognition have detrimental effects on judgment." [60]. As a consequence, it may be that in the current study, differences in the informant ratings of decision regulation may reflect subtle, indirect judgments of cognitive decline, more so than differences in motivation regulation.

The predictive ability of motivational abilities disappeared when controlling for the influence of cardiovascular risk factors. It can be assumed that cardiovascular risk might act as a mediator between motivational and cognitive abilities by translating motivational abilities into beneficial health outcomes. For instance, higher motivated individuals may engage more in activities that are promoting cardiovascular health, such as the increased engagement in physical activities, which are known to exert a beneficial effect on cognitive health in older age (e.g. [61]). How can it be explained that motivational abilities predict a more benign course of MCI? Analogous to the brain or cognitive reserve concepts [8–10, 28], we propose the motivational reserve concept, based upon the assumption that the increased use of certain brain areas promotes synapse formation and neuronal growth, which lead to higher efficiency within the brain, that in turn allows the compensation of impaired neuronal networks. By an increased activation of brain areas directly related to motivational abilities, such as the prefrontal cortex, the nucleus accumbens and the amygdala [62, 63], or indirectly related by the influence of motivation on stress, emotional health or cognition [30, 31], those areas become more efficient and are thus able to compensate for affected networks through brain plasticity. Our preliminary findings support the predictions drawn from the motivational reserve model by showing that higher motivational abilities at an early stage of MCI may exert a protective influence on the course of MCI. Future studies are needed to investigate the underlying mechanims (e.g. potential mediation by health behavior tendencies) in the translation of motivational abilities into better health outcomes in later life.

An unexpected finding was the meaningful, *negative* association between motivational abilities and education, as it was expected that a higher level of motivational abilities would be related to higher educational achievements (i.e., more years of education). When controlling for the impact of gender, this association disappears. The control for the influence of gender might in fact be relevant with regard to this relation: on one hand, in our sample, female gender was related to higher motivational abilities. On the other hand, Swiss women of the generation of our sample (cohorts 1930–1960) did not gain the same access to higher education as their male counterparts. This is also reflected in the significant difference in years of education between male and female participants. As of that, it may be that a (social) gender bias within our older sample might have obscured the expected meaningful association between motivational abilities and (years of) education.

A further unexpected finding of our study was the result of a lower risk for MCI conversion in individuals having fewer children. Given the fact that we included this variable as a control variable due to a significant difference between the two MCI subgroups, this inclusion was not led by theory. To the best of our knowledge, this finding is unprecedented. A higher number of children is an indirect indicator of lower parental intelligence [64] and socio economic status (SES). Thus, we speculate that those individuals having more children may have less protection against cognitive decline, as higher intelligence and SES have a preventive influence on pathological cognitive decline [9, 10, 65]. However, our data did not reveal a meaningful relation between number of children and intelligence or years of education (as a proxy for SES), neither for men nor women (all correlations are non-significant, data not shown). Another, though highly speculative explanation, may be found in the life history theory (LHT), that states that increased reproductive effort (i.e., a higher number of offspring), might come at the expense of tissue maintenance and thus accelerate aging [66]. For instance, in a study including older women (mean age of 75 years), it was found that a higher number of children was associated with shorter telomere length [67], a proxy for cellular aging that has previously been linked to dementia risk [68]. However, a recent, prospective study did not find a meaningful association between the number of children and maternal telomere length. Rather, mothers with fewer children had even shorter telomere lengths [69]. Again, this explanation is highly speculative and more research is needed to understand the unexpected finding in our study that a greater number of children was associated with higher risk for MCI conversion.

Our findings must be interpreted in the light of the following limitations. A limiting factor of our study is the use of current motivational abilities that have been rated by informants of the participants. The assessment of current motivational abilities is flawed by the fact that it can be argued that lower current motivational abilities may be an early sign of an underlying neuropathological process rather than a premorbid risk factor. In fact, pathological cognitive decline seems to impact motivational abilities. For instance, in an own study, we were able to show that individuals with mild AD displayed higher rates in the motivational construct 'delay discounting' over an observation period of 2 years which indicates decreasing self-control with progressive cognitive decline [70]. Brain areas related to motivational abilities, such as the prefrontal cortex, the nucleus accumbens and the amygdala [62, 63] can all be affected by AD neuropathological processes. It is as such a possibility that lower motivational abilities in our study do reflect some sort of cognitive decline. However, this may not completely undermine our hypothesis of a protective effect of higher motivational abilities on the course of MCI, as higher levels of motivational abilities may still act as a buffer against cognitive decline, even when impairment has already begun. Nonetheless, we may not completely exclude the argument that lower current motivational abilities reflect early AD disease processes.

The optimal predictor with regard to the research question of interest may have been the direct assessment of motivational abilities during midlife, i.e., decades before the first clinical signs of cognitive impairment appeared. Given that this was not feasible in the current study, other possibilities (besides the indirect assessment through estimates of motivational abilities on the basis of participants' occupational history, see [30]), were either the retrospective assessment, which, however, is flawed by recall bias, or the use of the rating by informants, which, as we were able to show in a previous study, can be biased by the caregiving burden [71].

A further essential limiting factor is the small sample size of our study, particularly with regard to the regression analyses. Those results have to be interpreted with caution. Due to the small sample size and the related low statistical power [72], it is both likely that we did not find significant effects of factors that were previously identified as risk (MCI subtype) or protective factors (i.e., education). It is also likely that due to the small sample size our significant finding of a protective effect of motivational abilities on the course of MCI may not mirror a true effect [72], i.e., could have been an overestimation. In combination, i.e., due to the fact that our independent variable might have been affected by ongoing underlying disease processes, in combination with the small sample size, the external validity of our findings is limited, and interpretations of our results should be done with caution.

What is more, we did not assess the time point of when the diagnoses of the patients were made for the first time, which could have been used as a standardized proxy of the onset of the clinical symptoms of MCI. While most of our participants were diagnosed in the months before recruitment for the study, we have no information with regard to how long MCI symptomatology persisted before participants presented themselves to a clinician and were then diagnosed with MCI. It could therefore be that patients with stable courses were those with the most recent onset of MCI. But given the fact that the pre-clinical biological changes related to AD might take years to decades before the clinical phase of AD [73], any 'starting point' could only ever be vaguely defined. Nonetheless, future studies should include duration of the clinical manifestation of the symptomology as a proxy. Future studies should also include the assessment of biomarkers, to increase the level of certainty of the AD diagnosis [2]. Also, the assessment of A*B* protein would have been useful as it has previously been proposed that A*B* negative MCI cases are unlikely to progress to AD [1]. Furthermore, our measure for 'health', i.e., a proxy for cardiovascular health, is limited. Future studies should include a broader indicator for physical health. Additionally, it is to be assumed that the participants (and their informants) show self-selection bias. Taking part in a relative extensive longitudinal study while being diagnosed with MCI may itself be a sign for higher motivational abilities. Therefore, it may be that our results are biased towards higher motivated, research interested participants, which might have affected our study on various levels (e.g. recruitment, data collection) and might thus reduce validity of our results. Also, the assessments of the diagnoses at follow-ups were carried out by a group of clinicians that might involve the same or other persons that carried out the diagnoses at baseline. However, this group of clinicians was *not* involved in the assessment of affective and motivational variables. It was strived for having the group of clinicians blinded for the previous MCI and AD diagnoses, however, this could not have been guaranteed for all participants. Finally, the observation period of 3 years is relatively short. It is thus of importance to replicate our findings in a study with a larger sample size that is followed up for a longer period of time.

Conclusions

Bearing in mind the preliminary nature of our results, this study provides first evidence for a protective effect of motivational abilities on the course of MCI. Given the modifiable nature of motivational abilities, future studies should investigate how those skills may best be trained in coaching courses, how they might be integrated into existing psychotherapeutic manuals for both older and younger individuals and whether such interventions are effective in increasing cognitive health in older age [31].

Abbreviations

AB: amyloid-beta; AD: Alzheimer's disease; CDR: Clinical Dementia Rating Scale; CERAD-NP: Consortium to Establish a Registry for Alzheimer's Disease – Neuropsychological Assessment; CR: Cognitive reserve; DSM-IV-TR: Diagnostic and Statistical Manual of Mental Disorders; GDS: Geriatric Depression Scale; LHT: Life history theory; MA: Motivational abilities; MCAR: Little's missing completely at random; MCI: Mild cognitive impairment; MMSE: Mini Mental State Examination; MoReA: Motivational Reserve as a Protective Factor in Mild Alzheimer's Dementia and Mild Cognitive Impairment; MR: Motivational reserve; N: Number; NINCDS-ADRDA: National Institute of Neurological and Communicative Disorders and Stroke-Alzheimer's Disease and Related Disorders Association; O*Net: Occupational Information Network; SES: Socio economic status; VCQ: Volitional Components Questionnaire

Acknowledgements
We thank D. Drobetz, S. Fankhauser, M. E. Mortby, L. Pfeifer for their assistance in this project.

Funding
This work was supported by grants from the Swiss National Science Foundation (SNSF, 100014-124535); the Velux Foundation; the Tropos Foundation; the Kurt Fries Foundation; and the Swiss Alzheimer's Association.

Authors' contributions
MVT was the major contributor in writing the manuscript. SF and AM conceived, planned and carried out the study and were in charge of overall direction and planning. RS, OK, FX, USG, AB, AR, GB-B helped in recruiting and diagnosis participants. DD assisted in performing the analytic calculations and contributed to the interpretation of the results. All authors provided critical feedback and helped shape the research, analysis and manuscript. All authors read and approved the final manuscript.

Competing interests
The authors declare that they have no competing interests.

Author details
[1]University of Zurich, Binzmuehlestr, 14, 8050 Zurich, Switzerland. [2]University Research Priority Program "Dynamics of Healthy Aging", University of Zurich, Zurich, Switzerland. [3]University of Siegen, Faculty II, Developmental Psychology, Adolf-Reichwein-Str. 2, 57068 Siegen, Germany. [4]Psychiatrische Klinik Zugersee, Zug, Switzerland. [5]Integrierte Psychiatrie Winterthur, Winterthur, Switzerland. [6]Present Address: Alterspsychiatrische Praxis, Buehlach, Switzerland. [7]Clienia Schloessli AG, Oetwil am See, Switzerland. [8]Praxis für Psychiatrie Rehalp, Zurich, Switzerland. [9]Psychiatrische Dienste Thurgau, Muensterlingen, Switzerland. [10]Sanatorium Kilchberg AG, Kilchberg, Switzerland. [11]Present Address: KMG – Kompetenz mentale Gesundheit GmbH, Baar, Switzerland. [12]Geriatric service of the city of Zurich, Zurich, Switzerland. [13]Psychopathology and Clinical Intervention, University of Zurich, Binzmuehlestr. 14/17, CH-8050 Zurich, Switzerland.

References
1. Albert MS, et al. The diagnosis of mild cognitive impairment due to Alzheimer's disease: recommendations from the National Institute on Aging Alzheimer's association workgroups on diagnostic guidelines for Alzheimer's disease. Alzheimers Dement. 2011;7(3):270–9.
2. McKhann GM, et al. The diagnosis of dementia due to Alzheimer's disease: recommendations from the National Institute on Aging-Alzheimer's Association workgroups on diagnostic guidelines for Alzheimer's disease. Alzheimers Dement. 2011;7(3):263–9.
3. Hardy J, Allsop D. Amyloid deposition as the central event in the aetiology of Alzheimer's disease. Trends Pharmacol Sci. 1991;12:383–8.
4. Mitchell AJ, Shiri-Feshki M. Rate of progression of mild cognitive impairment to dementia–meta-analysis of 41 robust inception cohort studies. Acta Psychiatr Scand. 2009;119(4):252–65.
5. Wolf H, Grunwald M, Ecke GM, Zedlick D, Bettin S, Dannenberg C, Gertz HJ. The prognosis of mild cognitive impairment in the elderly. In Alzheimer's Disease—From Basic Research to Clinical Applications. Vienna: Springer; 1998. pp. 31-50.
6. Haaksma ML, Leoutsakos JMS, Bremer JA, Aalten P, Ramakers IH, Verhey FR, Melis RJ. The clinical course and interrelations of dementia related symptoms. Int Psychogeriatr. 2018;30(6):859-66.
7. Scarmeas N, Stern Y. Cognitive reserve and lifestyle. J Clin Exp Neuropsychol. 2003;25(5):625–33.
8. Stern Y. What is cognitive reserve? Theory and research application of the reserve concept. J Int Neuropsychol Soc. 2002;8(3):448–60.
9. Valenzuela MJ, Sachdev P. Brain reserve and cognitive decline: a non-parametric systematic review. Psychol Med. 2006;36(8):1065–73.
10. Valenzuela MJ, Sachdev P. Brain reserve and dementia: a systematic review. Psychol Med. 2006;36(4):441–54.
11. Knopman DS, et al. Neuropathology of cognitively normal elderly. J Neuropathol Exp Neurol. 2003;62(11):1087–95.
12. Arenaza-Urquijo EM, Vemuri P. Resistance vs resilience to Alzheimer disease: clarifying terminology for preclinical studies. Neurology. 2018;90(15):695–703.
13. Allen JS, Bruss J, Damasio H. The aging brain: the cognitive reserve hypothesis and hominid evolution. Am J Hum Biol. 2005;17(6):673–89.
14. Stern Y. Cognitive reserve in ageing and Alzheimer's disease. Lancet Neurol. 2012;11(11):1006–12.
15. Heckhausen, J. and H. Heckhausen, Motivation and action: introduction and overview. 2008.
16. Brandtstädter J, Rothermund K. The life-course dynamics of goal pursuit and goal adjustment: a two-process framework. Dev Rev. 2002;22(1):117–50.
17. Baltes P, Baltes M. Psychological perspectives on successful aging: the model of selective optimization with compensation. Successful Aging. 1990;1(1):1–34.
18. Heckhausen J, Schulz R. A life-span theory of control. Psychol Rev. 1995; 102(2):284.
19. Oettingen G, Gollwitzer P. Goal setting and goal striving. In emotion and motivation. Blackwell; 2004.
20. Bandura A. Self-efficacy: the exercise of control. New York: Freeman; 1997.
21. Kuhl, J. and A. Fuhrmann, Decomposing self-regulation and self-control: the volitional components inventory. 1998.
22. Kruglanski AW, et al. To "do the right thing" or to "just do it": locomotion and assessment as distinct self-regulatory imperatives. J Pers Soc Psychol. 2000;79(5):793.
23. Judge TA, et al. An empirical investigation of the predictors of executive career success. Pers Psychol. 1995;48(3):485–519.
24. Bauman AE, et al. Toward a better understanding of the influences on physical activity: the role of determinants, correlates, causal variables, mediators, moderators, and confounders. Am J Prev Med. 2002;23(2):5–14.
25. Montalvo FT, Torres MCG. Self-regulated learning: current and future directions. Electron J Res Educ Psychol. 2004;2(1):1–34.
26. Braver TS, et al. Mechanisms of motivation–cognition interaction: challenges and opportunities. Cogn Affect Behav Neurosci. 2014;14(2):443–72.
27. Maercker A, Forstmeier S. Healthy brain ageing: the new concept of motivational reserve. Psychiatrist. 2011;35:175–7.
28. Katzman R, et al. Clinical, pathological, and neurochemical changes in dementia: a subgroup with preserved mental status and numerous neocortical plaques. Ann Neurol. 1988;23(2):138–44.
29. Fratiglioni L, Winblad B, von Strauss E. Prevention of Alzheimer's disease and dementia. Major findings from the Kungsholmen project. Physiol Behav. 2007;92(1–2):98–104.
30. Forstmeier S, Maercker A. Motivational reserve: lifetime motivational abilities contribute to cognitive and emotional health in old age. Psychol Aging. 2008;23(4):886–99.
31. Forstmeier S, et al. Motivational reserve: motivation-related occupational abilities and risk of mild cognitive impairment and Alzheimer disease. Psychol Aging. 2012;27(2):353–63.
32. Valentijn SA, et al. Memory self-efficacy predicts memory performance: results from a 6-year follow-up study. Psychol Aging. 2006;21(1):165.
33. Judge TA, Bono JE. Relationship of core self-evaluations traits—self-esteem, generalized self-efficacy, locus of control, and emotional stability—with job satisfaction and job performance: a meta-analysis. J Appl Psychol. 2001; 86(1):80.
34. Pruessner JC, et al. Self-esteem, locus of control, hippocampal volume, and cortisol regulation in young and old adulthood. Neuroimage. 2005;28(4): 815–26.
35. Peterson NG, Mumford MD, Borman WC, Jeanneret PR, Fleishman EA. An occupational information system for the 21st century: The development of O*NET. Washington, DC: American Psychological Association; 1999.
36. Peterson NG, et al. Understanding work using the occupational information network (O* NET): implications for practice and research. Pers Psychol. 2001; 54(2):451–92.
37. Palmer K, et al. Neuropsychiatric predictors of progression from amnestic-mild cognitive impairment to Alzheimer's disease: the role of depression and apathy. J Alzheimers Dis. 2010;20(1):175–83.

38. Starkstein SE, et al. Syndromic validity of apathy in Alzheimer's disease. Am J Psychiatr. 2001;158(6):872–7.
39. Hardt J, Rutter M. Validity of adult retrospective reports of adverse childhood experiences: review of the evidence. J Child Psychol Psychiatry. 2004;45(2):260–73.
40. Snow AL, et al. Accuracy of self-reported depression in persons with dementia. J Am Geriatr Soc. 2005;53(3):389–96.
41. Forstmeier, S. and A. Maercker, Motivational processes in mild cognitive impairment and Alzheimer's disease: results from the Motivational Reserve in Alzheimer's (MoReA) study. 2015.
42. Winblad B, et al. Mild cognitive impairment--beyond controversies, towards a consensus: report of the international working group on mild cognitive impairment. J Intern Med. 2004;256(3):240–6.
43. Folstein MF, Folstein SE, McHugh PR. "Mini-mental state". A practical method for grading the cognitive state of patients for the clinician. J Psychiatr Res. 1975;12(3):189–98.
44. Morris JC. The clinical dementia rating (CDR): current version and scoring rules. Neurology. 1993;43(11):2412–4.
45. American Psychiatric Association. Diagnostic and statistical manual of mental disorders. DSM-IV-TR. Washington, DC: American Psychiatric Publishing, Inc; 2000.
46. Storandt M, et al. Rates of progression in mild cognitive impairment and early Alzheimer's disease. Neurology. 2002;59(7):1034–41.
47. Biessels GJ, et al. Risk of dementia in diabetes mellitus: a systematic review. Lancet Neurol. 2006;5(1):64–74.
48. Gauggel S, Birkner B. Validität und Reliabilität einer deutschen Version der geriatrischen Depressionsskala (GDS). Z Klin Psychol. 1999;28(1):18–27.
49. Yesavage JA, et al. Development and validation of a geriatric depression screening scale: a preliminary report. J Psychiatr Res. 1983;17(1):37–49.
50. Stroop JR. Studies of interference in serial verbal reactions. J Exp Psychol Gen. 1992;121(1):15.
51. Little RJ. A test of missing completely at random for multivariate data with missing values. J Am Stat Assoc. 1988;83(404):1198–202.
52. Singer JD, Willett JB, Willett JB. Applied longitudinal data analysis: Modeling change and event occurrence. USA: Oxford university press; 2003.
53. Heck RH, Thomas SL, Tabata LN. Multilevel and Longitudinal Modeling with IBM SPSS. Quantitative Methodology Series. Second ed. New York: Routledge; 2014.
54. Maas CJ, Hox JJ. Sufficient sample sizes for multilevel modeling. Methodology. 2005;1(3):86–92.
55. McNeish DM, Stapleton LM. The effect of small sample size on two-level model estimates: a review and illustration. Educ Psychol Rev. 2016;28(2): 295–314.
56. Xu R. Measuring explained variation in linear mixed effects models. Stat Med. 2003;22(22):3527–41.
57. Bruscoli M, Lovestone S. Is MCI really just early dementia? A systematic review of conversion studies. Int Psychogeriatr. 2004;16(02):129–40.
58. Reid LM, Maclullich AM. Subjective memory complaints and cognitive impairment in older people. Dement Geriatr Cogn Disord. 2006;22(5–6):471–85.
59. Mortby ME, Maercker A, Forstmeier S. Midlife motivational abilities predict apathy and depression in Alzheimer disease: the aging, demographics, and memory study. J Geriatr Psychiatry Neurol. 2011;24(3):151–60.
60. Boyle PA, et al. Poor decision making is a consequence of cognitive decline among older persons without Alzheimer's disease or mild cognitive impairment. PLoS One. 2012;7(8):e43647.
61. Laurin D, et al. Physical activity and risk of cognitive impairment and dementia in elderly persons. Arch Neurol. 2001;58(3):498–504.
62. Cardinal RN, et al. Emotion and motivation: the role of the amygdala, ventral striatum, and prefrontal cortex. Neurosci Biobehav Rev. 2002;26(3):321–52.
63. Kalivas PW, Volkow ND. The neural basis of addiction: a pathology of motivation and choice. Am J Psychiatr. 2005;162(8):1403–13.
64. Rodgers JL, et al. Resolving the debate over birth order, family size, and intelligence. Am Psychol. 2000;55(6):599.
65. Sattler C, et al. Cognitive activity, education and socioeconomic status as preventive factors for mild cognitive impairment and Alzheimer's disease. Psychiatry Res. 2012;196(1):90–5.
66. Stearns SC. Life history evolution: successes, limitations, and prospects. Naturwissenschaften. 2000;87(11):476–86.
67. Gray KE, et al. Leukocyte telomere length and age at menopause. Epidemiology. 2014;25(1):139–46.
68. Grodstein F, et al. Shorter telomeres may mark early risk of dementia: preliminary analysis of 62 participants from the nurses' health study. PLoS One. 2008;3(2):e1590.
69. Barha CK, et al. Number of children and telomere length in women: a prospective, longitudinal evaluation. PLoS One. 2016;11(1):e0146424.
70. Thoma MV, Maercker A, Forstmeier S. Evidence for different trajectories of delay discounting in older adults with mild cognitive impairment and mild Alzheimer's disease. Journals of Gerontology Series B: Psychological Sciences and Social Sciences. 2016;72(6):956-65.
71. Pfeifer L, et al. Caregiver rating bias in mild cognitive impairment and mild Alzheimer's disease: impact of caregiver burden and depression on dyadic rating discrepancy across domains. Int Psychogeriatr. 2013;25(8):1345–55.
72. Button KS, et al. Power failure: why small sample size undermines the reliability of neuroscience. Nat Rev Neurosci. 2013;14(5):365–76.
73. Sperling RA, et al. Toward defining the preclinical stages of Alzheimer's disease: recommendations from the National Institute on Aging-Alzheimer's Association workgroups on diagnostic guidelines for Alzheimer's disease. Alzheimers Dement. 2011;7(3):280–92.

2

The start of caring for an elderly dependent family member: a qualitative metasynthesis

Lourdes Moral-Fernández*, Antonio Frías-Osuna, Sara Moreno-Cámara, Pedro A. Palomino-Moral and Rafael Del-Pino-Casado

Abstract

Background: The family often takes care of an elderly person who suddenly becomes dependent. This greatly affects different aspects of the caregivers' lives. The aim of this study is to explore the initial experiences, during the first year of care, of persons who suddenly become caregivers for elderly dependent relatives.

Methods: A search in CINAHL, PsycINFO, WOS, Medline, and Scopus and a metasynthesis of qualitative research were conducted including 19 articles.

Results: Three categories were developed to explain the process of becoming a caregiver 'taking on the role' (life changes, uncertainty and confusion, and acceptance or resistance); 'beginning to realise' (new needs, impact, and appraisal); and 'implementing strategies' (seeking help and self-learning, reordering family and social relationships, solving problems, and devising strategies to decrease negative emotions and stress).

Conclusions: The synthesis provides a comprehensive understanding of the experience of becoming a caregiver in order to help health-care professionals to adapt care plans to this situation.

Keywords: Family caregiver, Qualitative, Metasynthesis, Initial, Elderly dependent

Background

The world population has been experiencing a growth in the numbers of older people since the mid-twentieth century, a trend which will no doubt continue through the twenty-first century [1]. This increase in life expectancy is one of the greatest human achievements of recent times, but the fact of living longer carries the likelihood of suffering chronic and disabling diseases that involve increasing dependency [1].

At present, public policy offers low levels of formal long-term care provisions in most EU countries [2, 3]. As a result, family and friends—and especially women—are mitigating this shortcoming. Thus, the figure of the family caregivers appears, as 'a non-professional person who provides primary assistance with activities of daily living, either in part or in whole, towards a dependent person in his/her immediate circle' [2].

Taking care of a dependent person involves changes and assumption of new responsibilities by the caregivers, which change their lives significantly. They have to deal with activities of daily living that they previously did not have had to do [4]. Thus, many aspects of caregivers' physical and mental health, as well as their social and family lives are affected negatively by their caring role [5], causing them problems with their physical health, relationships, personal well-being, and finances [6, 7].

The pathologies that generate dependency can appear progressively or suddenly. The type of appearance of the illness affects the adaptation process of the caregivers [8]. Progressive appearance diseases make the adaptation process easier because of the smooth and gradual onset of the disease. Abrupt or acute appearance diseases require an immediate adoption of the task of caring, and thus, these bring a more sudden change for the caregivers and make the adaptation process more difficult [9]. In this adaptation process, several aspects are

* Correspondence: lmf00006@red.ujaen.es
Department of Nursing, School of Health Sciences, University of Jaén, Campus Las Lagunillas, s/n, 23071 Jaén, Spain

involved, among which are the needs, expectations, consequences, and feelings of family caregivers [8].

Research shows that the initial stage of caregiving is the worst, especially when the relative has become suddenly dependent [10].

Helping caregivers to adapt to their role may diminish the negative consequences of care [11, 12]. In order to help this adaptation by implementing the right caregivers' interventions, it is essential to know the process and characteristics that surround this change.

There are few studies that attempt to clarify the phases that a person goes through as a family caregiver at the beginning of her or his caregiver role, and those that do involve either theoretical research [13, 14] or they focus on specific issues and specific areas [15–18].

Thus, we have perceived a need for a reinterpretation of the whole process of suddenly taking on a caregiver role. The knowledge and in-depth and holistic understanding of the caregivers' experiences in the early stages will allow us to understand and identify the elements and dimensions involved in the process of becoming a family caregiver. With this, health-care professionals could be better informed and offer interventions that are better adapted to the situation faced by caregivers at the beginning of their caring role, ensuring the well-being of the caregiver and, therefore, of the care recipient as well.

Because there are several qualitative studies that offer an in-depth analysis of the beginning of the caring role, we decided to conduct a qualitative metasynthesis in order to expand the transferability of the results from this research. The aim of this metasynthesis is to explore the experiences during the early stages of a person becoming the caregiver of an elderly dependent relative who has suddenly experienced an acute illness. The specific aims were to identify qualitative research in this area, and through synthesis of the study findings, describe the characteristics and the process of becoming a caregiver.

Methods

Design, setting, and sample

We present a qualitative metasynthesis, following the procedures of Sandelowski and Barroso [19]: (a) literature search, (b) quality assessment, (c) analysis of findings, and (d) synthesis of findings. We examined the study findings using constant comparative analysis, and we coded, compared, and sorted conceptual categories, attempting to interpret each category in relation to each other across studies.

Literature search

To identify qualitative studies, we formulated a comprehensive search carried out from May 2018 to June 2018. To find all relevant studies, we used a multifaceted search strategy with several search strings without time limit for inclusion of the publications. In spite of the difficulties involved in the search for qualitative studies because of the richness and expressive variety of the titles of qualitative research, different alternative terms were searched for the description of the research subject (transition, new or become), following the recommendations of McKibbon, Wilczynski and Haynes [20] and Evans [21] to maximise sensitivity. MeSH (Medical Subject Headings) terms were also added where possible, in order to encompass the most widely used database search such as Medline (caregiver * or carer *).

The search string used was: (Caregiv* or carer*) AND (new caregiv* or become caregiv* or transition in caregiv* or new carer* or become carer* or (transition and carer*)) AND ((("semi-structured" or semistructured or unstructured or informal or "in-depth" or indepth or "face-to-face" or guide or guides) AND (interview* or discussion* or questionnaire*)) or ("focus group" or "focus groups" or qualitative OR ethnograph* or fieldwork or "field work" or "key informant" or "interviews as topic" or "focus groups" or narration or qualitative research or "personal narratives as topic")).

The five databases searched were: CINAHL, PsycINFO, WOS, Medline, and Scopus. We manually searched the bibliographies of the selected articles to capture relevant research articles that fell outside the identified search terms utilised, through which four more manuscripts were added.

The search resulted in a total of 5102 results, of which 3037 were duplicates. Of the 2065 remaining records, 1603 were not relevant to the topic and 462 could fit the inclusion criteria according to the title and/or abstract. The main author reviewed the complete texts of these 462 articles and discarded 447 (73 studies that were not qualitative one, 94 because they did not focus on family care, 101 because they did not study dependent elderly people and 179 because the researches did not occur at the beginning of care). As a result, a total of 15 articles that met the inclusion criteria were selected to be included in the metasynthesis. In addition, four more studies were included by reviewing the references of full texts revised (Fig. 1).

Study selection

Due to the difficulty of identifying relevant research by keyword searching alone, we manually searched for all the studies which met the inclusion criteria. Papers were reviewed first by title, then by abstract, and finally by full text whenever it was necessary. Inclusion criteria for the metasynthesis were: (a) new primary caregiver (b) caring for less than 1 year (c) for a dependent elderly relative who has suffered an abrupt or acute disease causing dependency; (c) research using qualitative methodology.

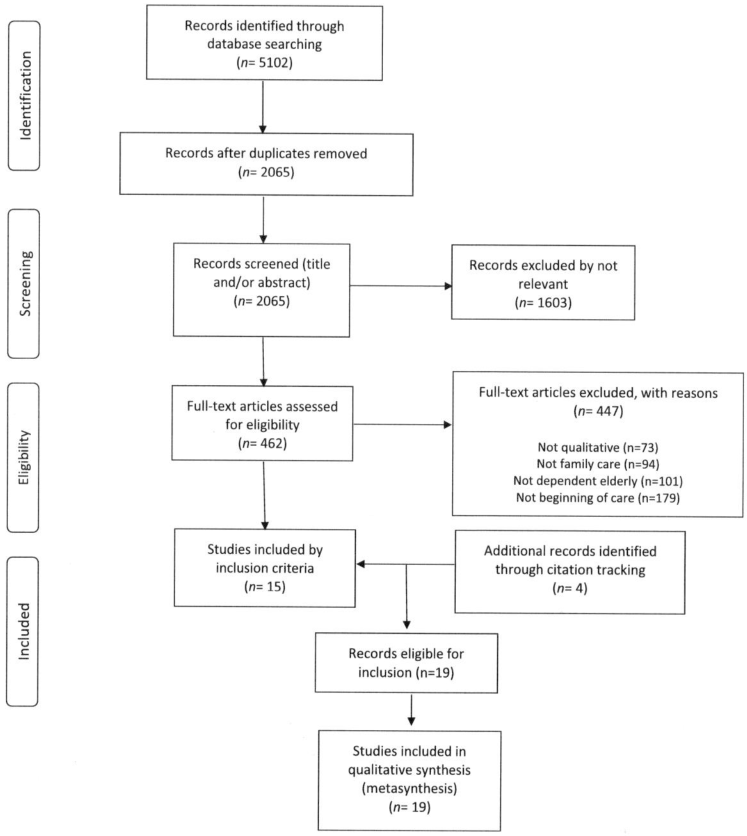

Fig. 1 PRISMA(*) flow diagram of the review process. (*) Moher D, Liberati A, Tetzlaff J, Altman DG, The PRISMA Group. The RISMA statement for reporting systematic reviews and meta-analyses of studies that evaluate health care interventions: explanation and elaboration. J Clin Epidemiol. 2009; 62: 1006–1012

Quality appraisal

According to Sandelowski and Barroso [19], although quality should not be a criterion used to exclude studies, it should be included in the comparative analysis of the design features of each study. For this, we used the Critical Appraisal Skills Programme (CASP) – Qualitative [22], following a prescriptive and comprehensive checklist appropriate for metasynthesis and widely extended in this type of research [23]. The tool consists of 10 questions relating to rigour and relevance, with an assessment system of "yes", "no" or "can't tell". This evaluation of the evidence is based on subjective and judicious discussions about the quality of the recovered evidence. The first two questions (yes / no) are mandatory questions. If the answer is affirmative in both questions, the remaining questions are assessed. The following seven questions are about the research design, data collection and analysis. The last question is about clinical applicability, so we did not use this question.

Data extraction

After the localisation and selection of the studies, the extraction of the findings from the primary sources was started through manual extraction in each manuscript, including the specific results presented by the researchers as subjects and the dialogues of the participants in the original. This allowed us to reduce the bias of erroneous extraction of data from primary sources [24]. To classify and summarise the studies, the descriptive data of each study were extracted, and the information of each article regarding its design and the characteristics of the sample were recorded in a customised form.

In total, we analysed interview fragments of 393 family caregivers, whose verbatim comments appear in the 19 included articles and are transcribed in 59 pages.

Data analysis

After the abstraction of data, two of the authors performed the analysis individually, developing categories and coding the data. A dynamic and iterative process of thought, induction, interpretation, theorisation and reflection (chosen against the method of integration and aggregation) were performed. The information was extracted and interpreted, and the findings were obtained through the taxonomic organisation of categories and subcategories, following axial, selective, in vivo, or imported encoding of the same. Everything was done with the help of memos, which arose from the writing of theoretical ideas about codes and their emerging relationships in the coding process [25].

Findings of the research have been introduced in the version 11 NVIVO software, developed by Qualitative Solutions and Research, which allows for the coding of texts in a series of categories that classify dimensions, properties and attributes. The study method and process are presented in detail below.

After a thorough reading of the interview fragments, 693 references resulted and 169 total codes were identified with the highest level of disaggregation. Secondly, we established the characteristics and relationships of the categories and subcategories grouped according to similarities and differences. As a result of this process, and after the consensus of the two researchers involved in the analysis, a total of 16 categories and 10 subcategories emerged.

Finally, a consensus was made between the two researchers involved in the analysis, in order to make the qualitative synthesis, guided by the grounded theory approach [26, 27] through the repeated use of the constant comparative method, for which we looked for similarities and differences in the information available. The memorandums were significant in the process of constant comparison, allowing for the design of the emergency map, and the identification of the concepts and their relationships.

To synthesize the categories, the research team relied on the discourses of the caregivers, repeatedly mentioning the existence of different stages of care. These discourses revealed an initial stage triggered by the illness of his relative and the great change that occurred in all aspects of his life as they began to become caregivers, causing feelings of uncertainty and confusion. From here, caregivers develop different ways of coping, leaving attention, avoiding facing or accepting it, beginning to realize this way of their new role as caregiver. During this phase, caregivers manifest new needs, different consequences of care and re-evaluate their situation with the intention of normalizing it. At this time, the caregivers implement strategies according to their resources, the relationship with the dependent person, the way in which they face their role as caregivers and the circumstances that surround them. Thus, to synthesize the findings, a process of becoming a caregiver with different moments and phases of care was proposed (Fig. 2).

In the last phase of the metasynthesis process, we determine a general conceptualization of the analysis among the researchers of the study, the adjustments of the matrix of each category, and the subcategory and the groups in an inductive manner. The findings were reduced in the coding process, regrouped into ten subcategories integrated into broader categories. This process was carried out according to the relationships of the axis and the care phases appeared in the caregivers' discourses, and finally three final categories were obtained. To complete the qualitative synthesis, the topics were discussed in several categories by the entire group and a diagram was made with the results of the process of becoming a family caregiver of an elderly dependent.

Validity

As suggested by Sandelowski and Barroso [19] or Maxwell [28], several procedures can be employed to

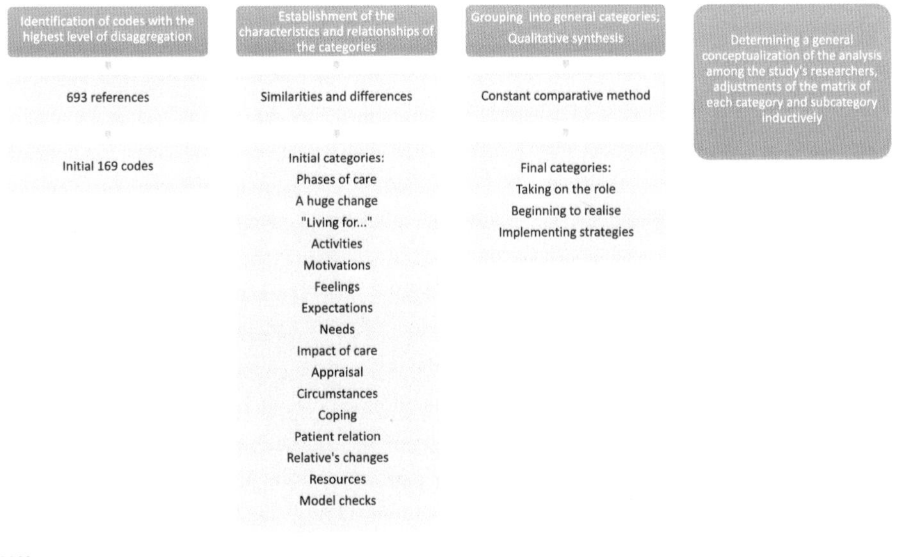

Fig. 2 Analysis process

improve the descriptive, interpretive and theoretical validity of qualitative research integrations.

The descriptive validity was maintained through a thorough search of research related to the subject of study and description of the information of each article included in this metasynthesis, as well as by a CASP quality score assigned by the research team.

Interpretive validity was maintained by team members who analysed the results of the individual studies and integrated them into consensus. In addition, notes were taken during meetings of the research team to maintain an audit trail in decision-making.

The theoretical validity was related to the theoretical constructs that were developed during the study, beyond the description and the interpretation of the primary studies.

Results

The 19 articles included a total of 393 family caregivers. Most caregivers were women (77%), usually wives and daughters, of various nationalities and with an average age of approximately 50 years. The people cared for were dependent elderly persons (average age of 72 years), with different types of health conditions: stroke, cancer, hip fracture, brain injury, accident, sepsis and transplant.

Of the 19 articles (Table 1), one was written in Portuguese but had translations in English and Spanish, one was written in Spanish, and the others were all written in English. Geographically, five of the articles were from the United States, one from Canada (Ontario), two from South America (Brazil), seven from Europe (Italy, Scotland, England, Spain and Portugal), two from Asia (China), and two from Australia.

The different methodological approaches found were: (a) phenomenological design (three works); (b) content analysis (one); (c) thematic content (three); (d) ethnographic design (one); (e) grounded theory (four); (f) constant comparative analyses (two); (g) theory based on data (one); (h) Van Manen's approach (one); and (i) method used not specified (three). The methods of collecting the information have been interviews and focus groups.

Regarding the methodological quality of the included studies, we found some weaknesses in the following questions: justification of the design used, adjustment of data collection method with the objective and methodology, and the analysis of authors' role in the research (Table 2).

First, the appearance of different moments or stages of care in the caregivers' discourses helped the researchers to classify the different categories around different stages of care: *"It has different stages, they change and each stage has its good and bad things. You have to adapt as you can to each situation"* [29].

According to this fact, and following the analysis, three categories appeared that involved the process of becoming a caregiver: 'Taking on the role' (including life changes, caregivers' uncertainty and confusion, and caregivers' acceptance or resistance); 'beginning to realise' (including caregivers' new needs, impact, and appraisal), and 'implementing strategies' (including seeking help and self-learning, reordering family and social relationships, solving problems, and devising strategies to decrease negative emotions and stress) (Fig. 3).

Taking on the role

Caregivers feel an initial shock associated with the illness and disability of their family members. Their lives are turned upside down due to the changes associated with becoming a caregiver [29–31].

They mention the new situation that they have to assume and describe the day of onset of their family member's illness as crucial to their lives and as unpredictable [32–34].

The transition in moving from the hospital to the home tends to be harder than they expected, as it contrasts with the joy they experience after discharge and being in their usual environment, where they find instead a concern and lack of preparation to provide necessary care to their family member [34–36].

Life changes

The changes in the lives of caregivers when they face an imminent situation of dependence of a family member are very large, since in most cases the dependent person has hitherto led an autonomous life and now, due to an illness or acute problem, suddenly finds him- or herself in a situation of dependence [29, 36–38]. *'This cancer has been a total disruption of my life. Your whole life changes in 24 hours.'* [30].

The caregiver must then leave his or her life aside and almost exclusively care for their relative. Normally, as the carers exercise their role, their daily activities are multiplied. As a result, caregivers have to cope with a huge amount of new responsibilities related to care.

Uncertainty and confusion

The changes and the assumption of new responsibilities of care cause diverse emotions for the caregivers, among which the following stand out: the uncertainty, the imprecision of the prognosis related to the illness, for the future that they have to face, and for the lack of information and preparation for the situation [32, 34, 37–41]. *'They just don't know—that is what is quite scary, it is the unknown. You just don't know what it is going to be like in a year's time... because... everybody is just so different.'* [40].

Table 1 Summary of articles included in the metasynthesis

Author (year), country	Purposes	Methods and sample	Main Results
Houldin (2007) [30] Philadelphia (EEUU)	To report on a descriptive study of patients newly diagnosed with advanced colorectal cancer.	Semi-structured interviews to 14 carers and thematic content analysis.	Findings revealed three domains: Experiencing total disruption of my life, Staying positive, and Attempting to keep family and children's routines as normal as possible.
Paiva et al. (2012) [31] Río de Janeiro (Brasil)	To discuss the relationship between the family and hospital discharge regarding manifestations, attitudes, feelings and practices.	Semi-structured interviews to 9 carers and theory based on data approach.	Findings reflected the categories: "Facing the unexpected," "Recognizing the need for care after discharge" and "Realizing one's importance in the recovery of the relative".
Plank et al. (2012) [32] Verona (Italy)	To explore and understand the experience of new informal carers in Italy during the transition from hospital to home.	In-depth interviews and focus groups to 18 carers and a qualitative phenomenological approach.	Family caregivers reflected their newly acquired role; the recipient's condition; and the support they required. The core concept of 'being responsible for everything' seemed to be a recurring theme running through these three subject matters.
Grimmer et al. (2004) [36] Australia	To describe the perceptions of people taking on a new or expanded caring role of an elderly patient recently hospitalised with a new or intensified health problem.	Semi-structured interviews to 24 carers (method used not specified).	The study highlighted carers' perceptions of being unprepared for their new tasks, and their frustrations at the long-term and frequently significant changes to their lives brought about by assuming a caring role.
Teschendorf et al. (2007) [41] EEUU	To describe informal cancer care provision from the perspective of the carer.	Focus groups to 63 carers and content analysis.	Providing supportive care introduced a balancing act in caregivers' lives as they attempted to address complex and overlapping roles. They felt alone in their decisions, were under-prepared for tasks they assumed, and tried to shield the care recipient
Nahm et al. (2010) [37] Baltimore (EEUU)	To explore informal carers' experiences with providing care to older adults over the first 6-month trajectory of hip fracture recovery and their support needs.	In-depth interviews to 10 carers and phenomenological approach.	Management of hospital bills and transitions between care settings were especially burdensome. The caregiving situation was viewed as an opportunity to spend more time with their loved ones. Findings revealed unmet support needs expressed by caregivers of older adult hip fracture patients.
Smith et al. (2004) [35] Glasgow (Scotland)	This paper reports on a study that aimed to describe the experience of caring for a stroke survivor at one year after stroke in Scotland.	Semi-structured interviews to 90 carers and thematic data.	Initially most carers found that they lacked the knowledge and skills to care for the stroke survivor at home and so they had to learn how to obtain the information and assistance required. Carers had to adapt to the changes that stroke effected in the stroke survivor and seek alternative ways of securing the resources they needed for managing their lives.
Pereira and Rebelo-Botelho (2011) [38] Portugal	The purpose of this qualitative study was to understand the lived experience of individuals taking on the role of informal adult carers after an unexpected event involving a relative.	Unstructured interviews to 14 carers and Van Manen's approach.	Four main themes were identified: losing control over time, feeling alone, failing expectations and taking over someone else's life.
Greenwood et al. (2009) [40] London (England)	To investigate the experiences of informal carers of stroke survivors over time.	Audio-taped in-depth inter views to 31 carers (method used not specified).	A central theme of uncertainty with a number of other interconnected themes were identified. Other themes including adopting routines and strategies, absolute and relative positives and questioning the future could be seen to both influence and be influenced by uncertainty.
Bakas et al. (2002) [39] Oklahoma (EEUU)	To determinate the self-reported needs, concerns, strategies, and advice of stroke carers during the first 6 months after hospital discharge.	Open questions by telephone to 14 carers (method used not specified).	Findings revealed five major categories of caregivers needs and concerns: information, emotions and behaviours, physical care, instrumental care, and personal responses to caregiving.
Weng et al. (2011) [42] Taiwan (China)	To explore the stress experienced by the primary family carer of the living-related liver transplantation patient during the postopera tive stage.	Face-to-face semi-structured interviews to 6 carers and the matic content analysis.	Participant stress was caused by the gap between expectations and primary caregiving experiences. In particular, the five themes that were identified: unstable sentiment towards liver transplantation; entanglement of burden; non-synchronized family interaction; distance

Table 1 Summary of articles included in the metasynthesis *(Continued)*

Author (year), country	Purposes	Methods and sample	Main Results
			from the healthcare professional; and concern about the protector role function.
Silva-Smith (2007) [43] Colorado (EEUU)	To describe the process associated with preparing for and beginning a new caring role following a family member's stroke.	Audio-taped interviews to 12 carers and grounded theory analysis.	Restructuring life for caregiving was associated with five dimensions: daily life, managing multiple roles, relationship with the stroke survivor, future hopes and plans, and time for self.
Brereton and Nolan (2002) [45] Sheffield (England)	To gain a better appreciation of the needs of new carers of stroke survivors and to consider how these needs change as their role develops.	Interviews to 14 carers and grounded theory analysis.	During the initial period carers engage in a number of different 'seeking' activities in order to try and ensure that they feel competent, confident and safe to provide care and that they understand the likely future demands they may face. Rather than being facilitated by staff, carers' efforts often go unnoticed or are overlooked, resulting in carers feeling that they are 'going it alone'.
Shyu (2000) [46] Taiwan (China)	This study explored the needs of family carers during the transition from hospital to home.	Face-to-face interviews to 16 carers and constant comparative analysis.	Role tuning was the process used by caregivers and care receivers to achieve a harmonious pattern of caregiving and care receiving during the transition from hospital to home.
Shaw et al. (2013) [33] Sidney (Australia)	To explore the experiences of family carers of people diagnosed with upper GI cancer after surgical intervention to (1) identify their unmet supportive care needs and (2) investigate how family carers perceive their role during this time.	Semi-structured telephone interviews to 15 carers and constant comparative analysis.	Family caregivers reported significant information and support needs, their distress was exacerbated by a lack of patient care knowledge. Access to support was limited by caregivers' lack of understanding of the health system and they view their role as part of their family responsibility.
Rodrigues et al. (2013) [44] Sao Paulo (Brasil)	To examine the transition of care in families caring for elderly persons who suffered the first episode of a cerebrovascular accident.	Interviews to 10 carers and instrumental ethnographic approach.	They describe the care process for the dependent elderly person, strategies for the care process and impact and acceptance of the limitations.
Abrahamson et al. (2017) [34] England	To explore the experiences of individuals who have had a severe traumatic brain injury (TBI) and their carers in the first month post-discharge from in-patient rehabilitation into living in the community.	Semi-structured interviews to 10 patients and nine carers, and thematic analysis.	Many patients and carers felt unsupported in the inpatient phase, during transitions; they struggled to accept a new reality of changed abilities, loss of roles and loss of autonomy, and early experiences post-discharge exacerbated fears for the future.
Giosa et al. (2014) [47] Ontario (Canada)	To explore informal family caregiver experiences in supporting care transitions between hospital and home for medically complex older adults.	Semi-structured interviews to 12 caregivers and grounded theory analysis.	They describe the theory "building capacity to care", which involves assessing a caregiver's unique family situation to tailor and provide relevant information, education, and training.
Moral-Fernández et al. (2018) [29] Jaén (Spain)	To describe the initial process through which people who imminently become caregivers of a dependent elderly relative.	In-depth interviews to 11 caregivers, and grounded theory analysis.	An initial phase of changes, in which the caregiver assumes new activities; a second phase full of emotions, in which the needs and consequences emerge; and a third phase that emphasises acceptance as a coping strategy and uncertainty as an expectation of the future.

Although uncertainty is present both in the present and in the future, family caregivers experience different feelings such as: concern about the care situation they must assume; suffering from seeing the discomfort of the family member they are caring for and the change they have undergone; impotence for not being able to do more or take better care of them; or guilt for failing to perform this task as they would consider appropriate or even for wanting to end that situation in any way [29, 32, 33, 38, 41].

Acceptance or resistance

Given all the problems and needs that family caregivers have, they show different ways of tackling the changes that occur when they begin caring for their relatives. Among these ways that can be adopted of tackling the issue, we find there is generally acceptance of or resistance to the care situation [31–33, 35, 40, 41].

However, other family caregivers are not located on either end, and they underline the lack of knowledge about how to deal with this situation [35]. *'You have to*

Table 2 Critical Appraisal Skills Program

	Answer 1	Answer 2	Answer 3	Answer 4	Answer 5	Answer 6	Answer 7	Answer 8	Answer 9
Houldin (2007) [30]	Yes	Yes	No	?	?	No	Yes	?	Yes
Paiva et al. (2012) [31]	Yes	Yes	No	Yes	?	No	Yes	Yes	Yes
Plank et al. (2012) [32]	Yes	Yes	Yes	Yes	Yes	?	Yes	Yes	Yes
Grimmer et al. (2004) [36]	Yes	Yes	No	No	?	No	Yes	No	Yes
Teschendorf et al. (2007) [41]	Yes	Yes	No	Yes	?	No	?	?	?
Shaw et al. (2013) [33]	Yes	Yes	No	Yes	?	?	Yes	?	Yes
Smith et al. (2004) [35]	Yes	Yes	No	Yes	Yes	?	Yes	Yes	Yes
Greenwood et al. (2009) [40]	Yes	Yes	No	No	?	No	Yes	Yes	Yes
Bakas et al. (2002) [39]	Yes	Yes	No	?	?	No	Yes	?	Yes
Weng et al. (2011) [42]	Yes	Yes	No	?	Yes	?	Yes	?	Yes
Silva-Smith (2007) [43]	Yes	Yes	No	?	?	No	Yes	Yes	?
Brereton and Nolan (2002) [45]	Yes	Yes	Yes	Yes	?	No	Yes	Yes	Yes
Shyu (2000) [46]	Yes	Yes	No	Yes	Yes	?	Yes	Yes	Yes
Rodrigues et al. (2013) [44]	Yes	Yes	?	Yes	?	No	Yes	No	Yes
Pereira and Rebelo-Botelho (2011) [38]	Yes	Yes	?	Yes	Yes	?	Yes	?	Yes
Nahm et al. (2010) [37]	Yes	Yes	No	?	Yes	No	Yes	No	?
Abrahamson (2016)	Yes	Yes	Yes	Yes	Yes	No	Yes	Yes	Yes
Giosa et al. (2014) [47]	Yes	Yes	Yes	Yes	Yes	No	Yes	Yes	Yes
Moral-Fernández et al. (2018) [29]	Yes	Yes	No	Yes	Yes	No	Yes	Yes	Yes
Yes	19	19	4	12	9	0	18	10	16
No +?	0	0	15	7	10	19	1	8	3
No	0	0	13	2	0	13	0	3	0
?	0	0	2	5	10	6	1	5	3

put up a barrier. I sort of just try to look at it as if it's not my husband. ... Learning to separate yourself from the patient. You get so emotionally involved.' [41].

Beginning to realise

Following the assumption of the role and the changes produced, and once in the home, family caregivers begin to realise what the care of their relative entails for their own lives. They begin to be aware of the situation of dependency of their family member, which they sometimes compare with young children, and the amount of care they require for, where possible, an improvement to occur [31, 32].

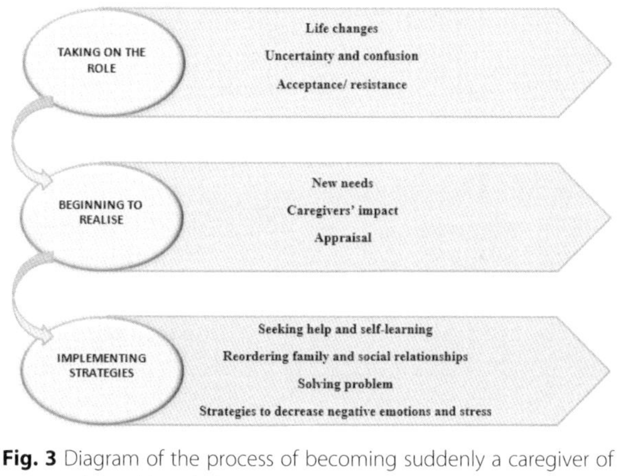

Fig. 3 Diagram of the process of becoming suddenly a caregiver of a dependent older relative

Carers' impact

With the development of caregiving, family caregivers begin to realise the difficulty of this task and the responsibility for be the well-being of their relative being in their hands. Many areas of their lives are altered as a result of their work as a caregiver, starting with their own personal life [33, 38]. *'We lost our personal life... most of it depends on my mother's schedule. For us, being still young, it's hard'* [38].

The performance of so many activities, with the reconciliation of their lives up to the present, presents a challenge to them, causing them stress, weight, and anxiety [29, 32, 37–39, 42]. *'I have been diagnosed with anxiety. I am nervous and get angry easily. The stress comes from inside myself and causes me to feel tremendous tension. This is a difficult time for me'* [42].

The difficulty in combining so many activities is also due to a lack of time. Continuous supervision of a relative is a great time constraint [29, 35, 43].

As a result of the development of care and restrictions of their time, some family caregivers have repercussions in their working life, and even have to leave their paid work in order to dedicate themselves to the care of their family member: *'End up abandoning my job, because there was nobody to care for my mother'* [44]. This, together with the economic impact of the development of an elderly person in a situation of dependency, also causes their economic situation to be negatively impacted [29, 35, 39–41, 43].

They do not have time for themselves, they cannot do the same activities they used to do, and even their sleep is affected, either because of concerns about the care situation and their family, or the person's needs for attention [29, 30, 32, 37, 40]. *'I'm sleeping less and less, because of all the problems regarding appropriate home environment'* [32].

This lack of sleep also affects the physical state of the caregiver, in addition to the mental state, which causes daily fatigue and exhaustion [29, 33, 37, 39, 41, 45]. *'I'm getting tired. 'Cause I need a holiday...I'm just a bit tired, emotionally drained actually'* [33].

Their social life is largely non-existent because they have to spend so much time taking care of their relative. Moreover, relationships between the dependent family member and the caregiver's nuclear family are affected in this situation, especially in the early stages, because there is a loss of privacy for the family or couple, which can cause family conflict [29, 30, 38, 39, 43, 45]. *'He never complained of anything, and suddenly he fell in the bathroom, it was such a fright... this situation had an impact on the family relationships, because of his limitations'* [44].

It is also worth mentioning that there are also discourses in which caregivers mention the personal growth and satisfaction that the care task reports to them, and how it helps them value day-to-day things [29, 40, 41]. *'You appreciate a lot of things, don't you when you can't do all the things you did? So I think you learn to know yourself a lot better... and then you think 'I can'... and there is a certain satisfaction, isn't there?'* [40].

New needs

The synthesis of the findings found in the articles on the first moments in the care of a dependent family shows that the main needs of the initial caregivers are the need for information, time, help, support, and instruction for care.

The need for information about the illness, care and prognosis of the family member, and the training to develop the necessary skills to perform the task of caring in the best possible way, is reflected in the requests of family caregivers to health personnel [29, 30, 32, 33, 35–37, 39–41, 43, 45–47]. *'We would like to know how ill she is; I think the hospital should give us a card and state what kind of disease the patient has, how well the disease has been treated, and whether there are any risks left, so the family can know what to expect.'* [46].

They emphasise expressions like, 'there was nobody there that could tell me', 'no one tells you anything', 'nobody really told me anything', from which the presence of personnel is glimpsed, without any offer of information or help.

They do not feel sufficiently prepared to take care of their relative with all the problems that the patient may present at any time [34, 41, 42, 47].

Caregivers also complain about the need for financial resources, because caring for a dependent person entails a lot of expenses and they do not normally have a paid job, or as stated in the previous category, they have had to leave a job because of the care [29, 35, 46].

They find it difficult to balance care with their other responsibilities, and for this reason they express that aid is one of the most important needs, whether at the professional level, by health personnel; or family, in many cases no other family member is involved in care [32, 33, 43, 45].

Family caregivers not only do not receive help in caring for their relatives, they do not receive support for themselves. Hence they express the need for someone to go and see them and talk to them to get their act together [29, 38, 46]. *'I feel like I am in a room with thousands of people and I am screaming out and no one is hearing me.'* [43].

Appraisal

According to Lazarus and Folkman [48], appraisal is a process by which a person evaluates the situation and makes changes in his or her behaviours or skills needed to cope with the stressful situation. In this case, family caregivers generally feel that they cannot cope with this task properly and need help in their functions and resources to continue in the right way [33, 36, 45]. *'It really battered me around... it really wears you down. I couldn't cope I had to get out...I'm tired of it.'* [35].

Implementing strategies

After assuming the role of caregiver and beginning to realise the consequences, caregivers try to adopt certain strategies that make this task of care more bearable for them.

Seeking help and self-learning

Among these strategies adopted, caregivers try to learn about the disease that affects their family and the dispensing of care required, thus seeking both formal and family help, and they try to learn care skills [36, 40, 45, 47]. *'I started reading a lot about what to expect. .. so I tried to understand what she is going to be changing into'* [40]. *"We were pulling it [looking for information] on our own because otherwise it was just a black hole ... you're kind of thirsting for information that whole time"* [47].

Reordering family and social relationships

As stated earlier, one of the consequences of taking on the carer role is the changing of their social and family relationships, so that caregivers seek to reorganise these relationships to normalise the situation. Thanks to this family organisation, the work is done as a routine that is divided into jobs for each member of the family, which creates a greater sense of family calm [40, 43]. *'I think that we're calming down, I can feel this too, I myself am much calmer! But I still think the insecurity affects us because it's all very new, you know? However, I feel, like my sisters, that we're restructuring...it's because time is passing.'* [43].

Solving problems

Following trying to normalise the situation of care, caregivers may adopt coping strategies focused on solving problems, which increases safety in the care they provide [29, 38, 40]. *'I think that every time we get a little bit further away, it makes us more secure. It is like dangerous waters and we are gradually sailing out of them'* [40].

Strategies to decrease negative emotions and stress

Finally, in the process of becoming a caregiver, they seek to reduce the negative effects by trying to take care of strategies to maintain emotional positivity and reduce stress levels such as talking to the family and letting go, taking things intentionally humorously, being positive and optimistic, and encouraging the person cared for to maintain spiritual support, among others [30, 31, 40]. *'One thing that – whatever happens, I always say that it is [the] best. Better. God never wants to harm you, it is your destiny. And there is always something positive – good.'* [40].

Discussion

The findings of the present metasynthesis respond to the objective proposed in the research and show that the process by which people suddenly become caregivers of an elderly relative in a situation of dependence is dynamic and progressive in time. It happens when a family member develops symptoms that make it difficult to carry out the activities of his daily life, and a person from his family environment helps him with the care needs that arise, until this person who takes on the caregiver's role begins to realise the consequences and tries to normalise his new role of caregiver.

There is no article that indicates the generic phases through which a caregiver passes to take care of a dependent family suffering an acute-onset illness, but we found articles that describe stages of this transition in dementia [15, 17, 18], research about the stages towards cohabitation [16], the process of adaptation to dependency in older adults and their families [49], some theoretical approaches [13], and another review about family care in terminally ill patients [50]. Firbank and Johnson [16], examine the paths that lead elderly people and their family caregivers to cohabiting. Bunn et al. [15] evaluate the qualitative evidence about how people accommodate and adapt to the diagnosis of dementia and its immediate consequences. Prorok et al. [18] try to understand the health-care experience of people with dementia and their carevigers. Gibbons et al. [17] try to understand the experience of family caregivers during the liminality phase. Finally, Martín et al. [50] reveal the experience of family caregivers who care for a terminally ill patient in their home. The results of these studies coincide roughly with our results, so that Firbank and Johnson [16], Bunn et al. [15], Gibbons et al. [17], and Martín et al. [50] first identified a health event that causes some kind of dependency in a family, which means that a family member takes over care, hence after diagnosis, the stage of change begins.

A common event in all phases of research dedicated to the process of becoming a caregiver is the changes. This research shows that the trigger with which the process of becoming a caregiver begins is the great change caused by a dependence situation in a family member. This is widely supported with various studies. Bunn et al. [15] and Moreno-Cámara et al. [11] describe these changes in a way that is similar the present research; during the first phase of care, when the family has been diagnosed with dementia and begins with a succession of changes that interfere with all areas of the lives of the caregiver, and to which they must adapt. Gibbons et al. [17], speaks about a pivotal event (disability or illness) in the pre-liminal phase that turns the lives of caregivers upside down and causes changes in the intermediate stage of care; in particular they highlight social changes. Prorok et al. [18] agree with our results that identify confusion and uncertainty early in the process, and identify changes in the last phase of the start of care, in which the caregiver must live with these changes. Changes are also a constant in most of the research on the early stages of care [9, 50–55]. In spite of 'change' being a category as such individually, it is also the precursory of other categories and influences in the development of them, not only because of its meaning but because all other categories that make up the process of becoming a caregiver happen with subsequent changes. For this reason, it is a dimension identified in the early stages of care.

In this first phase of assuming the role of caregiver, a range of emotions experienced by carers will accompany the changes, highlighting the uncertainty and suffering that coincide with those expressed by Gibbons et al. [17] in the liminal and post-liminal phase in their research about the beginning of caring, and by Moreno et al. [11]. These emotions have also consistently surfaced in several original studies and reviews about the beginning stage of care [54, 56] and they are widely developed in the studies of this metasynthesis, from comforting and satisfying emotions to emotions of fear and despair.

In the second stage, caregivers begin to realise their new role. In this way, new needs arise that are associated with the care of their relative, and they start to experience the consequences of exercising this role. The results of this metasynthesis resemble those found in Prorok's article [18], which identifies the need for information during the early stages of care, Bunn's article [15], which also describes the second phase of the start of care as a time when conflicts arise, and Firbank's research [16], which explains the elderly person's inability to perform activities of daily living and the children's needs in providing help to their parent. Also, the needs that emerge in the early stages of caring are matched in studies of caregivers of people who have had a stroke [56, 57], and the consequences coincide, to a large degree, with the results most commonly found in other research into the early stages of care [55, 58, 59].

During the third phase, which involves implementation of strategies to minimise the negative effects of care, the emotional consequences and stress occur. Caregivers seek to learn the skills to become more self-sufficient in care and finally reorganise relations for a better adaptation of both the family and social situation. Among these implemented strategies we can find coping strategies, which include seeking help and solving the problems that arise during care. The latest strategy is, according to Gottlieb and Wolfe [60], the most important and better coping strategy. This coincides roughly with the third stage proposed by Bunn et al. [15] where, as in this metasynthesis, the implementation of strategies that help to minimise the impact of care was located after the initial changes, and with Prorok's [18] and Moreno--Cámara's research [11], identifying self-learning as also being an important strategy of implementation. All these facts mark a new situation of normality for the family caregiver [17, 48], thus showing a sample of acceptance and normalization of her new role and culminating the process of conversion to caregiver.

It is interesting how significant differences were not found in relation to the different pathologies that the dependent person suffered, but to their level of dependence and the abilities of the caregiver to develop adequate coping strategies. The phases proposed in this research can be related to the common phases of a crisis, referred to as 'a temporary event with a start and an end that appears unexpectedly and whose course follows the following phases: impact phase, reaction phase and phase of reorientation' ([61] p. 51). In agreement with the results of the present research and the phases proposed by Ruiz [61], it could be determined that the people who become caregivers at first are impacted due to the unexpected character of their new role, stunning him and affecting him emotionally. This could correspond to a state of shock, which is characterised by a state of shock and blockage. The reaction phase is related to the awareness of the situation, which implies suffering and different emotional reactions. After that, the reorientation phase is characterised by the assimilation of the situation, whereby the caregiver begins to accept what has happened and is mobilised to face and overcome the situation, producing in this way a readjustment in their lives in search of a new stability.

The results of this metasynthesis help us to understand how a relative takes care of a dependent elderly person and how this care evolves until the caregiver begins to adapt to this role. Knowing the stages of the process of becoming a caregiver may be useful for health professionals in establishing interventions tailored to each stage in order to help caregivers to adapt to their new role and resolve their uncertainty and inexperience.

Because the first moments of care have a common succession of changes triggered after diagnosis, which causes feelings of confusion, suffering, and uncertainty, early interventions might be appropriate based on generic information about the disease that has led to the dependence of the older person, the care needs during the first moments of care, and information about available resources, in order to alleviate feelings of confusion and uncertainty experienced by caregivers. During the second and third stages, caregivers evaluate the caring situation and implement strategies to adapt to the caring situation; at this time, tailored interventions are needed to help caregivers in assuming their role, implementing better adaptive strategies, and solving care needs.

Limitations

The main limitation of this research is the lack of availability of the complete original transcripts of the primary studies, which hinders and influences the researchers' analysis of this metasynthesis. This research is based on fragments of caregiver discourses that the primary authors have selected as a reflection of their results. To try to solve this limitation, two different researchers have analyzed the discourses independently and unrelated to the interpretation of the original authors.

With respect to the quality of the studies included in metasynthesis, a good quality of the included studies has generally been observed. According to the CASP tool, a large number of responses are positive, although criteria related to the justification of the research design in relation to the aims of the research, the explanation of the data collection and the consideration of the relationships between the researcher and the study participants. Although the first two criteria are evaluated in a deficient manner, it is possible to observe the congruence of designs and data collection methods used in the included studies with the analysis of the initial experiences of persons who suddenly become caregivers for elderly dependent relatives, even though these issues are not specifically detailed in most of the articles of the present review. Thus, it would have a minimal impact of the low quality in the previous criteria on the review's quality. This possible minimal impact is based not only in previous reasoning but also in the assertion of Sandelowski and Barroso, which argued that the quality of the studies should not determine the integrity of the research [19].

Transferability

The analysis of qualitative information included in this metasynthesis, which comes from different cultural contexts and various caregiver profiles, means these results are useful for understanding the earliest stages of care for dependent elderly family members in different situations.

In addition, both the search strategy and the characteristics of each included study have been described in detail, which allows its replication, and may facilitate transferability to other similar situations.

Conclusions

The main contribution of this study is the identification of the process characterised through the stages of 'taking on the role', 'beginning to realise', and 'implementing strategies'. At the beginning stage of caring for a dependent family member, it is usual for the caregiver to experience changes that affect most aspects of the caregiver's life, such as the responsibilities they assume and the activities they must perform once they become carers. As they have to perform all the activities and meet all the needs that the patient cannot do for themselves, there is an increase in their own needs that is provoked by the new situation that they have to deal with regarding their caring role. All this entails some consequences for the caregiver, which often tend to be emotional, familial, and social. Finally, the carer of an elderly person who becomes dependent suddenly seeks strategies to normalise their situation as caregiver and reduce stress.

This study will allow us to learn more about the transition to the role of caregiver in order to propose a more detailed plan of care, with specific interventions during the early days of caring. Early interventions based on generic information may be needed at the beginning of the process in order to alleviate uncertainty, and tailored interventions may be needed later, depending on the evaluation of the caring situation, in order to help caregivers with implementing adaptive strategies.

We recommend that future research should include the development of studies that address the process of becoming a primary caregiver as a phenomenon of global study with primary data.

Abbreviations

CASP: Critical appraisal skills programme; GI cancer: Gastrointestinal cancer; MeSH: Medical subject headings; TBI: Traumatic brain injury

Funding

This research received no specific grant from any funding agency in the public, commercial, or not-for-profit sectors.

Authors' contributions

All authors have agreed on the final version and they were responsible for the conception and design of the study. MF, FO, MC, PM and DPC performed the collection of data, data analysis and interpretation by consensus. MF and FO were responsible for the drafting of the manuscript. MF, FO, MC, PM and DPC made critical revisions to the article for important intellectual content.

Competing interests

The authors declare that they have no competing interests.

References

References marked with an asterisk indicate studies included in the metasynthesis. The in-text citations to studies selected for metasynthesis are not preceded by asterisks

1. United Nations, Department of Economic and Social Affairs, Population division. World population ageing 2013. New York: United Nations; 2013.
2. Confederation of Family Organisations in the European Union. Charter for Family Carers. 2011. http://www.coface-eu.org/wp-content/uploads/2017/01/COFACE-Disability-CharterEN.pdf. Accessed 24 Jan 2017.
3. Verbakel E. How to understand informal caregiving patterns in Europe? The role of formal long-term care provisions and family care norms. Scand J Public Health. 2017 1. [Epub ahead of print].
4. Macleod M, Chesson RA, Blackledge P, Hutchison JD, Ruta N. To what extent are carers involved in the care and rehabilitation of patients with hip fracture? Disabil Rehabil. 2005;27(18–19):1117–22.
5. Schulz R, Sherwood PR. Physical and mental health effects of family caregiving. Am J Nurs. 2008;108(9 Suppl):23–7. https://doi.org/10.1097/01.NAJ.0000336406.45248.4c.
6. Brewin A. The quality of life of carers of patients with severe lung disease. Br J Nurs 2004 08/12; 13(15):906–912.
7. van Vliet D, de Vugt ME, Bakker C, Koopmans RTCM, Verhey FRJ. Impact of early onset dementia on caregivers: a review. Int J Geriatr Psychiatry. 2010;25(11):1091–100.
8. Rolland J. Families, illness and disability. New York: Basic Books; 1994.
9. Covelli V, Cerniauskaite M, Leonardi M, Sattin D, Raggi A, Giovannetti AM. A

qualitative study on perceptions of changes reported by caregivers of patients in vegetative state and minimally conscious state: the "time gap experience". Sci World J. 2014;2014:1–9.
10. Ducharme F, Lévesque L, Lachance L, Kergoat MJ, Coulombe R. Challenges associated with transition to caregiver role following diagnostic disclosure of Alzheimer disease: a descriptive study. Int J Nurs Stud. 2011;48(9):1109.
11. Moreno-Cámara S, Palomino-Moral PA, Moral-Fernández L, Frías-Osuna A, del-Pino-Casado R. Problemas en el proceso de adaptación a los cambios en personas cuidadoras familiares de mayores con demencia [problems in the process of adapting to change among the family caregivers of elderly people with dementia]. Gac Sanit. 2016;30(3):201–7.
12. Perren S, Schmid R, Wettstein A. Caregivers' adaptation to change: the impact of increasing impairment of persons suffering from dementia on their caregivers' subjective well-being. Aging Ment Health. 2006;10(5):539–48.
13. Montgomery R, Kosloski K. Caregiving as a process of changing identity: implications for caregiver support. Generations. 2009;33(1):47–52.
14. Schumacher KL, Jones PS, Meleis AI. Helping elderly people in transition: a framework for research and practice. In: Swanson EA, Tripp-Reimer T, editors. Life transitions in the older adult. Issues for nurses and other health professionals. New York: Springer; 1999. p. 1–23.
15. Bunn F, Goodman C, Sworn K, Rait G, Brayne C, Robinson L, et al. Psychosocial factors that shape patient and carer experiences of dementia diagnosis and treatment: a systematic review of qualitative studies. PLoS Med. 2012;9(10):e1001331. https://doi.org/10.1371/journal.pmed.1001331.
16. Firbank OE, Johnson-Lafleur J. Older persons relocating with a family caregiver: processes, stages, and motives. J Appl Gerontol. 2007;26(2):182–207.
17. Gibbons SW, Ross A, Bevans M. Liminality as a conceptual frame for understanding the family caregiving rite of passage: an integrative review. Res Nurs Health. 2014;37(5):423–36.
18. Prorok JC, Horgan S, Seitz DP. Health care experiences of people with dementia and their caregivers: a meta-ethnographic analysis of qualitative studies. CMAJ. 2013;185(14):E669–80. https://doi.org/10.1503/cmaj.121795.
19. Sandelowski M, Barroso J. Handbook for synthesizing qualitative research. New York: Springer; 2006.
20. McKibbon AK, Wilczynski NL, Haynes RB. Developing optimal search strategies for retrieving qualitative studies in PsyCinfo. Eval Health Prof. 2006;29(4):440–54.
21. Evans D. Database searches for qualitative research. J Med Libr Assoc. 2002; 90(3):290–3.
22. Critical Appraisa Skills Programme. CASP Qualitative Checklist. 2018. https://casp-uk.net/wp-content/uploads/2018/01/CASP-Qualitative-Checklist.pdf. Accessed 16 July 2017.
23. Walsh D, Downe S. Meta-synthesis method for qualitative research: a literature review. J Adv Nurs. 2005;50(2):204–11.
24. Whittemore R, Knafl K. The integrative review: updated methodology. J Adv Nurs. 2005;52(5):546–53.
25. Glaser BG. Theoretical sensitivity. Mill Valley: Sociology Press; 1978.
26. Glaser BG, Strauss AL. Discovery of grounded theory. Mill Valley: Sociology Press; 1967.
27. Strauss A, Corbin J. Bases de la investigación cualitativa. Técnicas y procedimientos para desarrollar la Teoría Fundamentada. Antioquía: Universidad de Antioquía; 2002.
28. Maxwell J. Understanding and validity in qualitative research. Harv Educ Rev. 1992;62(3):279–301.
29. Moral-Fernández L, Frías-Osuna A, Moreno-Cámara S, Palomino-Moral PA, Del-Pino-Casado R Primeros momentos del cuidado: el proceso de convertirse en cuidador de una familiar mayor dependiente. Aten Primaria. 2018;50(5):282–90.
30. *Houldin A. A qualitative study of caregivers' experiences with newly diagnosed advanced colorectal cancer. Oncol Nurs Forum. 2007;34(2):323–30.
31. *Paiva R, Valadares G, Silva J. The need to become family caregivers: grounded theory. OBJN. 2012;11(3):607-620.
32. *Plank A, Mazzoni V, Cavada L. Becoming a caregiver: new family carers' experience during the transition from hospital to home. J Clin Nurs. 2012; 21(13–14):2072–82. doi:https://doi.org/10.1111/j.1365-2702.2011.04025.x.
33. *Shaw J, Harrison J, Young J, Butow P, Sandroussi C, Martin D, Solomon M. Coping with newly diagnosed upper gastrointestinal cancer: a longitudinal qualitative study of family caregivers' role perception and supportive care needs. Support Care Cancer. 2013;21(3):749–56.
34. *Abrahamson JJ, Jensen J, Springett K, Sakel M. Experiences of patients with traumatic brain injury and their carers during transition from inpatient rehabilitation to the community: a qualitative study. Disabil Rehabil. 2017; 39(17):1683–94.
35. *Smith LN, Lawrence M, Kerr SM, Langhorne P, Lees KR. Informal carers' experience of caring for stroke survivors. J Adv Nurs. 2004;46(3):235–44. doi: https://doi.org/10.1111/j.1365-2648.2004.02983.x.
36. *Grimmer K, Moss J, Falco J. Becoming a carer for an elderly person after discharge from an acute hospital admission. IJAHSP. 2004;2(4):4.
37. *Nahm ES, Resnick B, Orwig D, Magaziner J, DeGrezia M. Exploration of informal caregiving following hip fracture. Geriatr Nurs. 2010;31(4):254–62.
38. *Pereira HR, Botelho MA. Sudden informal caregivers: the lived experience of informal caregivers after an unexpected event. J Clin Nurs. 2011;20(17–18):2448–57. doi:https://doi.org/10.1111/j.1365-2702.2010.03644.x.
39. *Bakas T, Austin J, Okonkwo K, Lewis R, Chadwick L. Needs, concerns, strategies and advice of stroke caregivers the first 6 months after discharge. JNeurosci Nurs. 2002;34(5):242.
40. *Greenwood N, Mackenzie A, Cloud GC, Wilson N. Informal primary carers of stroke survivors living at home – challenges, satisfactions and coping: a systematic review of qualitative studies. Disabil Rehabil. 2009;31(5):337–51.
41. *Teschendorf B, Schwartz C, Ferrans CE, O'Mara A, Novotny P, Sloan J. Caregiver role stress: when families become providers. Cancer Control. 2007; 14(2):183–9.
42. *Weng L, Huang H, Wang Y, Chang C, Tsai C, Lee W. Primary caregiver stress in caring for a living-related liver transplantation recipient during the postoperative stage. J Adv Nurs. 2011;67(8):1749–57. doi:https://doi.org/10.1111/j.1365-2648.2011.05625.x.
43. *Silva-Smith AL. Restructuring life preparing for and beginning a new caregiving role. J Fam Nurs. 2007;13(1):99.
44. *Rodrigues RA, Marques S, Kusumota L, Barros E, da Silva JR, Coelho SC. Transition of care for the elderly after cerebrovascular accidents: from hospital to the home. Rev Lat Am Enfermagem. 2013;21(spe):216–24.
45. *Brereton L, Nolan M. 'Seeking': a key activity for new family carers of stroke survivors. J Clin Nurs. 2002;11(1):22–31. doi:https://doi.org/10.1046/j.1365-2702.2002.00564.x.
46. *Shyu YIL. The needs of family caregivers of frail elders during the transition from hospital to home: a Taiwanese sample. J Adv Nurs. 2000;32(3):619–25.
47. *Giosa J, Stolee P, Dupuis S, Mock S, Santi S. Experiences during care transitions of older adults. Canadian Journal on Aging. 2014;33(2):137–53.
48. Lazarus RS, Folkman S. Stress, appraisal and coping. New York: Springer; 1984.
49. Abad-Corpa E, Gonzalez-Gil T, Martínez-Hernández A, Barderas-Manchado AM, De la Cuesta-Benjumea C, Monistrol-Ruano O, et al. Caring to achieve the maximum independence possible: a synthesis of qualitative evidence on older adults' adaptation to dependency. J Clin Nurs. 2012;21(21–22):3153–69.
50. Martín J, Olano-Lizarraga M, Saracíbar-Razquin M. The experience of family caregivers caring for a terminal patient at home: a research review. Int J Nurs Stud. 2016;64:1–12.
51. Lin H, Lin H, Lin W. Middle-aged female spouses of patients with metastatic cancer: lived experiences. J Nurs Res. 2015;23(2):135–44.
52. McConigley R, Halkett G, Lobb E, Nowak A. Caring for someone with high-grade glioma: a time of rapid change for caregivers. Palliat Med. 2010;24(5):473–9.
53. Pringle J, Hendry C, McLafferty E. A review of the early discharge experiences of stroke survivors and their carers. J Clin Nurs. 2008;17(18):2384–97.
54. Seal K, Murray CD, Seddon L. The experience of being an informal 'carer' for a person with cancer: a meta-synthesis of qualitative studies. Palliat Support Care. 2015;13(03):493–504.
55. Nalder E, Fleming J, Cornwell P, Foster M. Linked lives: the experiences of family caregivers during the transition from hospital to home following traumatic brain injury. Brain Impair, Special Issue. 2012;13(01):108–22.
56. Cecil R, Thompson K, Parahoo K, McCaughan E. Towards an understanding of the lives of families affected by stroke: a qualitative study of home carers. J Adv Nurs. 2013;69(8):1761–70.
57. Ågård AS, Egerod I, Tønnesen E, Lomborg K. From spouse to caregiver and back: a grounded theory study of post-intensive care unit spousal caregiving. J Adv Nurs. 2015;71(8):1892–903.
58. Bocchi SCM. Vivenciando a sobrecarga ao vir-a-ser um cuidador familiar de pessoa com acidente vascular cerebral (AVC): Análise do conhecimento. Revista Latino-Americana de Enfermagem. 2004;12(1):115–21.
59. Turner B, Fleming J, Cornwell P, Worrall L, Ownsworth T, Haines T, Kendall M, Chenoweth L. A qualitative study of the transition from hospital to home for individuals with acquired brain injury and their family caregivers. Brain Inj. 2007;21(11):1119–30.

3

Interventions to address social connectedness and loneliness for older adults

Hannah M. O'Rourke[1*], Laura Collins[2] and Souraya Sidani[2]

Abstract

Background: Older adults are at risk for loneliness, and interventions to promote social connectedness are needed to directly address this problem. The nature of interventions aimed to affect the distinct, subjective concepts of loneliness/social connectedness has not been clearly described. The purpose of this review was to map the literature on interventions and strategies to affect loneliness/social connectedness for older adults.

Methods: A comprehensive scoping review was conducted. Six electronic databases were searched from inception in July 2015, resulting in 5530 unique records. Standardized inclusion/exclusion criteria were applied, resulting in a set of 44 studies (reported in 54 articles) for further analysis. Data were extracted to describe the interventions and strategies, and the context of the included studies. Analytic techniques included calculating frequencies, manifest content analysis and meta-summary.

Results: Interventions were described or evaluated in 39 studies, and five studies described strategies to affect loneliness/social connectedness of older adults or their caregivers in a qualitative descriptive study. The studies were often conducted in the United States (38.6%) among community dwelling (54.5%), cognitively intact (31.8%), and female-majority (86.4%) samples. Few focused on non-white participants (4.5%). Strategies described most often were engaging in purposeful activity and maintaining contact with one's social network. Of nine intervention types identified, the most frequently described were One-to-One Personal Contact and Group Activity. Authors held divergent views of why the same type of intervention might impact social connectedness, but social contact was the most frequently conceptualized influencing factor targeted, both within and across intervention types.

Conclusions: Research to test the divergent theories of why interventions work is needed to advance understanding of intervention mechanisms. Innovative conceptualizations of intervention targets are needed, such as purposeful activity, that move beyond the current focus on the objective social network as a way to promote social connectedness for older adults.

Keywords: Loneliness, Social connectedness, Intervention, Scoping review, Older adult

Background

The interplay of health and contextual factors puts older adults at risk for loneliness [1], a negative feeling resulting from a perceived deficit in companionship, quantity or quality in one's relationships with either an attachment figure or a community [2–4]. Health factors include chronic disease experiences that interfere with functioning, and cognitive decline resulting in communication impairments [5] or inability to remember significant others or the recent interactions with them [6]. Contextual factors relate to lacking a confidant [7], relocation to a care facility as well as loss of loved ones due to death [2, 7, 8], and spending too much time alone [7] or idle [8], which yields feelings of separation from others. Loneliness may also be influenced by the number and structure of one's relationships (i.e. social network), frequency of interaction with others (i.e. social contact), or the types and amounts of assistance received from others (i.e. social support) [9, 10].

Lonely people are at risk for reduced health and well-being, including poor life satisfaction [11–15], depression [16, 17], low self-esteem [13], reduced hope [13], negative affect [18, 19], and impaired function in

* Correspondence: hannah.orourke@ualberta.ca
[1]Faculty of Nursing Level 3, Edmonton Clinic Health Academy, University of Alberta, 11405-87 Avenue, Edmonton, Alberta T6G 1C9, Canada
Full list of author information is available at the end of the article

activities of daily living [9, 17, 18]. The opposite of loneliness, social connectedness, is a basic human need [20] that may influence health and wellbeing for older adults, more than social contact, network or support [9]. Social connectedness is a positive subjective evaluation of the extent to which one has meaningful, close, and constructive relationships with other individuals, groups, or society indicated by: (1) feelings of caring about others and feeling cared about by others, such as love, companionship or affection and (2) feeling of belonging to a group or community [1].

Interventions to promote social connectedness/reduce loneliness among older adults have been analyzed and described in previous literature reviews in concert with interventions aimed at the distinct, but related, concept of social contact/isolation [21–26]. Intervention types were described by Dickens et al. (2011) based on their component activities and included "activities (social or physical programmes), support (discussion, counseling, therapy or education), internet training, home visiting, and service provision" [21] (p. 5). Other reviews categorized interventions based on a combination of the activities offered and the mode of delivery (e.g. group or one-to-one) [22–25]. Cattan et al. (2005) [22] described group (including activities of educational input or social support), one-to-one (including activities of home visits or telephone contact to provide information, services, or support), service provision (e.g. transport, medical intervention), and community development (e.g. social activities) interventions. Hagan et al. (2014) described group (including activities such as cognitive enhancement workgroups, adult day centre attendance, and gender-based social groups) and one-to-one interventions (including activities like befriending and mentoring programs, animal-assisted therapy, use of the internet, and contact with family or friends using a variety of technological approaches) [24]. Cohen-Mansfield et al. (2015) described group (educational, shared activity, or specific therapy techniques) and one-to-one activities (educational, sensory technological aids, and specific therapy techniques) [25]. Windle et al. (2011) described one-to-one interventions (befriending, mentoring, and gatekeeping), group services (day-centre services and social group schemes), and wider community engagement (participation in existing activities, outreach programmes, or volunteer schemes) [26]. Similarly, Findlay et al. (2003) identified group (tele-conferencing or discussion/support groups) and one-to-one (telephone support and gatekeeper programmes that connect socially isolated older adults with support services) interventions, as well as service provision (community support services) and use of the Internet.

Because interventions aimed to affect loneliness/social connectedness and isolation/social contact among older adults were reviewed and analyzed together in these previous reviews [21–26], which interventions actually addressed loneliness/social connectedness for this population is unclear. Isolation/social contact and loneliness/social connectedness are different concepts, the former objective and the latter subjective: one may be alone (i.e. isolated) and still feel a sense of social connectedness, or be surrounded by people (i.e. have social contact) and feel lonely [4, 8, 27]. The components and activities of interventions designed to target loneliness/social connectedness may differ in important ways from those designed to reduce isolation/increase social contact [28]. Furthermore, how the interventions addressed either the indicators of loneliness/social connectedness or its possible influencing factors is unclear. Conceptualization of the mechanisms by which interventions address loneliness/social connectedness, as opposed to isolation/contact, is needed [27, 29], responding to calls for theory-based interventions that are problem-specific [21, 22]. The purpose of this scoping review was to identify and describe the number and features of interventions that were designed to address loneliness/social connectedness among older adults. The aims were to: (1) describe and clarify the interventions' goals, components, activities, mode and dose of delivery and (2) shed light on the theoretical underpinnings of these interventions by assessing the extent to which their hypothesized mechanisms of effect mapped to factors that may influence social connectedness.

Methods

To identify and describe the nature of strategies and interventions designed to affect loneliness/social connectedness for older adults, scoping review procedures were applied to systematically search, screen, extract and synthesize this broad body of literature [30, 31]. Typical of scoping review methodology, quality appraisal was not conducted since our aim was not to assess intervention efficacy [30, 31]. Scoping review results are particularly useful to inform the design of future systematic reviews, which would include a transparent and rigorous quality appraisal process [30, 31]. The results of the current scoping review will identify types of interventions that are sufficiently homogenous in their components, activities, and theoretical underpinnings and evaluated across multiple studies, warranting assessment of their efficacy in future systematic reviews. Articles included in this scoping review reported on the: (i) design of an intervention; (ii) protocol or results of a quantitative study to evaluate an intervention; (iii) or findings of a qualitative study that explored older adults' or caregivers' strategies to promote social connectedness.

Search procedures

Six electronic databases—Psycinfo, Medline, Cumulative Index to Nursing and Allied Health Literature, Proquest Dissertations and Theses, Proquest Nursing, and Proquest

Social Service Abstracts —were searched in July 2015 from inception. Search strategies, using keywords and database-specific subject headings, were designed to capture the concepts of 'social connectedness' (using terms identified in collaboration with a health sciences librarian like social connectedness, connectedness, lonely, or loneliness) and 'intervention' or 'strategy' (using terms identified from a previous systematic review [32] like therapy, treatment, strategy, or intervention studies). The results were exported to Refworks and duplicates removed prior to screening. See Additional file 1 for full details of database-specific search strategies.

Inclusion/exclusion criteria

Broad selection criteria were used to be comprehensive. Articles were included if they: (i) described an intervention evaluated using any quantitative, qualitative or mixed methods design, or explored in a qualitative study the strategies used by older adults or caregivers to promote social connectedness; (2) identified loneliness/social connectedness or its indicators (i.e. feelings of caring for/about others or feelings of belonging) as a primary goal or outcome of the intervention or strategies; (3) targeted adults 55 years of age or older; and (4) were available in full text in either English or French. Studies were not excluded based on year made available or publication status. Standardized criteria were developed to clarify the inclusion/exclusion criteria and to guide the selection of articles. Two independent reviewers applied the criteria to screen a random selection of 9% ($n = 46$) of the full text articles, which resulted in good inter-rater agreement (kappa = 0.784, SE = 0.119). Reviewer discrepancies were discussed until consensus was reached.

Data extraction

Detailed data extraction instructions were developed to maintain consistency. The instructions clarified the data to be extracted, their possible locations in the articles, and the way to document them; illustrative examples were provided. Multiple reports of a single study were grouped together in the data extraction tables so that they would be counted once in the analysis, and so that all data about a single intervention was in one place.

Data extracted from all articles included name of first author, year published, and whether it was a peer-reviewed article, book chapter, or dissertation. For empirical quantitative or qualitative studies, the following additional information was documented: study design; contextual details (i.e. target population, country that the study was conducted in, cultural background of participants, and setting based on descriptions of the recruitment sites); and information about the sample (i.e. sample size, age, gender, level of cognitive impairment, marital status).

Data extracted from articles that described or evaluated an intervention also included the theoretical underpinnings of the intervention (i.e. any explicit guiding framework or theory, and the authors' more implicit conceptualizations from the rationale provided for why the intervention may affect loneliness/social connectedness), and details of the intervention. Pertinent details of an intervention include its goal, components and activities, and mode of delivery and dose [28]. The goal referred to what the intervention was set to achieve. Active ingredients were the components and the activities required to implement each component, as operationalized in the study. Delivery mode was the format for giving the intervention, and dose was the amount of the intervention to which participants were exposed. Additional data extracted from qualitative studies that explored strategies to promote social connectedness among older adults were the results that identified and / or described strategies to affect loneliness/social connectedness, and supporting descriptions if needed to clarify the nature of the strategy.

Analysis

Frequencies were calculated to describe the context (i.e. target populations and settings) in which the intervention was implemented. Strategies to affect loneliness/social connectedness extracted from qualitative studies were analyzed as follows: (i) an initial list of two indicators of social connectedness/loneliness (i.e., caring for and about others and feelings of belonging) and nine modifiable influencing factors (i.e., social network, social support, self-reported health, technology use, formal group memberships, mental and emotional well-being, community-based social participation, religious affiliation, and use of services such as home care) identified from a previous review [1] was used as the initial coding framework; (ii) the studies' findings were coded and grouped together when similar (i.e. manifest content analysis), and new codes created as needed, thereby adding the factors of keeping busy/purposeful activity and personal development to the initial list; and (iii) the frequency of indicators and factors addressed across studies was assessed (i.e. metasummary [33]). The first author completed this analysis, and the last reviewed the findings.

To analyze the interventions, manifest content analysis was used to group similar types of interventions, and identify and describe their components. The first author completed this analysis and the last reviewed the findings. The first and second authors then independently assessed the extent to which the authors' hypothesized mechanisms of effect (i.e., the theoretical underpinnings of the intervention) mapped to the indicators of and the list of factors that may influence social connectedness. Factors were not always explicitly stated in the articles, so this mapping involved making low-level inferences based on a careful review of the authors' descriptions and definitions of hypothesized mechanisms of effect. Having two independent reviewers complete this analysis improved credibility of the findings. Discrepancies were resolved through discussion and review of coded data until consensus was reached on a final list of factors targeted by each intervention.

Results

Search results

From 5530 titles/abstracts (the number after removal of duplicates), 424 full text articles were reviewed, and 44 separate studies (reported in 54 articles) met the inclusion criteria (Fig. 1). Studies were conducted primarily in the United States (38.6%) or in the Netherlands or other Nordic countries (22.7%). Most often, cultural background of the study sample or target population was not clearly reported (54.5%). Few studies included a majority of non-white participants (4.5%). Most of the studies focused on people who lived in the community, either independently, in assisted living, or 'living alone' (54.5%). The studies' samples were often described as cognitively intact (31.8%) or level of cognitive function was not reported (31.8%), and usually included a majority (i.e. ≥ 50%) of women (86.4%) (Table 1). A few qualitative studies explored strategies to impact older adults' loneliness/social connectedness from the perspective of older adults or their caregivers (11.4%); most of the studies described or evaluated an intervention (88.6%). Study details can be found in Additional file 2. Next, the synthesis of strategies from the qualitative studies is discussed, followed by the description of the core features of the interventions.

Strategies from qualitative studies

The most common strategies described were engaging in purposeful activity or keeping busy ($n = 5$ studies) [6, 34–38] and having contact with a social network

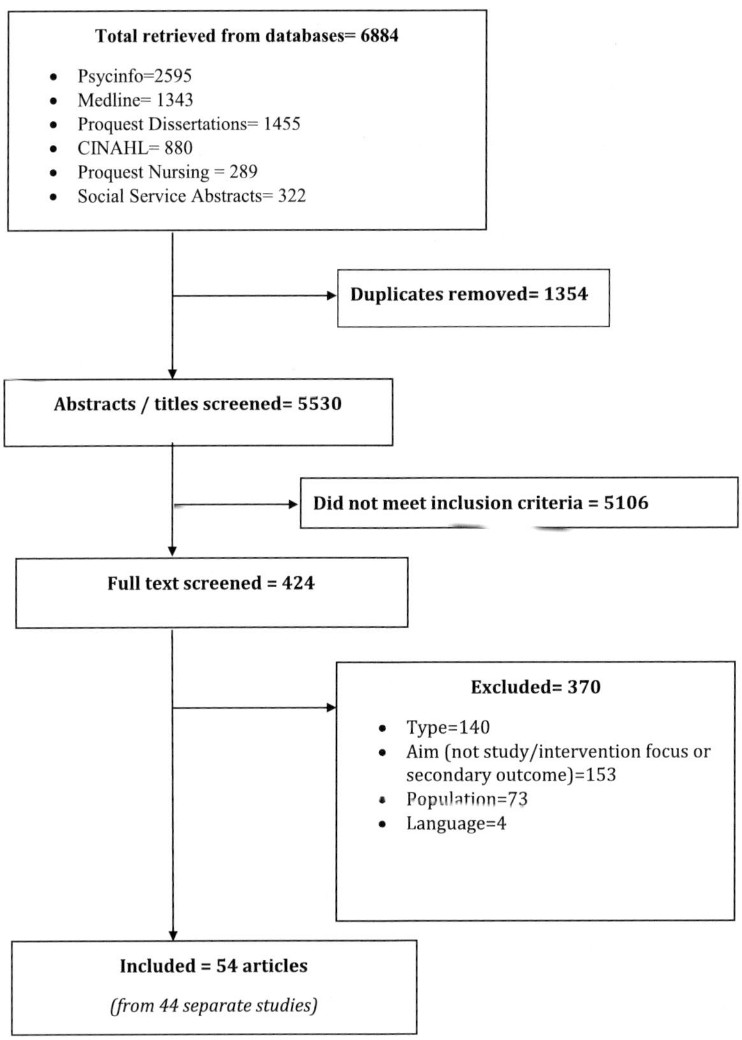

Fig. 1 Search results. Results of the search and screening process

Table 1 Key characteristics of included studies (*N* = 44)

Characteristic	% (N)
Country	
United States	38.6% (17)
The Netherlands / Nordic countries	22.7% (10)
Australia/New Zealand	13.6% (6)
the United Kingdom	9.1% (4)
Asian countries	6.8% (3)
Canada	6.8% (3)
Eastern Europe	2.3% (1)
Culture	
Not reported	54.5% (24)
More than 60% white or Caucasian participants	40.9% (18)
More than 50% non-white participants	4.5% (2)
Setting	
Community (i.e. *Lived independently, in assisted living or 'alone'*)	54.5% (24)
Residential care (i.e. *Nursing home or long term care facility*)	29.5% (13)
Mixed community/residential care	13.6% (6)
Not reported	2.3% (1)
Cognitive Impairment	
Cognitively intact	31.8% (14)
Not reported	31.8% (14)
Included some people with mild impairment	29.5% (13)
Majority cognitively impaired to a mild, moderate or severe degree	6.8% (3)
Gender	
50% or more of participants were women	86.4% (38)
Not reported	9.1% (4)
50% or more of participants were men	4.5% (2)

[6, 34–38] (n = 5). Purposeful activity/keeping busy was about engaging in pastimes or daily responsibilities, regardless of whether these involved contact with others and which were actually often solitary in nature, with the intent to pass the time or to accomplish something. Examples of activities included reading, listening to music, going for a walk, cleaning, cooking, and arts and crafts. All studies also described maintaining contact or interaction with a social network as an important strategy ($n = 5$) [6, 34–38]. Both in-person interactions and interactions occurring over the telephone or email were described. Of the five studies, three emphasized the importance of maintaining familiar relationships with family and friends, as opposed to making new contacts [6, 36, 37, 39].

Social participation, community-based activities that people choose and that have the potential to bring them into contact with others like volunteer work, joining clubs, or pursuing recreational activities [15], was discussed as a strategy in three studies [34, 35, 37–39]. One study described how people who had led active lives joined groups [34, 35], while another described how community-dwelling older adults watched television to feel connected to and engaged in the social world [37, 39]. Another study described how older adults who were part of a senior's club joined groups, went on bus trips, went dancing, or attended a senior's centre [38].

Just two studies explicitly described strategies that directly targeted the need to feel cared for, described as needing to have satisfying emotional relationships that result in feeling valued or affection from others [36] or seeking companionship from pets [37, 39]. All studies did emphasize having contact with *familiar* people (i.e. existing friends and family), which suggests that older adults may seek out the type of contact that results in feelings of being valued or cared for [6, 36, 37, 39].

Two studies described a strategy of personal development to change one's outlook on life or social relationships. In one study, the people described how personal growth could result in reframing their outlook on solitude to prevent loneliness [38]. In the other, people would feel better about their own situation when comparing themselves to those perceived as being worse off or more lonely than they were [34, 35]. Social support, which refers to receipt of different types of assistance from others [9], was only explicitly described in one study [37, 39]. Interestingly, in this instance, it was not receiving social support, but providing social support that was described as a strategy to ameliorate loneliness, because helping others made people feel needed. Finally, having a religious affiliation and belief in a higher power, regardless of church attendance, was identified in one study to provide strength to combat loneliness [38].

Interventions

Nine different intervention types, classified based on their components (i.e. active ingredients), were identified in 39 studies (Table 2). The mapping of theoretical underpinnings—the authors' descriptions or rationale for why an intervention would work—to indicators and factors that influence loneliness/social connectedness, by intervention type across all studies, is shown in Table 3 and summarized in-text, following the descriptions of the interventions' components. One-to-One Personal Contact (21%, $n = 8$) and Activity Group (18%, $n = 7$

Table 2 Intervention descriptions by type

Intervention Type	Components & Activities	Mode of Delivery	Doses Described
Personal Contact [17, 44–50] (8 studies/reports) Scheduled contact with another person.	1. Personal contact: Scheduled contact with someone from one's social network (e.g. a family member or friend) or a volunteer who may be similar to the recipient on some characteristics (e.g. age, gender, interests, culture). Discussions are unscripted and informal in nature. Personal contacts may be specifically trained to offer emotional support, and may or may not be permitted to provide instrumental support (e.g., transportation, shopping, minor housekeeping and repairs, letter writing/correspondence, or meal preparation).	• One-to-one • Face-to-face, phone, email, or videoconference • Researcher supports training with videoconference equipment	• Usually weekly • 5 min to 1 h or more per interaction • 3 to 36 months
Activity & Discussion Groups [51–61] (7 studies, 11 reports) Engagement with a new group of people in an activity and/or facilitated discussion.	1. Group Activity Participation: joining a new group, and engaging in an activity of interest (e.g. song-writing, gardening projects, painting, pottery, dance, music, poetry, drama, jewelry making, storytelling, therapeutic writing, exercise, etc.) 2. Group Discussion: joining a new group, and engaging in facilitated discussion focused on a pre-determined topic of interest to the participants (e.g. movie discussion, bible discussion, role of the retiree) sharing of personal experiences. Group members may be taught how to offer emotional support to one another. All interventions of this type either addressed component 1 [57, 58], component 2 [54, 55, 57, 59–61], or both components 1&2 [51–53]	• Group of 5 to 9 people • Face-to-face sessions held in a neutral location (e.g. an activity room). • Facilitated (e.g. by a health care provider, researcher, university student, professional artist) who guides discussion and provides resources (e.g. songbooks, painting supplies).	• Sessions once or twice per week • 90 min to 6 h per session • 3 to 72 weeks
Animal Contact [62–68] (6 studies, 7 reports) Scheduled contact with an animal	1. Animal Contact: contact with an animal, usually a cat or dogs; animal simulations have also been used (e.g. a robotic seal). Activity with the animal is self-guided and may include talking to, holding, petting, playing with, grooming, or walking the animal on a leash. A person's preference for animal type (e.g. cat or dog) as well as size (e.g. small or large) may be assessed in order to individualize the treatment. Sometimes, the person is assigned to one animal to have contact with for all sessions.	• Face-to-face • One-to-one in a person's private room OR to a group (size has ranged from 2 to 13) in a common space of a long-term care facility (e.g. activity room, garden, etc.). • A pet attendant brings and supervises animals	• 1 to 3 times per week • 30 to 90 min per session • 3 to 24 weeks OR • Animal lives at the long term care or assisted living facility and residents can seek out contact
Skills Course [69–76] (6 studies, 8 reports) Courses delivered to develop participants' personal skills.	1. Skills instruction: Instruction given to older adults to improve their ability to have contact with others and/or to enhance their existing friendships, or to make new friends. The activities differ depending on the type of skills that are taught. Skills taught have included: mindfulness-based stress reduction [76], use of a computer and internet [74, 75], those supporting friendship development (e.g. self-esteem, reflection on expectations of friendships, analysis of one's network, goal and boundary-setting) [69–72], and self-management (to meet needs of comfort, stimulation, affection, behavioral confirmation and status [73]).	• Face-to-face • Usually group (size has ranged from 5 to 15) (one study was one-to-one [75]) • Lead by trained clinicians, researchers, experienced instructors	• Usually weekly • 2 to 4 h per session • 3 to 12 lessons • Some also include skills practice at home

Table 2 Intervention descriptions by type *(Continued)*

Intervention Type	Components & Activities	Mode of Delivery	Doses Described
Varied/Non-Specific [40, 41, 77–80] (5 studies, 6 reports) Broad, multifaceted programs not focused on a single type of intervention	1. Service delivery or social assistance: These are usually multi-component interventions, but the different components are not clearly conceptualized or described, and are described broadly as improving service delivery within a community. Types of services offered in a single program to a community may be related to any combination of: increased fitness or arts programs, or other social/leisure activities; improved transportation; access to information or resources; and/or consultation with medical, nursing, counseling, financial or housing experts.	Unclear as to who delivered different services and/or how these were delivered	• Programs lasted for 6 months to 2 years • Unclear what individuals within a community would have received
Model of Care [81, 82] (2 studies/reports) Implementation of a new philosophy for care provision (i.e. the Eden Philosophy)	1. Increase spontaneous, resident-driven and purposeful interaction with plants, animals and children: the Eden philosophy is about creating a 'human habitat' by providing opportunity for residents to interact as desired with plants, animals and children in their daily life in order to address issues related to loneliness, boredom and helplessness experienced by residents of long-term care facilities. Both interventions described staff training to understand the philosophy. One intervention also stated that work teams were formed to increase the number of plants, animals and involvement with children in the facility by opening a day-care program [81].	Unclear who was trained, and what implementation of this philosophy looked like in practice.	Unclear what facilities actually did to implement the philosophy
Reminiscence [83, 84] (2 studies/reports) Recalling and discussing past memories and experiences	1. Reminiscence: A topic or theme is provided for the session (e.g. school days, holiday traditions, first house and anniversaries, family histories and life stories, etc.) and participants share with the group their recollections.	• Face-to face in a comfortable setting • Group (size not reported or ≤ 10) • Lead by facilitators trained in reminiscence therapy and who may have experience working with older adults	• 1 to 2 times per week • 1 to 1.5 h • 4 to 8 weeks
Support Group [85, 86] (2 studies/reports) Sharing personal challenges and receiving emotional or informational support.	1. Peer support group: Participants attend meetings where they select areas of discussion related to their needs and challenges that they face. Peer and professionals provide information resources and/or emotional support related to identified challenges.	• Face-to-face • Group (size range from 5 to 12) • Co-lead by peers who had strong interpersonal skills and professionals (e.g. nurse, minister, social worker, music therapist) experienced in working with older adults who face challenges (e.g. bereavement) or by staff who received training on the program components (e.g. activity aides)	• Weekly • 0.75 to 1.5 h • 12 to 20 weeks
Public Broadcast [87] (1 study/report) Listening to a generation-specific radio program.	1. Familiar music: Listening to music (primarily), serials and other segments of radio programs that were popular in the 1920–1950s. 2. Interactive style: programming delivered using a friendly and interactive style including birthday messages and 'cheerio' calls.	• to individuals • via a community radio station; free radio receiver provided, operated by a simple on/off switch	• Daily • 1 h • 3 months

studies) were the interventions that were most frequently explored or evaluated. In One-to-One Personal Contact, participants were paired with another individual, either a family member, friend or a volunteer for those with a more limited social network, and given the opportunity to have scheduled contact and

Table 3 Theoretical underpinnings: proportion of studies targeting each modifiable[a] factor and indicator, by type of intervention based on proposed mechanisms of action

	Intervention Type								
	Personal Contact [17, 44–50] (8 studies/reports)	Activity Group [51–61] (7 studies, 11 reports)	Animal Contact [62–68] (6 studies, 7 reports)	Skills Course [69–76] (6 studies, 8 reports)	Varied/ Non-Specific [40, 41, 77–80] (5 studies, 6 reports)	Model of Care [81, 82] (2 studies/reports)	Reminiscence [83, 84] (2 studies/reports)	Support Group [85, 86] (2 studies/reports)	Public Broadcast [87] (1 study/report)
Proportion of studies targeting each factor/indicator									
Caring	3/8	3/7	4/6	3/6		2/2		1/2	1/1
Belonging	1/8	1/7							
Social Network	8/8	4/7	4/6	4/6	5/5	2/2	1/2		
Social Support	6/8	1/7	3/6	1/6	2/5			2/2	
Personal development		1/7		4/6	2/5		1/2	1/2	
Technology use	2/8			2/6					1/1
Busy/Purposeful			1/6	1/6					1/1
Mental/Emotional				1/6			1/2		
Social participation		6/7			1/5				

[a]There are additional influencing factors that are non-modifiable or difficult to modify. These include marital status, age, living arrangement, cognitive ability, sex or gender, level of formal education, income, religious affiliation, family composition, ethnicity, and death of a spouse. All modifiable factors were identified in a previous literature review [1], except for keeping busy/purposeful activity and personal development, which were identified in the current review from the synthesis of strategies identified in qualitative studies. Modifiable factors of service use, self-reported health and group memberships were not targeted by any of the studies

interaction with that person. One-to-One Personal Contact was conceptualized as targeting five different indicators/factors, but most often social network ($n = 8$) and social support ($n = 6$), while caring, belonging, and technology use (e.g., phone, computer) were described in fewer than half of the studies.

The components of Activity Group interventions included engaging in an activity of interest, and facilitated discussion aimed at promoting the development of relationships that may be characterized by support, friendship or companionship among group members. Many different activities were used, both within and across studies (e.g. arts and music, topical discussion, or exercise). Across the seven studies, Activity Groups were described as targeting six different indicators/factors including: caring, belonging, social support, and personal development (each described in less than half of the studies); and social participation ($n = 6$) and social network ($n = 4$) (each described in more than half of the studies).

Animal Contact (15%, n = 6), Skills Course (15%, n = 6), and Varied/Non-Specific (13%, $n = 5$) interventions were also explored in multiple studies. In Animal Contact interventions, most often referred to as 'Animal Assisted Therapy,' participants were paired and allowed to interact with an animal, usually a dog or a cat, either at their own convenience or at a scheduled time. Animal Contact was described as targeting four indicators/factors, most often caring ($n = 4$) and social network (n = 4); social support and keeping busy/purposeful activity were also described, but in fewer than half of the studies. Skills Course interventions promoted the development of the person's personal characteristics or skills in order to address loneliness/social connectedness. These involved training participants to obtain computer skills to increase access to resources or interpersonal contacts ($n = 2$), to develop psychological skills, like expectations of friends, self-esteem, or self-management, needed to develop and maintain strong interpersonal relationships ($n = 3$), or mindfulness skills to re-frame how one thinks about social relationships ($n = 1$). Skills Course interventions were described as targeting seven indicators/factors, but most often social network ($n = 4$), personal development (n = 4) and caring (n = 3); the others described in less than half of the studies included social support, technology use, keeping busy/purposeful activity, and mental and emotional well-being (e.g., avoiding stress).

Interventions that were classified as Varied/Non-Specific referred to the implementation, usually by a public health or community organization, of a large and multifaceted program that employed a combination of different types of interventions that were poorly specified. For example, the 'Healthy Aging' program [40, 41] was broadly conceptualized as addressing loneliness using any one of a variety of activities (e.g. reminiscence, skills course, or group activity). Each community involved in the program received a different type of intervention under the umbrella of 'Healthy Aging'. Varied/Non-Specific interventions were conceptualized as addressing four factors, most often social network ($n = 5$), and social support, personal development and social participation in less than half of the studies.

Reminiscence (5%, $n = 2$), Support Group (5%, n = 2), Model of Care (5%, n = 2), and Public Broadcast (3%, $n = 1$) were each explored or evaluated in just one or two studies. Reminiscence referred to an intervention where the primary component was to prompt participants to reflect on past memories or experiences. One of these interventions also had participants consider the future in light of insights gained, while the other described communication facilitation techniques aimed at promoting positive interactions between participants in a group setting. Reminiscence was conceptualized as targeting three factors: social network ($n = 1$), personal development (n = 1), and mental and emotional well-being (n = 1).

Support Group interventions involved bringing together a group of people who shared some common characteristics or life experiences, and facilitating group members to provide emotional, informational, or appraisal support through exploration of issues that members experienced. Support Groups differed from Activity Groups in that the focus was on the promotion of social support, not on engagement in an activity or building other types of relationships with others. Support Groups were described as targeting the indicator of caring ($n = 1$) and the factors of social support ($n = 2$) and personal development (n = 1).

Model of Care interventions implemented a philosophy of care within a long-term care facility that was clearly described as targeting loneliness/social connectedness as a primary outcome. Both studies identified in this review described implementation of the Eden Alternative Model philosophy, which espoused development of close relationships between staff and long-term care residents, the integration of plants and animals into the everyday lives of residents, and promoting residents' active involvement in the day-to-day life at the long-term care facility. Model of Care interventions targeted the indicator of caring ($n = 2$) and the factor of social network (n = 2). The final intervention type was a Public Broadcast. In this intervention, participants were asked to listen to a radio program that played music that may be familiar to participants based on their age, was presented by a friendly radio announcer, and included some programming that used an interactive style. The Public Broadcast intervention targeted the indicator of caring ($n = 1$), technology use (n = 1), and keeping busy/purposeful activity (n = 1).

Discussion

This review identified nine distinct intervention types, classified based on their active ingredients, developed to address loneliness/social connectedness among older adults. Within each of the nine types of interventions, the studies' authors had different theories about what factors were targeted, signaling inconsistency in the literature regarding the mechanisms by which the interventions have been conceptualized to affect loneliness/ social connectedness. In addition, authors frequently conceptualized a single component of an intervention (e.g. contact with a relative or visitor) as targeting multiple factors (e.g. caring, belonging, social network, social support), but did not test the assumption that a single component affected multiple outcomes. Taken together, these two features of the literature make it unclear whether an intervention component really accomplishes all that it is theorized to. Research that would strengthen the evidence base includes theory-informed intervention evaluation that delineates the series of factors that are targeted by the intervention as immediate outcomes and examines effects of the intervention on each factor [28].

Findings from this review supported that the types of interventions that have been developed to date address, in theory, many of the key strategies identified by key stakeholders including contact, social participation, feeling cared for, personal development and social support [6, 34–38]. Contact, or development of one's structural social network, was described as a target in all but two intervention types (the exceptions were 'Social Support' and 'Public Broadcast'). Social participation was described as a target in 86% of 'Activity Group' interventions. Feeling cared for was described as a target in 67% of 'Animal Contact' and 100% of 'Model of Care' interventions. Personal development was described as a target in 67% of 'Skills Course' interventions, and social support was described as a target in 75% of Personal Contact and 100% of Social Support interventions. Of note, none of the interventions directly targeted the strategy of purposeful activity/keeping busy, the importance of which was emphasized by key stakeholders in all five qualitative studies [6, 34–38]. Development of interventions to address loneliness/social connectedness which target purposeful activity/keeping busy would address stakeholder priorities and is consistent with calls to develop a range of interventions that are responsive to characteristics of participants and to their needs and preferences [42].

Other reviews have found highly inconsistent results of intervention impact within each of the different categories of interventions, concluding that there was very limited evidence supporting effectiveness of the interventions [21–24]. However, there are two key conceptual issues that may have affected these reviews' findings [43]: (1) mixing the findings of effectiveness of heterogeneous interventions, which will lead to inconsistent findings across studies; and (2) analyzing studies of an intervention delivered using a single mode of delivery, which will lead to an incomplete synthesis. The categories of interventions identified in the present review address the above issues in two ways and may be useful to guide future systematic reviews to establish efficacy. First, interventions were only analyzed if they targeted loneliness/social connectedness (not other social concepts like isolation/contact). Second, interventions were grouped according to their active ingredients, not the mode of delivery. While two of the intervention types referred to in the present review do specify whether the activity occurred in a group (i.e. Group Activity) or one-to-one (i.e. One-to-One Personal Contact), in these instances, group and one-to-one delivery represent an active ingredient (i.e. an element of the intervention hypothesized to affect the outcome) rather than simply a mode of delivery (i.e. how participants are given the intervention). Other intervention types described in the present review (e.g. Animal Contact) could be delivered in a group or to an individual. Mode of delivery should be considered in reviews of intervention effectiveness, but may be more appropriately examined as a secondary aim (e.g. is Animal Contact as effective when delivered in a group or one-to-one?), rather than as a primary aim (e.g. are interventions delivered to groups effective?).

Limitations of this study included that only studies in English and French were reviewed; other interventions and strategies have likely been described but the reports made available in other languages. Strengths of the review included a comprehensive search, transparent and standardized data extraction and screening procedures, in-depth description and synthesis of data, and independent reviewers for coding the interventions' theoretical underpinnings, which was the most subjective part of the analysis.

Conclusion

The findings from this review identified the interventions that have been designed to address loneliness/social connectedness for older adults, and described their key features as well as the influencing factors that they have been conceptualized to target. As such, the findings provide a strong foundation for future research to advance theory-informed design and evaluation of interventions to affect loneliness/social connectedness. The interventions identified also aligned with many of the strategies that have been used by older adults or caregivers to address loneliness/social connectedness among older adults, highlighting their relevance to key stakeholders. Future research should include systematic reviews to examine effectiveness of the distinct types of interventions that target loneliness/social connectedness, studies to test the interventions' theorized mechanisms of action, and development of interventions that target purposeful activity as a way to ameliorate loneliness among older adults.

Acknowledgements
The authors acknowledge Jhonna Collins for her support to develop the standardized inclusion/ exclusion criteria.

Funding
The primary author was supported by a postdoctoral fellowship (Canadian Institutes of Health Research) to complete this work.

Authors' contributions
HMO conceptualized and designed the study, completed the search, screening of titles and abstracts, data extraction, and analysis, and wrote the manuscript. SS provided methodological expertise to design the study, assisted in the analysis of intervention components and features, and provided critical intellectual content during manuscript writing. LC completed the intervention mapping analysis, helped conceptualize the results and discussion sections of the manuscript, and provided critical feedback on the manuscript. All authors read and approved the final manuscript.

Competing interests
The authors declare that they have no competing interests.

Author details
[1]Faculty of Nursing Level 3, Edmonton Clinic Health Academy, University of Alberta, 11405-87 Avenue, Edmonton, Alberta T6G 1C9, Canada. [2]Daphne Cockwell School of Nursing, Ryerson University, 350 Victoria Street, Toronto, ON M5B 2K3, Canada.

References
1. O'Rourke HM, Sidani S. Definition, determinants and outcomes of social connectedness for older adults: a scoping review. J Gerontol Nurs. in press
2. El Sadr CB, Noureddine S, Kelley J. Concept analysis of loneliness with implications for nursing diagnosis. Int J Nurs Terminol Classif. 2009;20:25–33.
3. Weiss RS. Loneliness: the experience of emotional and social isolation. Cambridge: MIT Press; 1973.
4. de Jong Gierveld J. A review of loneliness: concept and defintions, determinants and consequences. Rev Clin Gerontol. 1998;8:73–80.
5. Ericsson I, Hellström I, Kjellström S. Sliding interactions: an ethnography about how persons with dementia interact in housing with care for the elderly. Dementia. 2011;10:523–38.
6. Moyle W, Kellett U, Ballantyne A, Gracia N. Dementia and loneliness: an Australian perspective. J Clin Nurs. 2011;20:1445–53.
7. Victor CR. Loneliness in care homes: a neglected area of research? Aging Health. 2012;8:637–46.
8. Brownie S, Horstmanshof L. The management of loneliness in aged care residents: an important therapeutic target for gerontological nursing. Geriatr Nurs. 2011;32:318–25.
9. Ashida S, Heaney CA. Differential associations of social support and social connectedness with structural features of social networks and the health status of older adults. J Aging Health. 2008;20:872–93.
10. Lee RM, Robbins SB. Measuring belongingness: the social connectedness and the social assurance scales. J Couns Psychol. 1995;42:232–41.
11. Easton-Hogg E. An investigation of the associations between social connectedness and internet usage for older adults. Louisville: Spalding University; 2013.
12. Kim H-J, Hong S, Kim M. Living arrangement, social connectedness, and life satisfaction among Korean older adults with physical disabilities: the results from the national survey on persons with disabilities. J Dev Phys Disabil. 2015;27:307–21.
13. Lee E. The impact of social and spiritual connectedness on the psychological well-being among older Americans. J Relig Spiritual Aging. 2014;26:300–19.
14. Pan S. Online communities and older adults: the potential of social networks formed in the online community in enhancing social support, social connectedness and subjective well-being among Chinese older adults. Los Angelas: University of Southern California; 2011.
15. Zelenka A. Modeling social participation as predictive of life satisfaction and social connectedness: scale or index? Denver: University of Denver; 2011.
16. Marshall G. Predictors associated with late-life depressive symptoms among older black Americans. Washington: University of Washington; 2011.
17. Van Orden KA, Stone DM, Rowe J, McIntosh WL, Podgorski C, Conwell Y. The senior connection: design and rationale of a randomized trial of peer companionship to reduce suicide risk in later life. Contemp Clin Trials. 2013; 35:117–26.
18. Ong AD, Allaire JC. Cardiovascular intraindividual variability in later life: the influence of social connectedness and positive emotions. Psychol Aging. 2005;20:476–85.
19. Stanley IH, Conwell Y, Bowen C, Van Orden KA. Pet ownership may attenuate loneliness among older adult primary care patients who live alone. Aging Ment Health. 2014;18:394–9.
20. Townsend KC, McWhirter BT. Connectedness: a review of the literature with implications for counseling, assessment, and research. J Couns Dev. 2005;83: 191–201.
21. Dickens A, Richards S, Greaves C, Campbell J. Interventions targeting social isolation in older people: a systematic review. BMC Public Health. 2011;11:647.
22. Cattan M, White M, Bond J, Learmouth A. Preventing social isolation and loneliness among older people: a systematic review of health promotion interventions. Ageing Soc. 2005;25:41–67.
23. Findlay RA. Interventions to reduce social isolation amongst older people: where is the evidence? Ageing Soc. 2003;23:647–58.
24. Hagan R, Manktelow R, Taylor BJ, Mallett J. Reducing loneliness amongst older people: a systematic search and narrative review. Aging Ment Health. 2014;18:683–93.
25. Cohen-Mansfield J, Perach R. Interventions for alleviating loneliness among older persons: a critical review. Am J Health Promot. 2015;29:e109–25.
26. Windle K, Francis J, Coomber C. Preventing loneliness and social isolation: interventions and outcomes. London: Social Care Institute for Excellence; 2011.
27. Andersson L. Loneliness research and interventions: a review of the literature. Aging Ment Heal. 1998;2:264–74.
28. Sidani S, Braden CJ. Design, evaluation, and translation of nursing interventions. West Sussex: John Wiley & Sons, Inc; 2011.
29. Masi CM, Chen H-Y, Hawkley LC, Cacioppo JT. A meta-analysis of interventions to reduce loneliness. Personal Soc Psychol Rev. 2011;15:219–66.
30. Arksey H, O'Malley L. Scoping studies: towards a methodological framework. Int J Soc Res Methodol. 2005;8:19–32.
31. Levac D, Colquhoun H, O'Brien KK. Scoping studies: advancing the methodology. Implement Sci. 2010;5:69.
32. Leeman J, Calancie L, Hartman MA, Escoffery CT, Herrmann AK, Tague LE, et al. What strategies are used to build practitioners' capacity to implement community-based interventions and are they effective?: a systematic review. Implement Sci. 2015;10:80.
33. Sandelowski MJ, Barroso J. Handbook for synthesizing qualitative research. New York: Springer Publishing Company; 2007.
34. Cattan M, Newell C, Bond J, White M. Alleviating social isolation and loneliness among older people. Int J Ment Health Promot. 2003;5:20–30.
35. Cattan M, Ingold K. Implementing change: the alleviation of social isolation and loneliness among older people in Leeds. J Ment Heal Promot. 2003;2:12–9.
36. Pettigrew S, Roberts M. Addressing loneliness in later life. Aging Ment Health. 2008;12:302–9.
37. Smith J. An exploration of loneliness in community dwelling older adults: Saint Louis University; 2010.
38. Hooper K. Perceptions of loneliness and strategies used by community-dwelling older adults who are also part of a seniors' club to prevent loneliness: Dalhousie University; 2003.
39. Smith JM. Toward a better understanding of loneliness in community-dwelling older adults. Aust J Psychol. 2012;146:293–311.
40. Honigh-de Vlaming R, Haveman-Nies A, Ziylan C, Renes RJ. Acceptability of the components of a loneliness intervention among elderly Dutch people: a qualitative study. Am J Heal Educ. 2013;44:136–45.
41. de Vlaming R, Haveman-Nies A, Van't Veer P, de Groot LC. Evaluation design for a complex intervention program targeting loneliness in non-

institutionalized elderly Dutch people. BMC Public Health. 2010;10:552.
42. PCORI Board of Governors. Patient-centered outcomes research institute: National priorities for research and research agenda. 2012. http://www.pcori.org/assets/PCORI-National-Priorities-and-Research-Agenda-2012-05-21-FINAL1.pdf. Accessed April 3, 2017.
43. Centre for Reviews and Dissemination. Systematic reviews: CDR's guidance for undertaking reviews in health care. York: York Publishing Services; 2009.
44. Andrews GJ, Gavin N, Begley S, Brodie D. Assisting friendships, combating loneliness: users views on a befriending scheme. Ageing Soc. 2003;23:349–62.
45. Cattan M, Kime N, Bagnall AM. The use of telephone befriending in low level support for socially isolated older people - an evaluation. Heal Soc Care Community. 2011;19:198–206.
46. Moses B. Technology as a means of reducing loneliness in the elderly: Walden University; 2003.
47. Schwindenhammer TM. Videoconferencing intervention for depressive symptoms. Normal: Illinois State University; 2014.
48. Tsai H-H, Tsai Y-F, Wang H-H, Chang Y-C, Chu HH. Videoconference program enhances social support, loneliness, and depressive status of elderly nursing home residents. Aging Ment Health. 2010;14:947–54.
49. Tsai H-H, Tsai Y-F. Changes in depressive symptoms, social support, and loneliness over 1 year after a minimum 3-month videoconference program for older nursing home residents. J Med Internet Res. 2011;13:e93.
50. van der Heide LA, Willems CG, Spreeuwenberg MD, Rietman J, de Witte LP. Implementation of CareTV in care for the elderly: the effects on feelings of loneliness and safety and future challenges. Technol Disabil. 2012;24:283–91.
51. Pitkala KH, Routasalo P, Kautiainen H, Tilvis RS. Effects of psychosocial group rehabilitation on health, use of health care services, and mortality of older persons suffering from loneliness: a randomized, controlled trial. J Gerontol. Ser. A Biol. Sci. Med Sci. 2009;64A:792–800.
52. Routasalo PE, Tilvis RS, Kautiainen H, Pitkala KH. Effects of psychosocial group rehabilitation on social functioning, loneliness and well-being of lonely, older people: randomized controlled trial. J Adv Nurs. 2009;65:297–305.
53. Savikko N, Routasalo P, Tilvis R, Pitkälä K. Psychosocial group rehabilitation for lonely older people: favourable processes and mediating factors of the intervention leading to alleviated loneliness. Int J Older People Nurs. 2010;5:16–24.
54. Baker FA, Ballantyne J. "You've got to accentuate the positive": group songwriting to promote a life of enjoyment, engagement and meaning in aging Australians. Nord. J Music Ther. 2013;22:7–24.
55. Cohen BGD. Research on creativity and aging : the positive impact of the arts on health and illness. Generations. 2006;30:7–15.
56. Cohen GD, Perlstein S, Chapline J, Kelly J, Firth KM, Simmens S. The impact of professionally conducted cultural programs on the physical health, mental health, and social functioning of older adults. Gerontologist. 2006;46:726–34.
57. Brown VM, Allen AC, Dwozan M, Mercer I, Warren K. Indoor gardening older adults: effects on socialization, activities of daily living, and loneliness. J Gerontol Nurs. 2004;30:34–42.
58. Winstead V, Yost EA, Cotten SR, Berkowsky RW, Anderson WA. The impact of activity interventions on the well-being of older adults in continuing care communities. J Appl Gerontol. 2014;33:888–911.
59. Andersson L. Intervention against loneliness in a group of elderly women: a process evaluation. Hum Relations. 1984;37:295–310.
60. Andersson L. Intervention against loneliness in a group of elderly women: an impact evaluation. Soc Sci Med. 1985;20:355–64.
61. Cohen-Mansfield J, Parpura-Gill A, Kotler M, Vass J, MacLennan B, Rosenberg F. Shared interest groups (SHIGs) in low-income independent living facilities. Clin Gerontol. 2007;31:101–12.
62. Banks M. The effects of animal-assisted therapy on loneliness in an elderly population in long-term care facilities: Louisaiana State University Medical Center; 1998.
63. Banks MR, Banks WA. The effects of animal-assisted therapy on loneliness in residents of long-term care facilities. Anthrozoös. 2005;18:396–408.
64. Banks MR, Banks WA. The effects of animal-assisted therapy on loneliness in an elderly population in long-term care facilities. J Gerontol A Biol Sci Med Sci. 2002;57:M428–32.
65. Wright P. The effects of animal-assisted therapy on loneliness in elderly residents of a long-term care facility utilizing Roy's adaptation model: University of Southern Mississippi; 1995.
66. Reed M. The mascot model of human/companion interaction: its effects on levels of loneliness and depression among residents of a nursing home: Western Seminary; 1986.
67. Robinson H, MacDonald B, Kerse N, Broadbent E. The psychosocial effects of a companion robot: a randomized controlled trial. J Am Med Dir Assoc. 2013;14:661–7.
68. Vrbanac Z, Zecević I, Ljubić M, Belić M, Stanin D, Bottegaro NB, et al. Animal assisted therapy and perception of loneliness in geriatric nursing home residents. Coll Antropol. 2013;37:973–6.
69. Martina CMS, Stevens NL. Breaking the cycle of loneliness? Psychological effects of a friendship enrichment program for older women. Aging Ment Health. 2006;10:467–75.
70. Stevens N. Combating loneliness: a friendship enrichment programme for older women. Ageing Soc. 2001;21:183–202.
71. Stevens NL, Martina CMS, Westerhof GJ. Meeting the need to belong: predicting effects of a friendship enrichment program for older women. Gerontologist. 2006;46:495–502.
72. Stevens N, van Tilburg T. Stimulating friendship in later life: a strategy for reducing loneliness among older women. Educ Gerontol. 2000;26:15–35.
73. Kremers IP, Steverink N, Albersnagel FA, Slaets JPJ. Improved self-management ability and well-being in older women after a short group intervention. Aging Ment Health. 2006;10:476–84.
74. Blažun H, Saranto K, Rissanen S. Impact of computer training courses on reduction of loneliness of older people in Finland and Slovenia. Comput Human Behav. 2012;28:1202–12.
75. Fokkema T, Knipscheer K. Escape loneliness by going digital: a quantitative and qualitative evaluation of a Dutch experiment in using ECT to overcome loneliness among older adults. Aging Ment Health. 2007;11:496–504.
76. Creswell JD, Irwin MR, Burklund LJ, Lieberman MD, Arevalo JMG, Ma J, et al. Mindfulness-based stress reduction training reduces loneliness and pro-inflammatory gene expression in older adults: a small randomized controlled trial. Brain. Behav. Immun. 2012;26:1095–101.
77. Bartlett H, Warburton J, Lui C-W, Peach L, Carroll M. Preventing social isolation in later life: findings and insights from a pilot Queensland intervention study. Ageing Soc. 2013;33(7):1–23.
78. Clarke M, Clarke SJ, Jagger C. Social intervention and the elderly: a randomized controlled trial. Am J Epidemiol. 1992;136:1517–23.
79. Ollonqvist K, Palkeinen H, Aaltonen T, Pohjolainen T, Puukka P, Hinkka K, et al. Alleviating loneliness among frail older people – findings from a randomised controlled trial. Int J Ment Health Promot. 2008;10:26–34.
80. Passmore T, Lindenmeier D, Tapps T, Gibson H. Impact of participation in community-based recreation program on reported loneliness and feelings of usefulness of individuals diagnoses with early stage Alzheimer's disease. Am J Recreat Ther. 2007;6:27–39.
81. Bergman-Evans B. Beyond the basics: effects of the Eden alternative model on quality of life issues. J Gerontol Nurs. 2004;30:27–34.
82. Parsons M. The impact of the Eden alternative on quality of life of nursing home residents: University of Nebraska; 2004.
83. Chiang K-J, Chu H, Chang H-J, Chung M-H, Chen C-H, Chiou H-Y, et al. The effects of reminiscence therapy on psychological well-being, depression, and loneliness among the institutionalized aged. Int J Geriatr Psychiatry. 2010;25:380–8.
84. Dammeyer M. Does social isolation among facility-dwelling elderly decrease using a reminscence group intervention? University of Wyoming; 2004.
85. Stewart M, Craig D, MacPherson K, Alexander S. Promoting positive affect and diminishing loneliness of widowed seniors through a support intervention. Public Health Nurs. 2001;18:54–63.
86. Theurer K, Wister A, Sixsmith A, Chaudhury H, Lovegreen L. The development and evaluation of mutual support groups in long-term care homes. J Appl Gerontol. 2014;33:387–415.
87. Travers C, Bartlett HP. Silver memories: implementation and evaluation of a unique radio program for older people. Aging Ment Health. 2011;15:169–77

4

Using different anthropometric indices to assess prediction ability of type 2 diabetes in elderly population: a 5 year prospective study

Jing Yang[1], Fei Wang[1], Jing Wang[1], Xu Han[1], Hua Hu[1], Caizheng Yu[1], Jing Yuan[1], Ping Yao[1], Xiaoping Miao[2], Sheng Wei[2], Youjie Wang[1], Weihong Chen[1], Yuan Liang[1], Huan Guo[1], Xiaomin Zhang[1], Dan Zheng[1], Yuhan Tang[1], Handong Yang[3] and Meian He[1*]

Abstract

Background: Emerging studies have investigated the association between different anthropometric indices with diabetes risk but the results were inconsistent. The aims of the study were to examine the associations of different anthropometric indices with incident diabetes risk and whether novel anthropometric indices improve diabetes prediction beyond traditional indices among elderly Chinese.

Methods: Nine thousand nine hundred sixty-two elderly individuals (age ≥ 60 years old) derived from the prospective Dongfeng-Tongji cohort were included. Hazard ratio (HR) and corresponding 95% confidence interval (CI) were evaluated by Cox proportional hazard model to examine the associations between traditional anthropometric indices (body mass index [BMI], waist circumference [WC], waist-to-height ratio [WHtR]), novel anthropometric indices (visceral adiposity index [VAI], a body shape index [ABSI], body roundness index [BRI]) and diabetes risk. Receiver operating characteristic (ROC) curve and area under curve (AUC) were applied to compare the novel anthropometric indices with the traditional indices in diabetes prediction.

Results: During mean 4.6 years of follow-up, 614 incident cases of type 2 diabetes (T2D) were identified. Significant positive associations were detected between BMI, WC, WHtR, VAI and BRI and incident T2D risk. For ABSI, no significant association was observed in either men or women. BMI was the strongest predictor in diabetes in men (AUC = 0.655) comparable with the other anthropometric indices ($P < 0.05$). Similar as men, BMI was the strongest predictor (AUC = 0.635) in women. Except for WC, the AUC of BMI was larger than WHtR, VAI, and BRI. In contrast, ABSI was not a good predictor in either men (AUC = 0.507) or women (AUC = 0.503).

Conclusions: In elderly Chinese, BMI, WC, WHtR, VAI and BRI were positively associated with incident T2D risk. Among them, BMI was the strongest predictor in both men and women.

Keywords: Anthropometric indices, Elderly Chinese, Epidemiology, Diabetes mellitus, Prediction ability

* Correspondence: hemeian@hust.edu.cn
[1]Department of Occupational and Environmental Health and State Key Laboratory of Environmental Health for Incubating, School of Public Health, Tongji Medical College, Huazhong University of Science and Technology, 13 Hangkong Rd, Wuhan 430030, Hubei, China
Full list of author information is available at the end of the article

Background

In recent decades, type 2 diabetes (T2D) has increased rapidly and become a serious public health problem worldwide [1]. In China, the prevalence of T2D has risen to be 11.6% and over 100 million adults were affected [2].

Obesity is well recognized to be an important risk factor for the development of T2D. In epidemiological studies, anthropometric indices have been used to evaluate obesity for their simplicity and usefulness. Body mass index (BMI) has been the most commonly used anthropometric measure for defining obesity recommended by World Health Organization (WHO) [3] .Subsequently, studies found that BMI, an estimate of general obesity, could not reflect abdominal fat. Therefore waist circumference (WC) and waist-to-height ratio (WHtR) were suggested as an indicator of central adiposity [4–6], although they could not discriminate visceral fat from subcutaneous fat. In recent years, novel anthropometric indices, such as visceral adiposity index (VAI), a body shape index (ABSI), and body roundness index (BRI) have been proposed to be alternative indicators of obesity. VAI, an indicator of visceral fat dysfunction, has been reported to distinguish visceral fat from subcutaneous fat [7]. Bozorgmanesh et al. found VAI has a good predictive performance on diabetes in Tehran people [8]. In 2012, Krakauer developed a new anthropometric index named ABSI, and found ABSI was significantly associated with mortality [9]. In the following years, Thomas et al. developed another new anthropometric index known as BRI [10]. A recent study demonstrated that BRI was a potential and alternative obesity measure in assessment of T2D [11]. However, till now no comprehensive consensus has been reached about which one as the best anthropometric index to evaluate the risk and the predictive ability of diabetes, especially in elderly population.

The World Health Organization estimated that there were 600 million people aged 60 years or older in 2000, and that this number will increase to 1.2 billion in 2025 [12]. It is known that aging was related to significant changes in body composition, but it is unclear which anthropometric index is the best one to evaluate obesity and predict diabetes risk [13]. In the present study, based on the ongoing prospective Dongfeng-Tongji cohort study, we aim to examine the associations of different anthropometric indices with diabetes risk and to investigate whether these novel anthropometric indices could improve predictive ability of diabetes beyond traditional indices in elderly population.

Methods

Study participants

The participants in the present study were derived from the Dongfeng-Tongji (DFTJ) cohort study, which has been described elsewhere [14]. In brief, DFTJ, initiated in 2008, is a dynamic cohort study including 27,009 retirees from the Dongfeng Motor Corporation. The participants completed an epidemiology questionnaire including socio-demographic, lifestyle and medical history at baseline. The first follow-up was conducted from April to October 2013. As shown in (Additional file 1: Figure S1), participants with age below 60 years old ($n = 7932$), prevalent diabetes ($n = 4344$), coronary heart disease ($n = 2607$), stroke ($n = 437$) or cancer ($n = 555$) at baseline were excluded. Additionally, individuals were also ruled out if they had missing information on BMI ($n = 292$), WC ($n = 56$), triglyceride (TG, $n = 766$) or high-density lipoprotein cholesterol (HDL-c, $n = 58$). After exclusion, a total of 5998 men and 3964 women were eligible for the present study.

Anthropometric measurement

Height and weight were measured without shoes and heavy clothes, using standard device and methods, recorded to the nearest 0.5 cm and 0.1 kg. WC was determined at midway level between the lower rib margin and the iliac-crest at minimal respiration. BMI was calculated as weight (kg) divided by height (m) squared. WHtR was calculated as dividing WC (cm) by height (cm). VAI was defined as the following formula [7]:

$$\text{Male}: VAI = \left(\frac{WC(cm)}{39.68 + (1.88 \times BMI)}\right) \times \left(\frac{TG(mmol/L)}{1.03}\right) \times \left(\frac{1.31}{HDL\text{-}c(mmol/L)}\right)$$

$$\text{Female}: VAI = \left(\frac{WC(cm)}{39.58 + (1.89 \times BMI)}\right) \times \left(\frac{TG(mmol/L)}{0.81}\right) \times \left(\frac{1.52}{HDL\text{-}c(mmol/L)}\right)$$

ABSI was defined as: $ABSI = WC(\text{m}) / (BMI^{2/3} \times height(\text{m})^{1/2})$. BRI was defined as: $BRI = 364.2 - 365.5 \times \{1 - [(WC(\text{m})/2\pi)/(0.5 \times height(\text{m}))]^2\}^{1/2}$.

Type 2 diabetes definition

Type 2 diabetes cases were defined as self-reported physician-diagnosed diabetes or taking diabetes medications (oral hypoglycemic agent or insulin) or fasting glucose concentration (FBG) ≥ 7.0 mmol/L according to the WHO criteria [15]. In the study, a total of 614 incident diabetes were diagnosed.

Covariates assessment

Overnight fasting blood specimens were obtained and FBG level was measured by Abbott Aroset analyzer. TG, TC, HDL-c and high-density lipoprotein cholesterol (LDL-c) levels were measured by ARCHITECT Ci8200 automatic analyzer (ABBOTT Laboratories. Abbott Park, Illinois, U.S.A). Smokers were defined as those who smoke at least one cigarette per day for more than half a year, and smoking status was classified as never smoking, current smoking, and former smoking. Similarly, drinkers were defined as those who drink at least once per week for more than half a year, and drinking status was classified as never drinking, current drinking, and former drinking. Physical activity was defined as those who exercise at least 20 min per time regularly over the past 6 months. Education status was categorized into two levels: low level (middle or primary school or below) and high level (high school or beyond). Hypertension was defined if blood pressure ≥ 140/90 mmHg, or using antihypertensive medication or self-reported physician-diagnosed hypertension. Hyperlipidemia was defined if TC > 5.72 mmol/L or TG > 1.70 mmol/L or using lipid-lowing medication, or self-reported physician-diagnosed hyperlipidemia.

Statistical analysis

Categorical variables were presented in number (percentage) and continuous variables in mean (SD) or median. Student's *t*-test, Mann-Whiney U test or Chi-square test

Table 1 Baseline characteristic of the study population

Variables	Non T2D cases ($n = 9348$)	Incident T2D cases ($n = 614$)	*P* value
Age (years)	66.81 ± 5.55	66.44 ± 5.16	0.083
Female (%)	3715(39.7)	249(40.6)	0.690
WC (cm)	83.01 ± 9.31	87.13 ± 9.62	< 0.001
WHtR	0.51 ± 0.06	0.54 ± 0.06	< 0.001
BMI (kg/m^2)	24.22 ± 3.32	25.86 ± 3.18	< 0.001
VAI	1.55 ± 1.31	1.93 ± 1.58	< 0.001
ABSI	0.078 ± 0.006	0.078 ± 0.006	0.441
BRI	3.69 ± 1.15	4.17 ± 1.21	< 0.001
Smoking (Yes, %)			
Current smoker	2300(24.8)	147(24.1)	
Former smoker	1319(14.2)	84(13.7)	
Never smoker	5672(61.0)	380(62.2)	0.854
Alcohol consumption (Yes, %)			
Current drinker	147(24.1)	169(27.5)	
Former drinker	84(13.7)	49(8.0)	
Never drinker	380(62.2)	396(64.5)	0.020
Physical activity (Yes, %)	8470(90.0)	547(89.1)	0.213
Education (High school or beyond, %)	3036(32.8)	186(30.5)	0.244
HDL-c (mmol/L)	1.40	1.35	0.001
TG (mmol/L)	1.15	1.36	< 0.001
TC (mmol/L)	5.10	5.17	0.019
SBP (mmHg)	129.76 ± 18.28	133.54 ± 17.72	< 0.001
DBP (mmHg)	77.35 ± 10.84	79.07 ± 10.81	< 0.001
Hypertention (Yes, %)	3739(40.0)	328(53.4)	< 0.001
Hyperlipidemia (Yes, %)	4229(45.2)	353(57.5)	< 0.001
FBG (mmol/L)	5.54 ± 0.56	6.05 ± 0.63	< 0.001
T2D family history (Yes, %)	169(1.8)	17(2.8)	0.090

Continuous variables were presented as mean ± SD or median. Categorical variables were presented as a number (percentage)

Abbreviations: *WC* waist circumstance, *WhtR* waist-to-height ratio, *BMI* body mass index, *VAI* visceral adiposity index, *ABSI* a body shape index, *BRI* body round index, *HDL-c* high-density lipoprotein cholesterol, *LDL-c* low-density lipoprotein, *SBP* systolic blood pressure, *DBP* diastolic blood pressure, *TG* triglyceride, *TC* total cholesterol, *FBG* fasting blood glucose, *T2D* type 2 diabetes

Table 2 Anthropometric indices and incident T2D risk in men and women

Variables	Cases/Total(n)	Incidence/1000 person-years	Model 1	Model 2	Model 3
Men ($n = 5998$)					
WC (cm)					
< 85	142/3356	9.79	1.00(Reference)	1.00(Reference)	1.00(Reference)
≥ 85	223/2642	19.57	1.75(1.42,2.16)	1.73(1.40,2.14)	1.43(1.14,1.78)
P value			< 0.001	< 0.001	< 0.001
WHtR					
< 0.5	106/2763	8.88	1.00(Reference)	1.00(Reference)	1.00(Reference)
≥ 0.5	259/3235	18.55	1.91(1.52,2.39)	1.88(1.50,2.36)	1.43(1.22,1.82)
P value			< 0.001	< 0.001	< 0.001
BMI (kg/m^2)					
< 24	98/2868	7.94	1.00(Reference)	1.00(Reference)	1.00(Reference)
24–27.9	179/2467	16.71	2.09(1.63,2.67)	2.10(1.64,2.70)	1.56(1.21,2.02)
≥ 28	88/633	30.82	4.18(3.14,5.58)	4.21(3.14,5.64)	2.59(1.91,3.53)
P for trend			< 0.001	< 0.001	< 0.001
VAI					
Tertile 1	78/2000	8.99	1.00(Reference)	1.00(Reference)	1.00(Reference)
Tertile 2	99/1999	11.41	1.24(0.92,1.67)	1.24(0.92,1.67)	1.17(0.86,1.58)
Tertile 3	188/1999	22.00	2.39(1.84,3.11)	2.40(1.84,3.13)	2.00(1.49,2.67)
P for trend			< 0.001	< 0.001	< 0.001
ABSI					
Tertile 1	119/1999	13.73	1.00(Reference)	1.00(Reference)	1.00(Reference)
Tertile 2	128/1999	14.76	0.88(0.68,1.23)	0.86(0.67,1.10)	0.80(0.62,1.03)
Tertile 3	118/2000	13.79	0.78(0.60,1.01)	0.76(0.59,0.99)	0.79(0.61,1.03)
P for trend			0.056	0.039	0.098
BRI					
Tertile 1	93/1999	10.79	1.00(Reference)	1.00(Reference)	1.00(Reference)
Tertile 2	109/2000	12.57	1.43(1.06,1.92)	1.42(1.06,1.91)	1.14(0.84,1.54)
Tertile 3	183/1999	21.26	2.32(1.77,3.05)	2.27(1.73,2.99)	1.60(1.20,2.13)
P for trend			< 0.001	< 0.001	< 0.001
Women ($n = 3964$)					
WC (cm)					
< 80	78/1899	9.50	1.00(Reference)	1.00(Reference)	1.00(Reference)
≥ 80	171/2065	18.96	1.67(1.28,2.18)	1.67(1.27,2.20)	1.46(1.11,1.92)
P value			< 0.001	< 0.001	< 0.001
WHtR					
< 0.5	49/1395	8.11	1.00(Reference)	1.00(Reference)	1.00(Reference)
≥ 0.5	200/2569	17.87	1.87(1.37,2.56)	1.85(1.34,2.54)	1.51(1.10,2.09)
P value			< 0.001	< 0.001	< 0.001
BMI (kg/m^2)					
< 24	66/1864	8.15	1.00(Reference)	1.00(Reference)	1.00(Reference)
24–27.9	121/1486	18.70	2.31(1.71,3.11)	2.29(1.69,3.10)	1.74(1.27,2.36)
≥ 28	62/614	23.30	2.78(1.97,3.94)	2.81(1.98,4.00)	2.01(1.41,2.87)
P for trend			< 0.001	< 0.001	< 0.001

Table 2 Anthropometric indices and incident T2D risk in men and women *(Continued)*

Variables	Cases/Total(n)	Incidence/1000 person-years	Model 1	Model 2	Model 3
VAI					
Tertile 1	50/1322	8.77	1.00(Reference)	1.00(Reference)	1.00(Reference)
Tertile 2	97/1320	16.79	1.90(1.35,2.67)	1.86(1.32,2.63)	1.80(1.28,2.55)
Tertile 3	102/1322	17.72	2.04(1.45,2.87)	2.01(1.43,2.83)	1.85(1.31,2.61)
P for trend			< 0.001	< 0.001	0.003
ABSI					
Tertile 1	85/1321	14.74	1.00(Reference)	1.00(Reference)	1.00(Reference)
Tertile 2	79/1321	13.77	0.79(0.58,1.07)	0.77(0.56,1.05)	0.73(0.53,1.00)
Tertile 3	85/1322	14.82	0.76(0.56,1.03)	0.74(0.54,1.01)	0.83(0.61,1.41)
P for trend			< 0.001	0.073	0.313
BRI					
Tertile 1	46/1323	8.02	1.00(Reference)	1.00(Reference)	1.00(Reference)
Tertile 2	82/1327	14.05	1.50(1.04,2.16)	1.42(0.98,2.05)	1.23(0.85,1.78)
Tertile 3	121/1314	21.38	2.18(1.54,3.08)	1.98(1.39,2.82)	1.73(1.21,2.46)
P for trend			< 0.001	< 0.001	0.001

Model 1 unadjusted model. Model 2 additionally adjusted for age, smoking, drinking, physical activity and education level. Model 3 additionally adjusted for hypertension, hyperlipidemia (except VAI), FBG (except VAI) and family history of T2D

were used for comparison between groups. In the present analysis, central obesity was defined as WC ≥85 cm in men and WC ≥ 80 cm in women. The cut-off point of WHtR was 0.5 [16]. According to the China criterion, BMI < 24 kg/m^2 was defined as normal, 24–27.9 kg/m^2 overweight, and BMI ≥ 28 kg/m^2 obesity. VAI, ABSI and BRI were stratified into sex-specific tertiles. Partial correlation was used to examine the linear relationship between various anthropometric indices after adjustment for age. Cox proportional hazard model was used to calculate hazard ratio (HR) and corresponding 95% confidence intervals (CIs) of incident diabetes for different anthropometric indices. Receiver operating characteristic (ROC) analysis was used to compare discrimination ability and determine optimal cut-off value. Sensitivity and specificity were calculated based on cut-off values, which were estimated using the maximized Youden index. The areas under the ROC curves (AUC) was compared by a non-parametric test [17]. Statistical analyses were performed with SPSS Statistics 23.0 (SPSS, Chicago, Illinois, USA), except for the ROC analysis, which was tested using MedCalc V.17.9 (MedCalc Software, Belgium). A two-side value of $P < 0.05$ was considered statistically significant.

Results

Characteristics of participants

During mean 4.6 years of follow-up, 365 incident cases of T2D in the 5998 men (14.09/1000 person-years) and 249 cases in the 3964 women (14.45/1000 person-years) were identified. Baseline characteristics of the 614 (6.2%) participants who did and 9348 (93.8%) who did not develop to T2D are shown in Table 1. The average age of participants who did and who did not develop to T2D was 66.44 and 66.81 years old respectively. As expected, participants who developed to T2D were more likely to have higher levels of WC, WHtR, BMI, VAI, BRI, diastolic blood pressure (DBP), systolic blood pressure (SBP), TG, FBG (all $P < 0.001$), TC ($P = 0.019$) and lower levels of HDL-c ($P = 0.001$). Moreover, the rate of drinking ($P = 0.02$) in participants who developed to T2D was higher than who did not. No significant difference was observed in ABSI ($P = 0.441$), smoking ($P = 0.854$), physical activity ($P = 0.213$), education level ($P = 0.244$), and family history of T2D ($P = 0.09$) between participants who did and who did not develop to T2D.

The correlation coefficients between various anthropometric indices are shown in (Additional file 1: Table S1). All anthropometric indices showed significant correlation with each other ($P < 0.001$). The strongest correlation coefficient was found between WHtR and BRI ($r = 0.87$ and $r = 0.83$) and the weakest one between BMI and ABSI ($r = -0.047$ and $r = -0.161$). Similar findings were observed in both men and women.

Association of anthropometric indices with incident T2D risk

The relationships between anthropometric indices including WC, WHtR, BMI, VAI, ABSI, and BRI and incident T2D risk in men and women are shown in Table 2. For ABSI, no significant association was observed in either men (P for trend = 0.098) or women (P for trend = 0.313).WC, WHtR, BMI, VAI, and BRI were significantly associated with increased risk of T2D in both men and women after adjustment for potential confounders including age, smoking, drinking, physical activity and education. Further adjustment for hypertension, hyperlipidemia (except VAI), FBG (except VAI) and family history of T2D reduced the associations but still remained significant. In men, the hazard risks (95% CI; top vs lowest) were 1.43 (1.14–1.78) for WC, 1.43 (1.22–1.82) for WHtR, 2.59 (1.91–3.53) for BMI, 2.00 (1.49–2.67) for VAI, 0.79(0.61, 1.03) for ABSI, and 1.60(1.20–2.13) for BRI. For women, the corresponding HRs (95% CI) were 1.46 (1.11–1.92), 1.51 (1.10–2.09), 2.01(1.41–2.87), 1.85 (1.31–2.61), 0.83(0.61, 1.41), and 1.73 (1.21–2.46) for WC, WHtR, BMI, VAI, ABSI and BRI respectively.

ROC analysis

Figure 1 and Table 3 presents the results of ROC analysis and AUC (95% CIs) for BMI, WC, WHtR, VAI, ABSI, and BRI. Comparison of AUC in different anthropometric

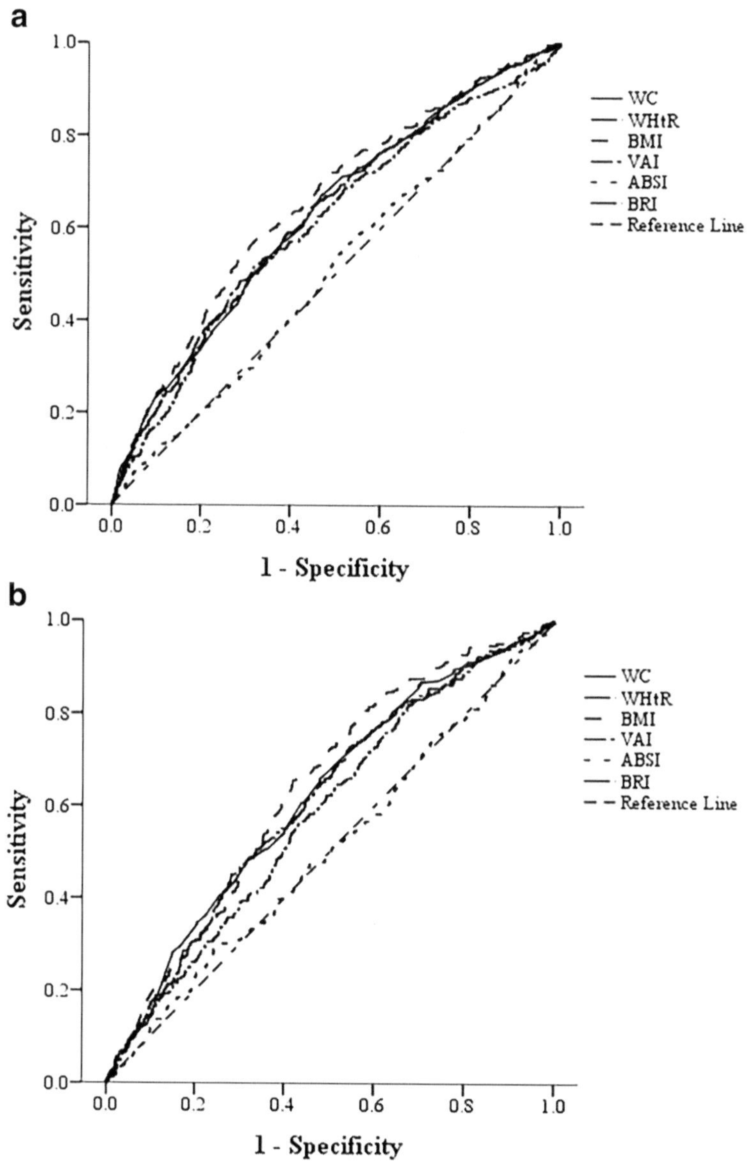

Fig. 1 ROC curves for WC, WHtR, BMI, VAI, ABSI and BRI in men (**a**) and women (**b**) The ROC curves were constructed for T2D as a response to each anthropometric index. In men (**a**): WC: AUC = 0.629 (95% CI: 0.600–0.659). WHtR: AUC = 0.629 (95% CI: 0.600–0.658). BMI: AUC = 0.655 (95% CI: 0.626–0.684). VAI: AUC = 0.609 (95% CI: 0.578–0.639). ABSI: AUC = 0.507 (95% CI: 0.477–0.538). BRI: AUC = 0.629 (95% CI: 0.600–0.658). In women (**b**): WC: AUC = 0.616 (95% CI: 0.581–0.651). WHtR: AUC = 0.609 (95% CI: 0.574–0.644). BMI: AUC = 0.635 (95% CI: 0.602–0.667). VAI: AUC = 0.582 (95% CI: 0.548–0.617). ABSI: AUC = 0.503 (95% CI: 0.465–0.540). BRI: AUC = 0.609 (95% CI: 0.574–0.644)

Table 3 AUC and corresponding 95% CI of anthropometric indices in men and women

Variables	Men ($n = 5998$)		Women ($n = 3964$)	
	AUC (95% CI)	*P* Value	AUC (95% CI)	*P* value
WC	0.629*(0.600,0.659)	< 0.001	0.616 (0.581,0.651)	< 0.001
WHtR	0.629*(0.600,0.658)	< 0.001	0.609**(0.574,0.644)	< 0.001
BMI	0.655 (0.626,0.684)	< 0.001	0.635 (0.602,0.667)	< 0.001
VAI	0.609*(0.578,0.639)	< 0.001	0.582* (0.548,0.617)	< 0.001
ABSI	0.507*(0.477,0.538)	0.631	0.503*(0.465,0.540)	0.882
BRI	0.629*(0.600,0.658)	< 0.001	0.609**(0.574,0.644)	< 0.001

AUC area under curve, *CI* confidence interval
*Compared with the AUC of BMI, $p < 0.05$
** Compared with the AUC of BMI, $p = 0.051$

indices is shown in (Additional file 1: Table S2). In men, ROC analysis revealed that BMI was the strongest predictor in diabetes (AUC = 0.655) comparable with the other anthropometric indices ($P < 0.05$) including WC (AUC =0.629), WHtR (AUC =0.629), VAI (AUC = 0.609) and BRI (AUC = 0.629). Similar as men, BMI was the strongest predictor (AUC = 0.635) in women. Except for WC (AUC = 0.616, $P = 0.165$ vs. BMI), the AUC of BMI was larger than other indices such as WHtR (AUC = 0.609, $P = 0.051$ vs. BMI), VAI (AUC = 0.582, $P = 0.017$ vs. BMI) and BRI (AUC = 0.609, $P = 0.051$vs. BMI). In contrast, ABSI was not a good predictor in either men (AUC = 0.507) or women (AUC = 0.503).

Optimal cutoff points of anthropometric indices in T2D risk prediction

Table 4 summarized the optimal cutoff points of the five significant anthropometric indices in prediction of T2D risk ($P < 0.05$ vs. AUC = 0.50). For men, optimal WC cut-off point was 84.90 cm in terms of Youden index; for women, the optimal cut-off point was 81.10 cm. The optimal cut-off point of BMI in men was 25.78 kg/m^2 and 24.86 kg/m^2 in women. The cut-off points for WHtR were similar in men (0.512) and women (0.514). For VAI, it was 1.34 in men and 1.23 in women. The optimal cut-off point of BRI in men was 3.58 and 3.62 in women.

Discussion

To the best of our knowledge, this is the largest prospective study to compare the novel anthropometric indices with the traditional indices in the risk prediction of T2D in elderly population. BMI, WC, WHtR, VAI, BRI were positively associated with incident T2D risk in the elderly, independent of the potential confounders. For ABSI, no significant association was observed in either men or women. BMI appeared to be the strongest predictor of incident T2D risk in both elderly men and women. In comparison with traditional anthropometric indices, novel anthropometric indices did not improve prediction of T2D in elderly population.

In the present study, BMI was the strongest predictor in both elderly men and women, while WC and WHtR showed similar prediction ability in men. These results were consistent with other studies. In Pima Indians, BMI was the best predictors of diabetes [18]. In the Health Professionals Follow-Up Study, BMI and WC showed similar associations with T2D in men aged 40–75 years; in contrast, WHR was the weakest predictor [19]. In the Atherosclerosis Risk in Communities (ARIC) Study, BMI, WC, and WHR showed similar associations in adults aged 40–64 years [20].

A large amount of studies examined the associations of novel anthropometric indices such as VAI, ABSI and BRI with diabetes risk and their performances on diabetes risk prediction. In cross-sectional [21, 22] and cohort studies [23, 24], VAI was associated with increased risk for T2D. The result was validated in the Tehran Lipid and Glucose cohort study [25]. Besides, researchers observed that VAI was a useful surrogate marker to identify risk of diabetes [23, 24], but whether the ability of the VAI to identify diabetes risk was superior to easily measurable anthropometric markers, such as BMI, WC, WHtR was still a matter of debate [22, 23, 25].

For ABSI, no significant association was observed in either men or women. ABSI was not a good discriminator of T2D in the present study. Some studies observed that ABSI was positively correlated with mortality from cardiovascular diseases and cancer [26]. Studies investigating the ABSI to predict T2D are scarce, especially in elderly population. Furthermore, until now studies have not shown

Table 4 Cutoff points for anthropometric indices in predicting type 2 diabetes

Variables	Men				Women			
	Cutoff	Sensitivity (%)	Specifity (%)	Youden index	Cutoff	Sensitivity (%)	Specifity (%)	Youden index
WC (cm)	84.90	67.1	53.2	0.203	81.10	65.9	52.1	0.180
BMI (kg/m^2)	25.78	54.2	71.3	0.255	24.86	65.5	58.2	0.237
WHtR	0.512	64.4	55.5	0.199	0.514	72.7	45.6	0.183
VAI	1.335	51.2	68.6	0.198	1.225	81.9	32.1	0.146
BRI	3.584	64.7	55.2	0.199	3.618	72.7	45.6	0.183

that ABSI is superior to BMI or waist circumference in predicting T2D.

BRI was significantly associated with increased risk of diabetes and potential for use as an alternative index in assessment of T2D, which was consistent with previous study [11]. Till now no comprehensive consensus has been reached which one is the best anthropometric index to evaluate the risk and the predictive ability of diabetes in elderly Chinese. Whereas, compared with other anthropometric indices, BMI was taken as a useful indicator for measuring obesity in epidemiological surveys for its simplicity [3]. Our study confirmed that increased BMI was associated with type 2 diabetes in elderly Chinese population, which could be useful in initiating early interventional measures including balanced diet and regular physical exercise to prevent overweight, obesity and type 2 diabetes in the elderly population [27].

Our study also proposed optimal cut-off points for these anthropometric indices. An obvious difference was observed in WC, VAI and BRI between men and women, suggesting that gender-specific reference values should be recommended in practice. The appropriate cutoff points to best identify T2D were not consistent among different age ranges and different population. Aging not only promotes increased body fat, but also changes its distribution. Furthermore, although numerous studies proposed alternative BMI criteria specific to Asian populations [28], no consistent findings were obtained. Our ROC analysis suggested that the ideal BMI cutoffs were 25.78 kg/m^2 and 24.86 kg/m^2 for identifying diabetes risk in Chinese elderly men and women, respectively. Besides, in the present study WC threshold was about 85 cm for men and 81 cm for women, similar as the findings from a meta-analysis in China with WC cut-off points of 85 cm in men and 80 cm in women. While in Japan the optimal WC cutoff for abdominal obesity in men and women was 85 and 90 cm [29]. Thus, WC cutoff points cannot be used universally across gender, race or different age ranges [30]. As for VAI or BRI, there was no study about its cutoff points previously. Therefore, the definition of obesity among the elderly is still a matter of debate and our findings still need further verification.

To our knowledge, it is the first prospective study focused on elderly Chinese to comparing the novel indices with the traditional indices for diabetes risk prediction. Moreover, a notable strength was its prospective design, sex-specific analysis and relative large sample size. The study also has some limitations. Firstly, the duration of follow-up (mean 4.6 years) was relatively short and limited T2D cases were identified. Secondly, although a variety of relevant confounding factors were controlled, residual confounders could not be eliminated.

Conclusions

In conclusion, significant associations were observed between BMI, WC, WHtR, VAI and BRI and incident risk of T2D in both elderly men and women. BMI was the strongest and best predictor of incident diabetes in elderly population. In comparison with traditional anthropometric indices, novel anthropometric indices did not improve prediction of T2D in elderly Chinese. Future studies should examine this issue in much larger samples and different population. The underlying mechanism also need to be further elucidated. Given that anthropometric indices are potentially modifiable factors, our findings may provide important public health implications for the prevention and management of T2D, especially in elderly population.

Abbreviations

ABSI: A body shape index; ARIC: Atherosclerosis Risk in Communities; AUC: Area under curve; BMI: Body mass index; BRI: Body round index; CI: Confidence interval; DBP: Diastolic blood pressure; EDTA: Ethylene diamine tetraacetic acid; FBG: Fasting glucose concentration; HDL-c: High-density lipoprotein cholesterol; HR: Hazard ratio; LDL-c: Low-density lipoprotein; OGTT: Oral glucose tolerance test; SBP: Systolic blood pressure; T2D: Type 2 diabetes; TC: Total cholesterol; TG: Triglyceride; VAI: Visceral adiposity index; WC: Waist circumstance; WHO: World Health Organization; WHtR: Waist-to-height ratio

Acknowledgements

The authors would like to thank all study subjects for participating in the present DFTJ cohort study as well as all volunteers for assisting in collecting the samples and data.

Funding

This work was supported by the grants from the National Natural Science Foundation (grants NSFC-81473051 and 81522040) and the Program for HUST Academic Frontier Youth Team. The funders were not involved in the design, conduct, or reporting of the study.

Authors' contributions

JY analyzed the data, interpreted the results, and wrote the manuscript. JY and FW conceptualized the research question and designed the study. JW, XH, HH and CZY provided consultation on methodology and helped with analysis interpretation. XPM and SW performed the statistical data analysis, and contributed to the interpretation of results. JY, PY, YJW, WHC, YL, HG, XMZ, DZ, YHT, HDY and MAH provided critical revisions to the manuscript. All authors read and approved the final manuscript.

Competing interests

The authors declare that they have no competing interests.

Author details

[1]Department of Occupational and Environmental Health and State Key Laboratory of Environmental Health for Incubating, School of Public Health, Tongji Medical College, Huazhong University of Science and Technology, 13 Hangkong Rd, Wuhan 430030, Hubei, China. [2]Department of Epidemiology and Biostatistics, School of Public Health, Tongji Medical College, Huazhong University of Science and Technology, Wuhan, China. [3]Dongfeng Central Hospital, Dongfeng Motor Corporation and Hubei University of Medicine, Shiyan, Hubei, China.

References

1. Chan JC, Malik V, Jia W, Kadowaki T, Yajnik CS, Yoon KH, et al. Diabetes in Asia: epidemiology, risk factors, and pathophysiology. JAMA. 2009;301:2129–40.
2. Xu Y, Wang L, He J, Bi Y, Li M, Wang T, et al. Prevalence and control of diabetes in Chinese adults. JAMA. 2013;310:948–59.
3. Misra A. Ethnic-specific criteria for classification of body mass index: a perspective for Asian Indians and American Diabetes Association position statement. Diabetes Technol Ther. 2015;17:667–71.
4. Daniels SR, Khoury PR, Morrison JA. Utility of different measures of body fat distribution in children and adolescents. Am J Epidemiol. 2000;152:1179–84.
5. Li C, Ford ES, McGuire LC, Mokdad AH. Increasing trends in waist circumference and abdominal obesity among US adults. Obesity (Silver Spring). 2007;15:216–24.
6. Esmaillzadeh A, Mirmiran P, Azizi F. Waist-to-hip ratio is a better screening measure for cardiovascular risk factors than other anthropometric indicators in Tehranian adult men. Int J Obes Relat Metab Disord. 2004;28:1325–32.
7. Amato MC, Giordano C, Galia M, Criscimanna A, Vitabile S, Midiri M, et al. Visceral adiposity index: a reliable indicator of visceral fat function associated with cardiometabolic risk. Diabetes Care. 2010;33:920–2.
8. Bozorgmanesh M, Hadaegh F, Azizi F. Predictive performance of the visceral adiposity index for a visceral adiposity-related risk: type 2 diabetes. Lipids Health Dis. 2011;10:88.
9. Krakauer NY, Krakauer JC. A new body shape index predicts mortality hazard independently of body mass index. PLoS One. 2012;7:e39504.
10. Thomas DM, Bredlau C, Bosy-Westphal A, Mueller M, Shen W, Gallagher D, et al. Relationships between body roundness with body fat and visceral adipose tissue emerging from a new geometrical model. Obesity (Silver Spring). 2013;21:2264–71.
11. Chang Y, Guo X, Chen Y, Guo L, Li Z, Yu S, et al. A body shape index and body roundness index: two new body indices to identify diabetes mellitus among rural populations in Northeast China. BMC Public Health. 2015;15:794.
12. Dodds RM, Roberts HC, Cooper C, Sayer AA. The epidemiology of sarcopenia. J Clin Densitom. 2015;18:461–6.
13. Michalakis K, Goulis DG, Vazaiou A, Mintziori G, Polymeris A, Abrahamian-Michalakis A. Obesity in the ageing man. Metabolism. 2013;62:1341–9.
14. Wang F, Zhu J, Yao P, Li X, He M, Liu Y, et al. Cohort profile: the Dongfeng-Tongji cohort study of retired workers. Int J Epidemiol. 2013;42:731–40.
15. Alberti KG, Zimmet PZ. Definition, diagnosis and classification of diabetes mellitus and its complications. Part 1: diagnosis and classification of diabetes mellitus provisional report of a WHO consultation. Diabet Med. 1998;15:539–53.
16. Ashwell M, Gunn P, Gibson S. Waist-to-height ratio is a better screening tool than waist circumference and BMI for adult cardiometabolic risk factors: systematic review and meta-analysis. Obes Rev. 2012;13:275–86.
17. DeLong ER, DeLong DM, Clarke-Pearson DL. Comparing the areas under two or more correlated receiver operating characteristic curves: a nonparametric approach. Biometrics. 1988;44:837–45.
18. Tulloch-Reid MK, Williams DE, Looker HC, Hanson RL, Knowler WC. Do measures of body fat distribution provide information on the risk of type 2 diabetes in addition to measures of general obesity? Comparison of anthropometric predictors of type 2 diabetes in Pima Indians. Diabetes Care. 2003;26:2556–61.
19. Wang Y, Rimm EB, Stampfer MJ, Willett WC, Hu FB. Comparison of abdominal adiposity and overall obesity in predicting risk of type 2 diabetes among men. Am J Clin Nutr. 2005;81:555–63.
20. Vazquez G, Duval S, Jacobs DR Jr, Silventoinen K. Comparison of body mass index, waist circumference, and waist/hip ratio in predicting incident diabetes: a meta-analysis. Epidemiol Rev. 2007;29:115–28.
21. Du T, Sun X, Huo R, Yu X. Visceral adiposity index, hypertriglyceridemic waist and risk of diabetes: the China health and nutrition survey 2009. Int J Obes. 2014;38:840–7.
22. Yang Y, Feng Y, Ma X, Chen K, Wu N, Wang D, et al. Visceral adiposity index and insulin secretion and action in first-degree relatives of subjects with type 2 diabetes. Diabetes Metab Res Rev. 2015;31:315–21.
23. Wang Y, He S, He J, Wang S, Liu K, Chen X. Predictive value of visceral adiposity index for type 2 diabetes mellitus: a 15-year prospective cohort study. Herz. 2015;40(Suppl 3):277–81.
24. Chen C, Xu Y, Guo ZR, Yang J, Wu M, Hu XS. The application of visceral adiposity index in identifying type 2 diabetes risks based on a prospective cohort in China. Lipids Health Dis. 2014;13:108.
25. Ghasemi A, Tohidi M, Derakhshan A, Hasheminia M, Azizi F, Hadaegh F. Cut-off points of homeostasis model assessment of insulin resistance, beta-cell function, and fasting serum insulin to identify future type 2 diabetes: Tehran lipid and glucose study. Acta Diabetol. 2015;52:905–15.
26. Dhana K, Kavousi M, Ikram MA, Tiemeier HW, Hofman A, Franco OH. Body shape index in comparison with other anthropometric measures in prediction of total and cause-specific mortality. J Epidemiol Community Health. 2016;70:90–6.
27. Olafsdottir E, Aspelund T, Sigurdsson G, Thorsson B, Benediktsson R, Harris TB, et al. Unfavourable risk factors for type 2 diabetes mellitus are already apparent more than a decade before onset in a population-based study of older persons: from the age, gene/environment susceptibility-Reykjavik study (AGES-Reykjavik). Eur J Epidemiol. 2009;24:307–14.
28. Misra A. Revisions of cutoffs of body mass index to define overweight and obesity are needed for the Asian-ethnic groups. Int J Obes Relat Metab Disord. 2003;27:1294–6.
29. Oda E. New criteria for 'obesity disease' in Japan. Circ J. 2006;70:150 author reply 150.
30. Misra A, Wasir JS, Vikram NK. Waist circumference criteria for the diagnosis of abdominal obesity are not applicable uniformly to all populations and ethnic groups. Nutrition. 2005;21:969–76.

5

Exploring the sensory screening experiences of nurses working in long-term care homes with residents who have dementia: a qualitative study

Fiona Höbler[1,2*], Xochil Argueta-Warden[3], Miriam Rodríguez-Monforte[4], Astrid Escrig-Pinol[1,5], Walter Wittich[6,7,8] and Katherine S. McGilton[1,3]

Abstract

Background: The prevalence of vision and hearing loss is higher amongst older individuals with dementia, as well as higher in long-term care settings than in the wider community. However, the incidence of sensory impairment is underreported and often goes untreated. In this study, we aimed to understand nurses' current experiences of screening and caring for long-term care residents who have dementia and sensory impairment.

Methods: As part of a larger study on the sensory screening of long-term care residents with dementia, an environmental scan was conducted with front-line healthcare providers. We report here on the findings from the content analysis of individual, semi-structured interviews with nurses working in two long-term care homes in Southern Ontario, Canada. Twenty regulated nurses, including designated resident assessment coordinators, working full- or part-time with individuals who have dementia, participated across the two sites. All interviews were transcribed, and their contents reviewed and coded for themes by means of inductive thematic analysis.

Results: Following a systematic and recursive approach, three analysts identified several themes relating to: 1) the sensory screening process, 2) communication strategies, and 3) quality of life, sensory loss, and dementia. Participants reported on the strengths and limitations of screening procedures, what improvements should be made, which informal strategies are effective, and the continued professional development that is needed.

Conclusions: Nurses demonstrated insight into the facilitators and barriers to effective screening and care of residents with dementia and sensory impairments, and expressed the need for further education, more suitable screening tools, and formalised accountability within the screening process for vision and hearing loss in these long-term care residents.

Keywords: Nursing, Long-term care, Dementia, Visual impairment, Hearing loss, Sensory loss, Screening

Background

Dementia is increasing in our aging population, and is directly reflected in growing incidence rates found in long-term care homes (LTCHs), as recorded in several countries worldwide. As LTCH residents tend to be older, they also tend to have higher levels and more severe physical and cognitive impairments than community-dwelling older adults [1]. The prevalence of dementia has been reported to be between 60 and 80% amongst residents in this setting [2, 3]. In addition, owing to its association with cognitive impairment, the prevalence of sensory impairment is also higher in this population [4]. More than 80% of residents have, at least, mild hearing loss and ~50% a moderate to severe hearing impairment [5–8]. Impaired vision is twice as high amongst LTCH residents as in the general older population, estimated at 30% to 57% [9–12]. Whereas, hearing and/or vision loss can affect over 60% of LTCH

* Correspondence: fiona.hobler@utoronto.ca
[1]Toronto Rehabilitation Institute-University Health Network, 130 Dunn Ave, Toronto M6K 2R7, Canada
[2]Rehabilitation Sciences Institute, University of Toronto, Toronto, ON, Canada
Full list of author information is available at the end of the article

residents; and estimates of combined vision and hearing impairment, known as dual sensory impairment (DSI), affects one third of LTCH residents [9]. Despite high prevalence rates, both dementia and sensory impairment are often undiagnosed, underreported or undocumented [3, 6, 13, 14].

Research of sensory screening measures in care settings, such as nursing homes [9], retirement homes [15], and LTCHs [16], has evidenced the need for assessment and intervention for this vulnerable population. In Canada and the United States, as in many countries across Europe and Australasia, the current standard for screening residents in these settings involves the Resident Assessment Instrument – Minimum Data Set 2.0 (RAI-MDS 2.0) [17]. This screening is advised to be carried out within two weeks of a resident's admission to the LTCH by a regulated nurse, either a Registered Nurse (RN) or Registered Practical Nurse (RPN), and coordinated with the appropriate health professionals [18]. The screening process has the purpose of identifying individuals with a probability of having a disease or condition, so that they can be referred for appropriate diagnostic testing [19], as well as detecting a change in the resident's status, to ensure their health, safety, and maximal functioning [20]. The RAI-MDS 2.0 comprises of subsections for vision and hearing, whereby data is gathered from observation, review of clinical records, care plans, and through interviews with the resident, as well as significant others and team members [21].

Assessment measures that rely on self-report or the observations of others have, however, been found to be less reliable [22–24] or accurate than standard objective techniques [25, 26]. Furthermore, individuals with dementia are often unable to complete hearing or vision screening self-report tests [27–29], due to communicative difficulties or problems understanding, and are less likely to be assessed than those without dementia [30]. This can create barriers to their access to necessary hearing and vision care from a specialist. Alongside residents with cognitive impairment, even LTCH residents with a single sensory impairment are more likely to be affected by communication problems, fatigue, balance problems, and sleep problems, than residents without impairment; with those who have dual impairment being at increased risk of faster cognitive decline [9].

With current methods of screening for sensory loss in LTCH residents reported as inadequate in sensitivity and appropriateness for older adults with dementia [31], a larger mixed-methods project was initiated to find the most effective vision and hearing screening tools suitable for this population [32]. As part of this investigation, an environmental scan was conducted with professionals working in hearing and vision care [33], as well as in nursing care, to identify tools, technologies, and strategies that are currently being used with clients who have dementia. Here, we report on the findings of our interviews with nurses who work with residents who have dementia in LTCHs, including nurses responsible for the sensory screening of these residents.

Methods

This study was originally guided by the broader research question seeking to identify the most effective measures and strategies used by healthcare professionals to screen for hearing and vision loss in persons with dementia. During data collection, the use of such screening measures in LTCHs was found to be limited, thus the research question was adjusted to also explore the experiences of nurses in caring for and screening residents with dementia and sensory impairment living in LTCHs.

All participants attended semi-structured, in-person interviews, conducted on site with a clinically trained member of the research team (FH, MSc, female). Participating nurses were asked about: their experiences with persons who have dementia, as well as hearing and vision loss; how they identify which residents have impairments; ways in which assessments could be improved, and key elements to include in a sensory screening package. The questions and protocol used to guide the interview are outlined in the Interview Guide (see Additional file 1), to which a semi-structured approach was applied to allow for probing and further exploration of participants' responses.

The study was conducted with the approval of the Research Ethics Boards of each LTC institution and in adherence to The Code of Ethics of the World Medical Association (Declaration of Helsinki) for experiments involving humans [34]. All participants provided informed written consent before participating in the study, and received compensation in-kind for their time and effort upon completion of their interview. The reporting of the study followed the published guidelines for qualitative research (see Additional file 2).

Study site and participants

In-person interviews took place across two LTCHs in Southern Ontario, Canada, which ranged in scale between 100 and 450 residents in their care, respectively. The larger facility also accommodated on-site, specialist services in audiology and ophthalmology; whereas, the smaller of the two homes referred residents to off-site clinics. This was the primary difference between the LTCHs, as both were for-profit institutions, with equivalent assimilation and ratio of staffing. These staffing models involved one nursing assistant for every nine residents during the day, with supervision provided by charge nurses (RPN or RN). These two homes were selected for this research as they had dedicated units for the care of residents with dementia, whilst providing for contrasting models of care in how specialist health services were provided to the residents in their care.

The principal investigator of the study (KMG, PhD) made initial contact with the Assistant Directors of Nursing (ADON) at each LTCH to inform them about the study and its purpose. The ADONs first approached potential participants, based on the provided eligibility criteria. Eligible participants were registered nurses (RNs) and registered practical nurses (RPNs), working full- or part-time with residents who have dementia, and were responsible for administering hearing and/or vision screening tests to residents as part of their duties, in the form of the RAI-MDS or otherwise. Each LTCH had one designated member of nursing staff who held the position of RAI coordinator, and so participation was extended to registered nurses involved in other areas of care and assessment of residents with dementia. A purposive sample of 20 nurses was interviewed across the two LTCHs ($N = 10$ at each site). Sampling was based on the qualitative research standards reported for this type of exploratory research [35].

The participant characteristics are summarised in Table 1. Participants ranged in their years of experience of working in LTC (from 7 months to 30 years), working with residents who have dementia (from limited interaction to 22 years), as well as in their experience of assessing residents with dementia. The designate RAI-MDS coordinator at each site was included in the sample for analysis. The majority of participants were female, had college level education, were practising as registered practical nurses, and worked full-time.

Data collection

The semi-structured interviews were conducted in-person and on-site [36] between January and May 2016. Identified eligible participants were invited to an individual, confidential interview in a quiet and convenient location, and at a time of their choice. Participants were first individually briefed about the study, its purpose, the voluntary basis of their participation, and received answers to any questions or concerns they had. Written informed consent was obtained from all participants prior to the interview. The semi-structured protocol for the interviews allowed for questions to be asked as appropriate to the participating nurse's role and experience, as well as to elaborate on information volunteered by the participant. Participants were encouraged to take adequate time to express their opinions, to do most of the talking, and advised that there was no right or wrong answer to any question. All interviews were audio-recorded, transcribed, proofed for completeness and accuracy, and anonymised prior to data analysis. Duration of interviews included in the analysis was a mean of 28 min 9 s [SD = 2.59].

Table 1 Summary of participant characteristics ($N = 20$)

Continuous Characteristics	Mean	[SD]
Years working in dementia care	9.63	[6.60]
Years working in LTC	10.48	[7.12]
Age [$N = 18$]	41.78	[7.52]
Categorical Characteristics	N	[%]
Registered Nurse	6	30
Employed full-time	14	70
Female	18	90

Data analysis

The data-driven analysis followed a thematic content approach as outlined by Graneheim and Lundman [37], and Braun and Clarke [38]. Table 2 outlines the methods employed for data analysis. The stepwise, recursive analysis began with three analysts (FH, MRM, XAW) familiarising themselves with the full data corpus (transcripts and audio recordings). Each of the 20 data sets were independently analysed by two members of the research team in the first level of coding [37]. The team met weekly to refine themes and to discuss disconfirming evidence emerging in the analysis. In this first level, the interview data were exhaustively coded into seven mutually exclusive themes [39]: LTC demographics, characteristics of participants, the process of care or screening, enablers of care, enablers of screening, barriers to care, and barriers to screening. Memos were made with analytical insights throughout this process.

On the second level of analysis, subthemes within the data from the four main categories of interest (i.e. enablers of care, enablers of screening, barriers to care, and barriers to screening) were identified inductively. Data from the remaining three themes were used to inform the background of the study (i.e. LTCH demographics, characteristics of participants, the process of care or screening). The subthemes reflected the prominent themes that characterised the participant's recommendations and concerns within the first level. These subthemes were then categorised into three main encompassing themes, which were used to present the results below (see Fig. 1 for Schematic chart of thematic development). Following the full content analysis, saturation of thematic data and supporting content information was assessed, which resulted in an agreed sample of the most richly informative citations, selected by the qualitative analysts, to represent the reported views and experiences of the interviewed participants [40, 41]

Results

In discussing the barriers to and enablers of care and screening of long-term care residents with sensory loss

Table 2 Phases of thematic analysis (adapted from Braun and Clarke, [38])

Phases of thematic analysis	Description of the process
1. Familiarization with the data	– The full corpus of interviews was transcribed and verified for accuracy. – The analysts first listened to, read and re-read all interviews to identify emerging trends and ideas in the data.
2. Generating initial codes	– Through group discussion and independent arbitration, the analysts agreed on initial codes: Barriers to Screening, Enablers of Screening, Barriers to Care, Enablers of Care, Process, LTC Demographics, and Participant Demographics. – The entire data set was systematically coded into exclusive categories of information. – Coding of data was reviewed by analysts and group consensus was reached. – Data was collated into each code manually.
3. Searching for themes	– The coded data were reviewed for common, emergent themes. – Thematic data was collated by each analyst manually.
4. Reviewing themes	– Themes were checked against all coded extracts, as well as against the entire data set for accuracy. – Identified themes were reviewed in group discussion with all three analysts and common links between the themes drawn.
5. Defining and naming themes	– Through recursive and independent review of full data sets, analysts verified the accuracy of the themes, and the overall story reported in the data. – Group discussion and a consensus approach was used for the generation of clear definitions and names for the main, overarching themes.
6. Producing the report	– Analysts selected representative and vivid extract examples to be included in the final report. – Final analysis of selected extracts was completed by relating the results of the analysis back to the research question and literature. – This scholarly report of the analysis was produced.

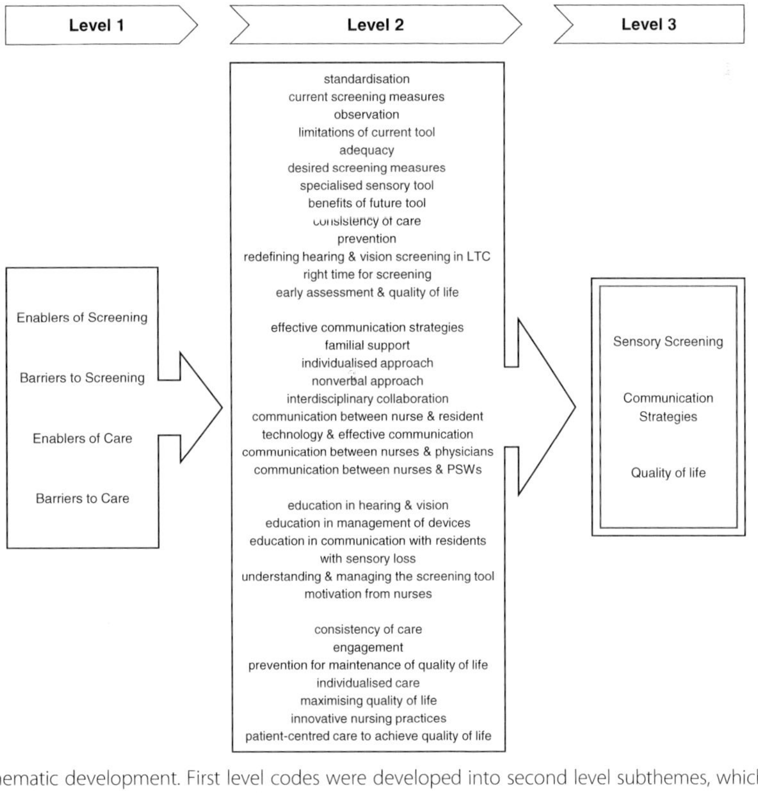

Fig. 1 Schematic chart of thematic development. First level codes were developed into second level subthemes, which were then categorised into three main encompassing themes at the final stage of thematic analysis.

and dementia, interviewed nurses provided insights into their experiences that were found to relate to three main themes. Interviewees described the current screening procedure across both sites in terms of its strengths and limitations, how screening measures should be more timely, suitable, and repeatable for residents with dementia, which informal screening strategies were being used instead, and what type of professional development was needed. Nurses also discussed how communication strategies were effectively used to circumvent gaps in the process, advocating for a person-centred approach and the effective application of interdisciplinary communication within the care team of the LTC setting. Ultimately, nurses highlighted that these implementations were essential for their quality of care and residents' quality of life, as untreated sensory loss could lead to social isolation or responsive behaviours. They recommended the maintenance of quality of life and maximisation of sensory abilities through use of appropriate intervention and assistive technologies. The nurses' comments on these topics are cited by reference to their LTC home (H#) and participant number (N#).

The sensory screening process

Across both LTCHs, a similar process of screening by use of the RAI-MDS was employed. Each facility had a designate member of nursing staff who was responsible for screening residents upon admission, at regular intervals (quarterly and annually), and tracking when residents were due to be screened again, e.g., if the resident's status changed. In the RAI-MDS, a section on "Hearing, Speech, and Vision" provides the examiner with two questions regarding the resident's hearing ability and hearing aid use, along with two questions on visual ability and corrective lenses use. To complete these questions, the examiner is instructed to ask the resident about their hearing and visual function, as well as "the resident's family, direct care staff, activities personnel," and speech or hearing specialists in the case of hearing. Examiners are also instructed to observe the resident in their verbal interactions, and to use a book or newspaper with varying sizes of print to evaluate the respective functions [42]. If concerns related to vision and/or hearing are detected during screening, the resident is referred to the respective ophthalmologic, optometric and/or or audiologic specialist for diagnostic assessment.

The barriers to and enablers of this process were outlined by nurses in terms of the baseline information that was provided, the suitability of the measure and manner of testing for residents with dementia, as well as their own developed strategies for overcoming current barriers.

Strengths and limitations of current screening measures

The current screening measure in use was identical across both LTCHs, and nurses who were familiar with the RAI-MDS and its screening protocol recognised both the advantages and limitations of the tool. Although some participants referred to the benefits of its simplicity in providing a "baseline" [H2N8] or a "snapshot of the resident"[H1N3] and their overall health status, as well as "a little bit of a framework to operate in" [H2N8], the same nurses also indicated an interest in learning about alternative measures that could be more beneficial to assessment.

H1N2: *"It's simple, and it works so far. So it's kind of something that it's handy"[...] "Maybe there's other tools that they use out there [...] so it'll be interesting to learn or... It'll be nice to know other useful tools that could be beneficial in doing some assessment."*

Where both facilities differed was the availability of on-site audiology and ophthalmology clinics at the larger LTCH (H2), to which residents could be referred upon admission or due to a suspected change in their status. Nurses here acknowledged that this was unique to their facility and described the advantages of the accessibility of this service to residents and their families.

H2N9: *"We're very fortunate here [...] that everything is just in the facility. So, they don't have to go out and families don't really feel like 'Oh, my gosh, I have to be there for this assessment' [...], then they're more inclined to say okay, go ahead, do the assessment, whatever you want."*

What was initially described as a snapshot of the resident's profile could be enhanced with added baseline information through specialist input, provided in an efficient manner, which also benefited the nurses' ability to care for their residents:

H2N9: *"And then once all the consults have been done, they're usually done really quickly anyways, especially for new admissions, so that we can get a baseline. We know where they're at, so we can care for them better."*

A need for more timely, suitable, and repeatable screening

For other nurses, the information provided by current screening measures was seen as insufficient, and suggestions for improvement were made. Participants sought additional questions for screening, supplemental responses that could be accepted for non-verbal residents, and repeatable measures, so that the influences of a resident's sensory and cognitive impairments could be distinguished.

H1N3: *"Oh, I love to change more. Put more questions in there. [...] Like asking, okay, the resident has impaired cognition, has dementia, and then you show this pen and the resident cannot recognize it. What's next? [...] Because the resident can't answer you accurately, [...] I cannot say that oh, the resident has impaired vision. It doesn't work that way. It should be like if there's impaired cognition, what are these questions to be asked in order to determine the resident has vision impairment or hearing impairment."*

Across both cohorts, differentiating between sensory and cognitive impairment in residents was reported as one of the nurses' greatest challenges, which called the suitability of current measures into question.

H2N4: "*That's actually one of the hardest assessments. [...] I mean, there's no way even for eyes and for hearing because they can't, they can't verbalize. That's a challenge*".

In addition to the need for tests to be better adapted to cognitively impaired individuals who are unable to provide a verbal response, several interviewees highlighted the importance of also considering the timing and repeatability of screening measures for these residents. These were also seen as not accommodated by the current screening schedule:

H1N9: "*You can't just assess somebody one day and say, well, look, he can't hear. You have to remember the status of the person" [...] "So with dementia maybe they will hear me today, and then tomorrow they won't. It depends on the person"; "[...] you don't wait for three months and five months [...] it takes a little bit for you to assess that person.*"

At the second LTCH, a nurse observed how repeated testing was implemented at their specialist clinics, and together with the knowledge of when the individual resident could perform at their best, a more reliable outcome could be measured.

H2N8: "*sometimes what they'll do, they'll have a recall, like another appointment another time to see if, okay, when they come and maybe they'll be in a better mood when they come back, and they cooperate. [...] But obviously you have to probably know the time of day that's best for the client, too. [...] You know, all these things you have to work in to get the most reliable tests in place, right?*"

Not only that the screening of residents should be scheduled at the optimal time of day for the individual, but nurses also highlighted the importance of early screening for timely detection of change or decline, calling for efficiencies in the screening and assessment process.

H2N8: "*You know, as I said it's just the key element is timing, really; [...] and making sure things are done in a certain amount of time in between so you catch, so things don't deteriorate quickly on you.*"

Throughout the interviews, nurses revealed conscientiousness and insight into the reality of the residents' well-being and experience of their cognitive status. Their developed familiarity with and sensitivity to the circumstances of residents in their care enabled them to understand the process from the individual's perspective and fully account for the range of adaptations to be made.

H2N8: "*I think with dementia you have to kind of go into their own little world with them. The reality of what they're feeling now is what they're feeling now, right? You can't really over-walk that reality, right? You have to go back, and they might feel one way this minute and the next minute they're totally compliant with what you're asking them to do. So when you get that compliant moment, then you go ahead with it, yeah.*"

Informal screening strategies

In the absence of suitable measures for residents with dementia, nurses described how they assumed the responsibility of further investigation, often by means of informal observation or self-developed strategies. One RAI Coordinator spoke of continuing the evaluation beyond that of the initial screening, to provide them with additional information on the resident's functioning:

H1N3: "*It's limited for only a few questions. It's in general. So based on the general question we have to create our own assessment or questions to go in details.*"

Enriched by their experience, nurses used informal observation and their developed intuition to effectively and reliably screen their residents for possible sensory loss. In the following, nurses from both homes describe strategies for the evaluation residents' hearing and vision, respectively:

H1N9: "*Because, remember, we are not here to diagnose anybody. Right? We're here to help them. [...] if I'm speaking to you right now and you can't hear me, you would show me signs that you can't hear me. You would say, "What did you say?" or you show me gesture, anything to ... for me to indicate that you can't hear me, right? [...] And then I would probably do it a couple more times, not the same day; maybe the next day or two days after, whatever. And then, after that, then we can report that you can't hear.*"

H2N2: "*It was just from experience. At least they know, they're familiar with the letters, if you put their name on it [...] they know. Like, if you [...] put the random letters they not really might engage. But [...] they know their names, they're engaged in it. They will know.*"

As well as repeating their evaluations for a more reliable result, nurses' strategies across both LTCHs involved the acceptance of meaningful responses and utilisation of meaningful stimuli, which were tailored by an individualised approach.

H2N4: "*For clients who have a certain stage of dementia; for end stage or who [don't] verbalise, I don't think that's appropriate [...].*"

H1N3: "*If it's non-verbal resident because of dementia, there should be a non-verbal assessment for observation.*"

H1N2: "*You have to kind of tweak it or change it a bit on how you approach them. [...] You don't use the same approach on every [...] resident*".

A call for standardised practice and professional development

Despite the reported insights into informal assessment strategies that had been used effectively, the knowledge and experiences of sensory screening as described by nurses were variable. Few nurses were not aware of the RAI-MDS instrument or any type of screening process being available to them. Due to a lack of awareness regarding the standard protocol, nurses would also rely on their intuition.

H2N8: *"I've never worked anywhere where they really have any set formalities for nurses to check for hearing and vision, you know".*

H2N4: *"...from my experience I've never conducted an official tool. Like it's just basing on your nursing assessment, let's say, the changes in behaviour, changes in the routine, but we don't have the tool, let's say, for the pain scale. We have a tool for skin assessment; we have a tool to use, but we don't have for the hearing and for the visual."*

However, with nurses' experience and their developed insights varying across interviewees, they did share the concern that not all staff could adopt an observational approach and that, owing to a lack of consistency in knowledge and experience, there was indeed a need for standardisation of these screening approaches.

H2N8: *"...because some people are [...] not observant, and people don't carry out stuff, but when there's a formal tool, then they have to be accountable for that formal tool, right?"*

Throughout the interviews, nurses expressed their desire to learn more about tools and strategies that can be used to better screen residents in their care. Nurses' education was also described across both LTCHs as an area with potential for development and improvement, in order for the screening competencies of LTC staff, as well as the screening process as a whole, to be ameliorated. Nurses suggested approaches and areas of focus for this improvement.

H2N5: *"I think education sessions or, you know, trainings for nurses, get updates. Like I think those will be like really helpful."*

H2N2: *"It can be improved, like, staff education ... should be like tell staff how to, like, take care of the hearing aid better like handling wise, sometimes you have to teach them. [...] some of them they bring new hearing aids from where we don't know it's - it's high tech. So - but they always have better education is always good; like the staff needs to be just you know, reminded."*

Education was reportedly provided by behavioural consultants to assist nurses in their understanding and management of responsive behaviours, which were recognised by one nurse participant as being impacted by underlying sensory impairments.

H2N4: *"Yeah, we do that and we're still doing it; [...] on how to speak with a client who has hearing impairment or vision impairment. [...] one of them also is the behavioural consult to see if they can give the nurses or the PSW, you know, tools or pointers on how to react, how to respond, what to see, what to expect."*

However, the knowledge and skill development required to carry out sensory screening was not reported to be currently offered or instructed through educational provision at either facility.

Communication strategies

Throughout the interviews at each LTC home, communication was often cited as a key facilitator or barrier to the care and assessment of residents with dementia. A person-centred approach was seen as an enabler of informal assessment and of better care provision, along with effective interdisciplinary communication also contributing to both. When interdisciplinary communication broke down, however, this would present itself as a formidable barrier to the screening process.

Person-centred communication

As evidenced in the informal strategies adopted by nurses in a screening context, interviewed participants also advocated for person-centredness in their everyday communications with residents:

H1N9: *"it's communication. That's the key thing. You have to talk to the resident, depending on their status, so he will understand what you're saying. [...] It depends on the individual how much they could understand, and if you were interviewing them at the - for the first time you have different strategies or different things that you would do to make sure that that person understand what you're saying. They have different barrier, like, language barrier. It depends on the individual [...]".*

When language or comprehension barriers existed, nurses described how going beyond verbal communication and using gesture was helpful in overcoming these and effectively connecting with their residents:

H2N9: *"communication is really hard, so you kind of use not just speech, but gestures and other tools that can help you communicate or get your, whatever you want to get across to them. More often than not, you really have to keep repeating yourself [...] I'll point to the ear, that this is for the ear, to help you. And then once it's on, then you can see that there's a change in their face and they start smiling and I guess, because they're already hearing what you're saying."*

H2N8: *"If their vision and hearing is poor, maybe you can demonstrate what you need to do, right? And if they can't see, it could be just taking their hands and putting the toothbrush in their hands and showing them that it's a toothbrush, if they can understand."*

Facilitative communication strategies consisted of simple language and environmental cues that helped engage residents who have dementia. At both sites, nurses shared their insights into using simple and effective communication strategies that were tailored to the individual.

H1N2: *"If they're legally blind, obviously they can't see you so you have to always have to introduce yourself to them and stuff. Even if they're not blind [...] you still have to introduce yourself."*

H1N8: *"First of all, it is very effective to introduce yourself every now and then, because they have dementia so they forget who you are [...] and then we using a simple words like can be answerable with yes or no".*

H2N9: *"...like simple, direct words, will help. And if you say it in, I guess, a more clear, concise manner and if you notice that they're sort of getting what you're saying then the hearing is okay, but it could be that, you know, cognitive impairment is at play",*

By these means, rapport with residents could be developed, as well as a better understanding of their cognitive abilities, and then a more valid assessment context could be enabled.

H1N2: *"I would say when someone has dementia and also have behaviour, you kind of have to talk to them first [...] you have to gain their trust first. And then you do – like once they're interactive and they're talking to you and stuff [...] That's kind of a way of, I would say, doing the assessment as well".*

H2N8: *"So it could be that, you know, they love a muffin. You know, you get a muffin and get a little coffee [...] So you have to figure out how you're going to approach somebody with this kind of stuff so you get the best possible result from them. So you can't just go, 'Okay, tell me what this means', you know?"*

Nurses' communication strategies considered the person's privacy, preferences, as well as impairments, and were individualised not only to the resident, but appropriate in their timing.

H1N8: *"Maybe you approach the resident in the wrong situation. Like maybe since lots of them they were incontinent, maybe something is bothering them like pain or sun-downing or they wanted to go to the washroom; so be sure before approaching the residents, you approach them on the right time."*

The benefits of interdisciplinary communication

Beyond communicative interactions with the LTC residents, nurses placed an emphasis on the enablement provided by consistency of care and how this, in turn, facilitated effective interdisciplinary communication. The exchange of effective strategies and important considerations that are unique to the resident could help nurses learn how to overcome the barriers to communicating with and screening residents with more severe dementia.

H2N4: *"It's, dementia - it's very hard, especially if they're not able to verbalise, if they don't really know what's happening to them. You really have to really get to know the clients. So therefore consistency is important for us [...] because I don't deal with the client, I only see them when I've been told by my PSW [...] So if there's a big change of staff, then there's no way they would be able to see that there's a change in that particular client. [...] So I think caring for a client with dementia, consistency is one of the key rule that we are, for us to see and do a proper assessment."*

The dependence upon the Personal Support Workers (PSWs), and their everyday familiarity with residents, was described as essential to the care and screening of residents by many nurses across both facilities. PSWs were highly regarded by nurses for having increased exposure to and heightened awareness of the residents who may experience a change of functional status.

H1N2: *"I don't do hands on with each residents and stuff, so I rely to my staff like the PSW who is there every day taking care of them, doing care with them. So it's just pretty much, I would say, communication has always had to be the key."*

This communication was viewed as a reciprocal and collaborative effort to enable more reliable screening of residents. These efforts also extended to the larger care team to enable the identification of problems, as well as the most appropriate solutions.

H1N9: *"...I find that you need to work with your partner on the day shift or even the night shift. That's how we work on this floor. If I'm not certain... because, as I said, we're not here to diagnose. So I will communicate with my partner and say, "Well, this is what I feel." And then, if she feels the same way, then we communicate together. Because, I said, I could be wrong, she could be wrong, so two heads is better than one."*

H2N8: *"So we have that forum. So that's why we have that status report that we meet with each other, we discuss issues and then we come up with solutions together. And then based on the solutions that we can use other team members, like other doctors, the social worker, other people get involved and help with solutions for the clients, you know?"*

This circle of care and collaboration was described as extending to the resident's family, social workers, as well as additional medical and healthcare staff working with the resident, and provided for a multi-faceted team approach.

H2N8: *"all the facets are there, and then everybody has input and they bring up all these problems. It could be just – you know, the family will say, 'I notice my mom is not seeing too well.' It's a good thing we have that family meeting because maybe we didn't notice that. So then it comes to our attention and then based on the rounds, we come together as a team again and say well, maybe we should not only the ophthalmology, maybe we should get something else done or a screening test or – you know? So that's how the support is there. You're just not left alone to solve the problem."*

Challenges to effective communication

A consistent and collaborative approach to care provision was seen as bridging the gap created by inexperience and unfamiliarity with the residents, as well as a valuable way of sharing information and strategies between staff on different schedules and different levels. However, communication was not always reported as effective and helpful. One participant described the sharing of information from ophthalmologists or audiologists to nurses at their facility as "not really communicated very well" [H2N5]. Assessment results and pertinent diagnoses were not always relayed to staff who worked closely with residents, and this information was sometimes difficult to retrieve.

H2N5: *"[...] once a referral is done or findings have been done I think it is also good for the nurses or the PSWs to know what's really going on. [...] Because sometimes that's also missed, [...] it goes like to the physician level already. [...] Unless you go, you know, go deep to the transcription reports and to problem lists and all that and the notes. [...] but then, you know, sometimes it's written like not in a laymen's term."*

Even with procedures in place, there was still variability in how these were adhered to by members of the resident's circle of care, and what was previously cited as enabling better screening became a barrier to the process instead:

H2N4: *"It can be improved. The reason why because sometimes there's a little bit of a disconnect in the clinic. Because there are still some doctors [...] I don't think they are required to input their data in our electronic system. So they use the handwriting. [...] sometimes it's missed, what's in there or they just write it in but they never tell us that there's another follow-up, unless you really look and read it. So it's still... it's a work in progress."*

Changes in status, in care and in diagnoses were seen as important points for communication amongst frontline healthcare providers, a process in which nurses assume a leading role. Nurse participants provided examples of how breakdowns in communication can be circumvented or improved upon to provide for better consistency and continuity of care, following the outcomes of assessment or its attempt.

H2N9: *"So our role as nurses is to communicate whatever we find, so that we can better care for residents, communicate it to the PSWs. So that is not only communicated verbally but it's also done through care planning and whatnot, and we let them know that, you know, this is what the suggestion was, let's try it, if it doesn't work, at least we tried, do another strategy; [...] The PSWs are very good. And they know their residents very well. Most of the times they would even suggest "Oh, let's try this instead of that" to nurses or to doctors. And we steer the frontline, so we have to listen to them too."*

Quality of life, sensory loss, and dementia

The most oft-cited concern of nurses in relation to residents in their care who had vision or hearing loss, as well as cognitive impairment, was the impact of these challenges on their quality of life. Nurses identified the risks of social isolation and further decline in affected residents. They recognised the frustration caused by sensory impairment, and how this could lead to the incidence of responsive behaviours. They also confirmed the need for sensory screening, so that impairments can be detected early, and residents' quality of life can thereby be maintained, as well as maximised, with appropriate interventions. The most effective, and often informal, means of doing so was through the provision of assistive devices.

Sensory loss and social isolation

Across the facilities, nurses recognised the impact of sensory loss on participation and engagement in LTCH communities, as well as its impact on the socialisation abilities and self-esteem of directly affected residents.

H1N8: *"You know, when you cannot hear anything you thought like everybody's talking about you and you're being isolated. [...] one resident is deaf. Like she thought she's being isolated or not being loved or appreciated. [...] It will promote their self-esteem and feeling of being more confident."*

H2N8: *"They tend to be a little bit more withdrawn. They're not hearing anything, they're probably not seeing anything. They may have the activity – they can't participate, they're just sitting there. To me it isolates them and it takes away from their quality of life, right, and engagement."*

Sensory screening was seen as a means to providing residents with the support and devices they needed. One participant described the role of nurses in supporting and encouraging residents at the time of assessment as being facilitative to the process.

H1N8: *"First you have to comfort them, like "It's okay; like if you are scared of going by yourself, I can accompany you." Like spending quality time with them to give them emotional support and assurance".*

Drawing the link between sensory loss and responsive behaviour

A link between sensory loss and responsive behaviour had previously been made by a participant on the subject of education; however, sensory screening for the purposes of early identification and appropriate intervention for such impairment was also noted as an important preventative factor of further decline and incidence of responsive behaviours:

H2N8: *"Maybe the person, they're not hearing and they're starting to get agitated, irritated. All these different, maybe responsive behaviours that come out of not seeing, not hearing, and then they don't cooperate because it complicates the cognitive impairments more. And all that distress that they would've gone through would've been alleviated or stopped or – you know, prevented then, right?"*

To support and enable detection of impairments that may influence such behaviours, the right sensory screening measures were seen as essential. Nurses showed an appreciation for the impact of sensory loss on their residents and their concern for the frustration this can cause.

H2N4: *"So, I mean, in order for you to really get to know what's causing the responsive behaviour, you need to have tools to do a proper assessment, right. Whether that could be a... let's say hearing impairment; "I'm frustrated", if you don't hear you, get frustrated; and if you can't see, you get frustrated. And like, is that one of the cause of their being aggressive or being frustrated would that be one? But it's something that's not actually... not seen though it's part of the care but it's not, you know, it's not seen."*

Maintaining and maximising quality of life

The nurses advocated for the maintenance of residents' independence and quality of life, and saw the need to achieve this in the care setting, as well as at later stages of life. The nurses advocated for their residents' right to access the activities that are enjoyable and stimulating to them.

H1N5: *"So they still have the rights to live, you know, as normal people. [...] So those residents that likes to read, we're still giving books to read, because ... in order that they enhance [...] their brains more and then they can still function".*

Participants described how both sensory impairment and dementia could negatively impact a resident's quality of life, and identified the provision of routine, enabling participation and socialisation, and thereby maintaining independence and enjoyment, as significant mitigators:

H2N2: *"...if you take them out of their routine they get upset. You know. So or if their routine is [...] since before they're reading their newspaper, even though they don't understand it, they know that they've been reading it, so if they - you don't give it to them they get upset. So, then your day is - their day's good, their day's not good and your day's not good."*

H1N3: *"We do the assessments – we have to, the 24 hour care planning from main habits, what they do before coming in, what they do, what their job before. Because it will help us to give or like to maintain what the really social aspect of their life, right? When they were in the community. So at least we can provide those. Like, if the resident is fond of music, so we're going to provide music. If the resident is dancing so we're going to put into music program."*

By detecting sensory loss through the initial screening, helpful diagnoses could be provided to the resident and family, as well as assistive intervention that enable residents to enjoy their daily activities at the LTCH.

H2N8: *"sometimes they find out that maybe they have glaucoma at that time, or maybe they really should have had glasses. Or maybe that's why they were falling, because they probably weren't seeing where they were going when they were at home, when the family wasn't really noticing that that's the reason why they were falling, you know? So that screening tool is very important. Then nursing on a whole, eventually after getting to know the clients we'll be able to notice changes and be able to generate maybe other further assessments, you know, in between in case there are deteriorations."*

Across both care homes, an appreciation of the significant contributions yielded by socialisation and sensory stimulation to residents was evident. Music programmes were reported as being especially impactful in providing positive engagement for residents with Alzheimer's disease. This nurse described her observation and perceived importance of residents having access to music and sensory experiences.

H2N8: *"So once they can – especially people with Alzheimer's, that music is so important. Music, and seeing colours and, you know, stuff like that. And so, if they can enjoy like even hearing music, it's so important and they can sing and clap. You can see a joy come over them. They enjoy it, you know? So, and then even they even love to do the little exercise thing, and if they can see what she's showing them, you know, it's really important, at least you maximize [...], or amplify whatever [...] And it really helps. I've seen people improve on their socialization skills like that."*

Assistive technologies as an important tool to enhance quality of life

Ultimately, assistive technology was deemed to be the greatest facilitator to residents with dementia and sensory loss engaging in activities and maintaining their quality of life at the LTCH. The successful outcome to sensory assessment was seen as the appropriate prescription of the most suitable assistive devices for the individual resident.

H1N3: *"So it's either we get an upgrade eye glasses for the vision or we going to get a new or upgrade the hearing aid. So based on the referral. And then they will come back with the... whatever the recommendation is. [...] Yeah, it's effective because the resident can see more than the previous, or can hear more, or... Like we have one who has a hearing aid but then the hearing aid sometimes doesn't work, so we change to pocket talker. So once the resident has a pocket talker she can respond more to the staff, can express more herself."*

H2N8: *"I think it's good. I've seen patients use it and it really helps. It really helps, it really helps, you know, with communication. They don't seem so isolated and they obviously cannot hear from a low tone, a pocket talker then, and they'll be involved in conversation and stuff like that."*

In the absence of specialised technologies, alternative sensory aids were reportedly used across the facilities. For the hearing impaired, the pocket talker was widely seen as highly assistive; and for vision, a magnifying glass was commonly used instead of prescription lenses:

H2N8: *"Sometimes they use [...] this big [magnifying glass]; and then for reading sometimes I see they have these big screens that they put a book under and they kind of amplify the words really bigger. I've seen residents enjoy that, but who likes – especially who likes to read before and then they can't read anymore, that's a good device to, um... especially for people with Alzheimer's or cognitive impairment."*

Such assistive devices were also found to be useful for testing purposes, and discriminating between sensory loss and other types of impairment.

H2N8: *"They may not sit long enough to do it but the amplifying glass, sometimes it'll work, too. Or if you write words on a big paper, you know, to show them toothbrush so it's big enough that you can see in case their vision is really off a bit."*

Discussion

The findings from this exploratory study demonstrate a recognition amongst nurses of the disconnect between current screening practices, with its limitations, and the complex reality for residents living with multiple impairments in LTCHs. In the absence of suitable screening tools or adaptable protocols, nurses provided insightful and instructive examples of how to overcome communication barriers or systemic constraints through person-centred and informal strategies in their care and assessment. Consistency of care and effective interdisciplinarity were found to be crucial to the success of these adapted procedures, but could not be relied upon under current circumstances, which brought participants back to the need for standardisation of and accountability for assessment practices.

The nurses in our study acknowledged, however, their wanting expertise in screening for hearing and vision loss; an area in which they have expressed a need and desire to be enabled by the provision of more effective screening tools that are suitable for individuals with dementia, and to be empowered to use these by means of more specialised professional development.

These results consolidate the findings from previous research, in which nurses have reported feeling inadequately trained to care for residents with sensory impairment [43], and frontline healthcare providers reported difficulties in distinguishing the relative contributions of sensory loss and dementia to breakdowns in communication [44, 45]. Despite the evidenced sensitivity and appropriateness of some sensory screening measures in older and non-communicative populations [27, 46–49], as well as the feasibility of in-service training for healthcare providers who are willing to engage in these [16], and its benefit to residents with cognitive and physical fragility [50], relevant evidence-based practice guidelines have not yet been adopted in these LTCH settings [51].

Even though the field of nursing has previously engaged in efforts to increase the awareness of sensory impairment in older adults in general, and has developed continuing education materials for this purpose [52, 53], nursing is not the only allied health profession that has encountered similar challenges where sensory abilities become relevant in health service delivery. Previous work in Canada, the US and the UK has highlighted the need for training on sensory screening and its rehabilitation by occupational therapists, and pointed out the absences of suitable training content on sensory abilities in educational curricula [54–57]. None of these efforts have yet advanced to a level where sensory and cognitive impairments are considered simultaneously during screening.

In this study, interviewed nurses notably acknowledged the relationship between hearing and vision, and quality of life (QoL), and how impairment in either can negatively influence the individual's functioning as a whole, as well as their access to social engagement and participation. Research has shown that even without cognitive impairment, the ability to perform activities of daily living (ADLs), along with the QoL of LTCH residents, is significantly related to the presence of eye disorders or visual impairment [47, 58–61]. Likewise, access to social opportunities and QoL, is negatively impacted by hearing impairments [62, 63]. As suggested by nurses in the current study, the active management of dementia and coexisting conditions through coordination of care, as well as participation in activities and care programs [3], can improve QoL at all stages of severity for individuals directly affected, as well as for their care providers [64–66]. While ophthalmologist end otolaryngologists are often implicated in the medical sensory care of residents with dementia, their primary focus is on anatomy and physiology. Therefore, services provided by audiologists and optometrists that focus on functional ability are likely to be of great importance when considering the impact of sensory loss in this population, as well as being beneficial to the provision of specialised education to healthcare staff in this setting.

By use of a semi-structured interview approach in this study, respondents were provided with opportunity and encouragement to elaborate on responses, as well as to volunteer relevant information not directly related to questions [38]. Employing a qualitative content analysis of these interviews enabled a broad and reflexive search across the full data corpus for identification of the most prominent themes and meanings, which, in turn, informed and allowed for revision of the research question in line with the exploratory findings [67]. This study was limited to two LTC sites in Southern Ontario, Canada; however, these varied in their size and provision of services to residents. The investigation thereby captured ranging levels of exposure to assessment procedures, as well as varying levels of training and experience in caring for residents with dementia amongst participants. Despite differences in the provision of specialist healthcare services provided to residents by audiologists and ophthalmologists in the two LTCHs, regulated nurses reported common experiences and views regarding current standard procedures, as well as a shared need for additional education and the provision of more suitable sensory screening tools for residents.

In the current study, nurses highlighted communication as an important consideration in both the care and assessment of residents, providing insightful and creative examples of how they are personalising their approaches to communication, because many residents with sensory and cognitive impairment struggle most in this area. In addition, nurses recognised that hearing aids and glasses are not the sole solution to these problems. Through experience and team collaboration, successful communication strategies are shared and developed upon, and a patient-centred approach to care is at the core of their practice. Although communication strategies and strengths were identified as facilitative in overcoming the limitations of current screening procedures and interventions, this study did not explore the current procedures for assessing communication abilities. Future research is warranted in investigating the relative influence of communication, cognitive, and sensory abilities on interactions within the LTCH setting and on residents' QoL, and which tools can enable nurses to more effectively identify relative impairments in LTC residents, which require appropriate intervention [68, 69].

Conclusions

LTCH nurses demonstrated insight into the facilitators and barriers to effective screening and care of residents with dementia and possible vision and/or hearing impairments. Nurses recognised the limitations of current screening procedures, and emphasised the need for more suitable sensory assessment measures for residents with dementia, as well as their own expressed need for further education in carrying these out. Growing research supports the need for more appropriate screening measures and protocols to detect sensory decline in this vulnerable population, yet to be implemented in LTCHs. The current study, along with reports from previous research and governing bodies highlight the practicability and value of additional specialised training for registered nurses to empower these healthcare professionals to better screen, as well as feasibly diagnose and treat residents with complex needs under their care. The advancement of nurses' roles and their potential to lead practice developments and service reform through staff education in managing sensory-related impairments and environmental modifications for residents has long been proposed [70–72]. To bridge the gap between such guidelines and current policies further curriculum development, continued professional education, as well as reinforcing on-site policies for training, knowledge translation and interdisciplinarity, is important for the enablement of nurses in the care and assessment of individuals with dementia and complex sensory needs, as underscored and called for by the nurses in this study.

Abbreviations

ADON: Assistant Directors of Nursing; LTC: Long-term care; LTCH: Long-term care home; MDS: Minimum Data Set; PSW: Personal Support Worker; QoL: Quality of Life; RAI: Resident Assessment Instrument; REB: Research Ethics Board; RN: Registered Nurse; RPN: Registered Practical Nurse

Acknowledgements

We would like to thank the long-term care nurses who volunteered to participate in this study, as well as the social workers and assistant directors of nursing at the long-term care homes who facilitated this research. We would also like to acknowledge the support of the Alzheimer Society of Canada, who have funded this study through the Alzheimer Society Research Programme (ASRP; RG 16-08).

Funding

This study has been supported by the Alzheimer Society Research Programme (ASRP), Alzheimer Society of Canada; grant number RG 16–08. Dr. McGilton is supported by the Walter and Maria Schroeder Institute for Brain Innovation & Recovery.

Authors' contributions

KMG and WW designed and planned the overall project, including this qualitative study. KMG, WW and FH designed the data collection tools (i.e. interview scripts). KMG monitored the data collection, the data analysis plan, and revised the paper. KMG is guarantor. FH collected the data, monitored the transcription of interviews, cleaned the data, analysed the data, and drafted and revised the paper. XAW cleaned the data, analysed the data, and revised the paper. MRM analysed the data and revised the paper. AEP planned and monitored the data analysis, and drafted and revised the paper. WW assisted in the data analysis, and drafted and revised the paper. All authors read and approved the final manuscript.

Competing interests

All authors have completed the International Committee of Medical Journal Editors' (ICMJE) uniform disclosure form at www.icmje.org/coi_disclosure.pdf and declare that they have no competing interests, financial or non-financial.

Author details

[1]Toronto Rehabilitation Institute-University Health Network, 130 Dunn Ave, Toronto M6K 2R7, Canada. [2]Rehabilitation Sciences Institute, University of Toronto, Toronto, ON, Canada. [3]Lawrence S. Bloomberg Faculty of Nursing, University of Toronto, 130 Dunn Ave, Toronto M6K 2R7, Canada. [4]FCS Blanquerna-Universitat Ramon Llull, Carrer de Padilla, 326-332, 08025 Barcelona, Spain. [5]Dalla Lana School of Public Health, University of Toronto, Toronto, ON, Canada. [6]School of Optometry, Université de Montréal, 3744, rue Jean-Brillant, 260-7, Montréal, Québec H3T 1P1, Canada. [7]CRIR/Centre de réadaptation MAB-Mackay du CIUSSS du Centre-Ouest-de-l'Île-de-Montréal, Montréal, Québec, Canada. [8]CRIR/Institut Nazareth et Louis-Braille du CISSS de la Montérégie-Centre, Longueuil, Québec, Canada.

References

1. Carpenter I, Hirdes JP. Using interRAI assessment systems to measure and maintain quality of long-term care. A Good Life in Old Age. 2013:93–139.
2. Seitz D, Purandare N, Conn D. Prevalence of psychiatric disorders among older adults in long-term care homes: a systematic review. Int Psychogeriatr. 2010;22(7):1025–39.
3. Gaugler J, James B, Johnson T, Scholz K, Weuve J. Alzheimer's disease facts and figures. Alzheimer's and Dementia. 2016;12(4):459–509.
4. O'Malley PG. Evolving insights about the impact of sensory deficits in the elderly. JAMA Intern Med. 2013;173(4):299.
5. Weinstein BE. Geriatric audiology. New York: Thieme; 2000.
6. Garahan MB, Waller JA, Houghton M, Tisdale WA, Runge CF. Hearing loss prevalence and management in nursing home residents. J Am Geriatr Soc. 1992;40(2):130–4.
7. Bingea RL, Raffin MJ, Aune KJ, Baye L, Shea SL. Incidence of hearing loss among geriatric nursing-home residents. The Journal of auditory research. 1982;22(4):275–83.
8. Schow RL, Nerbonne MA. Hearing levels among elderly nursing home residents. Journal of Speech and Hearing Disorders. 1980;45(1):124–32.
9. Yamada Y, Vlachova M, Richter T, Finne-Soveri H, Gindin J, van der Roest H, Denkinger MD, et al. Prevalence and correlates of hearing and visual impairments in European nursing homes: results from the SHELTER study. J Am Med Dir Assoc. 2014;15(10):738–43.
10. Owsley C, McGwin G, Scilley K, Meek GC, Dyer A, Seker D. The visual status of older persons residing in nursing homes. Arch Ophthalmol. 2007;125(7): 925–30.
11. Tielsch JM, Javitt JC, Coleman A, Katz J, Sommer A. The prevalence of blindness and visual impairment among nursing home residents in Baltimore. N Engl J Med. 1995;332(18):1205–9.
12. Woodruff ME, Pack G. A survey of the prevalence of vision defects and ocular anomalies in 43 Ontario residential and nursing homes. Canadian J Public Health. 1980;71(6):413–23.
13. Sinoo MM, Kort HS, Duijnstee MS. Visual functioning in nursing home residents: information in client records. J Clin Nurs. 2012;21(13–14):1913–21.
14. Cohen-Mansfield J, Taylor JW. Hearing aid use in nursing homes, part 1: prevalence rates of hearing impairment and hearing aid use. J Am Med Dir Assoc. 2004;5(5):283–8.
15. Corwin BC. Vision screening in nursing and retirement homes. Optometry & Vision Science. 1972;49(12):1008–11.
16. Labreche T, Stolee P, McLeod J. An optometrist-led eye care program for older residents of retirement homes and long-term care facilities. Canadian Geriatrics J. 2011;14(1):8–11.
17. InterRAI. Instruments: Long-Term Care Facilities. 2016. http://www.interrai.org/long-term-care-facilities.html. Accessed 7 Jul 2017.
18. American Speech-Language-Hearing Association, ASHA. Guidelines for audiology service delivery in nursing homes [Guidelines]. 1997. https://www.asha.org/policy/GL1997-00004.htm. https://doi.org/10.1044/policy.GL1997-00004. Accessed 7 July 2017.
19. American Speech-Language-Hearing Association, ASHA. Hearing screening. 2016. http://www.asha.org/public/hearing/Hearing-Screening. Accessed 7 Jul 2017.
20. Ammentorp W, Gossett KD. Quality assurance for long-term care providers. Newbury Park, CA: SAGE Publications, Incorporated; 1990.
21. Ontario Ministry of Health and Long-Term Care. RAI-MDS 2.0 LTC Homes – Practice Requirements. 2016. http://www.health.gov.on.ca/en/public/programs/ltc/docs/rai_mds_practice_requirements.pdf. Accessed 7 Jul 2017.
22. Haanes GG, Kirkevold M, Hofoss D, Eilertsen G. Discrepancy between self-assessments and standardised tests of vision and hearing abilities in older people living at home: an ROC curve analysis. J Clin Nurs. 2015;24(23–24):3380–8.
23. Cohen-Mansfield J, Infeld DL. Hearing aids for nursing home residents: current policy and future needs. Health policy. 2006;79(1):49–56.
24. Mahoney DF. Hearing loss among nursing home residents: perceptions and realities. Clin Nurs Res. 1992;1(4):317–32.
25. Swanson MW, McGwin G Jr, Elliott AF, Owsley C. The nursing home minimum data set for vision and its association with visual acuity and contrast sensitivity. J Am Geriatr Soc. 2009;57(3):486–91.
26. Swanson MW. Care plan assessment of visual status and evaluated vision among nursing home residents. Optom Vis Sci. 1995;72(3):151–4.
27. Burkhalter CL, Allen RS, Skaar DC, Crittenden J, Burgio LD. Examining the effectiveness of traditional audiological assessments for nursing home residents with dementia-related behaviors. J Am Acad Audiol. 2009;20(9):529–38.
28. Bédard E, Kergoat H, Kergoat MJ, Leclerc BS. Systematic review of vision-related quality of life questionnaires for older institutionalised seniors with dementia. Ophthalmic Physiol Opt. 2015;35(4):377–87.
29. Friedman DS, Munoz B, Massof RW, Bandeen-Roche K, West SK. Grating visual acuity using the preferential-looking method in elderly nursing home residents. Invest Ophthalmol Vis Sci. 2002;43(8):2572–8.
30. Keller BK, Hejkal T, Potter JF. Barriers to vision care for nursing home residents. J Am Med Dir Assoc. 2001;2(1):15–21.
31. Burnip LG, Erber NP. Staff knowledge regarding hearing loss and communication among nursing home residents. Australian J Ageing. 1997;16(1):40–3.
32. McGilton KS, Höbler F, Campos J, Dupuis K, Labreche T, Guthrie DM, et al. Hearing and vision screening tools for long-term care residents with dementia: protocol for a scoping review. BMJ Open. 2016;6(7):e011945.
33. Wittich W, Höbler F, Jarry J, McGilton KS. Recommendations for successful sensory screening in older adults with dementia in long-term care: a qualitative environmental scan of Canadian specialists. BMJ Open. 2018;8(1):e019451.
34. Williams JR. The declaration of Helsinki and public health. Bull World Health Organ. 2008;86(8):650–2.
35. Sibbald SL, McPherson C, Kothari A. Ontario primary care reform and quality improvement activities: an environmental scan. BMC Health Serv Res. 2013; 13(1):209.
36. Whiting LS. Semi-structured interviews: guidance for novice researchers. Nurs Stand. 2008;22(23):35–40.
37. Graneheim UH, Lundman B. Qualitative content analysis in nursing research: concepts, procedures and measures to achieve trustworthiness. Nurse Educ Today. 2004;24(2):105–12.
38. Braun V, Clarke V. Using thematic analysis in psychology. Qual Res Psychol. 2006;3(2):77–101.
39. Krippendorff K. Content analysis: an introduction to its methodology. London, UK: Sage Publications Ltd; 1980.
40. Silverman D. Interpreting qualitative data. 5th ed. California, US: SAGE Publications Ltd.; 2015.
41. O'Reilly M, Parker N. 'Unsatisfactory saturation': a critical exploration of the notion of saturated sample sizes in qualitative research. Qual Res. 2013;13(2):190–7.
42. Morris JN, Hawes C, Mor V, Phillipo C, Frieo BE, Nonemaker S, Murphy K. Resident assessment instrument (RAI) RAI-MDS 2.0 user's manual. Canadian version. Canadian Institute for Health Information: Ottawa, ON; 2010.
43. Heron R, Wharrad HJ. Prevalence and nursing staff awareness of hearing impairment in older hospital patients. J Clin Nurs. 2000;9(6):834–41.
44. Dupuis K, Pichora-Fuller MK, Chasteen AL, Marchuk V, Singh G, Smith SL. Effects of hearing and vision impairments on the Montreal cognitive assessment. Aging Neuropsychol Cognit. 2015;22(4):413–37.
45. Slaughter SE, Hopper T, Ickert C, Erin DF. Identification of hearing loss among residents with dementia: perceptions of health care aides. Geriatr Nurs. 2014;35(6):434–40.
46. Jupiter T. Cognition and screening for hearing loss in nursing home residents. J Am Med Dir Assoc. 2012;3(8):744–7.
47. Nilforoush MH, Nasr Esfahani AA, Ishaghi R, Sepehrnejad M. Comparison of nursing home hearing handicap index with audiological findings: a presbycusis study. J aging Research. 2012;2012.
48. Marx MS, Werner P, Cohen-Mansfield J, Feldman R. The relationship between low vision and performance of activities of daily living in nursing home residents. J Am Geriatr Soc. 1992;40(10):1018–20.
49. Voeks SK, Gallagher CM, Langer EH, Drinka PJ. Self-reported hearing difficulty and audiometric thresholds in nursing home residents. J Fam Pract. 1993;36(1):54–8.
50. Deremeik J, Broman AT, Friedman D, West SK, Massof R, Park W, et al. Low vision rehabilitation in a nursing home population: the SEEING study. J visual impairment & blindness. 2007;101(11):701.
51. Adams-Wendling L, Pimple C, Adams S, Titler MG. Nursing management of hearing impairment in nursing facility residents. J Gerontol Nurs. 2008;34(11):9–17.
52. Wallhagen MI, Pettengill E, Whiteside M. SENSORY IMPAIRMENT IN OLDER ADULTS: PART 1: HEARING LOSS: Hearing impairment is a significant, often debilitating, problem for many older adults, but assessment and intervention by nurses can help. AJN The American Journal of Nursing. 2006;106(10):40–8.

53. Whiteside MM, Wallhagen MI, Pettengill E. Sensory impairment in older adults: part 2: vision loss. AJN The American Journal of Nursing. 2006 Nov 1; 106(11):52–61.
54. Wittich W, Barstow EA, Jarry J, Thomas A. Screening for sensory impairment in older adults: Training and practice of occupational therapists in Quebec: Formation et pratique des ergothérapeutes du Québec dans le dépistage des troubles sensoriels chez les personnes âgées. Can J Occup Ther. 2015; 82(5):283–93.
55. Wittich W, Jarry J, Barstow E, Thomas A. Vision and hearing impairment and occupational therapy education: needs and current practice. Br J Occup Ther. 2017 Jun;80(6):384–91.
56. Deacy RM, Yuen HK, Barstow EA, Warren M, Vogtle LK. Survey of the low vision rehabilitation curricula in occupational therapy and occupational therapy assistant programs. Am J Occup Ther. 2012 Nov 1;66(6):e114–8.
57. Campion C, Awang D, Ward G. Broadening the vision: the education and training needs of occupational therapists working with people with sight loss. Br J Occup Ther. 2010;73(9):413–21.
58. Dev MK, Paudel N, Joshi ND, Shah DN, Subba S. Impact of visual impairment on vision-specific quality of life among older adults living in nursing home. Curr Eye Res. 2014;39(3):232–8.
59. Elliott AF, Dreer LE, McGwin Jr G, Scilley K, Owsley C. The personal burden of decreased vision-targeted health-related quality of life in nursing home residents. J Aging Health 2010;22(4),504–521.
60. Scilley K, Owsley C. Vision-specific health-related quality of life: content areas for nursing home residents. Qual Life Res. 2002;11(5):449–62.
61. Horowitz A. Vision impairment and functional disability among nursing home residents. The Gerontologist. 1994;34(3):316–23.
62. Pryce H, Gooberman-Hill R. 'There's a hell of a noise': living with a hearing loss in residential care. Age Ageing. 2012;41(1):40–6.
63. Tsuruoka H, Masuda S, Ukai K, Sakakura Y, Harada T, Majima Y. Hearing impairment and quality of life for the elderly in nursing homes. Auris Nasus Larynx. 2001;28(1):45–54.
64. Vickrey BG, Mittman BS, Connor KI, Pearson ML, Della Penna RD, Ganiats TG, et al. The effect of a disease management intervention on quality and outcomes of dementia care: a randomized, controlled trial. Ann Intern Med. 2006;145:713–26.
65. Voisin T, Vellas B. Diagnosis and treatment of patients with severe Alzheimer's disease. Drugs Aging. 2009;26:135–44.
66. Grossberg GT, Christensen DD, Griffith PA, Kerwin DR, Hunt G, Hall EJ. The art of sharing the diagnosis and management of Alzheimer's disease with patients and caregivers: recommendations of an expert consensus panel. Prim Care Companion J Clin Psychiatry 2010;12.PCC.09cs00833.
67. Fitzpatrick R, Boulton M. Qualitative methods for assessing health care. Quality in health care. 1994;3(2):107.
68. Kim ES, Bayles KA. Communication in late-stage Alzheimer's disease: relation to functional markers of disease severity. Alzheim Care Q. 2007;8(1):43–52.
69. Behrman S, Chouliaras L, Ebmeier KP. Considering the senses in the diagnosis and management of dementia. Maturitas. 2014;77(4):305–10.
70. Grinspun D, Harripaul-Yhap A, Jarvi K, Lenartowych T. Mind the safety gap in health system transformation: reclaiming the role of the RN. Toronto. Canada: Registered Nurses' Association of Ontario; 2011.
71. Tolson D. Age-related hearing loss: a case for nursing intervention. J Adv Nurs. 1997;26(6):1150–7.
72. Voeks SK, Gallagher CM, Langer EH, Drinka PJ. Hearing loss in the nursing home. An institutional issue. J Am Geriatr Soc. 1990;38(2):141–5.

6

Predictors of recovering ambulation after hip fracture inpatient rehabilitation

Francesca Cecchi[1], Silvia Pancani[1*], Desiderio Antonioli[1], Lucia Avila[1], Manuele Barilli[1], Massimo Gambini[1], Lucilla Landucci Pellegrini[1], Emanuela Romano[1], Chiara Sarti[1], Margherita Zingoni[1], Maria Assunta Gabrielli[1], Federica Vannetti[1], Guido Pasquini[1] and Claudio Macchi[1,2]

Abstract

Background: Despite progress in surgery and care, hip fracture (HF) remains a catastrophic event, burdened with high risk of mortality and disability. This study aims at identifying predictors of recovering ambulation after intensive inpatient rehabilitation within the Tuscany Region HF rehabilitation pathway.

Methods: All HF patients referred from acute care to the two Massa-Carrara Rehabilitation facilities January 2015–June 2017 were enrolled. Comorbidity Total Score (CIRS) defined high- or low-care setting referral. Recovery of ambulation, with or without aid, (assessed by SAHFE) was the primary outcome. Personal data, comorbidity, cognitive (MMSe) and pre-fracture function (mRANKIN) were recorded on admission. Outcomes included hospital readmission, length of stay (LOS) and home discharge. Urinary catheter, bedsores, disability (modified Barthel Index-mBI), communication disability (CDS), trunk control (TCT), pain (NRS), and ambulation were recorded (admission-discharge).

Results: Of 352 patients enrolled (age 83.9 ± 7.1; 80% women), 1 died and 6 were readmitted to acute-care hospital; 97% patients referred to high-care, and 64% referred to low-care, presented moderate-high comorbidity on admission. Median LOS was 22 days; 95% patients were discharged back home; daily functional gain (mBIscore/LOS) was 1.3 ± 0.7. Patients who recovered ambulation on discharge were 84%. Older age, higher comorbidity, bladder catheter, impaired trunk control, worse cognitive and functional status on admission, and pre-fracture disability were associated to poor outcome, but only higher comorbidity and impaired communication on admission predicted failure to recover ambulation on discharge.

Conclusion: In HF patients entitled to intensive inpatient rehabilitation, moderate-high comorbidity and impaired communication are frequent findings and predict rehabilitation failure.

Keywords: Hip fracture, Rehabilitation outcome, Predictors of ambulation

Background

The event of hip fracture (HF) in elderly persons, a continuously growing segment of the general population [1, 2], increases exponentially with age, with a worldwide annual incidence expected to reach 4.5 million by 2050 [3, 4]. HF often selects patients defined as frail [5], characterized by high complexity and high risk of incident disability or worsening of existing disability. Indeed, despite progress in surgery and clinical care, HF is still a catastrophic event, burdened with a high risk of mortality and residual disability: approximately one-third of HF patients are institutionalized, and half experience a permanent post-fracture disability [6]. Identifying therapeutic pathways that ensure maximum functional recovery, while containing direct and indirect HF costs, is therefore of vital importance.

Rehabilitation is crucial for the functional recovery of elderly patients with HF [7, 8]. The optimal setting, intensity, and duration of rehabilitation are current issues of debate, but the evaluation of rehabilitation performance is often confined to the variation of a single functional scale, undervaluing the contribution of care processes and of clinical complexity and nursing needs to a final functional outcome [9]. Furthermore, practice is still inconsistent across different facilities [10].

* Correspondence: spancani@dongnocchi.it
[1]Don Carlo Gnocchi Foundation, IRCSS, Via di Scandicci, 269, 50143 Florence, Italy
Full list of author information is available at the end of the article

In the Italian Tuscany region, in 2008, 7027, persons aged 65 and over were hospitalized for hip fracture, 1551 (22.1%) men and 5476 (77.9%) women, with 7.8 admissions per 1000 Tuscan residents over 64 (IC95% 7.7–8.0), 9.7 ‰ IC95% 9.4–10.0 women and 4.8 ‰, IC95% 4.6–5.1 men [11]. Based on these alarming data, the Regional Council appointed a panel of experts to develop an evidence-based HF clinical–rehabilitation pathway [7, 8], published in Tuscan regional Council resolution N 677 of 30-07-2012 and implemented thereafter. Recent data from 2017, confirm the impressive number of hip fractures affecting persons aged 65 and over in Tuscany: 7665 persons, 1992 man (26%), 5673 women (74%). The resolution stated appropriateness criteria for different rehabilitation settings and average rehabilitation intervention duration foreseen for each setting [12], thus ensuring homogenous standards for HF rehabilitation in Tuscany.

The purpose of this study is to prospectively identify predictors of failure to recover ambulation in HF patients from the Massa-Carrara area, who received inpatient intensive rehabilitation, according to the Tuscany Region pathway.

Methods

Regional resolution

The pathway defines appropriate timing of surgery (48 h from fracture) and to hospital discharge (4 days from surgery if the patient is clinically stable). Patients aged 65 and over who are unable to walk with aid, though allowed weight bearing, are referred to intensive inpatient rehabilitation; Length of Stay (LOS) is considered appropriate within 21 days [12]. Comorbidity is scored by the Cumulative Illness Rating Scale, Total Score (CIRS-TS), scoring both number of diseases (14 items) and severity of chronic comorbidity and of complications, range 13–69 [13]. Patients with moderate-high comorbidity (CIRS ≥ 19) are referred high-care intensive rehabilitation, while those with CIRS< 19 to low-care. In both cases, patients should be fit to at least 3 h of rehabilitation per day. Non-weight bearing patients are discharged home or to intermediate care until weight bearing is allowed. Cognitive impairment is screened by the Mini Mental State examination, range 30 best- 0 worst (MMSe, [14]); severely demented patients, scoring MMSe≤ 10, and previously non-ambulating patients (mRANKIN pre-fracture disability) are entitled to home counseling, and patients able to use a walker on discharge, with adequate home caregiving, to outpatient rehabilitation [7, 8].

Setting

The Rehabilitation facilities of Marina di Massa and Fivizzano, Fondazione Don Gnocchi, provide rehabilitation for all the Massa-Carrara area: Massa has 19 high-care and 5 low-care beds, Fivizzano 13 high-care and 19 low-care beds. High clinical care setting requires daily vital parameter and medical assessment, and 24 h MD availability.

Inpatient rehabilitation

Inpatient intensive rehabilitation, coordinated by a specialist in Physical and Rehabilitation Medicine, implies individualized interdisciplinary care [15], delivered by a team of physiotherapists, occupational therapists, nurses, social health professionals, psychotherapists, always including the patient and his/her caregiver. Physiotherapy, tailored to individual needs, aims at balance recovery, muscle strengthening, hip range of motion, pain control, and ambulation (from walker to cane, to no aid, when possible); occupational therapy is focused on activities of daily living training. Pain is routinely monitored, and treated, either pharmacologically or by physical/instrumental therapy. Psychological support is available for patients and caregivers. Technical advice on aids for autonomy and eventual home adjustments is provided. Neuropsychological/logopedics assessment and treatment is available if undiagnosed cognitive decline/dysphagia/aphasia are suspected. The program engages each patient for an average of 3 h per day 6 days a week and is periodically redefined throughout the stay.

Patients

From January 1st, 2015 to June 30th, 2017, all HF patients referred to the Don Gnocchi Rehabilitation facility of Massa and Fivizzano by the local public health specialists were consecutively enrolled. All patients provided written consent to anonymous treatment of their personal and clinical data. As this was notified by Don Gnocchi Foundation to the Ministry of Health as a prospective observational study, in agreement with national guidelines, no formal ethics approval was required (MD 20 March G.U. n. 76 del 31-3-2008, GU n76, 31/03/2008).

Measures

Outcomes included hospital readmission, death, length of stay (LOS) and a series of functional and clinical parameters. Personal data, comorbidity (CIRS), cognitive level (MMSe), and pre-fracture functional level, modified Rankin scale (mRankin, [16]), ranging 0-no symptom - 5-severe disability, were collected on admission. According to a comprehensive approach to rehabilitation quality assessment [17], rehabilitation outcomes included both functional and clinical parameters, recorded on admission and on discharge: urinary catheter, bedsores, ADL disability by the modified Barthel Index (mBI, [18]) ranging 100-no to 0-complete disability, disability in communication, by the Communicative Disability Scale (CDS, [19]), ranging 0-complete to 4-no disability in communication [19], trunk control, by the Trunk Control Test (TCT, [20]), ranging 0-no to 100-complete control, Pain, by the Numeric Rating Scale (NRS)-PAIN, ranging 0-no to 10-worst possible pain [20], and ambulation, by the Standardized Audit of Hip Fracture In Europe (SAHFE) [21]. The primary rehabilitation outcome was SAHFE, scoring 1-Independent outdoor ambulation, without help, 2-Outdoor ambulation with aid, 3-Indoor ambulation with aid (except walker), 4-Indoor ambulation with a walker, 5-Unable to walk/ using a wheelchair.

Statistical analysis

All statistical analyses were performed using IBM SPSS Statistics 23.0 for Windows [22]. Clinical and functional scores on admission and on discharge were compared. CIRS, TCT and mBI scores were compared through a paired t-test. A Wilcoxon signed rank test was used to compare NRS, CDS and SAHFE scores, while dichotomous variables were analyzed using a McNemar test.

Patients that recovered ambulation on discharge ("able to walk", SHAFE< 5) were compared to those who did not ("unable to walk", SAHFE = 5. Patients with missing data on discharge ($n = 28$) were excluded from further analysis. Of the remaining 324 patients, age and CIRS, Barthel, TCT and MMSe scores were compared by an independent t-test, while a Mann Whitney U test was used to analyze mRankin, CDS, and NRS scores. Gender, use of bladder catheter and presence of bedsores were compared using a Chi-Square test.

In a logistic regression analysis, parameters shown to be significantly different between the two groups ("able to walk" and "unable to walk") were considered independent variables. The recovery of walking function was used as a dependent variable while age and gender were assumed as confounding factors.

In all the analyses, level of significance was set at a p-value< 0.05.

Results

All 352 HF patients (80% women, 20% men; 318 low-, 34 high-care) accessing the two rehabilitation facilities were enrolled in the study. Characteristics of the studied sample are resumed in Table 1. Among them, one patient (0.003%) died, 4 (0.01%) were discharged to resident care, 6 (0.02%) were readmitted to an acute care Hospital, 6 (0.02%) were referred to intermediate care and 1 (0.003%) was referred to a different rehabilitation facility; the remaining 334 patients (95%) were discharged back home. Patients' mean age was 83.9 ± 7.1 years (range: 65–99 years) while LOS showed a median value of 22 days (IQR: 7 days).

Only 1 of 34 patients was referred to high care with CIRS< 19, while 226/318 (71%) patients referred to low care presented CIRS≥ 9. For the latter, clinical and nursing care were delivered according to high clinical care requirements. Patients with MMSe< 10 were 28 (8%); 50% of patients presented some degree of cognitive impairment (MMSe score < 21). As to pre-fracture disability, 74 (21%) reported moderate, 51 (14.5%) moderately severe, and 10 (2.8%) severe disability (bedridden before

Table 1 Patients' characteristics, clinical and functional scores measured at admission and discharge

Parameters	N	Admission		Discharge		p-value
		Mean Median Percentage	Std. Dev. (Interquartile Range)	Mean Median Percentage	Std. Dev. (Interquartile Range)	
Age (years)	352	83.9	7.1			
Gender (F %)	352	80%				
Hospitalization period (days)	352	22	(7)			
MMSe at admission (score)	266	19.6	7.1			
RANKIN	352	2.0	1.3			
CIRS	352	21.0	3.8	20.9	3.7	0.255
CDS	349	4	(0)	4	(0)	0.239
SAHFE	324	=5.0		3.9	0.7	< 0.001
Barthel index	352	29.5	17.8	58.7	22.9	< 0.001
TCT	352	41.2	24.8	68.2	23.1	< 0.001
NRS	345	3	(6)	0	(2)	< 0.001
Urinary catheter (%Y)	349	23%		10%		< 0.001
Bedsore (%Y)	352	33%		19%		< 0.001

Parameters characterized by a normal distribution are expressed as mean and standard deviation, parameters with a non-normal distribution as median and interquartile range, dichotomous parameters as a percentage
MMSe mini-mental state examination, *CIRS* cumulative illness rating scale, *CDS* communication disability scale, *SAHFE* Standardized Audit of Hip Fracture in Europe, *TCT* trunk control test, *NRS* numeric rating scale

fracture); 96 patients presented some degree of impairment in communication on admission (27.5%).

Table 1 shows also the comparison between patients' characteristics and clinical and functional scores measured on admission and on discharge. SAHFE, mBI, TCT and NRS scores were significantly improved. Significantly fewer patients had urinary catheter or bedsores on discharge: Average mBI delta score was 29.0 ± 14.7, that, divided by LOS provided a rehabilitation efficiency rate of 1.3 ± 0.7.

Characteristics of the patients excluded from the second analysis are reported in Table 2. Among the excluded patients 1 died, 6 were referred to an ER and the remaining had missing data on discharge in one or more scales. Excluded subjects were significantly different from those included in the further analysis in terms of older age ($p = 0.001$), lower MMSe ($p = 0.048$), mRankin ($p = 0.035$), CIRS and SDC scores (both at admission and discharge, $p < 0.001$) and SAHFE score at discharge ($p < 0.001$). They presented also a significantly higher percentage of bladder catheters both at admission and discharge ($p = 0.002$ and $p < 0.001$, respectively) and a higher number of bedsores at discharge ($p = 0.001$).

Table 3 shows ambulation according to SAHFE achieved upon discharge: 84% patients recovered ambulation, and about 7% were able to walk outdoors on discharge.

As can be seen from Table 4, patients "unable to walk" (SAHFE = 5 on discharge, $n = 51$, 16%) were significantly older and showed significantly worse CIRS, RANKIN, CDS, mBI, TCT and MMSe scores and more of them needed a urinary catheter, while no significant differences were found in gender, NRS-pain score, presence of bedsores and LOS compared to those "able to walk" on discharge (SAHFE< 5, $n = 273$, 84%).

Table 5 shows the results for the logistic regression: comorbidity (CIRS, $p = 0.001$) and disability in communication (CDS, $p = 0.013$) were independently associated with failure to recover ambulation. The model was statistically significant ($p < 0.001$) and explained the 24% of the variance in the dependent variable.

Discussion

Traditional methods of evaluation of rehabilitation performance are mainly focused on the admission-discharge variation of a disability scale score. In evaluating predictors of HF rehabilitation failure, we chose to consider both clinical and functional parameters, in the attempt to investigate the complex relationship that binds care needs and patient characteristics to final functional gain.

We verified that cognitive and pre-function referral criteria were aligned to pathway requirements: only 28 patients presented an MMSe score ≤ 10 on admission and only 10 (2.8%) were already unable to walk before

Table 2 Characteristics of patients ($N = 28$) excluded from second analysis. Clinical and functional scores measured at admission and discharge

Parameters	N	Admission		N	Discharge	
		Mean Median	Std. Dev. (Interquartile Range)		Mean Median	Std. Dev. (Interquartile Range)
		Percentage			Percentage	
Age (years)	28	88.1*	6.9			
Gender (F %)	28	75%				
Hospitalization period (days)	28	21.5	(13)			
MMSe (admission score)	14	16.0*	5.3			
RANKIN	28	2.6*	1.3			
CIRS	28	23.4*	3.3	28	23.6*	3.6
CDS	28	3*	(1)	25	3*	(1)
SAHFE	5	=5.0		15	4.9*	0.3
Barthel index	28	23.0	14.3	21	47.2	22.9
TCT	28	32.6	22.0	21	61.5	22.7
NRS	28	3	(4)	22	0	(1)
Urinary catheter (%Y)	28	46%*		28	39%*	
Bedsore (%Y)	28	43%		28	43%*	

Parameters characterized by a normal distribution are expressed as mean and standard deviation, parameters with a non-normal distribution as median and interquartile range, dichotomous parameters as a percentage

MMSe mini-mental state examination, *CIRS* cumulative illness rating scale, *CDS* communication disability scale, *SAHFE* Standardized Audit of Hip Fracture in Europe, *TCT* trunk control test, *NRS* numeric rating scale

*significantly different ($p < 0.005$) compared to patients included in the second analysis

Table 3 number [percentage] of patients presenting with SAHFE score = 5 at admission and with different SAHFE score at discharge

SAHFE score at discharge	Nr of patients [%]
1 Able to walk autonomously outdoor without aid	1 [0.3%]
2 Able to walk outdoor with aid	21 [6.5%]
3 Able to walk indoor with aid (except walker)	33 [10.2%]
4 Able to walk indoor with a walker	218 [67.3%]
5 Unable to walk, use of wheelchair	51 [15.7%]

fracture. On the contrary, we found a substantial discrepancy in the comorbidity index: while only 1 patient with low comorbidity entered high-care rehabilitation, up to 64% of "low-care" patients presented a moderate-high comorbidity score. In the specific cases, the clinical decision was to deliver high care, regardless of referral, but this is not always possible in clinical practice. From a broader perspective, we hypothesize that if an older, previously ambulating HF patient, does not recover walking with aid on the 4th–5th day after surgery, this is very likely to be accounted by either diagnosed or undiagnosed comorbidity, that must be addressed in the rehabilitation process. So, as our results suggest, we argue that all these geriatric patients should be regarded as possibly complex and referred to high-care rehabilitation settings [23].

The rehabilitation program was overall highly successful: we reported 1 death and 6 hospital readmissions, and only 6 patients were institutionalized, while 95% were discharged back home. Although median LOS was 1 day longer than that the pathway required, it was shorter than what reported in most similar studies (22 days vs 28–30) [6, 24–27]. We also found a significant reduction of pain, bedsores, and number of patients with urinary catheter on discharge: these conditions are rarely reported as HF rehabilitation outcomes, although they may impact on clinical complications as well as on functional gain [9, 28]. Improvement of mobility was high (29% mBI increase), and the daily functional gain (improve in functional score divided by LOS) was highly efficient [6, 25–27, 29]. Recovery of ambulation was also achieved by a very high percentage of patients (84%); a similar Korean study conducted on younger patients receiving on average 30 days of inpatient intensive rehabilitation, reported a 70% recovery [27].

We assessed rehabilitation outcome at the time of discharge from inpatient rehabilitation, although patients may have continued rehabilitation further. We chose this time as, on discharge, the patient returns to his/her natural environment and because inpatient rehabilitation accounts for the most relevant share of HF rehabilitation [25]. We could only collect data from patients referred to inpatient rehabilitation, and not from all HF patients in the Massa-Carrara area. This is the main limitation of our study, as we could neither evaluate the first part of the pathway (acute care and surgery) nor elaborate on what happened to those who were not referred to inpatient rehabilitation. Theoretically, this also led to a selection bias in the study population, but, actually, the characteristics of our sample were similar to Canadian, Israelian, Asian, and US studies [6, 25–27] as the pathway appropriateness criteria for referral were defined on evidence-based guidelines [7, 8].

Table 4 Parameters assessed at admission for those patients that recovered walking independence (able to walk) and those that did not (unable to walk)

Parameters assessed on admission	Able to walk (*n* = 273)		Unable to walk (*n* = 51)		*p*-value
	Mean Median Percentage	Std. Dev. (IQR)	Mean Median Percentage	Std. Dev. (IQR)	
Age (years)	83.2	7.1	85.3	6.6	0.055
Gender (%F)	80%		81%		0.974
CIRS (score)	20.6	3.6	23.2	4.1	< 0.001
RANKIN (score)	1.9	1.3	2.5	1.4	0.006
CDS (score)	3.7	0.7	3.3	0.8	< 0.001
mBI (score)	31.2	17.5	20.8	16.9	< 0.001
TCT (score)	43.8	23.8	29.8	27.1	< 0.001
NRS (score)	3	(6)	2	(4)	0.248
Bladder catheter (%Y)	17%		40%		< 0.001
Bedsore (%Y)	32%		36%		0.542
Hospitalization period (days)	22	(7)	22	(10)	0.854
MMSe (score)	20.3	7.0	17.2	7.1	0.015

Parameters characterized by a normal distribution are expressed as mean and standard deviation, parameters with a non-normal distribution as median and interquartile range (IQR), dichotomous parameters as a percentage

CIRS cumulative illness rating scale, *CDS* communication disability scale, *mBI* modified Barthel index, *TCT* trunk con-trol test, *NRS* numeric rating scale, *MMSe* mini-mental state examination

Table 5 Association between parameters measured at admission and ability to recover ambulation according to a Logistic Regression model

	B	S.E.	Sig.	Exp(B)	Nagelkerke R Square
Model			< 0.001		0.241
Constant	3.297	3.459	.341	27.023	
CIRS	−.175	.053	.001	.839	
RANKIN	−.035	.174	.839	.965	
CDS	.755	.303	.013	2.129	
Mbi	−.002	.018	.893	.998	
TCT	.018	.010	.088	1.018	
Urinary catheter	.778	.450	.084	2.177	
Gender	−.183	.536	.733	.833	
Age	−.029	.033	.382	.972	
MMSe	.045	.035	.197	1.047	

Analysis of predictors of response to treatment may provide relevant insight into rehabilitation practice [30, 31]. In our analysis, patients who did not recover ambulation, with or without aid (16%), were significantly older and showed a significantly higher comorbidity, pre-fracture disability, disability in mobility and communication, worse trunk control, and reduced cognitive ability, compared to those that recovered ambulation; further, more of them needed a urinary catheter on admission, while LOS did not differ between the two groups. In the regression analysis, only comorbidity (CIRS) and disability in communication (CDS) remained independent predictors of failure to recover ambulation. As to this secondary analysis, we must mention the exclusion of 28 patients, either due to death/acute care readmission or missing data. However, these patients presented lower SDC and higher comorbidity on admission and overall worse outcome, thus suggesting that their exclusion was not a substantial bias to our final results, that are in line with some [9, 27], but not all studies focusing on HF recovery [25, 26, 32, 33]. Indeed, we must also point out that our model, although significant, explained only 24% of the variance of the final outcome; as we already acknowledged, the lack of information on the first stages of care and on surgery (timing, type) is the main limitation of our study, and, probably, our model would have been empowered by including this information [24, 27]. On the other hand, as generally happens in clinical practice, we could focus on what can be detected and addressed in the rehabilitation setting, regardless of what happened before admission. A possible reason for our finding that pre-fracture functional level and cognition did not predict ambulation on discharge, might be the exclusion, by pathway criteria, of the extremes of the spectrum (either of those already able to walk on hospital discharge and of those who were already severely disabled in mobility and/or cognition before the fracture), but, again, this cannot be verified without the data from patients excluded from inpatient rehabilitation after surgery.

Comorbidity on admission, including both chronic and acute complications, was a powerful predictor of HF rehabilitation outcome, confirming that, in our sample, the functional gain was strictly related to individual medical-nursing complexity [34]. This result indirectly supports our previously expressed view that HF patients require high standard clinical and nursing care to obtain the highest possible functional gain [35]. Bernardini et al. already showed in a large sample of inpatient rehabilitation patients, including HF, that those with clinical complexity on admission presented a lower functional recovery than those without clinical complexity [9]; Kim et al. [27] showed that pre-fracture ambulatory capacity and combined medical disease predicted ambulatory capacity with walking aid, whereas MMSe and functional status on admission did not.

While the predictive value of comorbidity to HF outcome is in line with most of the literature, the predictive value of communication skill is a rather novel, if not unexpected, finding. The main reason for this is probably the fact that communication is not routinely screened or considered in HF patients. In our sample, 30% patients presented an impairment in communication on admission; CDS score was significantly improved from admission to discharge. The CDS was designed for rapid screening of communication skills. Evaluation is carried out in an informal, but minimally structured communication setting (for example, during the collection of the anamnesis and the execution of the objective examination, during the assistance maneuvers made by the nursing staff), thus it is can be very rapidly and easily administered also to severely compromised patients, which cannot be evaluated with formal neuropsychological tests [19]. The CDS depends on verbal skills, sensory abilities, relationship, and collaboration. It scores disability, independent of its cause/causes (neuropsychological, sensory or psychomotor disorder), that must be addressed by specific diagnosis and treatment. We found that both MMSe and CDS were significantly associated to a worse outcome, but, in the regression analysis, only CDS predicted failure to recover walking ability. At least in this sample, excluding severely demented patients, cognitive impairment seemed not to impact rehabilitation outcome directly, but rather, if so, through reduced communication abilities. These findings confirm those reported by Mc Gilton and by Resnick [6, 36], supporting the appropriateness of referring cognitively impaired persons to intensive inpatient rehabilitation, while suggesting dedicating specific attention to communication strategies. Communication impairment by any cause (be it aphasia, depression, deafness or any other possible cause) may indeed compromise therapeutic alliance and learning abilities which deeply affect rehabilitation [19]; on the other hand, impaired communication may also indirectly affect rehabilitation outcome, as it may be a symptom of additional comorbidity. The good news is that many communication problems, stemming either from neurological, clinical, sensorial, cultural or psychological problems, may often be successfully addressed by either modifying patient factors, environmental factors or style of communication. Although we cannot make inference on how optimal management of comorbidity and impairment of communication may modify the final outcome of HF rehabilitation, the results of our study suggest that high care of clinical-nursing complexity and screening and address of any communication problems are recommended for all HF patients referred to intensive rehabilitation, to improve care provision and, possibly, final functional outcome.

Conclusions

The outcome of HF patients referred to intensive inpatient rehabilitation was very successful, and the interdisciplinary rehabilitation provided proved to be highly efficient, with a 1.3 mBI score daily functional gain and 84% patients recovering ambulation on discharge. Moderate-high comorbidity was a frequent finding, also in patients referred to a low-care setting. Higher comorbidity and impairment in communication ability on admission predicted failure to recover ambulation, independent of pre-fracture disability, compromised functional status on admission, age and MMSe. These results support the importance of addressing nursing and clinical complexity and of screening, and eventually addressing, any-cause communication disability in HF rehabilitation.

Abbreviations

ADL: Activities of daily living; CDS: Communicative disability scale; CIRS: Cumulative illness rating scale, total score; HF: Hip fracture; IQR: Interquartile range; LOS: Length of stay; mBI: modified Barthel Index; MMSe: Mini Mental State examination; NRS: Numeric rating scale; SAHFE: Standardized Audit of Hip Fracture In Europe; TCT: Trunk control test; TS: Cumulative final score

Authors' contributions

Study concept and design: FC, CM, MAG, MB. Acquisition of subjects and/or data: DA, LA, MB, MG, LLP, ER, CS, MZ, MAG. Analysis and interpretation of data: FC, SP, FV, GP, DA, LA, MG, LLP, ER, CS, MZ, CM. Preparation of manuscript: FC, SP, MB, CM. All authors read and approved the final version of the manuscript.

Competing interests

The authors declare that they have no competing interests.

Author details

[1]Don Carlo Gnocchi Foundation, IRCSS, Via di Scandicci, 269, 50143 Florence, Italy. [2]Department of Experimental and Clinical Medicine, University of Florence, Florence, Italy.

References

1. The UK National hip Fracture Database National Report 2017.
2. Cauley JACD, Kassem AM, Fuleihan G-H. Geographic and ethnic disparities in osteoporotic fractures. Nat Rev Endocrinol. 2014;10(6):338–51.
3. Global Health and Ageing [http://www.who.int/ageing/publications/global_health.pdf]. Accessed 1 Jan 2018.
4. Dyer SM, Crotty M, Fairhall N, et al. A critical review of the long-term disability outcomes following hip fracture. BMC Geriatr. 2016;16(1):158. https://doi.org/10.1186/s12877-016-0332-0.
5. Fried LP, Tangen CM, Walston J, et al. Frailty in older adults: evidence for a phenotype. J Gerontol. 2001;56A:M146–56.
6. McGilton KS, Chu CH, Naglie G, et al. Factors influencing outcomes of older adults after undergoing rehabilitation for hip fracture. J Am Geriatr Soc. 2016;64(8):1601–9.
7. Hip fracture: management. Clinical guideline [CG124] The National Institute for Health and Care Excellence (NICE) Published date: June 2011. Last updated: May 2017.
8. Management of hip fracture in older people A national clinical guideline Scottish Intercollegiate Guidelines Network ISBN 978 1 905813 47 6. Published June 2009.
9. Bernardini B, Meinecke C, Pagani M, et al. Epidemiology of adverse clinical events as a dynamic measure of geriatric care management. Aging Clin Exp Res. 1995;7:191–3i.
10. Williams NH, Roberts JL, Din NU, et al. Developing a multidisciplinary rehabilitation package following hip fracture and testing in a randomised feasibility study: fracture in the elderly multidisciplinary rehabilitation (FEMuR). Health Technol Assess. 2017 Aug;21(44):1–528.
11. Gli anziani in Toscana con ictus e frattura di femore: epidemiologia, ospedalizzazione e riabilitazione nei periodi 2003–2005 e 2007–2010 (2012) Collana dei *Documenti ARS*, n 65.
12. Regione Toscana Giunta Regionale Delibera N 677 del 30-07-2012.
13. Linn BS, Linn MW, Gurel L. Cumulative illness rating scale. J Am Geriatr Soc. 1968;16:622–5.
14. Folstein MF, Folstein SE, McHugh PR. "Mini-mental state". A practical method for grading the cognitive state of patients for the clinician. J Psychiatr Res. 1975;12(3):189–98.
15. Piano di indirizzo per la riabilitazione. GU 2/3/2011.
16. Quinn TJ, Dawson J, Walters MR, et al. Exploring the reliability of the modified Rankin scale. Stroke. 2009;40(3):762–6.
17. IPER 2. Indicatori di Processo Esito in Riabilitazione Versione 2.Uno strumento per l'audit clinico e il controllo di gestione. In: Quaderni ARS Liguria; 2012.
18. Shah S, Vanclay F, Cooper B. Improving the sensitivity of the Barthel index for stroke rehabilitation. J Clin Epidemiol. 1989;42(8):703–9.
19. Meinecke C, Cappadonia C, Bernardini B. Validazione di una semplice scala di impairment comunicativo nell'anziano. XXIII Congresso Nazionale SIMFER. Valutazione e qualità dell'assistenza in Medicina Riabilitativa. Abstract book Ancona; 1995. p. 56–7.
20. Collin C, Wade D. Assessing motor impairment after stroke: a pilot reliability study. J Neurol Neurosurg Psychiatry. 1990;53(7):576–9. (2000) Glossary. Spine 25:3200–3202
21. Parker MJ. Standardized audit of hip fracture in Europe. Hip Int. 1998;8:10–5.
22. SPSS Inc, 233 S Wacker Dr, 11th Fl, Chicago, IL 60606.
23. Kristensen MT, Kehlet H. The basic mobility status upon acute hospital discharge is an independent risk factor for mortality up to 5 years after hip fracture surgery. Acta Orthop. 2018;89(1)
24. Castronuovo E, Pezzotti P, Franzo A, Di Lallo D, Guasticchi G. Early and late mortality in elderly patients after hip fracture: a cohort study using administrative health databases in the Lazio region, Italy. BMC Geriatrics. 2011;11(1):37.
25. Lieberman D, Friger M, Lieberman D. Inpatient rehabilitation outcome after hip fracture surgery in elderly patients: a prospective cohort study of 946 patients. Arch Phys Med Rehabil. 2006;87(2):167–71.
26. Hershkovitz A, Kalandariov Z, Hermush V, et al. Factors affecting short-term rehabilitation outcomes of disabled elderly patients with proximal hip fracture. Arch Phys Med Rehabil. 2007;88(7):916–21.
27. Kim JL, Jung JS, Kim SJ. Prediction of ambulatory status after hip fracture surgery in patients over 60 years old. Ann Rehabil Med. 2016;40(4):666–74.
28. Magny, et al. Pressure ulcers are associated with 6-month mortality in elderly patients with hip fracture managed in orthogeriatric care pathways. Arch Osteoporos. 2017;12(1):77.

29. Toyama, et al. Changes in Basic Movement Ability and Activities of Daily Living After Hip Fractures: Correlation Between Basic Movement Scale and Motor-Functional Independence Measure Scores. A J Phys Med Rehabil. 2017; Epub ahead of print
30. Cecchi F, Negrini S, Pasquini G, Paperini A, Conti AA, Chiti M, et al. Predictors of functional outcome in patients with chronic low back pain undergoing back school, individual physiotherapy or spinal manipulation. Eur J Phys Rehabil Med. 2012;48(3):371–8.
31. Cecchi F, Pasquini G, Paperini A, Boni R, Castagnoli C, Pistritto S, Macchi C. Predictors of response to exercise therapy for chronic low back pain: result of a prospective study with one year follow-up. Eur J Phys Rehabil Med. 2014;50(2):143–51.
32. Cree AK, Nade S. How to predict return to the community after fractured proximal femur in the elderly. Aust N Z J Surg. 1999;69:723–5.
33. Tang VL, Sudore R, Cenzer IS, et al. Rates of recovery to pre-fracture function in older persons with hip fracture: an observational study. J Gen Intern Med. 2017;32(2):153–8.
34. Gialanella, et al. Determinants of functional outcome in hip fracture: the role of comorbidity. Aging Clin Exp Res. 2017; https://doi.org/10.1007/s40520-017-0812-x. Epub ahead of print
35. Gleason LJ, Benton EA, Alvarez-Nebreda ML, et al. FRAIL questionnaire screening tool and short-term outcomes in geriatric fracture patients. J Am Med Dir Assoc. 2017;18(12):1082–6.
36. Resnick B, Beaupre L, McGilton KS, et al. Rehabilitation interventions for older individuals with cognitive impairment post-hip fracture: a systematic review. J Am Med Dir Assoc. 2016;17(3):200–5.

7

Disability, quality of life and all-cause mortality in older Mexican adults: association with multimorbidity and frailty

Ana Rivera-Almaraz[1], Betty Manrique-Espinoza[1*], José Alberto Ávila-Funes[2], Somnath Chatterji[3], Nirmala Naidoo[3], Paul Kowal[3,4,5] and Aarón Salinas-Rodríguez[1]

Abstract

Background: Multimorbidity and frailty are relevant conditions among older adult population. There is growing evidence about their association with poor health outcomes like disability, worst quality of life, and death. Nonetheless, the independent associations of both conditions have been studied, and few evidence exists about an interaction between them. Our aims were to assess the association of frailty and multimorbidity with the disability, quality of life and all-cause mortality as well as to analyze a potential interaction between these conditions.

Methods: Analytical samples included 1410 respondents for disability and quality of life, and 1792 for mortality. We performed a longitudinal analysis with older Mexican adults aged 50, using data collected from the WHO's Study on global AGEing and Adult Health Waves 1 and 2. Disability was measured using the World Health Organization Disability Assessment Schedule (WHODAS 2.0), and quality of life using the WHOQOL (WHO Quality of Life) instrument. All-cause mortality was determined by reviewing death certificates. Associations of frailty and multimorbidity with disability, quality of life and mortality were estimated using linear regression and Cox proportional hazards models.

Results: Multimorbidity assessed through three patterns (cardiopulmonary, vascular-metabolic, and mental-musculoskeletal) was associated with the three outcomes in this study. Cardiopulmonary and mental-musculoskeletal patterns increased the WHODAS mean score ($\beta = 5.05$; $p < 0.01$ and $\beta = 5.10$; $p < 0.01$, respectively) and decreased WHOQOL score ($\beta = -1.81$; $p < 0.01$ and $\beta = -2.99$; $p < 0.01$, respectively). Vascular-metabolic was associated with mortality (HR = 1.47; $p = 0.04$), disability ($\beta = 3.27$; $p < 0.01$) and quality of life ($\beta = -1.30$; $p = 0.02$). Frailty was associated with mortality (pre-frail: HR = 1.48; $p = 0.02$ and frail: HR = 1.68; $p = 0.03$), disability (pre-frail: $\beta = 5.02$; $p < 0.01$; frail: $\beta = 13.29$; $p < 0.01$) and quality of life (pre-frail: $\beta = -2.23$; $p < 0.01$; frail: $\beta = -4.38$; $p < 0.01$). Interaction terms of frailty and multimorbidity were not statistically significant.

Conclusions: Multimorbidity and frailty are important predictors of poor health outcomes. These results highlight the importance of carrying out health promotion and prevention actions as well as specific interventions aimed at older adults who suffer from multimorbidity and frailty, in such a way that deleterious effects on health can be avoided.

Keywords: Multimorbidity, Frailty, Mortality, Disability, Quality of life, Older adults

* Correspondence: bmanrique@insp.mx
[1]National Institute of Public Health, Avenida Universidad #655, Colonia Santa María Ahuacatitlán, ZC, 62100 Cuernavaca, Morelos, Mexico
Full list of author information is available at the end of the article

Background

The proportion of the world's population aged 60 and older is increasing rapidly. Within 35 years, it will have spiraled from 12% (in 2015) to 22% (in 2050). Virtually all the regions in the world are witnessing this population aging process [1]. From a public health perspective, older adults (OA) account for 23% of the global burden of disease, particularly as regards chronic diseases (CDs) such as cardiovascular, pulmonary, musculoskeletal, neurological, mental, and neoplastic conditions [2]. They have also been found to be at higher risk for multimorbidity and geriatric syndromes such as frailty [3].

Regarding multimorbidity, associations with greater use of health-care services and adverse health events such as polypharmacy, increased health expenditures, disability, a low quality of life, and even mortality have been reported [4–6]. However, multimorbidity research has traditionally focused on counting diseases, thus hindering the detection of co-occurrences. Notwithstanding, recent literature has highlighted the importance of taking into account the CDs combinations in OA health studies [7].

Frailty, on the other hand, defined as a biological syndrome resulting from cumulative declines across multiple physiologic systems, with impaired homeostatic reserve and a reduced capacity of the organism to withstand stress [8], has been identified as an independent predictor for adverse health outcomes including falls, a diminished quality of life, disability and death [9–14].

Although OA can suffer from multimorbidity and frailty simultaneously, a causal link has been suggested between them [15], empirical evidence has focused on the independent effects that they have on adverse health outcomes. Among the scarce evidence that has explored the joint effects of multimorbidity and frailty, one study with OA residents of Hong Kong found that combination of frailty and multimorbidity increased the risk of disability and death [16]. However, it is still pending to analyze this interaction effect on other outcomes such as health-related quality of life. Therefore, our main aim in this study was to estimate the independent associations of multimorbidity and frailty with three different outcomes: disability, quality of life and all-cause mortality. A secondary aim was to determine whether exist a significant interaction effect of the multimorbidity and frailty on those same outcomes.

Methods

Study design

We drew our data from the Study on global AGEing and adult health (SAGE), a longitudinal, multicenter study conducted by the World Health Organization (WHO) across six low- and middle-income countries: India, Ghana, Russia, Mexico, South Africa and China [17]. Based on a multistage, stratified and cluster design, SAGE provided nationally representative groups of adults aged 50 and older, disaggregated by rural/urban strata. It applied standardized instruments including household and individual-level questionnaires, as well as anthropometric and functionality measurements. The present study consisted of a longitudinal analysis of SAGE-Mexico data derived from the two measurements available to date (2009 and 2014).

Study sample

Baseline measurement

In 2009, Wave 1 performed baseline measurements with a sample size of 2306 adults aged 50 years and older and a smaller comparison group of 436 subjects aged 18–49 years.

Follow-up

The first follow-up (Wave 2), conducted in 2014, included all eligible subjects from Wave 1. In addition, the sample was refreshed with a sample of both age groups: one from 18 to 49 years, the other 50 years and older. A total response rate of 83.47% was achieved. Full interviews were administered to a larger number of participants than in Wave 1: 853 aged 18–49 years, and 4301 aged 50 and older.

Our analytical sample included Wave 1 respondents aged 50 and older as well as Wave 2 subjects who provided information on the variables of interest. Of the 2306 OA in Wave 1, 1595 were interviewed and 273 had died (14.61%). The remaining 438 (19%) either declined our invitation to participate in the study or were not located. Analytical samples of OA aged 50 and older included 1410 respondents for disability and quality of life, and 1792 for mortality (Fig. 1).

Outcomes. We analyzed three of the Wave 2 outcomes: disability, quality of life and all-cause mortality.

Disability We measured this variable according to the World Health Organization Disability Assessment Schedule (WHODAS 2.0) [18]. The WHODAS 2.0 scale is widely used to measure last-month limitations in activity and daily-life participation. It covers six domains explored through a total of 12 items (two per domain): (1) cognition and communication, (2) self-care, (3) mobility, (4) interpersonal relations, (5) life activities, and (6) participation. The results of the 12 items are summed up to obtain a global score expressed on a continuous scale from 0 (no disability) to 100 (full disability) [18].

Quality of life For this variable, we used the WHOQOL (WHO Quality of Life) instrument. This eight-item questionnaire covers the following core domains (two items per domain): physical, psychological, social and environmental. The results of the eight items are added up to obtain an overall WHOQOL score expressed on a scale from 0 to 100. The higher the score, the higher the quality of life [19].

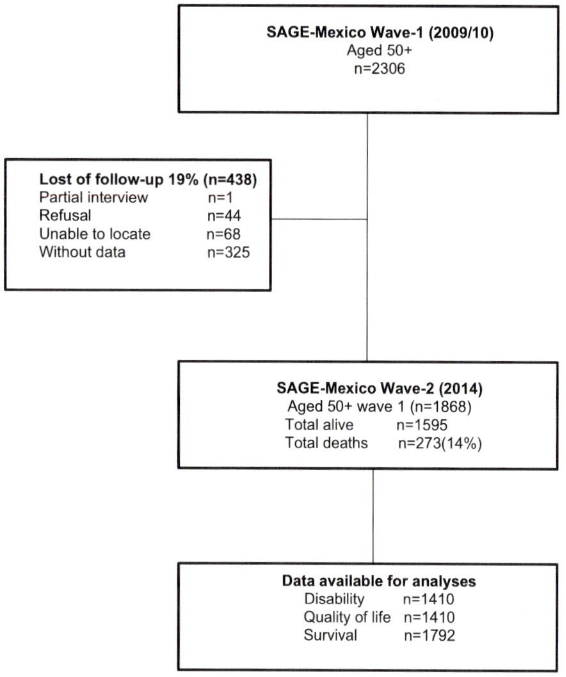

Fig. 1 Population study and analytical sample

All-cause mortality Data drawn from the Wave 2 interviews (2014) included information about death (for any cause) occurred between Waves 1 and 2 using a verbal autopsy. We recorded the date of death, which provided information on the interval between baseline and death.

Exposures

Multimorbidity

We used a nine CDs list that was included in the SAGE study. Three were measured according to self-reported medical diagnoses: diabetes, stroke, and cataracts. Five were estimated through algorithms for symptomatology and self-reported treatment: angina, arthritis, chronic obstructive pulmonary disease, asthma, and depression [20]. Finally, hypertension was determined by either blood pressure measurement and/or self-reported treatment. The CDs were assessed dichotomously (1 = presence, 0 = absence).

Frailty

For this variable, we used the frailty phenotype proposed by Fried et al. (2001), which covers five components: unintended weight loss, exhaustion, low physical activity, slow walking speed and weakness. Subjects considered frail presented three or more of these components; pre-frail one or two; and not frail, or robust, none. The results were thus expressed categorically: 0 = not frail, 1 = pre-frail, and 2 = frail [8]. Frailty components were assessed as follows:

(1) *Unintended weight loss* during the past year *was* determined according to a self-reported reduction of five kilograms or more in the past 12 months. Subjects with this condition were considered frail based on weight loss.

(2) *Exhaustion* was assessed according to a question from the World Health Organization World Mental Health Composite International Diagnostic Interview (WHO WMH-CIDI). The question took into account the definition and criteria for "depressive episode" diagnosis as specified in the International Statistical Classification of Diseases and Related Health Problems (ICD-10) and in the Diagnostic and Statistical Manual of Mental Disorders (DSM IV). It was used as a proxy for the depression-scale questions in the Center for Epidemiologic Studies Depression Scale (CES-D) used by Fried et al. in their definition of exhaustion. Subjects were specifically asked, "During the last 12 months, have you had a period lasting several days when you have been feeling your energy decreased or that you are tired all the time?" Those who gave a positive response were considered frail based on exhaustion.

(3) *Low physical activity* was determined according to the Global Physical Activity Questionnaire (GPAQ). It was measured by estimating the weekly caloric expenditure of respondents, stratified by sex. Those who fell within the fifth lowest percentile of weekly kilocalories, by sex, were considered frail based on physical activity.

(4) *Slow walking speed* was determined according to the time (seconds) it took participants to walk a distance of four meters at normal speed. Slow walking speed corresponded to a time span equal to or greater than the 80th percentile (in seconds), stratified by sex and median height.

(5) *Weakness* was measured with a dynamometer. Results were stratified by sex and quartiles of body mass index (BMI). We first considered maximum grip strength values, and then obtained quintiles for each BMI quartile. Low grip strength was equivalent to the lowest quintile in each BMI quartile by sex.

Covariates

Using the literature on factors associated with older adults' mortality and disability as a guide, risk factors were selected as potential covariates and then identified in the SAGE dataset. Covariates were categorized as follows: age, sex (1 = female), education (years of schooling), marital status (1 = with partner), place of residence (1 = rural), and household income using a continuous index based on household assets, where higher positive values indicated higher incomes.

Statistical analysis

We used bivariate analyses to examine the relationships between the independent variables (frailty and multimorbidity patterns) and the dependent variables (disability, quality of life and mortality). We employed the following tests: Chi-square for categorical variables and ANOVA or Kruskall-Wallis for continuous variables.

Multimorbidity patterns

As we were interested in the CDs combinations more than a simple count of them, we performed a principal-components analysis of the nine CDs mentioned above to identify possible multimorbidity patterns. Given that the CDs were coded dichotomously, we built a polychoric correlation matrix, with the optimal number of patterns (components) determined according to the rule of eigenvalues greater than one. Then each CD was assigned to the component where its coefficient yielded the highest factor loading (score).

Disability and quality of life

To assess the relationships of the multimorbidity patterns and frailty with (1) disability and (2) quality of life, we applied linear regression models.

Mortality

To analyze mortality, we explored participant survival time based on the Cox proportional hazards model. We performed exploratory analysis by estimating Kaplan-Meier curves for all categorical predictors, and log-rank test for equality of strata to assess the predictors in the final model. We selected model predictors according to the exploratory analysis and prior evidence on OA survival.

Finally, we assessed the interaction effects between frailty and each multimorbidity patterns. We tested the statistical significance of this potential interaction effect by including a multiplicative term between frailty and multimorbidity patterns into the three regression models.

Data were weighted using post-stratified individual probability weights based on the selection probability at each stage of selection. Differences were considered statistically significant if $p < 0.05$. All statistical analyses were performed using STATA version 15.1 software (StataCorp. 2017. College Station, TX.).

Results

Baseline characteristics

Table 1 presents the distribution of the study variables at baseline. Mean scores for WHODAS 2.0 and WHOQOL were 15.7 (SD = 16.3) and 47.4 (SD = 11.8) respectively. Meanwhile, prevalence rates for multimorbidity patterns were: 14.5% for cardiopulmonary, 68.3% for vascular-metabolic, and 21.5% for mental-musculoskeletal. Frailty prevalence was 7.9% and for pre-frailty was 58.0%.

Table 1 Baseline health and socio-demographic characteristics

	Mean/Percentage	S.D.
Outcomes		
Disability (WHODAS 2.0)[a]	15.7	16.3
Quality of life (WHOQOL)[b]	47.4	11.8
Main exposure variables		
Multimorbidity	34.5	
Multimorbidity patterns		
Pattern 1: Cardiopulmonary[c]	14.5	
Pattern 2: Vascular-metabolic[d]	68.3	
Pattern 3: Mental-musculoskeletal[e]	21.5	
Frailty		
Nonfrail	34.1	
Prefrail	58.0	
Frail	7.9	
Covariates		
Age (years)	63.0	10.6
Female	53.2	
Marital status (with partner)	73.0	
Education (years)	5.0	4.5
Residence (rural)	21.2	
Income	0.09	0.41

[a]WHODAS 2.0 (0 = no disability, 100 = total disability); [b]WHOQOL (0 = worst quality of life, 100 = best quality of life); [c]Pattern 1: chronic obstructive pulmonary disease, asthma and angina; [d]Pattern 2: diabetes, hypertension, stroke and cataracts; [e]Pattern 3: arthritis and depression

Multimorbidity patterns

We identified three multimorbidity patterns that explained 55% of the variance among the nine CDs analyzed. Pattern 1, cardiopulmonary conditions, included angina, chronic obstructive pulmonary disease, and asthma; Pattern 2, metabolic-vascular conditions, included diabetes, arterial hypertension, stroke and cataracts; and Pattern 3, mental-musculoskeletal conditions, included arthritis and depression (see Additional file 1: Figure S1 and Table S1).

Table 2 displays the bivariate associations of frailty and multimorbidity with disability, quality of life and all-cause mortality.

Disability

The presence of frailty was associated with disability, pre-frail and frail subjects indicating a higher average WHODAS score ($p < 0.001$). As regards multimorbidity patterns, cardiopulmonary conditions ($p < 0.001$) and mental-musculoskeletal conditions ($p < 0.001$) were also associated with greater disability.

Quality of life

Lower quality of life was observed in pre-frail and frail subjects ($p < 0.001$). Furthermore, the presence cardiopulmonary

Table 2 Bivariate associations of frailty and multimorbidity with disability, quality of life and all-cause mortality

Main exposure variables	Disability (WHODAS 2.0)[a] $n = 1410$		Quality of life (WHOQOL)[b] $n = 1410$		Mortality $n = 1792$	
	Mean	*p value*	Mean	*p value*	Percentage	*p value*
Frailty						
Nonfrail	8.7	*< 0.001*	56	*< 0.001*	4.3	*< 0.001*
Prefrail	19.4		51.1		10.2	
Frail	26.1		51.5		29.6	
Multimorbidity patterns						
Pattern 1: Cardiopulmonary[c]						
Presence	20.9	*< 0.001*	50.2	*< 0.001*	10.4	*0.966*
Absence	14.6		53.5		9.7	
Pattern 2: Vascular-metabolic[d]						
Presence	14.8	*< 0.001*	53.4	*0.004*	12.8	*< 0.001*
Absence	16.8		52.2		3.6	
Pattern 3: Mental-musculoskeletal[e]						
Presence	21.9	*< 0.001*	46	*< 0.001*	6.5	*0.751*
Absence	13.6		55.1		10.8	

[a]WHODAS 2.0 (0 = no disability, 100 = total disability); [b]WHOQOL (0 = worst quality of life, 100 = best quality of life); [c]Pattern 1: chronic obstructive pulmonary disease, asthma and angina; [d]Pattern 2: diabetes, hypertension, stroke and cataracts; [e]Pattern 3: arthritis and depression

conditions ($p < 0.001$) or mental-musculoskeletal conditions ($p < 0.001$) was associated with lower WHOQOL scores.

Mortality

Mortality was greater among frail (29.6%) and pre-frail (10.2%) OA as compared to those who were not frail (4.3%) ($p < 0.001$). Those exhibiting metabolic-vascular conditions had a higher mortality rate in comparison with those not suffering from these conditions: 12.8% versus 3.6% (< 0.001).

Table 3 shows the results of three regression models used to estimate the association between our main exposures (frailty and multimorbidity) and the three outcomes: disability, quality of life, and mortality.

Regarding disability, the results showed that pre-frailty and frailty increased the level of disability. Compared to non-frail, WHODAS score increased five points among pre-frail ($\beta = 5.02$; 95% CI 3.24; 6.80), and 13 points for frails individuals ($\beta = 13.29$; 95% CI 9.81; 16.78). For multimorbidity patterns, OA with cardiopulmonary and mental-musculoskeletal conditions had an increase in WHODAS scores ($\beta = 5.05$, and $\beta = 5.10$, respectively) and those with vascular-metabolic conditions had a slightly minor increase ($\beta = 3.27$) (Model 1).

For the quality of life, pre-frail and frail individuals had lowest scores in WHOQOL than non-frail subjects ($\beta = -2.2$, and $\beta = -4.3$, respectively). Similarly, the three morbidity patterns diminished the mean WHOQOL

Table 3 Adjusted associations of frailty and multimorbidity with disability, quality of life and all-cause mortality

	Model 1 Disability (WHODAS 2.0)[a]		Model 2 Quality of life (WHOQOL)[b]		Model 3 Mortality	
	β	(95% CI)	β	(95% CI)	HR	(95% CI)
Frailty						
Nonfrail	Reference		Reference		Reference	
Prefrail	5.02	(3.24,6.80)*	−2.23	(−3.23,-1.24)*	1.48	(1.05,2.09)*
Frail	13.29	(9.81,16.78)*	−4.38	(−6.32,-2.43)*	1.68	(1.06,2.68)*
Multimorbidity patterns						
Pattern 1: Cardiopulmonary[c]	5.05	(2.86,7.25)*	−1.81	(−3.04,-0.58)*	0.82	(0.58,1.14)
Pattern 2: Vascular-metabolic[d]	3.27	(1.40,5.13)*	−1.3	(−2.34,-0.26)*	1.47	(1.03,2.10)*
Pattern 3: Mental-musculoskeletal[e]	5.1	(2.98,7.22)*	−2.99	(−4.17,-1.81)*	0.72	(0.52,1.01)

*$p < 0.05$; β: beta coefficient; HR: hazard ratio; CI: confidence interval. [a]WHODAS 2.0 (0 = no disability, 100 = total disability); [b]WHOQOL (0 = worst quality of life, 100 = best quality of life). [c]Pattern 1: chronic obstructive pulmonary disease, asthma and angina; [d]Pattern 2: diabetes, hypertension, stroke and cataracts; [e]Pattern 3: arthritis and depression. All models were adjusted for age, sex, marital status, education (years), residence, and household income; only the Cox proportional model for mortality risk was adjusted for these variables plus disability (WHODAS 2.0 score)

scores. Musculoskeletal conditions had the greatest effect (β = – 2.99; 95% IC -4.17;-1.81), meanwhile cardiopulmonary conditions (β = – 1.81, 95% CI -3.04,-0.58), and vascular-metabolic conditions (β = – 1.30, 95% CI -2.34,-0.26) had a moderately minor impact (Model 2).

Related to mortality, results of the Cox models showed that pre-frail OA had a risk of death 48% higher than that non-frail (HR = 1.48; 95% CI 1.05; 2.09), and for the frail subjects that risk was 68% higher (HR = 1.68; 95% CI 1.06; 2.68). For the three morbidity patterns analyzed, only vascular-metabolic condition was associated with an increased risk of death (HR = 1.47; 95% CI 1.03; 2.10) (Model 3). Figure 2 depicts graphically the results of the Cox models for our two exposures, frailty and multimorbidity patterns.

Finally, results showed that none interaction term (between frailty and multimorbidity patterns) proved statistically significant (see Additional file 2: Table S2).

Discussion

The results of this study show that frailty and multimorbidity were independently associated with the disability, quality of life and mortality after 5-years follow-up among a national sample of older Mexican adults. Frailty and multimorbidity rose the mean scores of the WHODAS and WHOQOL and also increased the risk of death. However, no significant interactions between frailty and multimorbidity were found.

Our study identified three multimorbidity patterns in Mexican OA, which were: cardiopulmonary, vascular-metabolic and mental-musculoskeletal. The evidence related to multimorbidity patterns has led us to conclude that these patterns are composed of diseases sharing a number of similarities from a clinical perspective.

Regarding the first pattern, cardiopulmonary condition, comprised of asthma, chronic obstructive pulmonary disease (COPD), and angina, a clinical and molecular link had been previously established [21, 22]. For the second pattern identified, vascular-metabolic conditions, evidence support the relationship between metabolic syndrome (chronic inflammation, adiposity, etc.) and aging. This pattern includes CDs such as diabetes, arterial hypertension, stroke and cataracts [23, 24]. Finally, the third pattern, comprising arthritis and depression

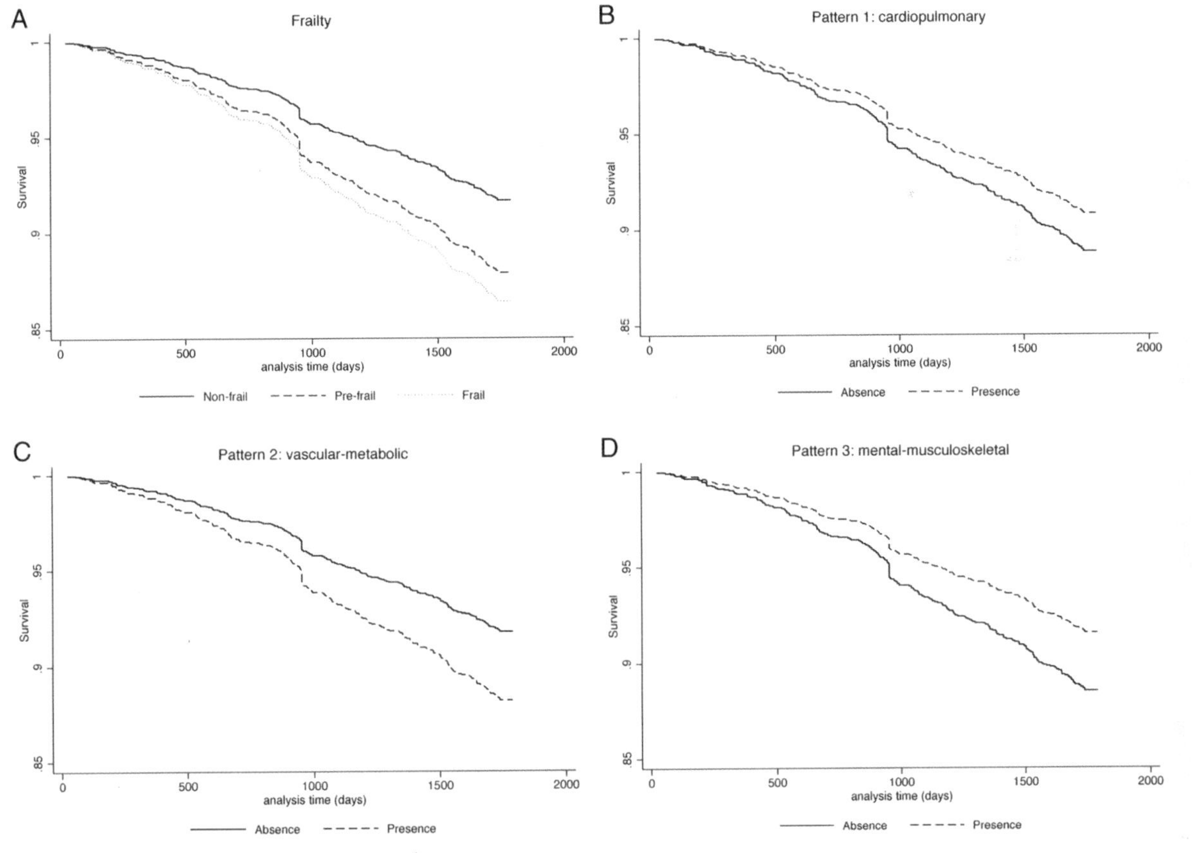

Fig. 2 Survival function for the Cox proportional hazard regression by (**a**) frailty categories (**b**) cardiopulmonary pattern; (**c**) vascular-metabolic pattern; and (**d**) mental-musculoskeletal pattern

(mental-musculoskeletal), can be explained by the link reported several decades ago between pain and mental illness, which suggests that they share a number of biological pathways [25–27].

Our findings indicate that the three multimorbidity patterns analyzed were independent predictors for increased disability among OA. These results are consistent with the studies that have analyzed this link taking multimorbidity patterns into account. Jackson et al. (2015) studied a cohort of older Australian women and found that patterns similar to mental-neurological and cardiopulmonary conditions were associated with higher levels of disability (measured by the basic and instrumental activities of daily life - ADL and IADL, respectively) [28]. Furthermore, Arokiasamy et al. reported an association between diabetes and hypertension combination and the presence of disability (+ 1 ADL) in adults 18 and older [5]. Otiniano et al. (2003) found that the combination of diabetes and stroke increased the risk of disability (1 + ADL and 1+ IADL) in Mexican-American OA aged 65 and older, at five-year follow-up [29]. Quinones et al. (2016) reported that the combination of arthritis, depression and hypertension in American OA was associated with higher levels of disability (combined ADL and IADL index) at two-year follow-up [30].

Frailty was also an independent predictor for disability. This finding is also consistent with those reported in the literature [9, 31], even allowing for different follow-up periods [8, 10, 32, 33]. In the Mexican context, at 11-year follow-up, the cohort of OA aged 60 years and older from the Mexican Health and Aging Study (MHAS) indicated that frailty was a predictor for disability as regards ADL, but not IADL, while pre-frailty was a predictor only for restricted mobility, but not for ADL or IADL [9]. Another study of urban OA aged 70 and older in the Mexican Coyoacan Cohort Study found that frailty increased ADL and IADL disability [31].

In our study disability was measured using the WHODAS 2.0, which traditionally has been done using ADL and IADL criteria in older adult population. The use of WHODAS allowed that functionality spectrum of OA was enhanced [34]. This means that vulnerability resulting from frailty in OA could affect other spheres beyond the physical dimension, inter alia, their interaction with others and their participation in society.

We also found that frailty and multimorbidity diminished the quality of life as measured in the follow-up study. These results are consistent with those of Arokiasamy et al., who reported that the combination of asthma and hypertension correlated with a diminished quality of life in adults aged 18 and older [5]. Moreover there is evidence that depression among OA is independently associated with a lower quality of life [35], and that adults with arthritis have a particularly high probability of suffering from a deteriorated quality of life [36].

Our results indicate that baseline frailty status were an independent predictor for a deteriorated quality of life in the follow-up. There is scarce longitudinal evidence of an association between frailty and quality of life [13, 37]. Even so, it has been hypothesized that this association could be bidirectional, baseline frailty could turns out to be predictive of a deteriorated quality of life, just as a low quality of life at baseline could be a predictor of frailty at follow-up [37]. Our results appears to provide support for the first scenario, which means that a decreased functionality among frail OA affects their satisfaction in various areas (physical and social) that are measured with instruments such as the WHOQOL [12, 13, 37]. However, this association must be deeply explored in future longitudinal studies with older adults.

Related to frailty and mortality, our results were consistent with previous studies that have identified frailty is an independent predictor for death. A systematic review and meta-analysis of longitudinal studies with OA using the frailty phenotype, found that frail subjects had a risk of dying two times higher than non-frail subjects. Pre-frailty also increased the risk of death, although the association was weaker [38]. For older Mexican adults, this association was also reported by various studies. Specifically, Mexican Health and Aging Study (*MHAS*) and 10/66 Dementia Study found that frailty was a predictor for death [9, 39].

Observed association between the metabolic-vascular pattern and mortality, supports the reported evidence on the relationship between metabolic syndrome and the likelihood of die [40], although recently it has been suggested that this association can be mediated by factors such as frailty [41, 42] and sleep disorders [43]. Nevertheless, even controlling for frailty, disability and other variables, it has been found that the metabolic-vascular combination has an independent effect on survival rate among OA.

A secondary objective of this study was to evaluate the potential interaction effects of multimorbidity and frailty. Although we did not find a significant interaction between these conditions, evidence suggests that a causal connection could exist, given they share common physiopathological mechanisms [15]. Even so, few studies have explored the possibility of a combined effect. Among them, Woo et al. (2014) found that combination of frailty and multimorbidity increased the risk of disability and death in OA [16]. Future research with OA that deeply explore on different combinations of chronic conditions will help to understand the potential interaction of frailty and multimorbidity and their effects on diverse health outcomes.

The results of our study should be interpreted taking into account the following limitations. First, the analysis of multimorbidity was confined to the nine high burden chronic conditions utilized in SAGE; it did not include diseases such as chronic kidney failure, cancer, cardiac conditions and dyslipidemia, all prevalent in older Mexican adults. Nevertheless, various studies using larger, equal or lower number of CDs, have found similar multimorbidity patterns. Second, potential selection bias may have resulted from differences between the analytical sample and excluded OA. Respondents in the study proved somewhat more affluent than respondents excluded (see Additional file 2: Table S3), it is not clear how this could affect our results, although it is possible that people with a higher economic level have greater knowledge about their health status, and then our prevalence of multimorbidity patterns could be underestimated. If the above were true, then our associations could be somewhat biased.

Conclusion

Our findings are consistent with previous evidence about the effects of frailty and multimorbidity on disability, quality of life, and risk of death. These results highlight the importance of carrying out health promotion and prevention actions as well as specific interventions aimed at older adults who suffer from multimorbidity and frailty, in such a way that deleterious effects on health can be avoided. Although a potential interaction effect between frailty and multimorbidity was hypothesized, this association was not statistically significant.

Abbreviations

ADL: Basic activities of daily life; BMI: Body mass index; CDs: Chronic diseases; CES-D: Center for Epidemiologic Studies Depression Scale; CI: Confidence Interval; COPD: Chronic obstructive pulmonary disease; DSM IV: Diagnostic and Statistical Manual of Mental Disorders; GPAQ: Global Physical Activity Questionnaire; HR: Hazard Ratio; IADL: Instrumental activities of daily life; ICD-10: International Statistical Classification of Diseases and Related Health Problems; MHAS: Mexican Health and Aging Study; NS: Not Statistically significant; OA: Older adults; SAGE: Study on global AGEing and adult health; SF-36: 36-Item Short Form Health Survey; WHO WMH-CIDI: World Health Organization World Mental Health Composite International Diagnostic Interview; WHO: World Health Organization; WHODAS 2.0: World Health Organization Disability Assessment Schedule 2.0; WHOQOL: WHO Quality of Life; β: Beta Coefficient

Funding

SAGE is supported by WHO and the US National Institute on Aging through Interagency Agreements (OGHA04034785, YA1323-08-CN-0020, and Y1-AG-1005-01) and competitive grant: R01AG034479.

Authors' contributions

ARA, BME and ASR conceived and designed the study; ARA and ASR carried out the analysis; ARA, and ASR drafted the manuscript. All authors reviewed, edited, and contributed to rewriting of the manuscript. All the authors granted final approval to the version submitted for publication.

Competing interests

The authors declare that they have no competing interests.

Author details

[1]National Institute of Public Health, Avenida Universidad #655, Colonia Santa María Ahuacatitlán, ZC, 62100 Cuernavaca, Morelos, Mexico. [2]Department of Geriatrics, Salvador Zubirán National Institute of Medical Sciences and Nutrition, Mexico City, Mexico. [3]Department of Health Statistics and Information Systems, World Health Organization, Geneva, Switzerland. [4]University of Newcastle Research Centre on Gender, Health and Ageing, Newcastle, Australia. [5]Chiang Mai University Research Institute for Health Sciences, Chiang Mai, Thailand.

References

1. United Nations, Department of Economic and Social Affairs PD. World Population Prospects: The 2015 Revision, Key Findings and Advance Tables. 2015. Report No.: ESA/P/WP.241. Available from: https://esa.un.org/unpd/wpp/publications/files/key_findings_wpp_2015.pdf
2. Prince MJ, Wu F, Guo Y, Gutierrez Robledo LM, O'Donnell M, Sullivan R, et al. The burden of disease in older people and implications for health policy and practice. Lancet. 2015:549–62.
3. Beard JR, Bloom DE. Towards a comprehensive public health response to population ageing. Lancet. 2015;385:658–61.
4. Marengoni A, Angleman S, Melis R, Mangialasche F, Karp A, Garmen A, et al. Aging with multimorbidity: a systematic review of the literature. Ageing Res Rev. 2011:430–9.
5. Arokiasamy P, Uttamacharya U, Jain K, Biritwum RB, Yawson AE, Wu F, et al. The impact of multimorbidity on adult physical and mental health in low- and middle-income countries: what does the study on global ageing and adult health (SAGE) reveal? BMC Med. 2015;13.
6. Salive ME. Multimorbidity in older adults. Epidemiol Rev. 2013;35:75–83.
7. Prados-Torres A, Calderón-Larrañaga A, Hancco-Saavedra J, Poblador-Plou B, Van Den Akker M. Multimorbidity patterns: a systematic review. J Clin Epidemiol. 2014:254–66.
8. Fried LP, Tangen CM, Walston J, Newman AB, Hirsch C, Gottdiener J, et al. Frailty in Older Adults: Evidence for a Phenotype. Journals Gerontol Ser A Biol Sci Med Sci [Internet]. 2001;56:M146–57. Available from: https://academic.oup.com/biomedgerontology/article-lookup/doi/10.1093/gerona/56.3.M146
9. Aguilar-Navarro SG, Amieva H, Gutiérrez-Robledo LM, Avila-Funes JA. Frailty among Mexican community-dwelling elderly: a story told 11 years later. The Mexican health and aging study. Salud Publica Mex. 2015;57:S62–9.
10. Vermeulen J, Neyens JC, Van Rossum E, Spreeuwenberg MD, De Witte LP. Predicting ADL disability in community-dwelling elderly people using physical frailty indicators: a systematic review. BMC Geriatr. 2011;11.
11. Shamliyan T, Talley KMC, Ramakrishnan R, Kane RL. Association of frailty with survival: a systematic literature review. Ageing Res Rev. 2013:719–36.
12. Kojima G, Iliffe S, Morris RW, Taniguchi Y, Kendrick D, Skelton DA, et al. Frailty predicts trajectories of quality of life over time among British community-dwelling older people. Qual Life Res. 2016:1743–50.
13. Moreno-Aguilar M, García-Lara JMA, Aguilar-Navarro S, Navarrete-Reyes AP, Amieva H, Avila-Funes JA. the Phenotype of Frailty and Health-Related Quality of Life. J Frailty Aging. 2013;2:1–6.
14. Kojima G. Frailty as a predictor of future falls among community-dwelling older people: a systematic review and meta-analysis. J Am Med Dir Assoc. 2015:1027–33.
15. Fried LP, Ferrucci L, Darer J, Williamson JD, Anderson G. Untangling the Concepts of Disability, Frailty, and Comorbidity: Implications for Improved Targeting and Care. Journals Gerontol Ser A Biol Sci Med Sci [Internet]. 2004;59:M255–63. Available from: https://academic.oup.com/biomedgerontology/article-lookup/doi/10.1093/gerona/59.3.M255
16. Woo J, Leung J. Multi-morbidity, dependency, and frailty singly or in combination have different impact on health outcomes. Age (Omaha). 2014;36:923–31.
17. Kowal P, Chatterji S, Naidoo N, Biritwum R, Fan W, Ridaura RL, et al. Data resource profile: the world health organization study on global ageing and adult health (SAGE). Int J Epidemiol. 2012;41:1639–49.
18. Ustün TB, Chatterji S, Kostanjsek N, Rehm J, Kennedy C, Epping-Jordan J, et al. Developing the World Health Organization Disability Assessment Schedule 2.0. Bull World Health Organ. 2010;88:815–823. PMCID: PMC2971503. Available from: http://www.who.int/bulletin/volumes/88/11/09-067231/en/.

19. Skevington SM, Lotfy M, O'Connell KA. The World Health Organization's WHOQOL-BREF quality of life assessment: psychometric properties and results of the international field trial a report from the WHOQOL group. Qual Life Res. 2004:299–310.
20. Garin N, Koyanagi A, Chatterji S, Tyrovolas S, Olaya B, Leonardi M, et al. Global multimorbidity patterns: a cross-sectional, population-based, multi-country study. Journals Gerontol - Ser A Biol Sci Med Sci. 2016;71:205–14.
21. Sin DD. Asthma-COPD overlap syndrome: what we know and what we don't. Tuberc. Respir. Dis (Seoul). 2017;80:11–20.
22. Rothnie KJ, Yan R, Smeeth L, Quint JK. Risk of myocardial infarction (MI) and death following MI in people with chronic obstructive pulmonary disease (COPD): a systematic review and meta-analysis. BMJ Open. 2015.
23. Morley JE. The metabolic syndrome and aging. J Gerontol A Biol Sci Med Sci. 2004 [cited 2018 mar 21];59:139–42. Available from: https://academic.oup.com/biomedgerontology/article/59/2/M139/610275.
24. Denys K, Cankurtaran M, Janssens W, Petrovic M. Metabolic syndrome in the elderly: an overview of the evidence. Acta Clin Belg. 2009;64:23–34.
25. Von Korff M, Simon G. The relationship between pain and depression. Br J Psychiatry. 1996;168:101–8.
26. Salazar A, Dueñas M, Ojeda B, Failde I. Association of painful musculoskeletal conditions and migraine headache with mental and sleep disorders among adults with disabilities, Spain, 2007–2008. Prev Chronic Dis. 2014;11:E30. Available from: https://www.ncbi.nlm.nih.gov/pmc/articles/PMC3938964/.
27. Bair MJ, Robinson RL, Katon W, Kroenke K. Depression and pain comorbidity: a literature review. Arch Intern Med. 2003:2433–45.
28. Jackson CA, Jones M, Tooth L, Mishra GD, Byles J, Dobson A. Multimorbidity patterns are differentially associated with functional ability and decline in a longitudinal cohort of older women. Age Ageing. 2015;44:810–6.
29. Otiniano ME, Du XL, Ottenbacher K, Markides KS. The effect of diabetes combined with stroke on disability, self-rated health, and mortality in older Mexican Americans: Results from the Hispanic EPESE. Arch Phys Med Rehabil [Internet]. 2003;84:as0003999303049419. Available from: https://www.sciencedirect.com/science/article/pii/S0003999302049419?via%3Dihub.
30. Quiñones AR, Markwardt S, Botoseneanu A. Multimorbidity combinations and disability in older adults. Journals Gerontol - Ser A Biol Sci Med Sci. 2016;71:823–30.
31. Avila-Funes JA, Medina-Campos RH, Tamez-Rivera O, Navarrete-Reyes AP, Amieva H, Aguilar-Navarro S. Frailty is associated with disability and recent hospitalization in community-dwelling elderly: the Coyoacan cohort. J frailty aging. 2014;3:206–10 Available from: http://www.ncbi.nlm.nih.gov/pubmed/27048858.
32. Papachristou E, Wannamethee SG, Lennon LT, Papacosta O, Whincup PH, Iliffe S, et al. Ability of self-reported frailty components to predict incident disability, falls, and all-cause mortality: results from a population-based study of older British men. J Am Med Dir Assoc. 2017;18:152–7.
33. Makizako H, Shimada H, Doi T, Tsutsumimoto K, Suzuki T. Impact of physical frailty on disability in community-dwelling older adults: a prospective cohort study. BMJ Open. 2015;5.
34. Cieza A, Sabariego C, Bickenbach J, Chatterji S. Rethinking Disability. BMC Med. 2018;16.
35. Sivertsen H, Bjørkløf GH, Engedal K, Selbæk G, Helvik AS. Depression and quality of life in older persons: a review. Dement Geriatr Cogn Disord. 2015: 311–39.
36. Senra H, Rogers H, Leibach G, Altamar MLP, Plaza SLO, Perrin P, et al. Health-related quality of life and depression in a sample of Latin American adults with rheumatoid arthritis. Int J Rheum Dis. 2014.
37. Kojima G, Iliffe S, Jivraj S, Walters K. Association between frailty and quality of life among community-dwelling older people: a systematic review and meta-analysis. J Epidemiol Community Health. 2016:716–21.
38. Chang S-F, Lin P-L. Frail phenotype and mortality prediction: a systematic review and meta-analysis of prospective cohort studies. Int J Nurs Stud [Internet]. 2015;52:1362–74 Available from: http://linkinghub.elsevier.com/retrieve/pii/S0020748915001066.
39. At J, Bryce R, Prina M, Acosta D, Ferri CP, Guerra M, et al. Frailty and the prediction of dependence and mortality in low- and middle-income countries: a 10/66 population-based cohort study. BMC Med. 2015;13:138.
40. Forti P, Pirazzoli G. Metabolic syndrome and all-cause mortality in older men and women. Eur J. 2012;42:1000–9. Available from: https://onlinelibrary.wiley.com/doi/abs/10.1111/j.1365-2362.2012.02688.x.
41. Kane AE, Gregson E, Theou O, Rockwood K, Howlett SE. The association between frailty, the metabolic syndrome, and mortality over the lifespan. GeroScience. 2017;39:221–9.
42. Hoogendijk EO, Huisman M, van Ballegooijen AJ. The role of frailty in explaining the association between the metabolic syndrome and mortality in older adults. Exp Gerontol. 2017;91:5–8.
43. Fernandez-Mendoza J, He F, LaGrotte C, Vgontzas AN, Liao D, Bixler EO. Impact of the metabolic syndrome on mortality is modified by objective short sleep duration. J Am Heart Assoc. 2017;6.

8

A mixed methods case study exploring the impact of membership of a multi-activity, multicentre community group on social wellbeing of older adults

Gabrielle Lindsay-Smith[1*], Grant O'Sullivan[1], Rochelle Eime[1,2], Jack Harvey[1,2] and Jannique G. Z. van Uffelen[1,3]

Abstract

Background: Social wellbeing factors such as loneliness and social support have a major impact on the health of older adults and can contribute to physical and mental wellbeing. However, with increasing age, social contacts and social support typically decrease and levels of loneliness increase. Group social engagement appears to have additional benefits for the health of older adults compared to socialising individually with friends and family, but further research is required to confirm whether group activities can be beneficial for the social wellbeing of older adults.

Methods: This one-year longitudinal mixed methods study investigated the effect of joining a community group, offering a range of social and physical activities, on social wellbeing of adults with a mean age of 70. The study combined a quantitative survey assessing loneliness and social support ($n = 28$; three time-points, analysed using linear mixed models) and a qualitative focus group study ($n = 11$, analysed using thematic analysis) of members from Life Activities Clubs Victoria, Australia.

Results: There was a significant reduction in loneliness ($p = 0.023$) and a trend toward an increase in social support ($p = 0.056$) in the first year after joining. The focus group confirmed these observations and suggested that social support may take longer than 1 year to develop. Focus groups also identified that group membership provided important opportunities for developing new and diverse social connections through shared interest and experience. These connections were key in improving the social wellbeing of members, especially in their sense of feeling supported or connected and less lonely. Participants agreed that increasing connections was especially beneficial following significant life events such as retirement, moving to a new house or partners becoming unwell.

Conclusions: Becoming a member of a community group offering social and physical activities may improve social wellbeing in older adults, especially following significant life events such as retirement or moving-house, where social network changes. These results indicate that ageing policy and strategies would benefit from encouraging long-term participation in social groups to assist in adapting to changes that occur in later life and optimise healthy ageing.

Keywords: Ageing, Social support, Social engagement, Friendship, Loneliness, Retirement, Group activity

* Correspondence: gabrielle.lindsaysmith@live.vu.edu.au
[1]Institute for Health and Sport, Victoria University, Melbourne, Australia
Full list of author information is available at the end of the article

Background

Ageing population and the need to age well

Between 2015 and 2050 it is predicted that globally the number of adults over the age of 60 will more than double [1]. Increasing age is associated with a greater risk of chronic illnesses such as cardio vascular disease and cancer [2] and reduced functional capacity [3, 4]. Consequently, an ageing population will continue to place considerable pressure on the health care systems.

However, it is also important to consider the individuals themselves and self-perceived good health is very important for the individual wellbeing and life-satisfaction of older adults [5]. The terms "successful ageing" [6] and "healthy ageing" [5] have been used to define a broader concept of ageing well, which not only includes factors relating to medically defined health but also wellbeing. Unfortunately, there is no agreed definition for what exactly constitutes healthy or successful ageing, with studies using a range of definitions. A review of 28 quantitative studies found that successful ageing was defined differently in each, with the majority only considering measures of disability or physical functioning. Social and wellbeing factors were included in only a few of the studies [7].

In contrast, qualitative studies of older adults' opinions on successful ageing have found that while good physical and mental health and maintaining physical activity levels are agreed to assist successful ageing, being independent or doing something of value, acceptance of ageing, life satisfaction, social connectedness or keeping socially active were of greater importance [8–10].

In light of these findings, the definition that is most inclusive is "healthy ageing" defined by the World Health Organisation as "the process of developing and maintaining the functional ability (defined as a combination of intrinsic capacity and physical and social environmental characteristics), that enables well-being in older age" (p28) [5].This definition, and those provided in the research of older adults' perceptions of successful ageing, highlight social engagement and social support as important factors contributing to successful ageing, in addition to being important social determinants of health [11, 12].

Social determinants of health, including loneliness and social support, are important predictors of physical, cognitive and mental health and wellbeing in adults [12] and older adults [13–15]. Loneliness is defined as a perception of an inadequacy in the quality or quantity of one's social relationships [16]. Social support, has various definitions but generally it relates to social relationships that are reciprocal, accessible and reliable and provide any or a combination of supportive resources (e.g. emotional, information, practical) and can be measured as perceived or received support [17]. These types of social determinants differ from those related to inequality (health gap social determinants) and are sometimes referred to as 'social cure' social determinants [11]. They will be referred to as 'social wellbeing' outcome measures in this study.

Unfortunately, with advancing age, there is often diminishing social support, leading to social isolation and loneliness [18, 19]. Large nationally representative studies of adults and older adults reported that social activity predicted maintenance or improvement of life satisfaction as well as physical activity levels [20], however older adults spent less time in social activity than middle age adults.

Social wellbeing and health

A number of longitudinal studies have found that social isolation for older adults is a significant predictor of mortality and institutionalisation [21–23]. A meta-analysis by Holt-Lunstadt [12] reported that social determinants of health, including social integration and social support (including loneliness and lack of perceived social support) to be equal to, or a greater risk to mortality as common behavioural risk factors such as smoking, physical inactivity and obesity. Loneliness is independently associated with poor physical and mental health in the general population, and especially in older adults [13–15]. Adequate perceived social support has also been consistently associated with improved mental and physical health in both general and older adults [20, 24–29]. The mechanism suggested for this association is that social support buffers the negative impacts of stressful situations and life events [30]. The above research demonstrates the benefit of social engagement for older adults; in turn this highlights the importance of strategies that reduce loneliness and improve social support and social connectedness for older adults.

Socialising in groups seems to be especially important for the health and wellbeing of older adults who may be adjusting to significant life events [26, 31–33]. This is sometimes referred to as social engagement or social companionship [26, 30, 31]. It seems that the mechanism enabling such health benefits with group participation is through strengthening of social identification, which in turn increases social support [31, 34, 35]. Furthermore, involvement in community groups can be a sustainable strategy to reduce loneliness and increase social support in older adults, as they are generally low cost and run by volunteers [36–39].

Despite the demonstrated importance of social factors for successful ageing and the established risk associated with reduced social engagement as people age, few in-depth studies have longitudinally investigated the impact of community groups on social wellbeing. For example, a non-significant increase in social support and reduction in depression was found in a year-long randomised controlled trial conducted in senior centres in

Norway with lonely older adults in poor physical and mental health [37]. Some qualitative studies have reported that community groups and senior centres can contribute to fun and socialisation for older adults, however social wellbeing was not the primary focus of the studies [38, 40, 41]. Given that social wellbeing is a broad and important area for the health and quality of life in older adults, an in-depth study is warranted to understand how it can be maximised in older adults. This mixed methods case study of an existing community aims to: i) examine whether loneliness and social support of new members of Life Activities Clubs (LACs) changes in the year after joining and ii) conduct an in-depth exploration of how social wellbeing changes in new and longer-term members of LACs.

Methods

Design

A mixed methods study was chosen as the design for this research to enable an in-depth exploration of how loneliness and social support may change as a result of joining a community group. A case study was conducted using a concurrent mixed-methods design, with a qualitative component giving context to the quantitative results. Where the survey focused on the impact of group membership on social support and loneliness, the focus groups were an open discussion of the benefits in the lived context of LAC membership. The synthesis of the two sections of the study was undertaken at the time of interpretation of the results [42].

The two parts of our study were as follows:

a) a longitudinal survey (three time points over 1 year: baseline, 6 and 12 months). This part of the study formed the quantitative results;
b) a focus group study of members of the same organisation (qualitative).

Ethics approval to conduct this study was obtained from the Victoria University Human Research Ethics Committee (HRE14–071 [survey] and HRE15–291 [focus groups]) All participants provided informed consent to partake in the study prior to undertaking the first survey or focus group.

Setting and participants

Life activities clubs Victoria

Life Activities Clubs Victoria (LACVI) is a large not-for-profit group with 23 independently run Life Activities Clubs (LACs) based in both rural and metropolitan Victoria. It has approximately 4000 members. The organisation was established to assist in providing physical, social and recreational activities as well as education and motivational support to older adults managing significant change in their lives, especially retirement.

Survey

Eighteen out of 23 LAC clubs agreed to take part in the survey study. During the sampling period from May 2014 to December 2016, new members from the participating clubs were given information about the study and invited to take part. Invitations took place in the form of flyers distributed with new membership material.

Inclusion/ exclusion criteria Community-dwelling older adults who self-reported that they could walk at least 100 m and who were new members to LACVI and able to complete a survey in English were eligible to participate. New members were defined as people who had never been members of LACVI or who had not been members in the last 2 years.

To ensure that the cohort of participants were of a similar functional level, people with significant health problems limiting them from being able to walk 100 m were excluded from participating in the study.

Once informed consent was received, the participants were invited to complete a self-report survey in either paper or online format (depending on preference). This first survey comprised the baseline data and the same survey was completed 6 months and 12 months after this initial time point. Participants were sent reminders if they had not completed each survey more than 2 weeks after each was delivered and then again 1 week later.

Focus groups

Two focus groups (FGs) were conducted with new and longer-term members of LACs. The first FG ($n = 6$) consisted of members who undertook physical activity in their LAC (e.g. walking groups, tennis, cycling). The second FG ($n = 5$) consisted of members who took part in activities with a non-physical activity (PA) focus (e.g. book groups, social groups, craft or cultural groups). LACs offer both social and physical activities and it was important to the study to capture both types of groups, but they were kept separate to assist participants in feeling a sense of commonality with other members and improving group dynamic and participation in the discussions [43]. Of the people who participated in the longitudinal survey study, seven also participated in the FGs.

The FG interviews were facilitated by one researcher (GLS) and notes around non-verbal communication, moments of divergence and convergence amongst group members, and other notable items were taken by a second researcher (GOS). Both researchers wrote additional notes after the focus groups and these were used in the analysis of themes. Focus groups were recorded and later transcribed verbatim by a professional transcriptionist, including identification of each participant speaking. One researcher (GLS) reviewed each transcription to check for any errors and made any required modifications before importing the transcriptions into NVivo for analysis. The transcriber identified each focus group participant so themes for individuals or other age or gender specific trends could be identified.

Dependent variables

Social support

Social support was assessed using the Duke–UNC Functional Social support questionnaire [44]. This scale specifically measures participant perceived functional social support in two areas; i) confidant support (5 questions; e.g. chances to talk to others) and ii) affective support (3 questions; e.g. people who care about them). Participants rated each component of support on a 5-item likert scale between *'much less than I would like'* (1 point) to *'as much as I would like'* (5 points). The total score used for analysis was the mean of the eight scores (low social support = 1, maximum social support = 5). Construct validity, concurrent validity and discriminant validity are acceptable for confidant and affective support items in the survey in the general population [44].

Loneliness

Loneliness was measured using the de Jong Gierveld and UCLA-3 item loneliness scales developed for use in many populations including older adults [45]. The 11-item de Jong Gierveld loneliness scale (DJG loneliness) [46] is a multi-dimensional measure of loneliness and contains five positively worded and six negatively worded items. The items fall into four subscales; feelings of severe loneliness, feelings connected with specific problem situations, missing companionship, feelings of belongingness. The total score is the sum of the items scores (i.e. 11–55): 11 is low loneliness and 55 is severe loneliness. Self-administered versions of this scale have good internal consistency (> = 0.8) and inter-item homogeneity and person scalability that is as good or better than when conducted as face-to face interviews. The validity and reliability for the scale is adequate [47]. The UCLA 3-item loneliness scale consists of three questions about how often participants feel they lack companionship, feel left out and feel isolated. The responses are given on a three-point scale ranging from hardly ever (1) to often (3). The final score is the sum of these three items with the range being from lowest loneliness (3) to highest loneliness (9). Reliability of the scale is good, (alpha = 0.72) as are discriminant validity and internal consistency [48]. The scale is commonly used to measure loneliness with older adults ([49] – review), [50, 51].

Sociodemographic variables

The following sociodemographic characteristics were collected in both the survey and the focus groups: age, sex, highest level of education, main life occupation [52], current employment, ability to manage on income available, present marital status, country of birth, area of residence [53]. They are categorised as indicated in Table 2.

Health variables

The following health variables were collected: *Self-rated general health (from SF-12)* [54] and *Functional health (ability to walk 100 m- formed part of the inclusion criteria)* [55]. See Table 2 for details about the categories of these variables.

Analysis

Survey

The effects of becoming a member on quantitative outcome variables (i.e. Social support, DJG loneliness and UCLA loneliness) were analysed using linear mixed models (LMM). LMM enabled testing for the presence of intra-subject random effects, or equivalently, correlation of subjects' measures over time (baseline, 6-months and 12 months). Three correlation structures were examined: independence (no correlation), compound symmetry (constant correlation of each subjects' measures over the three time points) and autoregressive (correlation diminishing with increase in spacing in time). The best fitting correlation structure was compound symmetry; this is equivalent to a random intercept component for each subject. The LMM incorporated longitudinal trends over time, with adjustment for age as a potential confounder. Statistical analyses were conducted using SPSS for windows (v24).

UCLA loneliness and social support residuals were not normally distributed and these scales were Log10 transformed for statistical analysis.

Analyses were all adjusted for age, group attendance (calculated as average attendance at 6 and 12 months) and employment status at baseline (Full-time, Part-time, not working).

Focus groups

Focus group transcripts were analysed using thematic analysis [56, 57], a flexible qualitative methodology that can be used with a variety of epistemologies, approaches and analysis methods [56]. The transcribed data were analysed using a combination of theoretical and inductive thematic analysis [56]. It was theorised that membership in a LAC would assist with social factors relating to healthy ageing [5], possibly through a social identity pathway [58], although we wanted to explore this. Semantic themes were drawn from these codes in order to conduct a pragmatic evaluation of the LACVI programs

[56]. Analytic rigour in the qualitative analysis was ensured through source and analyst triangulation. Transcriptions were compared to notes taken during the focus groups by the researchers (GOS and GLS). In addition, Initial coding and themes (by GLS) were checked by a second researcher (GOS) and any disagreements regarding coding and themes were discussed prior to finalisation of codes and themes [57].

Results

Survey

Sociodemographic and health characteristics of the 28 participants who completed the survey study are reported in Table 1. The mean age of the participants was 66.9 and 75% were female. These demographics are representative of the entire LACVI membership. Education levels varied, with 21% being university educated, and the remainder completing high school or technical certificates. Two thirds of participants were not married. Some sociodemographic characteristics changed slightly at 6 and 12 months, mainly employment (18% in paid employment at baseline and 11% at 12-months) and ability to manage on income (36% reporting trouble managing on their income at baseline and 46% at 12 months). Almost 90% of the participants described themselves as being in good-excellent health.

Types of activities

There were a variety of types of activities that participants took part in: physical activities such as walking groups ($n = 7$), table tennis ($n = 5$), dancing class ($n = 2$), exercise class ($n = 1$), bowls ($n = 2$), golf ($n = 3$), cycling groups ($n = 1$) and non-physical leisure activities such as art and literature groups ($n = 5$), craft groups ($n = 5$), entertainment groups ($n = 12$), food/dine out groups ($n = 18$) and other sedentary leisure activities (e.g. mah jong, cards),($n = 4$). A number of people took part in more than one activity.

Frequency of attendance at LACVI and changes in social wellbeing

At six and 12 months, participants indicated how many times in the last month they attended different types of activities at their LAC. Most participants maintained the same frequency of participation over both time points. Only four people participated more frequently at 12 than at 6 months and nine reduced participation levels. The latter group included predominantly those who reduced from more than two times per week at 6 months to 2×/week at 6 months to one to two times per week ($n = 5$) or less than one time per week ($n = 2$) at 12 months. Average weekly club attendance at six and 12 months was included as a covariate in the statistical model.

Outcome measures

Overall, participants reported moderate social support and loneliness levels at baseline (See Table 2). Loneliness, as measured by both scales, reduced significantly over time. There was a significant effect of time on the DJG loneliness scores ($F(2, 52) = 3.83$, $p = 0.028$), with Post-Hoc analysis indicating a reduction in DJG loneliness between baseline and 12 months ($p = 0.008$). UCLA loneliness scores (transformed variable) also changed significantly over time ($F(2, 52) = 4.08$, $p = 0.023$). Post hoc tests indicated a reduction in UCLA loneliness between baseline and 6 months ($p = 0.007$). There was a small non-significant increase in social support ($F(2, 53) = 2.88$, $p = 0.065$) during the first year of membership (see Table 2 and Figs. 1 and 2).

Focus groups

In total, 11 participants attended the two focus groups, six people who participated in PA clubs (four women) and five who participated in social clubs (all women). All focus group participants were either retired ($n = 9$) or semi-retired ($n = 2$). The mean age of participants was 67 years (see Table 2 for further details). Most of the participants (82%) had been members of a LAC for less than 2 years and two females in the social group had been members of LAC clubs for 5 and 10 years respectively.

Analysis of the focus group transcripts identified two themes relating to social benefits of group participation; i) Social resources and ii) Social wellbeing (see Fig. 3). Group discussion suggested that membership of a LAC provides access to more social resources through greater and diverse social contact and opportunity. It is through this improvement in social resources that social wellbeing may improve.

Social resources

The social resources theme referred to an increase in the availability and variety of social connections that resulted from becoming a member of a LAC. The social nature of the groups enabled an expansion and diversification of members' social network and improved their sense of social connectedness. There was widespread agreement in both the focus groups that significant life events, especially retirement, illness or death of spouse and moving house changes one's social resources. Membership of the LAC had benefits especially at these times and these events were often motivators to join such a club. Most participants found that their social resources declined after retirement and even felt that they were grieving for the loss of their work.

> *"I just saw work as a collection of, um, colleagues as opposed to friends. I had a few good friends there. Most were simply colleagues or acquaintances ....*

Table 1 Sociodemographic and health characteristics of survey and focus group respondents at baseline

Sociodemographic characteristics		Survey respondents ($n = 28$)	Focus groups ($n = 11$)
Age in years, mean (SD)		66.9 (9.0)	67.1 (5.9)
Sex, n (%)	Male	7 (25)	2 (18)
	Female	21 (75)	9 (82)
Highest level of education, n (%)	Completed primary school	0 (0)	1 (9)
	Up to year 12	10 (36)	3 (27)
	Technical studies/ trade certificate	10 (36)	4 (36)
	Tertiary studies	6 (21)	3 (27)
	Missing	2 (7)	0
Main life occupation, n (%)	Manager	4 (14)	2 (18)
	Professional	10 (36)	4 (3)
	Clerical	9 (32)	5 (45)
	Trade, production or labour	5 (18)	0
Current employment, n (%)	Full-time	2 (7)	0
	Part-time/casual	3 (11)	2 (18)
	Not in paid employment	23 (82)	9 (81)
Ability to manage on Income, n (%)	Very difficult	2 (7)	0
	Somewhat difficult	8 (29)	3 (27)
	Not difficult	18 (64)	8 (18)
Present marital status, n (%)	Not married	17 (61)	8 (73)
	Married/defacto	11 (40)	3 (27)
Country of birth, n (%)	Australia	23 (82)	8 (73)
	Other	5 (18)	3 (27)
Area of residence, n (%)	Urban	23 (82)	9 (82)
	Rural	5 (18)	2 (18)
Health			
General health, n (%)	Very good- excellent	16 (57)	NA
	Good	9 (32)	NA
	Fair	3 (11)	NA
Functional health (Walking limitation), n (%)	Some limitation	2 (7)	NA
	No limitation	26 (93)	NA

Table 2 Means and standard errors for social wellbeing variables over time

Variable	Baseline ($n = 28$)	6 months ($n = 27$)	12 months ($n = 28$)	p-value
Duke social support[a]	3.83 (0.2)	4.08 (0.2)	4.09 (0.2)	0.065[d]
DJG loneliness[b]	27.95 (1.94)	26.18 (1.94)	25.17 (1.94)	0.028*
UCLA loneliness[c]	5.31 (0.39)	4.64 (0.39)	4.93 (0.39)	0.023*[d]

*significant effect of time for the indicated variable at $p < 0.05$
All analyses are adjusted for age, employment at baseline, and mean weekly LAC attendance
[a]Duke_UNC functional social support scale. Range 1–5. High social support = 5. p-value represents the p-value for the log-transformed variable
[b]De Jong Gierveld loneliness scale. Scored as a 5 item likert scale from Yes!, yes, more or less, no, No! Range = 11–55. Highest loneliness = 55.
[c]UCLA 3-item loneliness scale. Range = 3–9. Highest loneliness = 9
[d]p-value presented here are log-transformed variable analyses

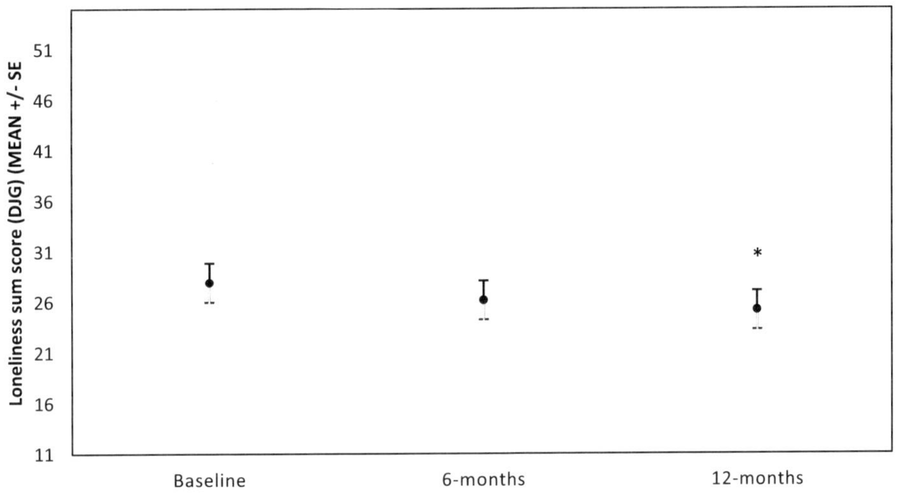

Fig. 1 DJG loneliness for all participants over first year of membership at LAC club ($n = 28$). *Represents significant difference compared to baseline ($p < 0.01$)

[interviewer- Mmm.] ..Okay, you'd talk to them every day. You'd chatter in the kitchen, oh, pass banter back and forth when things are busy or quiet, but... Um, in terms of a friendship with those people, like going to their home, getting to know them, doing other things with them, very few. But what I did miss was the interaction with other people. It had simply gone..... But, yeah, look, that, the, yeah, that intervening period was, oh, a couple of months. That was a bit tough.... But in that time the people in LAC and the people in U3A.... And the other dance group just drew me into more things. Got to know more people. So once again, yeah, reasonable group of acquaintances." (Male, PAFG)

Group members indicated general agreement with these two responses, however one female found she had a greater social life following retirement due to the busy nature of her job.

Within the social resources theme, three subthemes were identified, *i) Opportunity for social connectedness, ii) Opportunity for friendships, and iii) Opportunity for social responsibility/leadership*. Interestingly, these subthemes were additional to the information gathered in the survey. This emphasises the power of the inductive nature of the qualitative exploration employed in the focus groups to broaden the knowledge in this area.

The most discussed and expanded subtheme in both focus groups was *Opportunity for social connectedness*, which arose through developing new connections, diversifying social connections, sharing interests and experiences with others and peer learning. Participants in both focus groups stated that being a member of LAC

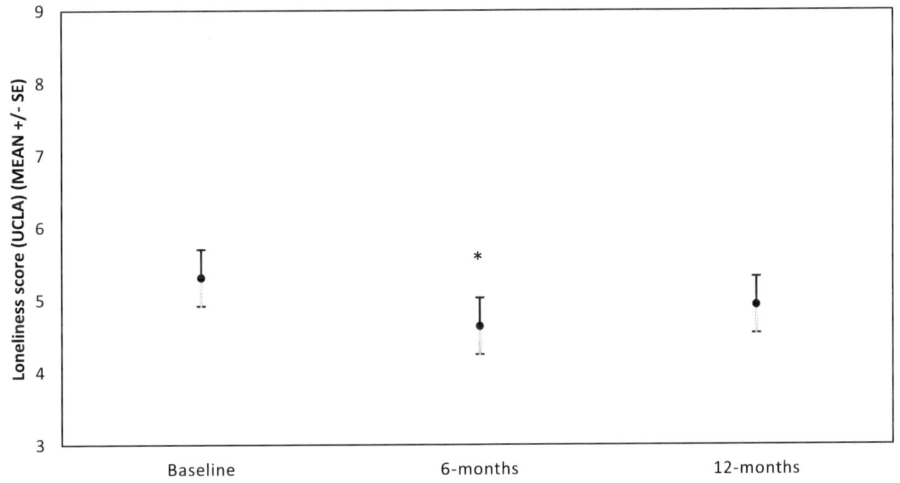

Fig. 2 UCLA loneliness score for all participants over first year of membership at LAC club ($n = 28$). *Indicates log values of the variable at 6-months were significantly different from baseline ($p < 0.01$)

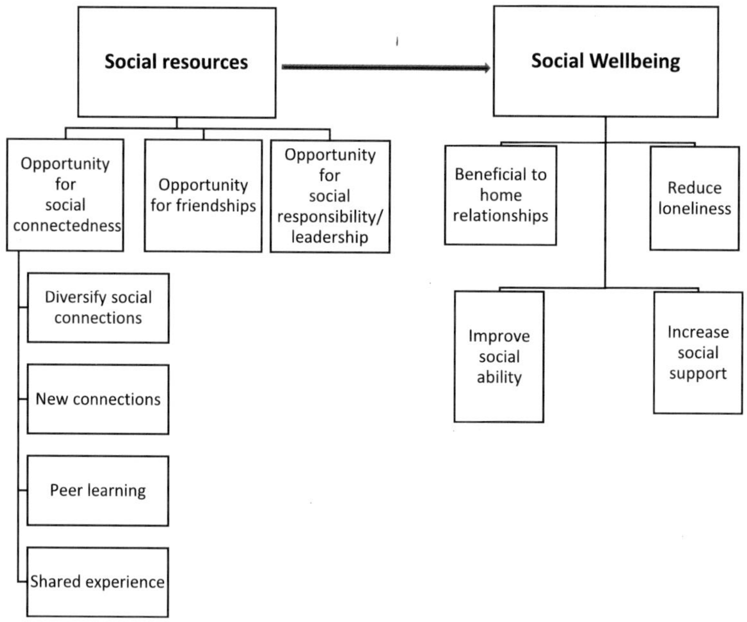

Fig. 3 Themes arising from focus group discussion around the benefits of LAC membership

facilitated their socialising and connecting with others to share ideas, skills and to do activities with, which was especially important through times of significant life events. Furthermore, participants in each of the focus groups valued developing diverse connections:

> *"Yeah, I think, as I said, I finished up work and I, and I had more time for wa-, walking. So I think a, in meeting, in going to this group which, I saw this group of women but then someone introduced me to them. They were just meeting, just meeting a new different set of people, you know? As I said, my work people and these were just a whole different group of women, mainly women. There's not many men. [Interviewer: Yes.]..... Although our leader is a man, which is ironic and is about, this man out in front and there's about 20 women behind him, but, um, so yeah, and people from different walks of life and different nationalities there which I never knew in my work life, so yeah. That's been great. So from that goes on other things, you know, you might, uh, other activities and, yeah, people for coffee and go to the pictures or something, yeah. That's great." (Female, PAFG)*

Simply making new connections was the most widely discussed aspect related to the opportunity for social connectedness subtheme, with all participants agreeing that this was an important benefit of participation in LAC groups.

> *"Well, my experience is very similar to everybody else's.......: I, I went from having no social life to a social life once I joined a group." (Female, PAFG)*

There was agreement in both focus groups that these initial new connections made at a LAC are strengthened through development of deeper personal connections with others who have similar demographics and who are interested in the same activities. This concurs with the Social Identity Theory [58] discussed previously.

> *"and I was walking around the lake in Ballarat, like wandering on my own. I thought, This is ridiculous. I mean, you've met all those groups of women coming the opposite way, so I found out what it was all about, so I joined, yeah. So that's how I got into that.[Interviewer: Yeah.] Basically sick of walking round the lake on my own. [Interviewer: Yeah, yeah.] So that's great. It's very social and they have coffee afterwards which is good."* (female, PAFG)

The subtheme *Opportunity for development of friendships* describes how, for some people, a number of LAC members have progressed from being just initial social connections to an established friendship. This signifies the strength of the connections that may potentially develop through LAC membership. Some participants from each group mentioned friendships developing, with slightly more discussion of this seen in the social group.

"we all have a good old chat, you know, and, and it's all about friendship as well." (female, SocialFG)

The subtheme *Opportunity for social responsibility or leadership* was mentioned by two people in the active group, however it was not brought up in the social group. This opportunity for leadership is linked with the development of a group identity and desiring to contribute meaningfully to a valued group.

"with our riding group, um, you, a leader for probably two rides a year so you've gotta prepare for it, so some of them do reccie rides themselves, so, um, and also every, uh, so that's something that's, uh, a responsibility." (male, PAFG)

Social wellbeing

The social resources described above seem to contribute to a number of social, wellbeing outcomes for participants. The sub themes identified for Social wellbeing were, *i) Increased social support, ii) Reduced loneliness, iii) Improved home relationships* and *iv) Improved social skills.*

Increased social support

Social support was measured quantitatively in the survey (no significant change over time for new members) and identified as a benefit of LAC membership during the focus group discussions. However, only one of the members of the active group mentioned social support directly.

'it's nice to be able to pick up the phone and share your problem with somebody else, and that's come about through LAC. ......'Cos before that it was through, with my family (female, PAFG)

There was some agreement amongst participants of the PA group that they felt this kind of support may develop in time but most of them had been members for less than 2 years.

"[Interviewer: Yeah. Does anyone else have that experience? (relating to above quote)*]" There is one lady but she's actually the one that I joined with anyway. [Interviewer: Okay.] But I, I feel there are others that are definitely getting towards that stage. It's still going quite early days. (female1, PAFG) [Interviewer: I guess it's quite early for some of you, yeah.] "yeah" (female 2, PAFG)*

Social support through sharing of skills was mentioned by one participant in the social group also, with agreement indicated by most of the others in the social focus group.

Discussion in the focus groups also touched on the subthemes *Reduced loneliness* and *Improved home relationships,* which were each mentioned by one person. And focus groups also felt that group membership *Improved social skills* through opening up and becoming more approachable (male, PAFG) or enabling them to become more accepting of others' who are different (general agreement in Social FG).

Discussion

This case study integrated results from a one-year longitudinal survey study and focus group discussions to gather rich information regarding the potential changes in social wellbeing that older adults may experience when joining community organisations offering group activities. The findings from this study indicate that becoming a member of such a community organisation can be associated with a range of social benefits for older adults, particularly related to reducing loneliness and maintaining social connections.

Loneliness

Joining a LAC was associated with a reduction in loneliness over 1 year. This finding is in line with past group-intervention studies where social activity groups were found to assist in reducing loneliness and social isolation [49]. This systematic review highlighted that the majority of the literature explored the effectiveness of group activity interventions for reducing severe loneliness or loneliness in clinical populations [49]. The present study extends this research to the general older adult population who are not specifically lonely and reported to be of good general health, rather than a clinical focus. Our findings are in contrast to results from an evaluation of a community capacity-building program aimed at reducing social isolation in older adults in rural Australia [59]. That program did not successfully reduce loneliness or improve social support. The lack of change from pre- to post-program in that study was reasoned to be due to sampling error, unstandardised data collection, and changes in sample characteristics across the programs [59]. Qualitative assessment of the same program [59] did however suggest that participants felt it was successful in reducing social isolation, which does support our findings.

Changes in loneliness were not a main discussion point of the qualitative component of the current study, however some participants did express that they felt less lonely since joining LACVI and all felt they had become more connected with others. This is not so much of a contrast in results as a potential situational issue. The lack of discussion of loneliness may have been linked to the common social stigma around experiencing loneliness outside certain accepted circumstances (e.g. widowhood), which may lead to underreporting in front of others [45].

Overall, both components of the study suggest that becoming a member of an activity group may be associated with reductions in loneliness, or at least a greater sense of social connectedness. In addition to the social nature of the groups and increased opportunity for social connections, another possible link between group activity and reduced loneliness is an increased opportunity for time out of home. Previous research has found that more time away from home in an average day is associated with lower loneliness in older adults [60]. Given the significant health and social problems that are related to loneliness and social isolation [13–15], the importance of group involvement for newly retired adults to prevent loneliness should be advocated.

Social support

In line with a significant reduction in loneliness, there was also a trend ($p = 0.056$) toward an increase in social support from baseline to 12 months in the survey study. Whilst suggestive of a change, it is far less conclusive than the findings for loneliness. There are a number of possible explanations for the lack of statistically significant change in this variable over the course of the study. The first is the small sample size, which would reduce the statistical power of the study. It may be that larger studies are required to observe changes in social support, which are possibly only subtle over the course of 1 year. This idea is supported by a year-long randomised controlled trial with 90 mildly-depressed older adults who attended senior citizen's club in Norway [37]. The study failed to see any change in general social support in the intervention group compared to the control over 1 year. Additional analysis in that study suggested that people who attended the intervention groups more often, tended to have greater increases in SS ($p = 0.08$). The researchers stated that the study suffered from significant drop-out rates and low power as a result. In this way, it was similar to our findings and suggests that social support studies require larger numbers than we were able to gain in this early exploratory study. Another possible reason for small changes in SS in the current study may be the type of SS measured. The scale used gathered information around functional support or support given to individuals in times of need. Maybe it is not this type of support that changes in such groups but more specific support such as task-specific support. It has been observed in other studies and reviews that task-specific support changes as a result of behavioural interventions (e.g. PA interventions) but general support does not seem to change in the time frames often studied [61–63].

There were many social wellbeing benefits such as increased social connectivity identified in focus group discussion, but the specific theme of social support was rarely mentioned. It may be that general social support through such community groups may take longer than 1 year to develop. There is evidence that strong group ties are sequentially positively associated between social identification and social support [34], suggesting that the connections formed through the groups may lead increased to social support from group members in the future. This is supported by results from the focus group discussions, where one new member felt she could call on colleagues she met in her new group. Other new members thought it was too soon for this support to be available, but they could see the bonds developing.

Other social wellbeing changes

In addition to social support and loneliness that were the focus of the quantitative study, the focus group discussions uncovered a number of other benefits of group membership that were related to social wellbeing (see Fig. 3). The social resources theme was of particular interest because it reflected some of the mechanisms that appeared enable social wellbeing changes as a result of being a member of a LAC but were not measured in the survey. The main social resources relating to group membership that were mentioned in the focus groups were social connectedness, development of friendships and opportunity for social responsibility or leadership. As mentioned above, there was wide-spread discussion within the focus groups of the development of social connections through the clubs. Social connectedness is defined as "the sense of belonging and subjective psychological bond that people feel in relation to individuals and groups of others." ([25], pp1). As well as being an important predecessor of social support, greater social connectedness has been found to be highly important for the health of older adults, especially cognitive and mental health [26, 32, 34, 35, 64]. One suggested theory for this health benefit is that connections developed through groups that we strongly identify with are likely to be important for the development of *social identity* [34], defined by Taifel as: *"knowledge that [we] belong to certain social groups together with some emotional and value significance to [us] of this group membership" (Tajfel, 1972, p. 31 in [58] p 2).* These types of groups to which we identify may be a source of "personal security, social companionship, emotional bonding, intellectual stimulation, and collaborative learning and......allow us to achieve goals." ([58] p2) and an overall sense of self-worth and wellbeing. There was a great deal of discussion relating to the opportunity for social connectedness derived through group membership being particularly pertinent following a significant life event such as moving to a new house or partners becoming unwell or dying and especially retirement. This change in their social circumstance is likely to have triggered the need to renew their social identity by joining a community group. Research with university students has shown that new group identification can assist in transition for university students who have lost their old groups of friends because of starting university [65]. In an example relevant to older adults, maintenance or increase in number of group memberships at the time of retirement reduced mortality risk 8 years later compared to people who reduce their number of group activities in a longitudinal cohort study [66]. This would fit with the original Activity Theory of ageing; whereby better ageing experience is achieved when levels of social participation are maintained, and role replacement occurs when old roles (such as working roles) must be relinquished [67]. These connections therefore appear to assist in maintaining resilience in older adults defined as "the ability to maintain or improve a level of functional ability (a combination of intrinsic physical and mental capacity and environment) in the face of adversity" (p29, [5]). Factors that were mentioned in the focus groups as assisting participants in forming connections with others were shared interest, learning from others, and a fun and accepting environment. It was not possible to assess all life events in the survey study. However, since the discussion from the focus groups suggested this to be an important motivator for joining clubs and potentially a beneficial time for joining them, it would be worth exploring in future studies.

Focus group discussion suggested that an especially valuable time for joining such clubs was around retirement, to assist with maintaining social connectivity. The social groups seem to provide social activity and new roles for these older adults at times of change. It is not necessarily important for all older adults but maybe these ones identify themselves as social beings and therefore this maintenance of social connection helps to continue their social role. Given the suggested importance of social connectivity gained through this organisation, especially at times of significant life events, it would valuable to investigate this further in future and consider encouragement of such through government policy and funding. The majority of these types of clubs exist for older adults in general, but this study emphasises the need for groups such as these to target newly retired individuals specifically and to ensure that they are not seen as 'only for old people'.

Strengths and limitations

The use of mixed –methodologies, combining longitudinal survey study analysed quantitatively, with a qualitative exploration through focus group discussions and thematic analysis, was a strength of the current study. It allowed the researchers to not only examine the association between becoming a member of a community group on social support and loneliness over an extended period, but also obtain a deeper understanding of the underlying reasons behind any associations. Given the variability of social support definitions in research [17] and the broad area of social wellbeing, it allowed for open exploration of the topic, to understand associations that may exist but would have otherwise been missed. Embedding the research in an existing community organisation was a strength, although with this also came some difficulties with recruitment. Voluntary coordination of the community groups meant that informing new members about the study was not always feasible or a priority for the volunteers. In addition, calling for new members was innately challenging because they were not yet committed to the club fully. This meant that so some people did not want to commit to a year-long study if they were not sure how long they would be a member of the club. This resulted in slow recruitment and a resulting relatively low sample size and decreased power to show significant statistical differences, which is a limitation of the present study. However, the use of Linear Mixed Models for analysis of the survey data was a strength because it was able to include all data in the analyses and not remove participants if one time point of data was missing, as repeated measures ANOVAs would do. The length of the study (1 year) is another strength, especially compared to previous randomised controlled studies that are typically only 6–16 weeks in length. Drop-out rate in the current study is very low and probably attributable to the benefits of working with long-standing organisations.

The purpose of this study was to explore in detail whether there are any relationships between joining existing community groups for older adults and social wellbeing. The lack of existing evidence in the field meant that a small feasibility-type case study was a good sounding-board for future larger scale research on the topic, despite not being able to answer questions of causality. Owing to the particularistic nature of case studies, it can also be difficult to generalise to other types of organisations or groups unless there is a great deal of similarity between them [68]. There are however, other types of community organisations in existence that have a similar structure to LACVI (Seniors centres [36, 40], Men's Sheds [38], University of the Third Age [34, 69], Japanese salons [70, 71]) and it may be that the results from this study are transferable to these also. This study adds to the literature around the benefits of joining community organisations that offer social and physical activities for older adults and suggests that this engagement may assist with reducing loneliness and maintaining social connection, especially around the time of retirement.

Directions for future research

Given that social support trended toward a significant increase, it would be useful to repeat the study on a larger scale in future to confirm this. Either a case study on a similar but larger community group or combining a number of community organisations would enable recruitment of more participants. Such an approach would also assist in assessing the generalisability of our findings to other community groups. Given that discussions around social benefits of group membership in the focus groups was often raised in conjunction with the occurrence of significant life events, it would be beneficial to include a significant life event scale in any future studies in this area. The qualitative results also suggest that it would be useful to investigate whether people who join community groups in early years post retirement gain the same social benefits as those in later stages of retirement. Studies investigating additional health benefits of these community groups such as physical activity, depression and general wellbeing would also be warranted.

Conclusion

With an ageing population, it is important to investigate ways to enable older adults to age successfully to ensure optimal quality of life and minimisation of health care costs. Social determinants of health such as social support, loneliness and social contact are important contributors to successful ageing through improvements in cognitive health, quality of life, reduction in depression and reduction in mortality. Unfortunately, older adults are at risk of these social factors declining in older age and there is little research investigating how best to tackle this. Community groups offering a range of activities may assist by improving social connectedness and social support and reducing loneliness for older adults. Some factors that may assist with this are activities that encourage sharing interests, learning from others, and are conducted in a fun and accepting environment. Such groups may be particularly important in developing social contacts for newly retired individuals or around other significant life events such as moving or illness of loved ones. In conclusion, ageing policy and strategies should emphasise participation in community groups especially for those recently retired, as they may assist in reducing loneliness and increasing social connections for older adults.

Abbreviations

FG: Focus group; LAC: Life Activities Club; LACVI: Life Activities Clubs Victoria; LMM: Linear mixed model; PA: Physical activity; WHO: World Health Organisation

Funding

The primary author contributing to this study (GLS) receives PhD scholarship funding from Victoria University. The other authors were funded through salaries at Victoria University.

Authors' contributions

GLS, RE and JVU made substantial contributions to the conception and design of the study. GLS and GOS supervised data collection for the surveys (GLS) and focus groups (GOS and GLS). GLS, GOS, RE, JH and JVU were involved in data analysis and interpretation. All authors were involved in drafting, the manuscript and approved the final version.

Competing interests

The authors declare that they have no competing interests.

Author details

[1]Institute for Health and Sport, Victoria University, Melbourne, Australia.
[2]School of Health and Life Sciences, Federation University, Ballarat, Australia.
[3]Department of Movement Sciences, Physical Activity, Sports and Health Research Group, KU Leuven - University of Leuven, Leuven, Belgium.

References

1. United Nations. In: P.D. Department of Economic and Social Affairs, editor. World Population Ageing 2015. New York: United Nations; 2015.
2. World Health Organisation. Global Health and Ageing. 2011 [cited 2014 March 25]; Available from: http://www.who.int/ageing/publications/global_health/en/.
3. Balogun JA, et al. Age-related changes in balance performance. Disabil Rehabil. 1994;16(2):58–62.
4. Singh MAF. Exercise comes of age: rationale and recommendations for a geriatric exercise prescription. J Gerontol Ser A Biol Med Sci. 2002;57(5): M262–82.
5. World Health Organisation. World report on ageing and health. Geneva: World Health Organisation; 2015.
6. Rowe JW, Kahn RL. Successful Aging1. The Gerontologist. 1997;37(4):433–40.
7. Depp CA, Jeste DV. Definitions and predictors of successful aging: a comprehensive review of larger quantitative studies. Am J Geriatr Psychiatry. 2006;14(1):6–20.
8. Song M, Kong E-H. Older adults' definitions of health: a metasynthesis. Int J Nurs Stud. 2015;52(6):1097–106.
9. Tate RB, Lah L, Cuddy TE. Definition of successful aging by elderly Canadian males: the Manitoba follow-up study. The Gerontologist. 2003;43(5):735–44.
10. Phelan EA, et al. Older Adults' views of "successful aging"—how do they compare with Researchers' definitions? J Am Geriatr Soc. 2004;52(2):211–6.
11. Haslam SA, et al. Social cure, what social cure? The propensity to underestimate the importance of social factors for health. Soc Sci Med. 2018;198:14–21.
12. Holt-Lunstad J, Smith TB, Layton JB. Social relationships and mortality risk: a meta-analytic review. PLoS Med. 2010;7(7):e1000316.
13. Richard A, et al. Loneliness is adversely associated with physical and mental health and lifestyle factors: results from a Swiss national survey. PLoS One. 2017;12(7):1–18.
14. Luo Y, et al. Loneliness, health, and mortality in old age: a national longitudinal study. Soc Sci Med. 2012;74(6):907–14.
15. Luo Y, Waite LJ. Loneliness and mortality among older adults in China. J Gerontol B Psychol Sci Soc Sci. 2014;69(4):633–45.
16. de Jong Gierveld J, Van Tilburg T, Dykstra PA. Loneliness and social isolation. In: Vangelisti A, Perlman D, editors. Cambridge handbook of personal relationships. Cambridge: Cambridge University Press; 2006. p. 485-500.
17. Williams P, Barclay L, Schmied V. Defining social support in context: a necessary step in improving research, intervention, and practice. Qual Health Res. 2004;14(7):942–60.
18. Valtorta N, Hanratty B. Loneliness, isolation and the health of older adults: do we need a new research agenda? J R Soc Med. 2012;105(12):518–22.
19. Jylhä M. Old age and loneliness: cross-sectional and longitudinal analyses in the Tampere longitudinal study on aging. Can J Aging La Revue can du vieil. 2010;23(2):157–68.

20. Huxhold O, Miche M, Schüz B. Benefits of having friends in older ages: differential effects of informal social activities on well-being in middle-aged and older adults. J Gerontol B Psychol Sci Soc Sci. 2014;69(3):366–75.
21. Berkman L, Syme S. Social networks, host resistance and mortality: a nine year follow-up study of alameda county residents. Am J Epidemiol. 1979; 185(11):1070–88.
22. House JS, Landis KR, Umberson D. Social relationships and health. Science. 1988;241(4865):540–5.
23. Pynnonen K, et al. Does social activity decrease risk for institutionalization and mortality in older people? J Gerontol B Psychol Sci Soc Sci. 2012;67(6):765–74.
24. Broadhead WE, et al. The epidemiologic evidence for a relationship between social support and health. Am J Epidemiol. 1983;117(5):521–37.
25. Haslam C, et al. Social connectedness and health. Encyclopedia of geropsychology. 2017:2174–82. https://doi.org/10.1007/978-981-287-080-3_46-1.
26. Haslam C, Cruwys T, Haslam SA. "The we's have it": evidence for the distinctive benefits of group engagement in enhancing cognitive health in aging. Soc Sci Med. 2014;120:57–66.
27. Uebelacker LA, et al. Social support and physical activity as moderators of life stress in predicting baseline depression and change in depression over time in the Women's Health Initiative. Soc Psychiatry Psychiatr Epidemiol. 2013;48(12):1971–82.
28. Tajvar M, et al. Social support and health of older people in middle eastern countries: a systematic review. Australas J Ageing. 2013;32(2):71–8.
29. Dalgard OS, Bjork S, Tambs K. Social support, negative life events and mental health. Br J Psychiatry. 1995;166(1):29–34.
30. Cohen S, Wills TA. Stress, social support, and the buffering hypothesis. Psychol Bull. 1985;98(2):310–57.
31. Gilmour H. Social participation and the health and well-being of Canadian seniors. Health Rep. 2012;23(4):1B.
32. Glei DA, et al. Participating in social activities helps preserve cognitive function: an analysis of a longitudinal, population-based study of the elderly. Int J Epidemiol. 2005;34(4):864–71.
33. Lee SH, Kim YB. Which type of social activities may reduce cognitive decline in the elderly?: a longitudinal population-based study. BMC Geriatr. 2016;16(1):165.
34. Haslam C, et al. Group ties protect cognitive health by promoting social identification and social support. J Aging Health. 2016;28(2):244–66.
35. Haslam C, et al. Groups 4 health: evidence that a social-identity intervention that builds and strengthens social group membership improves mental health. J Affect Disord. 2016;194:188–95.
36. Bøen H. Characteristics of senior Centre users -- and the impact of a group programme on social support and late-life depression. Norsk Epidemiologi. 2012;22(2):261–9.
37. Bøen H, et al. A randomized controlled trial of a senior Centre group programme for increasing social support and preventing depression in elderly people living at home in Norway. BMC Geriatr. 2012;12:20.
38. Golding BG. Social, local, and situated: recent findings about the effectiveness of older Men's informal learning in community contexts. Adult Educ Q. 2011;61(2):103.
39. Life Activities Clubs. Life Activities Clubs. About Us. . 2014 [cited 2014 January 13, 2014]; Available from: http://www.life.org.au/aboutus.
40. Hutchinson SL, Gallant KA. Can senior Centres be contexts for aging in third places? J Leis Res. 2016;48(1):50–68.
41. Millard J. The health of older adults in community activities. Work Older People. 2017;21(2):90–9.
42. Creswell JW, Plano-Clark VL. Designing and conducting mixed methods research. Thousand Oaks, Calif: SAGE Publications; 2007. p. c2007.
43. Loeb S, Penrod J, Hupcey J. Focus groups and older adults: tactics for success. J Gerontol Nurs. 2006;32(3):32–8.
44. Broadhead W, et al. The Duke-UNC functional social support questionnaire: measurement of social support in family medicine patients. Med Care. 1988; 26(7):709–23.
45. De Jong Gierveld J, Van Tilburg T. Living arrangements of older adults in the Netherlands and Italy: Coresidence values and behaviour and their consequences for loneliness. J Cross Cult Gerontol. 1999;14(1):1–24.
46. de Jong-Gierveld J, Kamphuls F. The development of a Rasch-type loneliness scale. Appl Psychol Meas. 1985;9(3):289–99.
47. Tilburg Tv, Leeuw Ed. Stability of scale quality under various data collection procedures: a mode comparison on the 'De Jong-Gierveld loneliness scale. Int J Public Opin Res. 1991;3(1):69–85.
48. Hughes ME, et al. A short scale for measuring loneliness in large surveys - results from two population-based studies. Res Aging. 2004;26(6):655–72.
49. Dickens AP, et al. Interventions targeting social isolation in older people: a systematic review. BMC Public Health. 2011;11:647.
50. Hawkley LC, et al. Loneliness predicts increased blood pressure: 5-year cross-lagged analyses in middle-aged and older adults. Psychol Aging. 2010;25(1):132.
51. Netz Y, et al. Loneliness is associated with an increased risk of sedentary life in older Israelis. Aging Ment Health. 2013;17(1):40–7.
52. Australian Bureau of Statistics. Australian and New Zealand Standard Classification of Occupations, 2013, Version 1.2. Canberra: Australian Bureau of Statistics; 2013.
53. Australian Bureau of Statistics, Australian Standard Geographical Classification (ASGC). Canberra: Australian Bureau of Statistics; 2011.
54. Ware JE, Kosinski M, Keller SD. A 12-item short-form health survey - construction of scales and preliminary tests of reliability and validity. Med Care. 1996;34(3):220–33.
55. Sanson-Fisher RW, Perkins JJ. Adaptation and validation of the SF-36 health survey for use in Australia. J Clin Epidemiol. 51(11):961–7.
56. Braun V, Clarke V. Using thematic analysis in psychology. Qual Res Psychol. 2006;3(2):77–101.
57. Patton MQ. Qualitative research & evaluation methods. 4 ed. Thousand Oaks, California: Sage Publications; 2015.
58. Haslam SA, et al. Social identity, health and well-being: an emerging agenda for applied psychology. Appl Psychol. 2009;58(1):1–23.
59. Bartlett H, et al. Preventing social isolation in later life: findings and insights from a pilot Queensland intervention study. Ageing Soc. 2013;33(07):1167–89.
60. Petersen J, et al. Time out-of-home and cognitive, physical, and emotional wellbeing of older adults: a longitudinal mixed effects model. PLoS One. 2015;10(10):e0139643.
61. Lindsay Smith G, et al. The association between social support and physical activity in older adults: a systematic review. Int J Behav Nutr Phys Act. 2017;14(1):56.
62. Sallis JF, et al. The development of scales to measure social support for diet and exercise behaviors. Prev Med. 1987;16(6):825–36.
63. Oka R, King A, Young DR. Sources of social support as predictors of exercise adherence in women and men ages 50 to 65 years. Womens Health Res Gender Behav Policy. 1995;1:161–75.
64. Greenaway KH, et al. From "we" to "me": group identification enhances perceived personal control with consequences for health and well-being. J Pers Soc Psychol. 2015;109(1):53–74.
65. Iyer A, et al. The more (and the more compatible) the merrier: multiple group memberships and identity compatibility as predictors of adjustment after life transitions. Br J Soc Psychol. 2009;48(4):707–33.
66. Steffens NK, et al. Social group memberships in retirement are associated with reduced risk of premature death: evidence from a longitudinal cohort study. BMJ Open. 2016;6(2):e010164.
67. Havighurst RJ. Successful aging. Gerontol. 1961;1:8–13.
68. Yin R. Case study research: design and methods. Beverly Hills, CA: Sage publishing; 1994.
69. Merriam SB, Kee Y. Promoting community wellbeing: the case for lifelong learning for older adults. Adult Educ Q. 2014;64(2):128–44.
70. Hikichi H, et al. Social interaction and cognitive decline: results of a 7-year community intervention. Alzheimers Dement: Translat Res Clin Interv. 2017; 3(1):23–32.
71. Hikichi H, et al. Effect of a community intervention programme promoting social interactions on functional disability prevention for older adults: propensity score matching and instrumental variable analyses, JAGES Taketoyo study. J Epidemiol Community Health. 2015;69(9):905–10.

An anticholinergic burden score for German prescribers: score development

Esther Katharina Kiesel[1*], Yvonne Marina Hopf[1] and Michael Drey[2]

Abstract

Background: Anticholinergic drugs put elderly patients at a higher risk for falls, cognitive decline, and delirium as well as peripheral adverse reactions like dry mouth or constipation. Prescribers are often unaware of the drug-based anticholinergic burden (ACB) of their patients. This study aimed to develop an anticholinergic burden score for drugs licensed in Germany to be used by clinicians at prescribing level.

Methods: A systematic literature search in pubmed assessed previously published ACB tools. Quantitative grading scores were extracted, reduced to drugs available in Germany, and reevaluated by expert discussion. Drugs were scored as having no, weak, moderate, or strong anticholinergic effects. Further drugs were identified in clinical routine and included as well.

Results: The literature search identified 692 different drugs, with 548 drugs available in Germany. After exclusion of drugs due to no systemic effect or scoring of drug combinations ($n = 67$) and evaluation of 26 additional identified drugs in clinical routine, 504 drugs were scored. Of those, 356 drugs were categorised as having no, 104 drugs were scored as weak, 18 as moderate and 29 as having strong anticholinergic effects.

Conclusions: The newly created ACB score for drugs authorized in Germany can be used in daily clinical practice to reduce potentially inappropriate medications for elderly patients. Further clinical studies investigating its effect on reducing anticholinergic side effects are necessary for validation.

Keywords: Anticholinergic, Geriatrics, Anticholinergic scales, Anticholinergic burden, Germany, Expert opinion, Potentially inappropriate medicine

Background

Studies show that over 50% of elderly patients take five or more drugs, both prescription and over-the-counter [1]. A cross-sectional study in Germany revealed further that 62% of people aged 65 or older suffer from multimorbidity [2]. This combination of multimorbidity and polypharmacy leads to a higher risk for drug-drug interactions and adverse drug reactions (ADRs) [3, 4]. Hence, the use of drugs should be considered carefully in geriatric patients. Part of this consideration should be to avoid potentially inappropriate medications.

Drugs with anticholinergic properties are part of inappropriate medications for geriatric patients [5, 6]. Anticholinergic activity of multiple drugs add up to the so-called anticholinergic burden (ACB). Older patients are more prone to anticholinergic side effects than younger patients [5, 6]. Due to reduced metabolic capacity and slowed elimination in older patients, drugs are eliminated slower, in addition to age-related reductions in cholinergic transmissions [5, 6]. The permeability of the blood-brain-barrier increases which leads to a higher drug concentration in the central nervous system [7]. Central nervous ADRs may especially increase the risk of falls, e.g. blurred vision, confusion, or tremors [6]. More severe anticholinergic side effects are tachyarrhythmia, hallucinations, delirium, and cognitive impairment [6]. Other ADRs like dry mouth, constipation, and urinary retention might reduce the quality of life [6]. Several reviews indicate a higher risk for falls, cognitive decline and delirium with an increased ACB of older patients [8–12].

Despite these apparent risks it is estimated that approximately 50% of elderly people take anticholinergic medications [13, 14]. Qualitative studies demonstrated

* Correspondence: esther.kiesel@med.uni-muenchen.de
[1]Department of Pharmacy, University Hospital, LMU Munich, Munich, Germany
Full list of author information is available at the end of the article

that very few prescribers are aware of the anticholinergic properties of drugs and of the nature of anticholinergic side effects [15]. Even if they know about the negative impact of anticholinergic medications, they hesitate to deprescribe or change those drugs as they do not feel responsible or lack time, knowledge, and resources [16]. In clinical practice there is rarely a registration, documentation and/or conscious reduction of the ACB [15, 17].

Worldwide studies identified over 100 different drugs as having anticholinergic properties [9, 10, 18–33]. Depending on study population, method, and setting, there are different drug lists and different scales to calculate the ACB [18, 19]. The variety of scales and systems complicates the implementation in practice.

Therefore, the current study aimed to develop an anticholinergic burden score specifically for the German healthcare system. This, in turn, can help German prescribers identify and reduce drugs with anticholinergic properties in geriatric patients in order to facilitate easy application in the daily clinical setting. To our knowledge a specific ACB score for Germany is not yet available.

Methods

To identify appropriate tools, PubMed was searched for systematic reviews on tools to quantify anticholinergic drug burden. The search terms were "review AND anticholinergic burden AND (scale OR list OR tool)" without a date limitation. The search was conducted on December 1, 2016. The search and identification process is presented in Fig. 1. Articles were excluded if they were not systematic reviews on tools to quantify anticholinergic drug burden or the language was not English. Three systematic reviews [11, 18, 34] were included identifying 12 tools to quantify anticholinergic burden [10, 20–26, 32, 33, 35, 36]. Tools were excluded because the scoring system was not comparable to the other tools [33, 36], the tool was outdated, [35] there was an updated version published [32], or the scoring was solely based on serum assays [25]. Literature reviews and meta-analysis failed to show an association of serum anticholinergic activity and anticholinergic effects [37], whereas there is an association shown for anticholinergic drug scores mainly based on expert opinion [8–12, 27]. To avoid missing relevant tools, the excluded articles were reviewed regarding more tools as they all evaluated the association of anticholinergic drugs and negative outcomes in patients [9, 19, 27, 38, 39]. These reviews identified four further tools, all ineligible for inclusion because (1) it was impossible to access the drug list despite contacting the authors [28, 31], (2) the scoring system was not comparable to other drug lists [29], and (3) the study assessed the overall medication of patients not specific drugs [30]. The included anticholinergic drug lists were summarized and reduced to drugs available in Germany

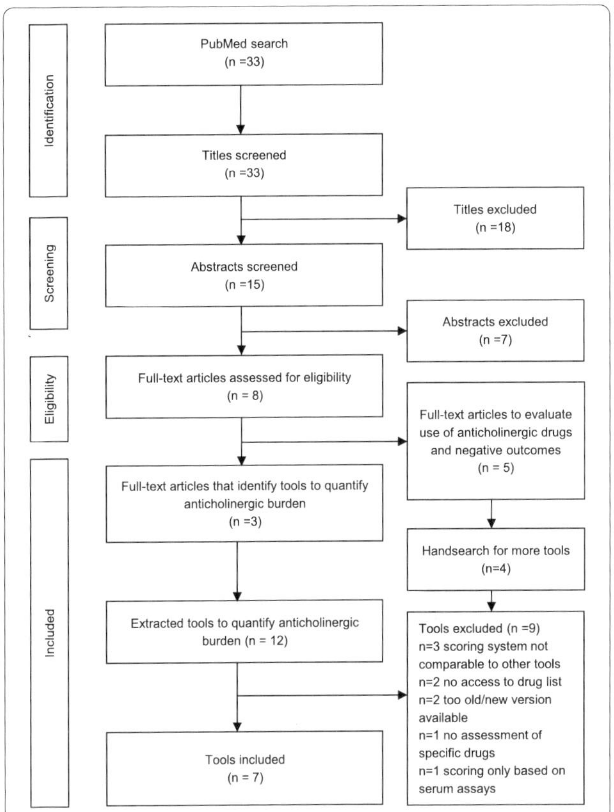

Fig. 1 Identification of tools

[10, 20–24, 26]. For Boustani et al. an updated version was included [10, 40].

The approach to merge the identified scales was similar to the approach of Duran et al. [18]. For all scales, quantitative grading scores proposed by the authors were extracted. Most lists used scores ranging from 0 to 3, one was modified according to Duran et al. so that its 0–4 scale was comparable to 0–3 scales [18, 24]. Topical, ophthalmic, otic and nasal drugs were excluded, while oral, parenteral, inhalative and transdermal drugs were included as these are more likely to show systemic effects [41]. As these lists have only low to moderate concordance, the algorithm depicted in Fig. 2 was used to get a consistent scoring.

Where further evaluation was needed as existing lists scored them differently or only one of the scores evaluated that specific drug., one researcher (EK) looked at the mechanism of action and the ADRs as reported in the German Summary of Product Characteristics and DRUGDEX® (expert-reviewed database for detailed drug information) to assess the anticholinergic properties of the respective drug. This assessment, the existing scores and the scoring by Duran et al. [18] were discussed in a multidisciplinary team of one geriatrician and two clinical pharmacists. This discussion led to a final score. Each drug was coded according to the Anatomical,

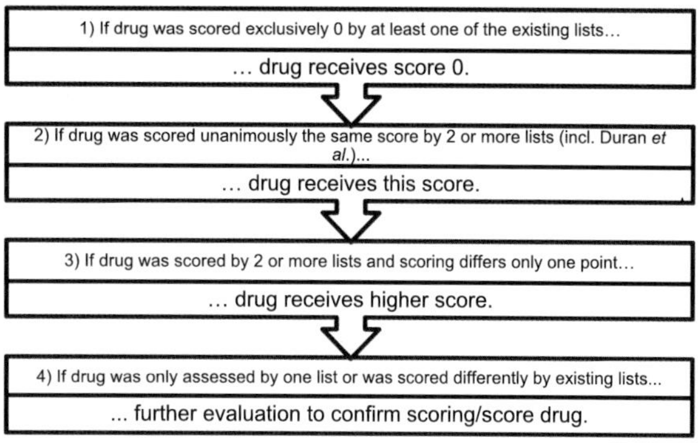

Fig. 2 Algorithm for consistent scoring

Therapeutic and Chemical (ATC) Classification from the World Health Organization. If there were discrepancies in rating within the same drug class, we reconsidered some ratings as well.

In order to tailor the ACB list to the clinical setting a retrospective evaluation of admission and discharge medication on an acute geriatric ward identified a range of further drugs. Consecutive patients for two 6-week-periods were included, which meant the admission and discharge medication of 34 patients was evaluated. The patients were prescribed a total of 235 drugs at admission and 276 drugs at discharge. All drugs thus identified that were not mentioned in the reviewed scales were evaluated for their anticholinergic properties as described above. Based on our final anticholinergic drug list, we designed a pocket-sized guideline for prescribers with information on anticholinergic drugs, anticholinergic side effects and recommendations how to assess and handle the ACB of patients on ward. The recommendation was based on the approach of Boustani et al. and is presented in Fig. 3 [10].

The anticholinergic scores of all drugs used by a patient were calculated in total. If one drug scored 3 or the patient had a summated score of 3 or higher, it was recommended to switch to alternative drugs with a lesser ACB score in order to reduce the summated score to < 3 [10]. If discontinuation or switching was not possible, a dose reduction and/or monitoring for ADRs were advised. Through the upper limit of score 3, the suggested ceiling effect of the ACB is included [19]. This means that at a high ACB, drug effects are assumed to reach a plateau even when the number of anticholinergic drugs further increases [19].

Results

The summary of existing anticholinergic drug lists [20–24, 26, 40] resulted in a list of 692 different drugs with 548 available in Germany (for excluded, international drugs see Additional file 1: Table S1). In total, 67 drugs were excluded because they were rated for topical, nasal,

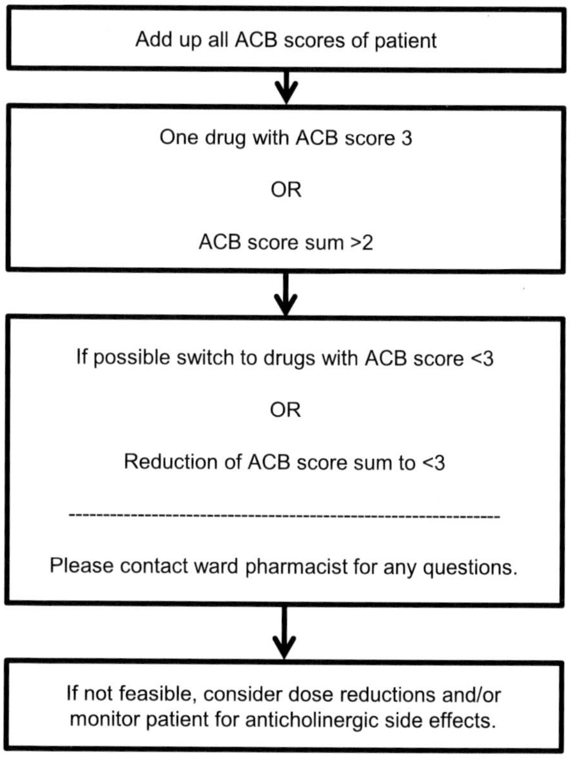

Fig. 3 Recommendation for prescribers on pocket-card based on Boustani et al. [10]

ophthalmic, or otic application only, or were drug combinations (Additional file 1: Table S2).

In terms of effect, 334 of the drugs were categorised as having no anticholinergic effects (ACB score = 0), 77 of the drugs were scored as displaying weak anticholinergic effects (ACB score = 1), 10 as moderate anticholinergic effects (ACB score = 2) and 27 as strong anticholinergic effects (ACB score = 3). These anticholinergic drugs are displayed in Table 1. Drugs rated as having no anticholinergic effects are available in the supplementary material.

Further evaluation was required for 35 drugs. After consideration of adverse drug reactions and mechanism of action, we scored one drug with no anticholinergic effects (ACB score = 0), 22 drugs with weak anticholinergic effects (ACB score = 1), eight as moderate anticholinergic effects (ACB score = 2), and four as having strong anticholinergic effects (ACB score = 3). See Table 2 for specific drugs.

During the retrospective evaluation, 26 drugs were identified that were not yet scored by these already existing scores. Parallel to drugs with inconsistent scores, the adverse drug reactions and the mechanism of action were reviewed and the drugs discussed by three researchers to score the drugs. Five drugs were scored as weak anticholinergic effects (ACB score = 1) and 21

Table 1 Anticholinergic drugs with concordant ratings of sores

Drug	ATC-Code	Carnahan 2006 USA [20]	Ancelin 2006 France [21]	Rudolph 2008 USA [22]	Han 2008 USA [23]	Ehrt 2010 Norway modified [24]	Sittironnarit 2011 Australia [26]	Boustani 2012 USA [40]	Duran 2013 [18]
Weak anticholinergic effects ACB score 1									
Ampicillin	J01CA01	1							0 or 1
Aripiprazole	N05AX12						0	1	
Atenolol	C07AB03	0			1	0	0	1	0
Azathioprine	L04AX01	1							0 or 1
Benazepril	C09AA07	0			1				0 or 1
Betaxolol	C07AB05				1		0		0 or 1
Bisacodyl	A06AB02	0					1		0 or 1
Bromocriptine	N04 BC01	1				0			weak(1–2)
Bupropion	N06AX12	0			1			1	0 or 1
Captopril	C09AA01	1				0	0	1	0 or 1
Celecoxib	M01AH01	0					1		0 or 1
Chlordiazepoxide	N05BA02	1			1				weak(1–2)
Chlorthalidone	C03BA04	1					0	1	0 or 1
Ciclosporin	L04 AD01	1							0 or 1
Citalopram	N06AB04	0				1	1		weak(1–2)
Clindamycin	J01FF01	1							0 or 1
Clonazepam	N03AE01	1					1		weak(1–2)
Dexamethasone	H02AB02	1					0		0 or 1
Dextromethorphan	R05DA09	0			1				0 or 1
Diazepam	N05BA01	1			1	1	1	1	weak(1–2)
Digitoxin	C01AA04	1				1			weak(1–2)
Diltiazem	C08DB01	1					0		0 or 1
Dipyridamole	B01AC07	1				0		1	0 or 1
Domperidone	A03FA03						1		weak(1–2)
Entacapone	N04BX02	0		1					weak(1–2)
Escitalopram	N06AB10	0					1		0 or 1
Famotidine	A02BA03	1					0		0 or 1
Fentanyl	N02AB03	1						1	weak(1–2)
Flunitrazepam	N05CD03					1			0 or 1
Fluoxetine	N06AB03	1			1	1	1		weak(1–2)
Flurazepam	N05CD01	1							0 or 1
Fluvoxamine	N06AB08	1				1	1	1	weak(1–2)
Gentamicin	J01GB03	1							0 or 1
Guaifenesin	R05CA03	0			1				0 or 1
Hydralazine	C02DB02	1					0	1	0 or 1
Hydrocortisone	H02AB09	1						1	0 or 1
Isosorbide dinitrate	C01DA08	1				0	0		0 or 1
Isosorbide mononitrate	C01DA14	1					0		0 or 1
Ketorolac	M01AB15				1				weak(1–2)
Lansoprazole	A02BC03	0				1	0		0 or 1
Levodopa	N04BA01	0		1	1	0	0 or 1		0 or 1
Lithium	N05AN01	0					1		weak(1–2)
Lorazepam	N05BA06	1							0 or 1

Table 1 Anticholinergic drugs with concordant ratings of sores *(Continued)*

Drug	ATC-Code	Carnahan 2006 USA [20]	Ancelin 2006 France [21]	Rudolph 2008 USA [22]	Han 2008 USA [23]	Ehrt 2010 Norway modified [24]	Sittironnarit 2011 Australia [26]	Boustani 2012 USA [40]	Duran 2013 [18]
Metformin	A10BA02	0					1		0 or 1
Methotrexate	L04AX03	0					1		0 or 1
Methylprednisolone	H02AB04	1					0		0 or 1
Metoprolol	C07AB02	0			1	0	0	1	0
Midazolam	N05CD08	1							0 or 1
Mirtazapine	N06AX11	0		1					weak(1–2)
Morphine	N02AA01	1			1			1	weak(1–2)
Naratriptan	N02CC02						1		0 or 1
Nifedipine	C08CA05	1				0	0	1	0
Oxazepam	N05BA04	1				0	1		0 or 1
Oxycodone	N02AA05	1			1		1		weak(1–2)
Pancuronium	M03 AC01	1							0 or 1
Phenobarbital	N03AA02	0			1	1			0 or 1
Piperacillin	J01CA12	1							0 or 1
Pramipexole	N04 BC05	0		1		0			0 or 1
Prednisolone	A07EA01	1				0	0		0 or 1
Prednisone	A07EA03	1						1	
Quinidine	C01BA01	0						1	
Risperidone	N05AX08	0		1	1		1	1	weak(1–2)
Selegiline	N04BD01	0		1		0			0 or 1
Sertraline	N06AB06	1			1	0	0		0
Sumatriptan	N02CC01						1		0 or 1
Temazepam	N05CD07	1					1		weak(1–2)
Trandolapril	C09AA10	0			1		0		0 or 1
Trazodone	N06AX05	0		1	1			1	weak(1–2)
Triamcinolone	H02AB08	1					0		0 or 1
Triamterene	C03DB02	1					0	1	0 or 1
Triazolam	N05CD05	1			1				weak(1–2)
Valproic acid	N03AG01	1					0		0 or 1
Vancomycin	J01XA01	1							0 or 1
Venlafaxine	N06AX16	0			1	0	1	1	0
Warfarin	B01AA03	1				0	0	1	0
Ziprasidone	N05AE04			1					0 or 1
Zolmitriptan	N02CC03						1		0 or 1
Moderate anticholinergic effects ACB score 2									
Amantadine	N04BB01	1		2				2	weak(1–2)
Cimetidine	A02BA01	2		2				1	weak(1–2)
Loperamide	A07DA03	1		2	1		1	1	weak(1–2)
Loxapine	N05AH01	2						2	weak(1–2)
Methadone	N07 BC02				2				weak(1–2)
Oxcarbazepine	N03AF02	2						2	weak(1–2)
Pimozide	N05AG02	2						2	weak(1–2)
Ranitidine	A02BA02	2		1	2	1	1	1	weak(1–2)
Theophylline	R03DA04	1	2			1	2	1	weak(1–2)
Tramadol	N02AX02	1			2		2		weak(1–2)

Table 1 Anticholinergic drugs with concordant ratings of sores *(Continued)*

Drug	ATC-Code	Carnahan 2006 USA [20]	Ancelin 2006 France [21]	Rudolph 2008 USA [22]	Han 2008 USA [23]	Ehrt 2010 Norway modified [24]	Sittironnarit 2011 Australia [26]	Boustani 2012 USA [40]	Duran 2013 [18]
Strong anticholinergic effects ACB score 3									
Amitriptyline	N06AA09	3	3	3	3	3	3	3	Strong(3)
Atropine	A03BA01	3		3	3		3	3	Strong(3)
Chlorpheniramine	R06AB04	3	3	3	3		3	3	Strong(3)
Clemastine	R06AA04	3						3	Strong(3)
Clomipramine	N06AA04	3	3					3	Strong(3)
Clozapine	N05AH02	3		2		3		3	Strong(3)
Cyproheptadine	R06AX02	2		3			3	2	Strong(3)
Darifenacin	G04BD10	3						3	Strong(3)
Dimenhydrinate	A04AB02	3						3	Strong(3)
Diphenhydramine	A04AB05	3		3	3			3	Strong(3)
Doxepin	N06AA12	3			3	3	3	3	Strong(3)
Flavoxate	G04BD02	3						3	Strong(3)
Hydroxyzine	N05BB01	3	3	3				3	Strong(3)
Imipramine	N06AA02	3	3	3	3		3	3	Strong(3)
Levomepromazine	N05AA02	2	3					2	Strong(3)
Nortriptyline	N06AA10	3		2	3	2		3	Strong(3)
Orphenadrine	N04AB02	3	3			3		3	Strong(3)
Oxybutynin	G04BD04	3	3	3		3	2	3	Strong(3)
Procyclidine	N04AA04	3							Strong(3)
Scopolamine	A04AD01	3			3			3	Strong(3)
Thioridazine	N05 AC02	3		3	3	3		3	Strong(3)
Tizanidine	M03BX02			3					Strong(3)
Tolterodine	G04BD07	3		2	3		3	3	Strong(3)
Trihexyphenidyl	N04AA01	3	3		3	3		3	Strong(3)
Trimipramine	N06AA06	3	3			3		3	Strong(3)

Drugs are sorted by their assigned score and then alphabetical

drugs were categorised as having no anticholinergic effects (ACB score = 0). See Table 3 for specific drugs.

Table 4 shows all drugs scored sorted by their score. Additional file 1: Table S3 shows all drugs scored 0.

Discussion

To our knowledge, this is the first ACB score developed especially for prescribers in Germany. There have been similar international publications [18, 27]. The drugs most commonly used in Germany differ from other countries especially England, USA, and Australia, where many published studies on anticholinergic drugs were conducted. Our ACB score did not only summarize existing scores but re-evaluated the drugs, especially those with discrepancies, and reduced the list to those authorized in Germany. This saves valuable time and effort for clinicians trying to evaluate anticholinergic burden in patients.

The scores used were identified via a systematic literature search in pubmed. This systematic approach should ensure a replicable and complete choice of peer-reviewed and published ACB scores, although it was not a systematic literature review conducted in different databases. All included scores were previously validated. Drug evaluation was based on expert opinion which was previously preferred to measuring serum assays [18, 27]. This expert review of the drugs by three different people (one geriatrician and two clinical pharmacists) based on clinical experience and literature data on method of action and ADRs strengthens the development of this score. Scoring was confirmed by the expert committee not only for drugs with discrepancies, but also for drugs that were only scored by one of the existing scores. Being rated by only one score is not necessarily a limitation as the individual selection of drugs is always depending on the country, the setting, and other specifics of the score development.

Table 2 Scoring of drugs with discrepant ratings (=ratings differed more than 1 score) or only one previous scoring

Drug	ATC-Code	Carnahan 2006 USA [20]	Ancelin 2006 France [21]	Rudolph 2008 USA [22]	Han 2008 USA [23]	Ehrt 2010 Norway modified [24]	Sittironnarit 2011 Australia [26]	Boustani 2012 USA [40]	Duran 2013 [18]
No anticholinergic effects ACB score 0									
Colchicine	M04 AC01	0	3				0	1	discrepant
Weak anticholinergic effects ACB score 1									
Alprazolam	N05BA12	1	3		1		1	1	discrepant
Asenapine	N05AH05							1	
Baclofen	M03BX01	0		2	2				1 or 2
Cetirizine	R06AE07	0		2	2		2	1	1 or 2
Clorazepate	N05BA05	1	3					1	discrepant
Codeine	R05DA04	1	2		1	0	1	1	1 or 2
Desloratadine	R06AX27							1	
Digoxin	C01AA05	1	3			1	1	1	discrepant
Doxylamine	R06AA09						0	3	
Fexofenadine	R06AX26	0			2		2	0	1 or 2
Fluphenazine	N05AB02	1		3			3		3
Furosemide	C03CA01	1	3			1	0	1	discrepant
Ipratropium inhalative	R03BB01	0				3			3
Levocetirizine	R06AE09							1	
Loratadine	R06AX13	0		2	1		1	1	1 or 2
Methocarbamol	M03BA03			1	1			3	1 or 2
Metoclopramide	A03FA01	0		1	3	0	1		discrepant
Paliperidone	N05AX13							1	
Perphenazine	N05AB03	1		3	2	0		3	discrepant
Promethazine	R06AD02	3		3			0	3	3
Pseudoephedrine	R01BA02	0					2		0 oder 1
Tiotropium inhalative	R03BB04						0		
Moderate anticholinergic effects ACB score 2									
Carbamazepine	N03AF01	2			1	0	0	2	1 or 2
Haloperidol	N05 AD01	0		1		0	2	1	1 or 2
Maprotiline	N06AA21		3						discrepant
Pethidine	N02AB02	2				0		2	1 or 2
Olanzapine	N05AH03	1		2	1	2		3	1 or 2
Opipramol	N06AA05		3						discrepant
Paroxetine	N06AB05	1		1	2	2	2	3	1 or 2
Quetiapine	N05AH04	0		1	2	1		3	1 or 2
Strong anticholinergic effects ACB score 3									
Fesoterodine	G04BD11							3	
Propiverine	G04BD06							3	
Solifenacin	G04BD08						0	3	
Trospium	G04BD09							3	

Drugs are sorted first by their assigned score and then alphabetical

As our score is based on previously published ACB scores and drugs within our hospital during a retrospective evaluation, we do not claim this list to be comprehensive. There are over 2000 drugs approved in Germany, so there are potentially more anticholinergic drugs not yet considered in this list. There were few drugs found in our retrospective evaluation that had not been rated by previously published ACB scores. Potential reasons for those

Table 3 Drugs added during retrospective evaluation

Drug	ATC-Code
No anticholinergic effects ACB score 0	
Agomelatine	N06AX22
Apixaban	B01FAF02
Colecalciferol	A11CC05
Dabigatran	B01AE07
Dulaglutide	A10BJ05
Edoxaban	B01AF03
Empagliflozin	A10BK03
Fenoterol inhalative	R03AC04
Formoterol inhalative	R03AC13
Metamizole	N02BB02
Saccharomyces boulardii	A07FA02
Phenprocoumon	B01AA04
Pipamperone	N05 AD05
Piritramide	N02 AC03
Rivaroxaban	B01AF01
Sevelamer	V03AE02
Sitagliptin	A10BH01
Teriparatide	H05AA02
Thiamazole	H03BB02
Tilidine/Naloxone	N02AX51
Vemurafenib	L01XE15
Weak anticholinergic effects ACB score 1	
Aclidinium inhalative	R03BB05
Dimetindene	R06AB03
Etoricoxib	M01AH05
Glycopyrronium inhalative	R03BB06
Rotigotine patch	N04 BC09

Drugs are sorted by their assigned score and then alphabetical

drugs missing could be that the drugs were mainly used in Germany and not internationally, e.g. Metamizol sodium, or that the drugs were new on the market and not previously analysed, e.g. Apixaban. To address missing and potentially new anticholinergic drugs, updates are planned in follow-up projects.

The validity of selection of drugs with anticholinergic activity and the grading can be questioned. Among the selected scores there is a great variety in study design and setting. Different methods to assess and rate anticholinergic activity were used: product information, specialised literature on ADRs, review of literature, expert opinion as well as serum radio receptor assay, dissociation constant for cholinergic receptor and other laboratory data [10, 18–24, 26, 40]. We worked with that variety by comparing different scores. As final decision on inclusion and rating of anticholinergic drugs was mainly a subjective decision of experts and not based on clinical outcomes, the ratings may be discussed further. Nevertheless, there is no approved methodology to measure the ACB and expert rating is preferred to measuring serum assays [27]. The list did not include topical, ophthalmic, otic or nasal drugs. It cannot be excluded that there might be systemic or local anticholinergic effects with these application routes.

The distinction of anticholinergic potency from 0 to 3 might not be the best method to quantify anticholinergic burden, but as most existing scores used this or a similar rating it was the only way to work with the existing lists [18, 19]. Through the upper limit of score 3, the suggested ceiling effect of the ACB was included [19]. This means that at a high ACB, drug effects are assumed to reach a plateau even when the number of anticholinergic drugs further increases [19]. For a more accurate evaluation of anticholinergic burden a finer distinction in some drug classes would be useful. Drug classes like tricyclic antidepressants or anticholinergics for urinary incontinence were all scored with a strong ACB (ACB = 3). Although those drugs all have a strong anticholinergic burden, some are more problematic than others. For example, Trospium should have less central reactions than other anticholinergics for urinary incontinence because of its quaternary chemical structure, but it still shows anticholinergic adverse effects and was rated having strong anticholinergic properties by Boustani et al. [40]. Another method to further refine the evaluation of ACB would be to consider the dosages of anticholinergic drugs via the Drug Burden Index [33]. A recently published cohort study of German older outpatients found a significant association of the drug Burden Index with Mini-Mental State Examination Score, Barthel index, Falls and use of laxatives [42]. We did not use this approach as it is more complicated and time-consuming to use in daily routine and it is not compatible with the scores used [11]. Our decision to apply the higher score (Fig. 2 step 3) might be questioned due to the automatic application of a higher anticholinergic rating. We decided to take this approach in order to avoid missing any drugs with anticholinergic properties.

Although a high anticholinergic burden should be avoided if possible, the deprescribing of anticholinergic drugs is not always possible. Some indications like for example urinary incontinence or some psychiatric indications require anticholinergic medications that cannot be easily subsidised by other non-anticholinergic drugs due to clinical reasons. While urinary incontinence can be handled well with non-pharmacological options, if pharmacological treatment is required anticholinergic drugs are the best options. Thus, this list should be considered as decision support for the prescriber rather than as a strict deprescribing directive.

Table 4 Overview of all drugs scored. Caution: This list does not contain necessarily all drugs with anticholinergic properties

ACB score = 1			ACB score = 2	ACB score = 3
Aclidinium[inh]	Entacapone	Mirtazapine	Amantadine	Amitriptyline
Alprazolam	Escitalopram	Morphine	Carbamazepine	Atropine
Ampicillin	Etoricoxib	Naratriptan	Cimetidine	Chlorpheniramine
Aripiprazole	Famotidine	Nifedipine	Haloperidol	Clemastine
Asenapine	Fentanyl	Oxazepam	Loperamide	Clomipramine
Atenolol	Fexofenadine	Oxycodone	Loxapine	Clozapine
Azathioprine	Flunitrazepam	Paliperidone	Maprotiline	Cyproheptadine
Baclofen	Fluoxetine	Pancuronium	Methadone	Darifenacin
Benazepril	Fluphenazine	Perphenazine	Olanzapine	Dimenhydrinate
Betaxolol	Flurazepam	Phenobarbital	Opipramol	Diphenhydramine
Bisacodyl	Fluvoxamine	Piperacillin	Oxcarbazepine	Doxepin
Bromocriptine	Furosemide	Pramipexole	Paroxetine	Fesoterodine
Bupropion	Gentamicin	Prednisolone	Pethidine	Flavoxate
Captopril	Glycopyrronium[inh]	Prednisone	Pimozide	Hydroxyzine
Celecoxib	Guaifenesin	Promethazine	Quetiapine	Imipramine
Cetirizine	Hydralazine	Pseudoephedrine	Ranitidine	Levomepromazine
Chlordiazepoxide	Hydrocortisone	Quinidine	Theophylline	Nortriptyline
Chlorthalidone	Ipratropium[inh]	Risperidone	Tramadol	Orphenadrine
Ciclosporin	Isosorbide dinitrate	Rotigotine patch		Oxybutynin
Citalopram	Isosorbide mononitrate	Selegiline		Procyclidine
Clindamycin	Ketorolac	Sertraline		Propiverine
Clonazepam	Lansoprazole	Sumatriptan		Scopolamine
Clorazepate	Levocetirizine	Temazepam		Solifenacin
Codeine	Levodopa	Tiotropium[inh]		Thioridazine
Desloratadine	Lithium	Trandolapril		Tizanidine
Dexamethasone	Loratadine	Trazodone		Tolterodine
Dextromethorphan	Lorazepam	Triamcinolone		Trihexyphenidyl
Diazepam	Metformin	Triamterene		Trimipramine
Digitoxin	Methocarbamol	Triazolam		Trospium
Digoxin	Methotrexate	Valproic acid		
Diltiazem	Methylprednisolone	Vancomycin		
Dimetindene	Metoclopramide	Venlafaxine		
Dipyridamole	Metoprolol	Warfarin		
Domperidone	Midazolam	Ziprasidone		
Doxylamine		Zolmitriptan		

[inh]inhalative

Conclusion

Although anticholinergic burden is only one factor of many to consider in multimorbid geriatric patients, it is important to discuss anticholinergic burden and its effects. This list can be used in Germany and countries with similar drugs approved to assess the anticholinergic burden of geriatric patients. It is valuable for prescribers to use in the daily clinical setting as only drugs available in Germany are listed and data from different studies is merged into one table so that a quick overview is possible. Further cluster-randomised studies investigating whether the implementation of the list reduces anticholinergic side effects, falls or delirium are necessary for its validation.

Abbreviations

ACB: Anticholinergic burden; ADR: Adverse drug reaction; ATC: Anatomical, Therapeutic and Chemical

Acknowledgements

We thank Carla Widman for language editing of the manuscript and all original authors for providing us with their drug lists. This research was supported within the interprofessional PhD-program Clinical Pharmacy, LMU Munich.

Funding

This research was co-funded by the Friedrich-Baur-Stiftung and the Stiftung Patient und Klinische Pharmazie, Munich, Germany.

Authors' contributions

All authors (EKK, YMH, MD) conceived the idea for conducting the study. EKK conducted the database searches, extracted and summarized existing scores. All authors (EKK, YMH, MD) were involved in the evaluation process as outlined in the methods section. The final manuscript was written, checked, and approved by all authors (EKK, YMH, MD).

Competing interests

EKK and MD declare that they have no competing interests. YMH received a research grant from the Friedrich-Baur-Stiftung.

Author details

[1]Department of Pharmacy, University Hospital, LMU Munich, Munich, Germany. [2]Department of Medicine IV, University Hospital, LMU Munich, Munich, Germany.

References

1. Kaufman D, Kelly J, Rosenberg L, Anderson T, Mitchell A. Recent patterns of medication use in the amulatory adult population of the United States. JAMA. 2002;287:337–44.
2. van den Bussche H, Schaefer I, Koller D, Hansen H, von Leitner E-C, Scherer M, Wegscheider K, Glaeske G, Schoen G. Multimorbidity in the German elderly population - part 1: prevalence in ambulatory medical care. ZFA (Stuttgart). 2012;88(9):365–71.
3. Field TS, Gurwitz JH, Harrold LR, Rothschild J, DeBellis KR, Seger AC, Auger JC, Garber LA, Cadoret C, Fish LS, et al. Risk factors for adverse drug events among older adults in the ambulatory setting. J Am Geriatr Soc. 2004;52(8): 1349–54.
4. Maher RL, Hanlon J, Hajjar ER. Clinical consequences of polypharmacy in elderly. Expert Opin Drug Saf. 2014;13(1):57–65.
5. Feinberg M. The problems of anticholinergic adverse effects in older patients. Drugs Aging. 1993;3(4):335–48.
6. Mintzer J, Burns A. Anticholinergic side-effects of drugs in elderly people. J R Soc Med. 2000;93:457–62.
7. Schliebs R, Arendt T. The cholinergic system in aging and neuronal degeneration. Behav Brain Res. 2011;221(2):555–63.
8. Fox C, Smith T, Maidment I, Chan WY, Bua N, Myint PK, Boustani M, Kwok CS, Glover M, Koopmans I, et al. Effect of medications with anti-cholinergic properties on cognitive function, delirium, physical function and mortality: a systematic review. Age Ageing. 2014;43(5):604–15.
9. Ruxton K, Woodman RJ, Mangoni AA. Drugs with anticholinergic effects and cognitive impairment, falls and all-cause mortality in older adults: a systematic review and meta-analysis. Br J Clin Pharmacol. 2015;80(2):209–20.
10. Boustani M, Campbell N, Munger S, Maidment I, Fox C. Impact of anticholinergics on the aging brain: a review and practical application. Aging Health. 2008;4(3):311–20.
11. Cardwell K, Hughes CM, Ryan C. The association between anticholinergic medication burden and health related outcomes in the 'oldest old': a systematic review of the literature. Drugs Aging. 2015;32(10):835–48.
12. Marcum ZA, Wirtz HS, Pettinger M, LaCroix AZ, Carnahan R, Cauley JA, Bea JW, Gray SL. Anticholinergic medication use and falls in postmenopausal women: findings from the women's health initiative cohort study. BMC Geriatr. 2016;16:76.
13. Best O, Gnjidic D, Hilmer SN, Naganathan V, McLachlan AJ. Investigating polypharmacy and drug burden index in hospitalised older people. Intern Med J. 2013;43(8):912–8.
14. Fox C, Richardson K, Maidment ID, Savva GM, Matthews FE, Smithard D, Coulton S, Katona C, Boustani MA, Brayne C. Anticholinergic medication use and cognitive impairment in the older population: the medical research council cognitive function and ageing study. J Am Geriatr Soc. 2011;59(8): 1477–83.
15. Mayer T, Haefeli WE, Seidling HM. Vorgehen bei der Erkennung, Bewertung und Vermeidung anticholinerger Nebenwirkungen - eine Querschnittsbefragung unter Ärzten. Krankenhauspharmazie. 2017;38(2):111.
16. Kouladjian L, Gnjidic D, Reeve E, Chen TF, Hilmer SN. Health care Practitioners' perspectives on Deprescribing anticholinergic and sedative medications in older adults. Ann Pharmacother. 2016;50(8):625–36.
17. Navila C. Using a "MAP" to steer patients away from medicines-related falls. Clin Pharm. 2013;5:119–21.
18. Duran CE, Azermai M, Vander Stichele RH. Systematic review of anticholinergic risk scales in older adults. Eur J Clin Pharmacol. 2013;69(7): 1485–96.
19. Mayer T, Haefeli WE, Seidling HM. Different methods, different results--how do available methods link a patient's anticholinergic load with adverse outcomes? Eur J Clin Pharmacol. 2015;71(11):1299–314.
20. Carnahan RM, Lund BC, Perry PJ, Pollock BG, Culp KR. The anticholinergic drug scale as a measure of drug-related anticholinergic burden: associations with serum anticholinergic activity. J Clin Pharmacol. 2006;46(12):1481–6.
21. Ancelin ML, Artero S, Portet F, Dupuy AM, Touchon J, Ritchie K. Non-degenerative mild cognitive impairment in elderly people and use of anticholinergic drugs: longitudinal cohort study. BMJ. 2006;332(7539):455–9.
22. Rudolph JL, Salow MJ, Angelini MC, McGlinchey RE. The anticholinergic risk scale and anticholinergic adverse effects in older persons. Arch Intern Med. 2008;168(5):508–13.
23. Han L, Agostini JV, Allore HG. Cumulative anticholinergic exposure is associated with poor memory and executive function in older men. J Am Geriatr Soc. 2008;56(12):2203–10.
24. Ehrt U, Broich K, Larsen JP, Ballard C, Aarsland D. Use of drugs with anticholinergic effect and impact on cognition in Parkinson's disease: a cohort study. J Neurol Neurosurg Psychiatry. 2010;81(2):160–5.
25. Chew ML, Mulsant BH, Pollock BG, Lehman ME, Greenspan A, Mahmoud RA, Kirshner MA, Sorisio DA, Bies RR, Gharabawi G. Anticholinergic activity of 107 medications commonly used by older adults. J Am Geriatr Soc. 2008; 56(7):1333–41.
26. Sittironnarit G, Ames D, Bush AI, Faux N, Flicker L, Foster J, Hilmer S, Lautenschlager NT, Maruff P, Masters CL, et al. Effects of anticholinergic drugs on cognitive function in older Australians: results from the AIBL study. Dement Geriatr Cogn Disord. 2011;31(3):173–8.
27. Salahudeen MS, Duffull SB, Nishtala PS. Anticholinergic burden quantified by anticholinergic risk scales and adverse outcomes in older people: a systematic review. BMC Geriatr. 2015;15:31.
28. Aizenberg D, Sigler M, Weizman A, Barak Y. Anticholinergic burden and the risk of falls among elderly psychiatric inpatients: a 4-year case-control study. Int Psychogeriatr. 2002;14(3):307–10.
29. Minzenberg MJ, Poole JH, Benton C, Vinogradov S. Association of anticholinergic load with impairment of complex attention and memory in schizophrenia. Am J Psychiatry. 2004;161(1):116–24.
30. Whalley LJ, Sharma S, Fox HC, Murray AD, Staff RT, Duthie AC, Deary IJ, Starr JM. Anticholinergic drugs in late life: adverse effects on cognition but not on progress to dementia. J Alzheimers Dis. 2012;30(2):253–61.
31. Cancelli I, Valentinis L, Merlino G, Valente M, Gigli GL. Drugs with anticholinergic properties as a risk factor for psychosis in patients affected by Alzheimer's disease. Clin Pharmacol Ther. 2008;84(1):63–8.
32. Han L, McCusker J, Cole M, Abrahamowicz M, Primeau F, Élie M. Use of medications with anticholinergic effect predicts clinical severity of delirium symptoms in older medical inpatients. Arch Intern Med. 2001;161(8):1099.
33. Hilmer SN, Mager DE, Simonsick EM, Cao Y, Ling SM, Windham BG, Harris TB, Hanlon JT, Rubin SM, Shorr RI, et al. A drug burden index to define the functional burden of medications in older people. Arch Intern Med. 2007; 167(8):781–7.
34. Villalba-Moreno AM, Alfaro-Lara ER, Perez-Guerrero MC, Nieto-Martin MD, Santos-Ramos B. Systematic review on the use of anticholinergic scales in poly pathological patients. Arch Gerontol Geriatr. 2016;62:1–8.
35. Summers WK. A clinical method of estimating risk of drug induced delirium. Life Sci. 1978;22(17):1511–6.
36. Dauphinot V, Faure R, Omrani S, Goutelle S, Bourguignon L, Krolak-Salmon P, Mouchoux C. Exposure to anticholinergic and sedative drugs, risk of falls, and mortality: an elderly inpatient, multicenter cohort. J Clin Psychopharmacol. 2014;34(5):565–70.
37. Salahudeen MS, Chyou TY, Nishtala PS. Serum anticholinergic activity and cognitive and functional adverse outcomes in older people: a systematic review and meta-analysis of the literature. PLoS One. 2016;11(3):e0151084.
38. Collamati A, Martone AM, Poscia A, Brandi V, Celi M, Marzetti E, Cherubini A, Landi F. Anticholinergic drugs and negative outcomes in the older population: from biological plausibility to clinical evidence. Aging Clin Exp Res. 2016;28(1):25–35.
39. Kersten H, Wyller TB. Anticholinergic drug burden in older people's brain - how well is it measured? Basic Clin Pharmacol Toxicol. 2014;114(2):151–9.
40. Aging Brain Program: Anticholinergic Cognitive Burden Scale 2012 Update. https://www.uea.ac.uk/documents/3306616/10940915/Anticholinergics/088bb9e6-3ee2-4b75-b8ce-b2d59dc538c2. Last accessed 3 Oct 2018.
41. Singh S, Loke YK, Enright P, Furberg CD. Pro-arrhythmic and pro-ischaemic effects of inhaled anticholinergic medications. Thorax. 2013;68(1):114–6.
42. Mayer T, Meid AD, Saum KU, Brenner H, Schottker B, Seidling HM, Haefeli WE. Comparison of nine instruments to calculate anticholinergic load in a large cohort of older outpatients: association with cognitive and functional decline, falls, and use of laxatives. Am J Geriatr Psychiatry. 2017;25(5):531–40.

Association between cognitive function and life-space mobility in older adults: results from the FRéLE longitudinal study

François Béland[1,2,3*], Dominic Julien[1,4,5], Nathalie Bier[6,7], Johanne Desrosiers[8,9], Marie-Jeanne Kergoat[6,10] and Louise Demers[6,7]

Abstract

Background: Cross-sectional and longitudinal studies show conflicting results regarding the association between cognition and life-space mobility, and little is known regarding the mediators and moderators of the association. The aim of this study was to investigate the association between cognition and life-space mobility in older adults, as well as the intervening variables modifying the relationship.

Methods: Community-dwelling older adults aged 65 years and older ($N = 1643$) were assessed at three time points over a period of 2 years. Growth mixture models with mediation and moderation analysis were utilised to investigate association between cognitive function and life-space mobility. The potential mediators and moderators were depressive symptoms, locus of control, gait speed and grip strength. Analysis was controlled for age, sex, education, annual income, number of chronic illnesses, and living site.

Results: The direct association between initial scores of cognitive function and life-space was mediated by initial scores of depressive symptoms and gait speed, and moderated by initial scores of grip strength. No direct association between change in cognitive function and change in life-space mobility was found; the scores were mediated by change in depressive symptoms.

Conclusions: We conclude that the relationship between change in cognitive function and life-space mobility in older adults is not well-defined over an observation period of 2 years.

Keywords: Cognition, Life-space, Mediation, Moderation, Aging

Background

The concept of life-space mobility is receiving growing attention in the field of aging. It defines a spectrum of geographic areas that extend from domicile to distant destinations [1]. Constricted life-space mobility has been associated with adverse health outcome, including illness, poor self-rated health, difficulty in basic and instrumental activities of daily living, [1] depressive symptoms, [1, 2] frailty, and death [2].

* Correspondence: francois.beland@umontreal.ca
[1]Groupe de recherche Solidage, CSSS de la Montagne, site Metro, 1801, boulevard de Maisonneuve Ouest, bureau 600, Montréal, Québec H3H 1J9, Canada
[2]École de santé publique, Département d'administration de la santé, Université de Montréal, C.P. 6128, succ. Centre-Ville, Montréal, Québec H3C 3J7, Canada
Full list of author information is available at the end of the article

Webber and colleagues have presented a comprehensive framework illustrating variables associated with life-space mobility [3] (Webber framework). Five categories of determinants of life-space mobility were hypothesized: (i) cognitive determinants are relevant for reaching distant destinations; (ii) psychosocial determinants affects the motivation to be mobile; (iii) physical performance reflects the influence of strength and balance; (iv) environmental context reflects the influence of the built environment; and (v) financial resources, which influences activities, access to mobility aids and modes of transportation. According to the Webber framework, all categories of determinants are influenced by age, culture, and personal life history.

The association between cognition and life-space mobility has been investigated in the literature, but the direction of the relationship remains unsettled. Although mobility may stimulate cognition, high levels of cognitive function may be a prerequisite for being mobile. Mobility is a complex activity requiring high levels of physical and cognitive function, especially when venturing beyond one's domicile [4]. A decline in higher-order cognitive abilities might be followed by a decline in the more complex aspects of life-space mobility, such as driving [5]. Older adults can also adjust their mobility behavior in a way that reflects their cognitive skills [6].

Empirically, cross-sectional studies have reported significant association between higher cognition and an expansive life-space, [2, 7–10] although discrepant findings were reported [11–13]. To our knowledge, three longitudinal studies have investigated whether baseline cognitive function was associated with future life-space mobility, all with mixed results [14–16].

Determinants may influence each other and interact to shape mobility, as suggested in the Webber framework. This opens the possibility that intervening variables mediate or moderate [17] the association between cognition and life-space mobility. Studies have shown that psychosocial determinants (depression or locus of control) and physical determinants (grip strength or walking speed) are related to cognition [9, 18–20] and to life-space mobility [1, 2, 8, 9, 11]. These determinants are legitimate, intervening variables in change in both cognition and mobility. However, with few exceptions, [9] the role of psychosocial and physical determinants as mediators or moderators in the association between cognition and life-space mobility has not been investigated.

Using the Webber framework, the current study examines the association between cognition and life-space mobility in community-dwelling older adults. It also focusses on the role of depressive symptoms and locus of control as psychosocial determinants, and the role of gait speed and grip strength as physical determinants. Both determinants are considered to be proximate forces modifying the association of change in cognition and physical mobility. Other determinants in the Webber framework are considered control variables. Specifically, the main research questions are:

1. Is change in cognition associated with change in physical mobility?
2. Do depression, locus of control, gait speed, and grip strength intervene in the association of change between cognition and mobility? If so,
   a. Do they play intervening roles along the continuum of values of the measurement instruments, from the lower to the higher end?
   b. Or, is there a threshold at which they start to intervene?

The first question pertains to the main issue raised within the Webber framework. The second question identifies four proximate intervening variables, while questions 2.a and 2.b specify the mechanisms – mediation and moderation - through which these variables act. Figure 1 models the relationship among the six variables, including control variables. Mediation is illustrated by using psychological determinants, and moderation by using the physical determinants.These research questions were examined using data from a longitudinal study of frailty – FRéLE (*Fragilité: étude longitudinale de ses expressions* [21]). Growth mixture models were used, simultaneously testing the association among the set of variables at baseline, or at a fixed state, and the association over time, or the rate of change [22].

Methods

Participants and design

The FRéLE study sampled community-dwelling older adults (aged 65 and over) from three locations in the province of Québec, Canada: a metropolitan area (Montréal); a mid-sized city (Sherbrooke); and a small town and surroundings (Victoriaville). Participants were recruited in 2010 by a random sample drawn from the Québec Medicare database. The sample was stratified by sex, age, and location to secure a sufficient number of participants presenting with frailty. Individuals with significant hearing problems, or inability to speak either French or English were excluded. From the database, 4915 individuals were identified and 432 were excluded based on the study screening criteria. Of the 4483 qualified individuals, 52.2% refused to participate. Of the remaining 2141 individuals, 20% dropped out of the survey before T0 (baseline), 2% could not be contacted, and 1.3% did not complete the questionnaire, leaving a total of 1643 participants in the study (see Additional file 1: Part 1 for sample characteristics and Additional file 5).

Participants underwent a series of functional and psychosocial measurements carried out by trained health professionals at baseline (T0), and two annual follow-ups (T1, T2). When moderate to severe cognitive issues were suspected, the consent of a trustee or fiduciary was obtained. The research protocol was approved by the Research Ethics Committee of the Jewish General Hospital (#15–182). Preliminary analysis revealed that the sociodemographic characteristics and health status of FRéLE participants reflected the community-dwelling elderly population across the province [23].

Measures

Predictor variable

Cognitive function **(MoCA)** Cognitive function was measured using the Montreal Cognitive Assessment

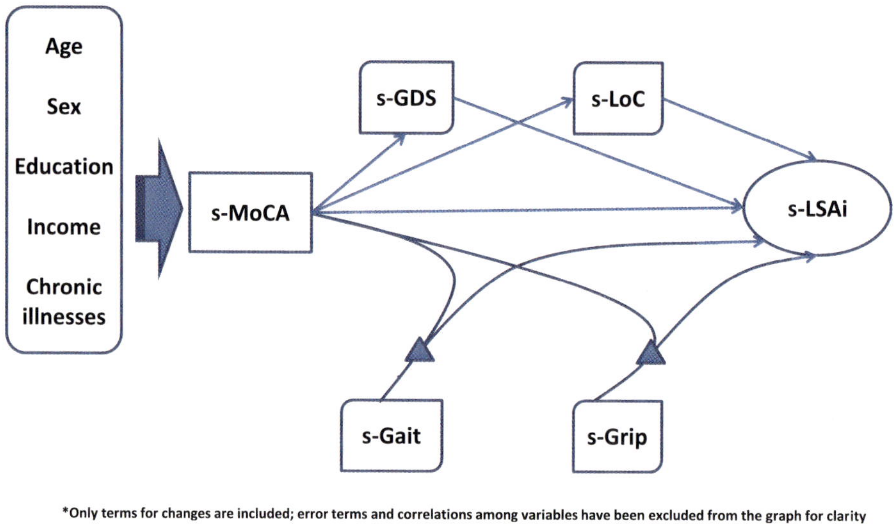

Fig. 1 Theoretical Model*

instrument [24]. MoCA scores ranged from 0 to 30, with lower scores representing greater cognitive impairment. The test-retest reliability of the MoCA is high, along with its internal consistency [24]. FRéLE respondents with scores above 23 on the Mini-Mental State Evaluation [25] were given the MoCA. The 66 respondents excluded from taking the MoCA were considered to have a lower cognitive status. They were not excluded from the analysis and were censured to the left. In the current study, continuous MoCA scores were used.

Predicted variable

***Life-space mobility* (LSA)** The Life-Space Assessment index [1] was used to investigate life-space mobility. In the LSA, five different types of life-space are assessed: within-home, around home, neighborhood, town and outside of town. For each type of life-space, participants reported the frequency of movement during the previous 4 weeks, and whether assistance was needed. LSA scores ranged from 0 to 120, with higher scores reflecting greater life-space mobility. The LSA shows excellent test-retest reliability over a two-week period [1].

Intervening variables

***Depressive symptoms* (GDS)** Depressive symptoms were assessed using the 15-item version of the *Geriatric Depression Scale* [26]. GDS scores ranged from 0 to 15, with higher scores indicating higher levels of depressive symptoms. In order to align GDS scores with other time-varying variables scores, they were transformed: high scores indicated lower depressive symptoms. Continuous GDS scores were used in this study.

***Locus of control* (LoC)** The Personal Mastery Scale [27] is a seven-item scale assessing the extent of the belief that one is able to control or influence outcomes. For each item, scores ranged from 1 (strongly agree) to 4 (strongly disagree), with higher scores reflecting a higher level of control.

***Gait speed* (gait)** Walking speed (cm/sec) was assessed by recording the time required to walk 4, 3, or 2.44 m (according to the space available in the participant's home) [28].

***Grip strength* (grip)** Handgrip strength was measured using the hand Baseline vigorimeter, following American Society of Hand Therapists recommendations [29]. Three measures for each hand were taken, alternating between the dominant and non-dominant hand. For the current study, the variable represented the average score in KiloPascal (KPa) of the three measures from the strongest hand.

Control variables

Control variables were assessed by a series of items on sex, age, education, annual income, number of chronic illnesses, and living site (metropolitan area, mid-sized city, small town) [30].

Statistical analysis

Modelling change on time-varying variables

The predictor variable (MoCA), the predicted variable (LSA), and the four intervening variables (Gait, Grip, GDS, and LoC) are time-varying indicators, as is one of the control variables (number of chronic illnesses). Change in each of the seven variables over the three observed time periods was modelled using growth modelling [31] with non-ignorable dropout cases [32]. At each period, the average of the time-varying variables at T0 was subtracted from the corresponding score. LSA, MoCA, gait speed, and grip strength scales were transformed by dividing each by a constant in order to align the range of variance values among all variables [22].

Observed scores for LSA (Lsam_t0; Lsam_t1; Lsam_t2) at the three time periods are shown in Fig. 2 with rectangles; above the rectangles, linked with arrows, are the associated standard errors (not shown). Over three time periods, the variables are patterned by two parameters: their intercepts (*iL6*-type), representing state or cross-sectional results; and the slope (*sL6-type*), representing change (increase, decrease, or stability). Coefficients for intercept with observed scores at each period are fixed to "1", and for slope to "0", "1" and "2" [31]. Change parameters for T0 are fixed to zero for identification purposes. Inasmuch as non-null standard errors are associated with intercept, respondent scores vary. Though slope may signal changes, the standard errors may not be significantly different from zero, inasmuch as the amount of change is not different among respondents. In this case, the cohort of respondents changes collectively in the same way from one time period to another.The first step in the analysis estimates the growth model parameters for each predicted and predictor variable and for the intervening time-varying variables, adjusting for control variables. Level of significance was set at $\alpha \leq 0.05$. The set of non-statistically significant growth model coefficients is then fixed to zero and tested to examine whether they can be excluded from further analysis using bootstrap likelihood ratio test (BLRT) and Bayesian information criterion (BIC).

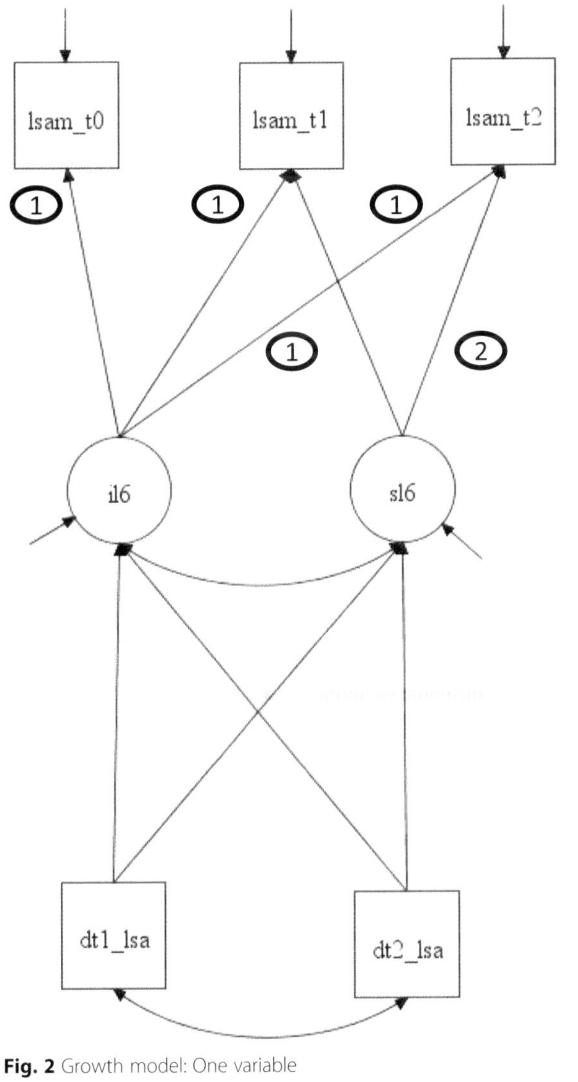

Fig. 2 Growth model: One variable

Pattern-mixture modelling (PMM) is used to model non-ignorable dropout cases (Fig. 2) [32, 33]. PMM does not explore causal effects of observed variables on dropout [32]. Rather, sources of variation in the outcome variables are identified.

Modelling change in LSA and MoCA

The association of MoCA with LSA, adjusting for control variables, is estimated using three terms: the regression of the intercept of LSA (*iLSA*) on 1) the intercept of MoCA (*iMoCA*); and the regression of the slope of LSA (*sLSA*) on 2) *iMoCA* and 3) *sMoCA*.

Parameter estimates for MoCA and for LSA growth models (Table 1) may change with the regression of LSA on MoCA. For example, the coefficient for dropout may lose statistical significance, inasmuch as MoCA and LSA contribute to loss of respondents between panels.

Muthén and Muthén [22] proposed the decomposition of complex models into parts, integrating the parts using resulting estimated parameters as starting values. This strategy was used in building the model to test our main hypotheses (Fig. 1). As in Cheong et al., [34] shapes of the growth trajectory for each intervening variable were investigated.

Mediating and moderating the association of MoCA with LSA

The direct association of MoCA with LSA, and the mediation and moderation of psychosocial characteristics and physical performance between MoCA and LSA are estimated with the Muthén and Asparouhov [31] web of hypotheses found in Fig. 3. The terms in Fig. 3 were derived from the expected value of LSA conditional on MoCA, and on the intervening variables [31]. Thus, the expected value of LSA is conditional based on:

Table 1 Parameter estimates for growth models

		Bootstrap CI			Bootstrap CI		
		Coef.	CI<0,95	CI>0,95	Coef.	CI<0,95	CI>0,95
A. Predictor and predicted variables							
		LSA/10			MoCA/2		
Fixed							
Average (i)		0.42	-0.03	0.87	0.02	-0.65	0.72
Growth rate (s)		-0.28*	-0.52	-0.08	0.57***	0.34	0.83
Random							
Average (i)		2.55*	2.23	2.93	4.57***	3.78	5.54
Growth rate (s)		0.21*	0.06	0.32	0.38**	0.07	0.64
(i) x (s)		-0.23*	-0.42	-0.04	0.16	-0.16	0.55
Pattern-Mixture: Missing not at random							
(i) Time_1		0.07	-0.29	0.43	-0.30	-0.76	0.12
(i) Time_2		-0.42**	-0.70	-0.11	-0.63**	-1.07	-0.23
(s) Time_1		-0.15	-0.37	0.01	-0.11	-0.40	0.12
(s) Time_2		-0.15	-0.37	0.01	-0.11	-0.40	0.12
Observed variables residual variances							
@t0		1.58*	1.21	1.97	1.08*	0.59	1.64
@t1		1.33*	1.14	1.56	1.36*	0.93	1.77
@t2		1.11*	0.77	1.43	1.41*	0.69	2.31
		LL	# of par.	BIC	LL	# of par.	BIC
Log-likehood	Model: H1[1]	-16244.00	36	32751	-16778.00	36	33824
	Model: H0[2]	-16245.20	34	32738	-16779.50	34	33850
	-2(LL[H1]-LL[H0]]	2.40	2	13	3.00	2	-26
B. Intermediate variables							
		Gait speed/10			Grip Strenght/10		
Fixed							
Average (i)		0.84*	0.35	1.31	-0.13	-0.45	0.20
Growth rate (s)		-0.12	-0.31	0.08	-0.14*	-0.26	-0.03
Random							
Average (i)		4.49*	4.04	5.14	1.99*	1.82	2.24
Growth rate (s)		0.18	-0.03	0.40	0.02	-0.06	0.10
(i) x (s)		-0.23	-0.51	0.02	-0.01	-0.09	0.08
Pattern-Mixture: Missing not at random							
(i) Time_1		0.01	-0.38	0.36	-0.05	-0.32	0.20
(i) Time_2		-0.64*	-0.94	-0.33	-0.09	-0.29	0.14
(s) Time_1		-0.13	-0.32	0.06	-0.16*	-0.29	-0.02
(s) Time_2		-0.13	-0.32	0.06	-0.16*	-0.29	-0.02
Observed variables residual variances							
@t0		2.37*	1.94	2.89	0.92*	0.76	1.01
@t1		1.63*	1.39	1.90	0.40*	0.32	0.49
@t2		1.02*	0.62	1.47	0.56*	0.41	0.73
		LL	# of par.	BIC	LL	# of par.	BIC
Log-likehood	Model: H1[1]	-16841.60	36	33950	-14848.00	36	29963
	Model: H0[2]	-16844.20	31	33918	-14852.60	30	29927

Table 1 Parameter estimates for growth models *(Continued)*

		Bootstrap CI			Bootstrap CI		
		Coef.	CI<0,95	CI>0,95	Coef.	CI<0,95	CI>0,95
	-2(LL[H1]-LL[H0]	5.20	5	32	9.20	6	36
		GDS			Locus of control		
Fixed							
Average (i)		0.00	-0.48	0.46	-0.24	-0.78	0.37
Growth rate (s)		-0.33*	-0.57	-0.13	0.06	-0.21	0.35
Random							
Average (i)		4.06*	3.62	4.70	6.06*	5.32	7.03
Growth rate (s)		0.54*	0.33	0.76	0.87*	0.59	1.23
(i) x (s)		-0.32*	-0.58	-0.07	-0.78*	-1.22	-0.43
Pattern-Mixture: Missing not at random							
(i) Time_1		0.19	-0.19	0.53	-0.25	-0.69	0.19
(i) Time_2		0.64*	0.34	0.92	-0.40	-0.71	0.01
(s) Time_1		0.05	-0.14	0.24*	0.04	-0.27	0.29
(s) Time_2		0.05	-0.14	0.24	0.04	-0.27	0.29
Observed variables residual variances							
@t0		1.32*	0.85	1.80	2.80*	2.12	3.50
@t1		1.87*	1.64	2.14	3.82*	3.48	4.29
@t2		0.74*	0.32	1.17	2.45*	1.80	3.16
		LL	# of par.	BIC	LL	# of par.	BIC
Log-likehood	2003Model: H1[1]	-16797.80	36	33862	-18108.40	36	36484
	Model: H0[2]	-16798.70	33	33841	-18109.30	32	36455
	-2(LL[H1]-LL[H0]	1.80	3	21	1.80	4	29

* $p \leq 0,05$; ** $p \leq 0,01$; *** $p \leq 0,001$
[1]H1: Models with all coefficients estimated
[2]H0: Models with non-significant coefficients fixed to 0
[3]LSA and Grip Strength scores were divided by 10; MoCA by 2

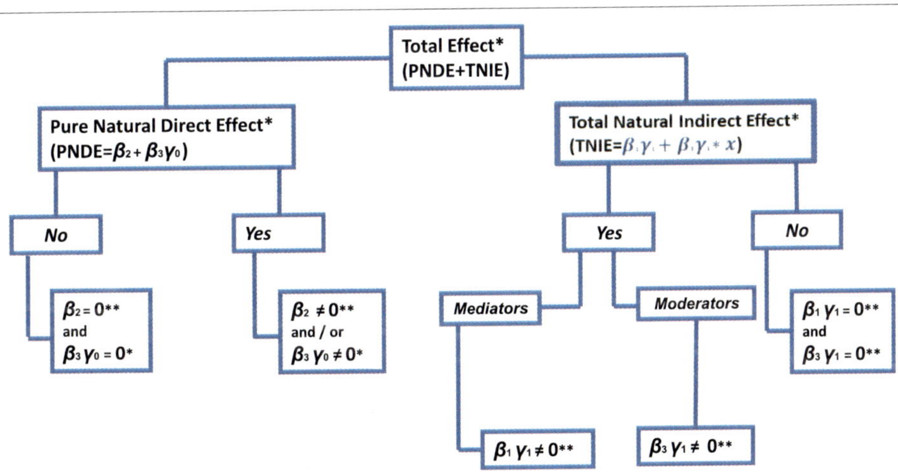

Fig. 3 Direct effects, mediators and moderators: A web of hypotheses

1. The coefficient of MoCA: β_2. This is the Baron and Kenny [17] estimation of the direct effect of MoCA on LSA;
2. The product of the coefficient of a mediator and MoCA with the coefficient of LSA and this mediator: $\beta_1\Upsilon_1$. This is the Baron and Kenny [17] formulation of the mediation hypothesis, with extensions by MacKinnon et al. [35] and Preacher et al.; [36]
3. The term for moderators: $\beta_3\Upsilon_1$. This is homologous with the Hayes index [37] of moderated mediation when the interaction involves the predictor and a mediator variable. In the Baron and Kenny scheme, [17] the interaction term β_3 alone defines moderation; [38]
4. The term $\beta_3\Upsilon_0$. Because Υ_0 is not involved in the association of MoCA with intervening variables, [31] $\beta_3\Upsilon_0$ does not contribute to indirect association, but to direct association. Thus, even though $\beta_2 = 0$, the direct association of MoCA with LSA can be significant.

Modeling intercept and slope introduces restrictions among the associations. Slope represents change occurring across all observation points, while intercept involves observations at baseline only. Thus, slope cannot predict intercept, but intercept can predict slope. The Parallel Process Latent Growth model [34] is an example. This model has been extended to include: [39] 1) the intercept-only model, where intercepts are sole mediators; 2) the slope-only model, where slopes are sole mediators; and 3) the multiple mediation model, where both intercepts and slopes are mediators. Intercepts are not mediators for other intercepts in any of these models. Thus, in these models, the structure of association among the intercepts is considered ignorable [40]. The FRéLE design is observational and longitudinal. Two data generating processes are proposed as expressions of the theoretical model of change originating from the Webber framework: 1) observations at baseline resulting from the cumulative operation of the model over the life-course, and 2) changes during the longitudinal observational period (2 years). This two-way process requires that the mediation and moderation structure is imposed on both intercepts and slopes.

Null hypotheses, as shown in Fig. 3, were tested using the Mplus constraint procedure [22]. Standard errors in the indicators for mediator and moderator were bootstrapped for all models, except for the model with two interaction terms. The bootstrap procedure could not be applied in this latter case, as the computer time required to obtain estimates became unwieldy on a 2-Xeon-based machine with 32 threads.

Results

At baseline, the average score on the LSA original scale was 62.6, decreasing somewhat over time. The MoCA score was below the threshold of 26 for normal cognitive functioning, [24] but increasing from baseline to T1. Grip strength was the only intervening variable with a continuing, decreasing trend. Gait speed was slightly above the cut-off point for acceptable functioning (8 cm/sec), with an average of 8.8 cm/sec. Gait speed and both psychosocial determinants were stable.

Estimating change in time-varying variables

Preliminary analysis was conducted to ensure that change observed in time-varying variables could not be confounded by unstable, unreliable measurements. Results suggested that change could not be attributed to measurement errors (Additional file 2: Part 2).

Table 1 provides the parameter estimates of modelling change for each of the intervening variables, adjusted for control variables. There were significant variations in respondent scores. Growth rates were negative on LSA, gait speed, grip strength, and GDS, and positive on MoCA. Dropouts had lower scores than respondents who remained in the study at T1, suggesting that the estimated positive values of growth rate on MoCA may be a survival effect. Though growth rate for LoC did not change significantly between periods, variations in respondent growth rates were obtained. Finally, except for MoCA, residual errors were smaller at T2 than at T0, indicative of a decrease in the heterogeneity of respondents (Additional file 3: Part 3).

Regression of MoCA and LSA

The coefficients for the regression of MoCA and LSA, with control variables included in the model, are shown in Table 2. The growth rates for MoCA and LSA and their random terms were more or less in the same range as estimates in Table 1. However, the association of *iMoCA* with *sMoCA* lost statistical significance. Only the regression coefficients of the LSA intercept (*iLSA*) on MoCA intercept (i*MoCA*) were significant. Thus, if life-space increased with MoCA, a change in life-space was not sensitive to levels and change in MoCA.

Estimating interactions

Following the Muthén and Muthén procedure, [22] interactions among the intervening variables and MoCA were grouped in six parts, one for each intervening variable intercept and slope with significant standard error (Table 3). Interaction was defined by the rule that *iLSA* cannot be regressed on slope terms for MoCA and intervening variables, and intervening variable intercept terms cannot be regressed on s*MoCA*. Intervening variable intercept terms were accepted as potential

Table 2 Regression of LSA on MoCA[a]

		Bootstrap CI		
		Coef.	CI < 0,95	CI > 0,95
Fixed				
LSA	Intercept (iLSA)	0.356*	0.031	0.684
	Growth rate (sLSA)	−0.284***	−0.432	−0.107
MoCA	Intercept (iMoCA)	0.086	−0.612	0.777
	Growth rate (sMoCA)	0.484***	0.359	0.619
Pattern-Mixture: Missing not at random				
LSA	(i) Time_1	0.000	[NS]	[NS]
	(i) Time_2	−0.294**	−0.522	− 0.073
	(s) Time_1	0.000	[NS]	[NS]
	(s) Time_2	0.000	[NS]	[NS]
MoCA	(i) Time_1	0.000	[NS]	[NS]
	(i) Time_2	−0.807***	−1.149	−0.499
	(s) Time_1	0.000	[NS]	[NS]
	(s) Time_2	0.000	[NS]	[NS]
Random				
LSA	Intercept (iLSA)	2.507***	2.180	2.860
	Growth rate (sLSA)	0.271***	0.114	0.426
	(iLSA) x (sLSA)	−0.297**	−0.477	−0.099
MoCA	Intercept (iMoCA)	4.633***	3.906	6.604
	Growth rate (sMoCA)	0.397*	0.125	0.642
	(iMoCA) x (sMoCA)	0.128	−0.196	0.474
Regression: LSA				
iLSA on	iMoCA	0.168***	0.123	0.217
sLSA on	iMoCA	− 0.002	−0.012	0.028
sLSA on	sMoCA	0.040	−0.231	0.216

*$p \leq 0{,}05$; ** $p \leq 0{,}01$; *** $p \leq 0{,}001$

[a]Control variables included

moderators between *sMoCA* and *sLSA* inasmuch as their association with *sMoCA* was not statistically significant. Latent interaction terms were obtained with the "xwith" operator in Mplus, [22] as in Luo et al. [41]. No interaction terms involving GDS and LoC were significant (Table 3, Part 2). The interaction of gait speed (*iGait*), and grip strength (*iGrip*) with *iMoCA* was significant (Table 3, Part 1) Interaction of *iGrip* with *sMoCA* almost reached significance for *sLSA* at the 0.05 level. Significant interaction terms, plus interaction of *iGrip* with *sMoCA* for *sLSA*, were introduced in a model including control variables, and the predictor, intervening, and predicted variables (Table 4). Interaction terms for *iLSA* were statistically significant when tested one at a time, but their BIC statistics were nearly equal to BIC for the model without interaction (Table 4, Part A.1). Also the null hypothesis for the interaction term for *sLSA* could not be rejected (Table 4, Part A.1). Both interaction terms for *iLSA* were entered in a model (Table 4, Part B.1), and the contribution of each examined. The contribution of *iGait* was not significant, while the null hypothesis for the interaction term with *iGrip* was rejected (Table 4, Part B.2). Finally, the significance of the interaction involving *iGrip* was tested against a new null model including the term for *iGrip*. The null hypothesis of no interaction was rejected (Table 4, Part B.3) and the interaction term of *iMoCA* with *iGrip* for *iLSA* was the only interaction retained in the final model.

Introducing intervening variables

A single model was set up that simultaneously included all statistically significant parameters from the above analytical steps. Parameters were excluded if both the estimates and the associated log likelihood ratio tests did not reach statistical significance. Results are shown in Figs. 4, 5 and 6. These figures are organized based on MoCA and LSA intercept and slope terms for clarity. Also, only the significant structural parameters involving association among intercept and slope for *MoCA*, the intervening variables, and LSA are shown. Control variables and residuals have been excluded from these figures for greater clarity.

The model for the association of *iMoCA* with *iLSA* is shown is Fig. 4. Though the direct association between the two is not significant, it was included in the model because of the *iMoCA-iGrip* interaction terms. Thus, the possibility that *iGrip* is a moderator was examined. All intervening variables were shown to be associated with *iMoCA* and all, except *iLoC*, were associated with *iLSA*. *iGDS*, *iGait* and *iGrip* were tested as mediators. Estimated regression parameters involving *sLSA* and *iMoCA* are shown in Fig. 5. *sLSA* was associated with *iGait* and *sGDS*. Only *iGait* may have a mediator relationship with *iMoCA* and *sLSA*. Finally, in Fig. 6, the terms for change are emphasized to enhance the association among *sMoCA* and *sLSA*, and the intervening variables. No direct association was found between the two variables. Also, *sMoCA* is associated with *sGait*, *sGrip* and *sGDS*. As the *sGait* and *sGrip* standard errors were fixed to zero, no association with sLSA could be estimated. In this case, only *sGDS* could be considered to be a mediator. In summary, the set of our main hypothesized mediations, except for LoC, was potentially retained for mediation involving intercept only. *iGrip* was retained as a moderator between iMoCA and *iLSA*. The term for change on LSA (*sLSA*) was not related to the intercept or slope for MoCA. *sGDS* and *iGait* were associated with *sLSA*, and *sGDS* almost reached statistical significance as a mediator between *sMoCA* and *sLSA*.

Statistical significance of mediator and moderator terms

The term for direct effect ($\beta_3\Upsilon_0$) was not statistically significant. All mediator and moderator relations shown in

Table 3 Interactions of intermediate variables with cognitive impairments

	Coef.	s.e.	*P*-level	Coef.	s.e.	*P*-level
Part 1: Physical performance		Gait speed [iGait]			Grip strength [iGrip]	
iLSA1 on interaction of iMoCA2 with:	−0,019**	0.007	0.008	−0,027*	0.011	0.014
sLSA1 on interaction of iMoCA2 with:	0.003	0.004	0.452	0.001	0.006	0.905
sLSA1 on Interaction of sMoCA2 with:	−0.029	0.019	0.121	−0.049	0.026	0.057
	-2LL	# of free Parameters	BIC	-2LL	# of free parameters	BIC
With interaction: [LLh1]	−33,550.4	66	67,589	−31,759.1	67	64,014
Without interaction: [LLh0]	−33,556.3	63	67,579	−31,764.9	64	64,004
−2*(LLh0-LLh1)	11,7*	3	−10	11,7**	3	−10
Part 2: Pyschosocial GDS [iGDS] GDS [sGDS]		GDS [iGDS]			GDS [sGDS]	
iLSA1 on interaction of iMoCA2 with:	0.005	0.008	0.514	N.A.**	N.A.**	N.A.**
sLSA1 on interaction of iMoCA2 with:	−0.037	0.061	0.542	0.006	0.023	0.803
sLSA1 on Interaction of sMoCA2 with:	0.165	0.260	0.526	0.187	0.380	0.623
	-2LL	# of free parameters	BIC	-2LL	# of free parameters	BIC
With interaction: [LLh1]	−33,586.5	71	67,699	−33,585.9	70	676
Without interaction: [LLh0]	−33,587.2	68	67,678	−33,585.6	68	67,678
−2*(LLh0-LLh1)	1.5	3	−21	−0.6	2	67,002
		Locus of control [iLoC]			Locus of control [sLoC]	
iLSA1 on interaction of iMoCA2 with:	−0.006	0.006	0.321	N.A.**	N.A.**	N.A.**
sLSA1 on interaction of iMoCA2 with:	< 0,001	0.003	0.914	−0.01	0.012	0.369
sLSA1 on Interaction of sMoCA2 with:	−0.033	0.027	0.222	−0.052	0.088	0.557
	-2LL	# of free parameters	BIC	-2LL	# of free parameters	BIC
With interaction: [LLh1]	−35,006.1	70	70,530	−35,007.3	69	70,525
Without interaction: [LLh0]	−35,008,0	67	70,512	−35,008,0	67	70,512
−2*(LLh0-LLh1)	3.7	3	−18	1.4	2	−13

*$p \leq 0,05$
**Not available

Figs. 4, 5 and 6 were statistically significant, except for the mediation of *iGrip* between *iMoCA* to *iLSA*. However, *iGrip* remained a statistically significant moderator (table not shown).

Figure 7 shows three regression lines for standardized *iLSA* scores on standardized *iMoCA* scores. The association of *iMoCA* with *iLSA* is progressively headed toward zero as *iGrip* scores increase. *iGrip* appears to compensate for the association of *iMoCA* with *iLSA* at lower scores on *iMoCA*. Thus, the association of *iMoCA* with *iLSA* is significant only for low *iGrip* scores. However, statistical significance is not a measure of association. Statistically significant coefficients in this study were small (Additional file 4: Part 4).

The weighted distribution of the number of FRéLE respondents on the *iMoCA* continuum is shown in Fig. 7 as shaded bars. The modification of the association of *iMoCA* with *iLSA* at low levels of *iGrip* concerns a minority of respondents.

Discussion

The aim of this study was to examine the longitudinal association between cognitive decline and change in life-space mobility in community-dwelling older adults, and to investigate the impact of moderators and mediators on this association. Based on the Webber framework, two questions were asked. The first examined the extent that change in cognitive function was associated with change in life-space mobility. In a model with cognition as the sole predictor, including controlled variables, the direct association was not significant. To our knowledge, no other studies have examined associations between change in cognitive function and change in life-space mobility. In our study, the direct association between the two variables was significant at baseline, suggesting an accumulation of reciprocal effects throughout the life course. Yet, with the introduction of intermediate psychosocial and physical performance variables, this direct association fell into the non-statistically significant

Table 4 Testing interactions of Cognitive Impairments with Gait Speed and Grip Strength in the final model

	# of free			Gait speed [iGait[3]]			Grip strength [iGrip[4]]		
	-2LL	Parameters	BIC	Coef.	s.e.	*P*-level	Coef.	s.e.	*P*-level
Part A.1: Testing interactions one at a time:									
Without interaction: [LLh4]	−58,867.3	115	118,586						
iLSA[1] on iGrip + Int[iGrip][5]: [LLh5]	−58,858.9	117	118,584				−0.033***	0.010	0.001
−2*(LLh4-LLh5)	16.84***	2	-2						
iLSA[1] on iGait + Int[iGait][6]: [LLh6]	−58,862.6	116	118,584	−0.018*	0.007	0.014			
−2*(LLh4-LLh6)	9.46**	1	-2						
sLSA[1] on iGrip + Int[sGrip][7]: [LLh7]	−58,865.0	117	118,596				−0.051	0.031	0.095
−2†(LLh4-LLh7)	4.48	2	10						
Part B.1: Testing simultaneously, for iLSA, Int[iGrip] & Int[iGait]									
iLSA on iGrip + Int[iGrip] + Int[iGait]: [LLh8]	− 58,858.7	118	118,591	−0.011	0.008	0.141	−0.026*	0.011	0.020
−2†(LLh4-LLh8)	17.09***	3	5						
Part B.2: Testing the significance of Int[iGrip] and Int[iGait]									
Excluding Int[iGait]: [LLLh9]	−58,858.9	117	118,584						
−2†(LLh9-LLh8)	0.25	1	−7						
Excluding Int[iGrip]: [LLh10]	−58,862.6	116	118,584						
−2†(LLh10-LLh8)	7.63*	2	7						
Part B.3: Testing the significance of Int[iGrip]									
Without interaction + [iGrip]: [LLh11]	−58,865.7	116	118,590						
−2†(LLh11-LLh5)	13.69***	1	-6						

$^{*}p \leq 0{,}05$; $^{**}p \leq 0{,}01$; $^{***}p \leq 0{,}001$

†Interactions are not defined for changes in moderators with the LSA intercept

(1) iLSA: intercept for LSA; sLSA: Slope for LSA

(2) iMoCA: intercept for MoCA; sMoCA: Slope for MoCA

(3) iGait: intercept for Gait speed

(4) iGrip: intercept for Grip strenght

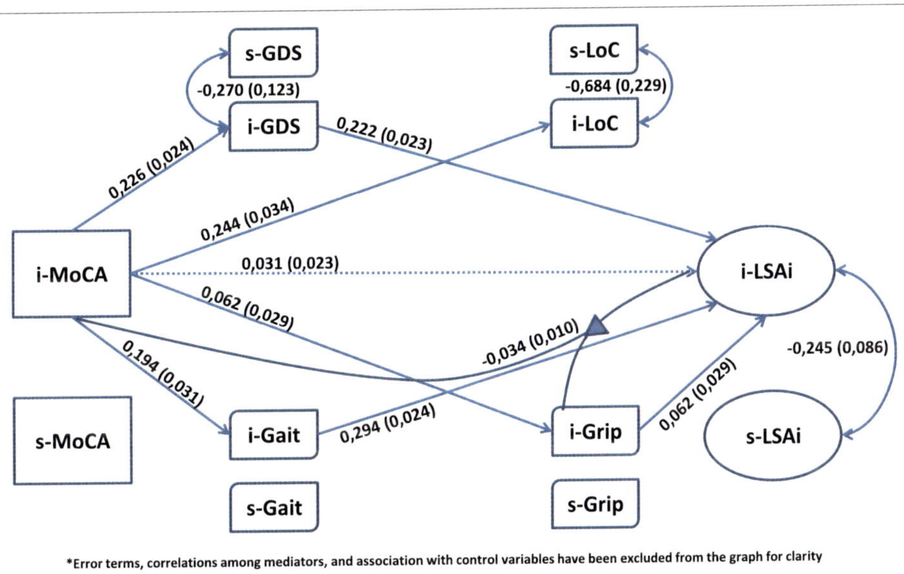

Fig. 4 Mediators and Moderators: MoCA's intercept & LSA's intercept*

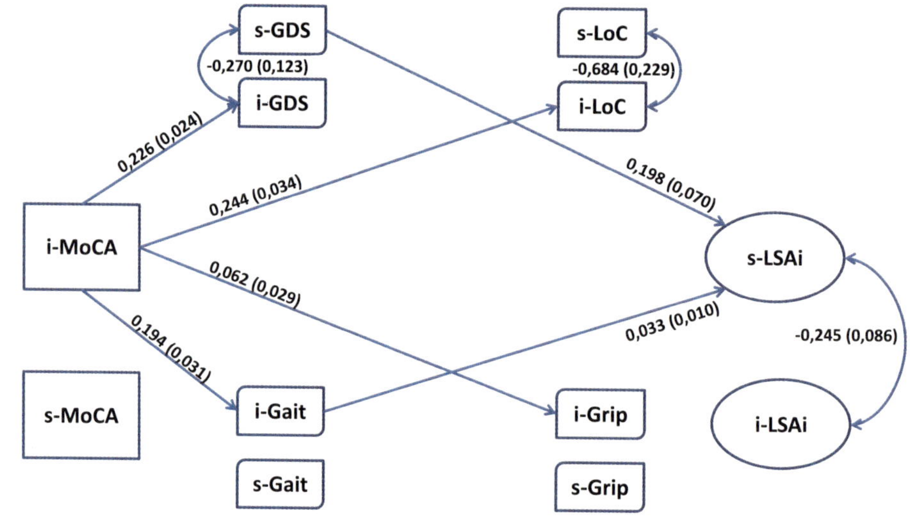

*Error terms, correlations among mediators, and association with control variables have been excluded from the graph for clarity

Fig. 5 Mediators and moderators: MoCA's intercept & LSA's slope*

range. Some studies did not report cross-sectional associations between cognition and life-space mobility, [11–13] while others showed a relationship [2, 7–10]. Discrepancies between these findings may be explained by heterogeneity in samples (e.g., Canadians, Americans female, Mexican Americans), sample size (ranging from 300 to 2737), age of respondents (e.g., 65 years and older, 75 years and older, 65–74 years), and country in which the studies were conducted (USA, Canada, Brazil, Columbia, Finland). That is, associations between cognition and life-space mobility may be influenced by individual as well as sociocultural factors.

The second question dealt with the mediation and mediator roles of psychosocial variables (depression and Locus of Control) and physical performance variables (gait speed and grip strength), and their potential to affect the association between change in cognitive function and life-space mobility. Our results showed a weak mediating effect for change in depression. Locus of control was not associated with change in life-space mobility; it had no mediating nor moderating roles. In contrast, one study reported that locus of control moderated association between cognition and life-space mobility at baseline [9]. Baseline values on gait speed were related with change in life-space mobility. Though change was observed at the cohort level in gait speed and grip strength, the change rate did not vary among individuals. The association of change in gait speed and

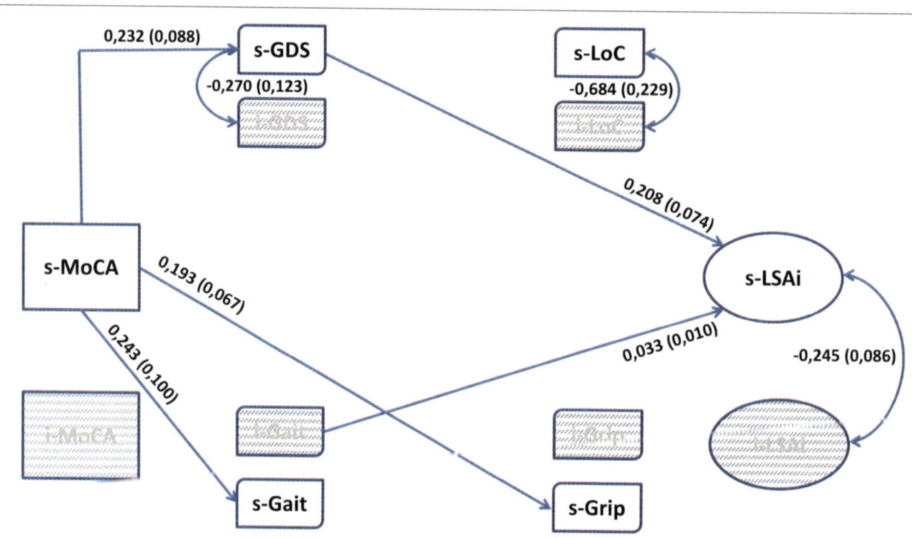

*Error terms, correlations among mediators, and association with control variables have been excluded from the graph for clarity

Fig. 6 Mediators and moderators: MoCA's slope & LSA's slope*

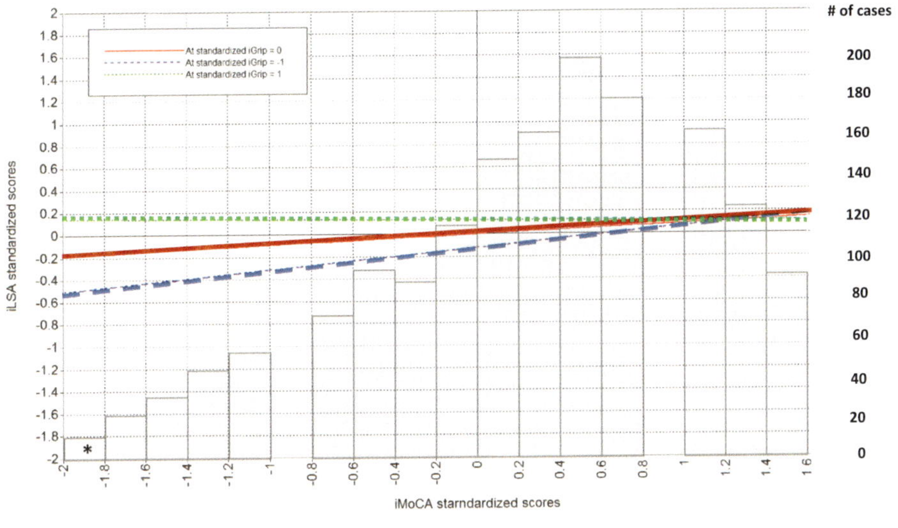

Fig. 7 Averages standardized iLSA scores predicted by iMoCA at three levels of standardized scores for iGrip

grip strength with change in life-space mobility could not be estimated.

At baseline, gait speed played a mediating role in the association between cognition and life-space mobility. Examined separately, interactions of gait speed and grip strength with cognition were statistically significant. However, only the interaction of grip strength remained statistically significant when both were entered simultaneously in the structural equation. Grip strength played a moderating role at baseline only: the association of cognition with life-space mobility decreased with increasing grip strength up to a point where the association had no statistical significance. Of the psychosocial variables, baseline depression showed a trend towards mediating association between cognitive function and life-space mobility. Locus of control was not associated with life-space mobility. Our results, at baseline, thus replicate those of studies reporting an association between higher depressive symptoms and lower life-space mobility [1, 2, 8].

Changes were observed in this study over a two-year period, a short period of time by any standard. Nonetheless, change in cognition and life-space mobility has been observed. Locus of control did not change at the population level, but change in individuals was observed. Grip strength decreased chronologically at the same level across the entire FRéLE sample.

To sum up our results, in persons aged 65 and over, change in life-space mobility occurs slowly and is not related to cognition at the population level. Only change in depression and gait speed at baseline was associated with change in life-space mobility. A low level of association was obtained between the Webber framework determinants and life-space mobility.

Our results support the fact that slow change, observed over time throughout the aging process is complex and not well-understood. Our results also suggest that the process of change in life-space mobility extends over a long period of time, including the entire life course. Thus, from a population health perspective, persons aged 65 and over cumulate life-long social, psychosocial, and health experiences, and any change in health status, from then on, depends on their life course. Whether or not conclusions can be drawn on the efficacy of population health interventions on slowly changing issues observed at a population level is a difficult topic. Whether public health interventions or policies on physical performance at the population level could affect the process of change in life-space mobility, given changes in cognitive ability, is still an unanswered question within the framework of this paper. Mobility in itself is a determinant of health [42]. Indeed, mobility is essential to create and maintain relationships and to participate socially [43]. Social participation has been associated with benefits to physical, cognitive and mental health of seniors [44]. Therefore, future studies should focus on a better understanding of the impact of determinants of health on mobility as well as the impact of mobility on health in seniors, in light of the Webber framework.

There are some limitations to the current study. First, although longitudinal, the study was not designed to determine the direction of causal processes in cognitive deficit, life space, psychosocial characteristics, or physical function, but rather to estimate the source of variations of change in life-space mobility within the Webber framework. Our research questions were legitimate, given our use of growth curve modelling and our understanding of causality in an observation-based longitudinal study design. Causality was not examined, but we tested and used null hypotheses for parameters derived from a structural equation model to get insight on the absence of causality in the set of predictor, intermediate, and predicted variables.

Second, association and interaction among the intermediate variables have not been considered. Also, it could be argued that some of the controlled variables should have been considered for moderation effects. Modeling these associations and interactions would have increased the already complex structural models tested in this paper, pushing to the limit our ability to obtain reliable parameter estimates.

Third, FRéLE was not designed to be representative of the older population in the three locations. However, the distribution of FRéLE characteristics does reflect the elderly population across Quebec.

Fourth, respondents lost to follow-up had lower scores on predictor, intermediate, and predicted variables, than those who remained in the study. However, these sources of variations attributable to non-ignorable missing cases were included in models. Fifth, only changes occurring in a short period of time were observed in the FRéLE study. However, significant changes in cognition and life-space, and psychosocial variables were observed over a two-year period. The variables in this study may require an observation period of longer than 2 years for their association in change to appear. We have not been able to identify latent classes for change in life-space mobility, suggesting that patterns of change are uniform in FRéLE respondents, whatever their age. It is possible that latent classes for change in the predictor and intermediate variables exist. However, estimating latent classes for change on multiple variables introduces complexity in the modelling of the structural equations, in the interpretation of results, and in the estimation procedures. Future work in this direction is under consideration (Additional file 5).

Conclusions

In conclusion, differences in respondents at baseline may have resulted from sequences of multiple processes over their life course: resilience, recovery, improvement or sustained decline [45]. The baseline variables of association, mediation and moderation could be considered as a starting point to examine life course processes. The type of processes that individuals, population subgroups, and whole populations experience could have resulted in different population health states, at baseline and over the course of our study. The FRéLE study was not set up to identify these processes. Nonetheless, locating FRéLE baseline results within a life course perspective opens up opportunities for new studies. In a life course perspective [46] where the baseline model (Fig. 4) can be considered the result of cumulative processes, a strong case can be made in retaining a mediating hypothesis for physical performance variables and depression, and a moderating hypothesis for grip strength. Though the *iGait* interaction term was not significant when it was considered with *iGrip*, difficulties in estimating multiple interaction terms in structural equation models suggest caution before rejecting the moderation hypothesis for *iGait* in future studies. Finally, correlated change in cognitive process and life-space at the population level seems to occur at a low level over all ages, 65 and older. A two-year period may be too short to capture these changes. Also, the association of cognition with life-space mobility seems to be limited to a small proportion of people, as suggested by the moderator role of grip strength. In effect, association of cognition with mobility was limited to lower scores on grip strength, while the sample grip strength scores were skewed toward middle and high scores. Finally, baseline results can be considered a cross-sectional sample, while growth-modeling results are derived from a longitudinal design. In any case, the cross-sectional data and longitudinal data in the FRéLE sample did not yield the same results.

Additional files

Additional file 1: Part 1 Characteristics of respondents. Describes the characteristics of the FRéLE sample.

Additional file 2: Part 2 Reliability of the time-varying variables. Examines the reliability of the time-varying variables to ensure that change observed in these variables was not confounded by unstable reliability of the measures.

Additional file 3: Part 3 Estimating change in each of the time-varying variables. Describes change in each of the time-varying variables.

Additional file 4: Part 4 Statistical significance and strength of association. Describes change in the predicted variable based on a 1-unit change in the predictor variable.

Additional file 5: Table S1. Characteristics of FRéLE participants. Table presenting descriptives of the FRéLE sample.

Abbreviations

BIC: Bayesian information criterion; BLRT: Bootstrap likelihood ratio test; FRéLE: Fragilité: étude longitudinale de ses expressions [Frailty: A longitudinal study of its expression]; Gait: Gait speed; GDS: Geriatric depression scale; Grip: Grip strength; *i*: Intercept; KPa: KiloPascal; LoC: Locus of control; LSA: Life-space assessment; MOCA: Montreal cognitive assessment; PMM: Pattern-mixture modelling; *s*: Slope

Acknowledgements

The authors wish to thank Claude Galand and John Fletcher for data management, and Rebecca Rupp for administrative support.

Funding

The FRéLE study was supported by the Canadian Institutes of Health Research – Instituts de recherche en santé du Canada (FRN# 82945). Additional funding was obtained from the Réseau québécois de recherche sur le vieillissement (Québec Research Network on Aging), Fonds de recherche du Québec – Santé (FRQS) (FRN# 3/31/2014). NB is supported by funding from the FRQS (Bursary # 29032).

The funding sources had no role in the design of the study, in collection, analysis, and interpretation of data, and in writing the manuscript.

Authors' contributions

NB, DJ, LD and JD: Drafting the introduction; FB: Operationalizing the theoretical model, testing statistical models, responsible for the method and results sections; DJ: Involved in writing the methods section; FB, NB, DJ and LD: Responsible for the discussion section. All authors made substantial contributions to the study concept, development of the theoretical model, interpretation of results, and manuscript revision for intellectual content. All approved the final version and agreed to be accountable for aspects regarding accuracy and integrity of the work.

Competing interests

The authors declare that they have no competing interests.

Author details

[1]Groupe de recherche Solidage, CSSS de la Montagne, site Metro, 1801, boulevard de Maisonneuve Ouest, bureau 600, Montréal, Québec H3H 1J9, Canada. [2]École de santé publique, Département d'administration de la santé, Université de Montréal, C.P. 6128, succ. Centre-Ville, Montréal, Québec H3C 3J7, Canada. [3]Faculté de médecine, Division de médecine gériatrique, Université McGill, Hôpital général juif, 3755, chemin de la Côte-Ste-Catherine, Montréal, Québec H3T 1E2, Canada. [4]Département de psychologie, Université de Montréal, Pavillon Marie-Victorin, C. P. 6128, succ. Centre-Ville, Montréal, Québec H3C 3J7, Canada. [5]Centre de recherche, Institut universitaire en santé mentale de Montréal, 7331, rue Hochelaga, Montréal, Québec H1N 3V2, Canada. [6]Centre de recherche, Institut Universitaire de Gériatrie de Montréal, 4545, Chemin Queen Mary, Montréal, Québec H3W 1W5, Canada. [7]Faculté de médecine, École de réadaptation, Université de Montréal, C.P. 6128, succ. Centre-Ville, Montréal, Québec H3C 3J7, Canada. [8]École de réadaptation, Faculté de médecine et des sciences de la santé, Université de Sherbrooke, 3001, 12e Avenue Nord, Sherbrooke, Québec J1H 5N4, Canada. [9]Centre de recherche sur le vieillissement, Centre intégré universitaire de santé et de services sociaux de l'Estrie, Centre hospitalier universitaire de Sherbrooke, 1036, rue Belvédère Sud, Sherbrooke, Québec J1H 4C4, Canada. [10]Faculté de médecine, Département de médecine, Université de Montréal, C.P. 6128, succ. Centre-Ville, Montréal, Québec H3C 3J7, Canada.

References

1. Baker PS, Bodner EV, Allman RM. Measuring life-space mobility in community-dwelling older adults. J Am Geriatr Soc. 2003;51(11):1610–4.
2. Xue Q-L, Fried LP, Glass TA, Laffan A, Chaves PH. Life-space constriction, development of frailty, and the competing risk of mortality: the Women's health and aging study I. Am J Epidemiol. 2007;167(2):240–8.
3. Webber SC, Porter MM, Menec VH. Mobility in older adults: a comprehensive framework. The Gerontologist. 2010;50(4):443–50.
4. Wettstein M, Wahl HW, Shoval N, Oswald F, Voss E, Seidl U, Frolich L, Auslander G, Heinik J, Landau R. Out-of-home behavior and cognitive impairment in older adults: findings of the SenTra project. J Appl Gerontol. 2015;34(1):3–25.
5. O'connor ML, Edwards JD, Wadley VG, Crowe M. Changes in mobility among older adults with psychometrically defined mild cognitive impairment. J Gerontol B Psychol Sci Soc Sci. 2010;65((3):306–16.
6. Ball K, Owsley C. Increasing mobility and reducing accidents of older drivers. In: Schaie KW, Pietrucha M, editors. Mobility and transportation in the elderly. New York: Springer Publishing Company, Inc.; 2000. p. 213–51.
7. Barnes LL, Wilson RS, Bienias JL, Mendes de Leon CF, Kim H-JN, Buchman AS, Bennett DA. Correlates of life space in a volunteer cohort of older adults. Exp Aging Res. 2007;33(1):77–93.
8. Peel C, Sawyer Baker P, Roth DL, Brown CJ, Brodner EV, Allman RM. Assessing mobility in older adults: the UAB study of aging life-space assessment. Phys Ther. 2005;85(10):1008–119.
9. Sartori AC, Wadley VG, Clay OJ, Parisi JM, Rebok GW, Crowe M. The relationship between cognitive function and life space: the potential role of personal control beliefs. PsycholAging. 2012;27(2):364–74.
10. Rantakokko M, Iwarsson S, Portegijs E, Viljanen A, Rantanen T. Associations between environmental characteristics and life-space mobility in community-dwelling older people. J Aging Health. 2015;27(4):606–21.
11. Al Snih S, Peek KM, Sawyer P, Markides KS, Allman RM, Ottenbacher KJ. Life-space mobility in Mexican Americans aged 75 and older. J Am Geriatr Soc. 2012;60(3):532–7.
12. Curcio C-L, Alvarado BE, Gomez F, Guerra R, Guralnik J, Zunzunegui MV. Life-space assessment scale to assess mobility: validation in Latin American older women and men. Aging Clin Exp Res. 2013;25(5):553–60.
13. Silberschmidt S, Kumar A, Raji MM, Markides K, Ottenbacher KJ, Al Snih S: Life-space mobility and cognitive decline among Mexican Americans aged 75 years and older. J Am Geriatr Soc 2017:Epub ahead of print.
14. Allman RM, Baker PS, Maisiak RM, Sims RV, Roseman JM. Racial similarities and differences in predictors of mobility change over eighteen months. J Gen Intern Med. 2004;19(11):1118–26.
15. Poranen-Clark T, von Bonsdorff MB, Rantakokko M, Portegijs E, Eronen J, Kauppinen M, Eriksson JG, Rantanen T, Viljanen A: Executive function and life-space mobility in old age. Aging Clin Exp Res 2017:Epub ahead of print.
16. Shah RC, Maitra K, Barnes LL, James BD, Leurgans S, Bennett DA. Relation of driving status to incident life space constriction in community-dwelling older persons: a prospective cohort study. J Gerontol A: Biomed Sci Med Sci. 2012;67(9):984–9.
17. Baron RM, Kenny DA. The moderator–mediator variable distinction in social psychological research: conceptual, strategic, and statistical considerations. J Pers Soc Psychol. 1986;51(6):1173–82.
18. Atkinson HH, Rapp SR, Williamson JD, Lovato J, Absher JR, Gass M, Henderson VW, Johnson KC, Kostis JB, Sink KM. The relationship between cognitive function and physical performance in older women: results from the women's health initiative memory study. J Gerontol A Biomed Sci Med Sci. 2009;65((3):300–6.
19. Watson N, Rosano C, Boudreau R, Simonsick E, Ferrucci L, Sutton-Tyrrell K, Hardy S, Atkinson H, Yaffe K, Satterfield S. Executive function, memory, and gait speed decline in well-functioning older adults. J Gerontol A Biomed Sci Med Sci. 2010;65((10):1093–100.
20. Yaffe K, Blackwell T, Gore R, Sands L, Reus V, Browner WS. Depressive symptoms and cognitive decline in nondemented elderly women: a prospective study. Arch Gen Psychiatry. 1999;56(5):425–30.
21. Galand C, Béland F, Fletcher J. FRéLE team: FRéLE : une étude québécoise sur la fragilité [FRéLE: a study on fraily in Quebec]. In: Béland F, Michel H, editors. La fragilité des personnes âgées: définitions, controverses et perspectives d'action [Fraily in older adults: definitions, controversies, and perspectives of action]. Rennes: Presses de l'EHESP; 2013. p. 177–204.
22. Muthén LK, Muthén BO: Mplus User's guide, 7th edition edn. Los Angeles, CA: Muthén & Muthén; 1998-2017.
23. Provencher V, Béland F, Demers L, Desrosiers J, Bier N, Avila-Funes JA, Galand C, Julien D, Fletcher J, Trottier L, et al. Are frailty components associated with disability in specific activities of daily living in community-dwelling older adults? A multicenter Canadian study. Arch Gerontol Geriatr. 2017;73:187–94.
24. Nasreddine ZS, Phillips NA, Bedirian V, Charbonneau S, Whitehead V, Collin I, Cummings JL, Chertkow H. The Montreal cognitive assessment, MoCA: a brief screening tool for mild cognitive impairment. J Am Geriatr Soc. 2005; 53(4):695–9.
25. Folstein MF, Folstein SE, McHugh PR. "mini-mental state": a practical method for grading the cognitive state of patients for the clinician. J Psychiatr Res. 1975;12(3):189–98.
26. Yesavage JA, Sheikh JI. 9/geriatric depression scale (GDS) recent evidence and development of a shorter version. Clin Gerontol. 1986;5(1–2):165–73.
27. Pearlin LI, Menaghan EG, Lieberman MA, Mullan JT. The stress process. J Health Soc Behav. 1981:337–56.
28. Guralnik JM, Simonsick EM, Ferrucci L, Glynn RJ, Berkman LF, Blazer DG, Scherr PA, Wallace RB. A short physical performance battery assessing lower extremity function: association with self-reported disability and prediction of mortality and nursing home admission. J Gerontol. 1994;49(2):M85–94.
29. Fess EE. Grip strength. In: Casanova JS, editor. Clinical assessment recommendations. 2nd ed. Chicago: American Society of Hand Therapist; 1992. p. 41–5.
30. Groll DL, To T, Bombardier C, Wright JG. The development of a comorbidity index with physical function as the outcome. J Clin Epidemiol. 2005;58(6):595–602.
31. Muthén B, Asparouhov T. Causal effects in mediation modeling: an

introduction with applications to latent variables. Struct Equ Model Multidiscip J. 2015;22(1):12–23.
32. Muthén B, Asparouhov T, Hunter AM, Leuchter AF. Growth modeling with nonignorable dropout: alternative analyses of the STAR* D antidepressant trial. Psychol Methods. 2011;16(1):17–33.
33. Demirtas H, Schafer JL. On the performance of random-coefficient pattern-mixture models for non-ignorable drop-out. Stat Med. 2003;22(16):2553–75.
34. Cheong J, MacKinnon DP, Khoo ST. Investigation of mediational processes using parallel process latent growth curve modeling. Struct Equ Model. 2003;10(2):238–62.
35. MacKinnon DP, Lockwood CM, Hoffman JM, West SG, Sheets V. A comparison of methods to test mediation and other intervening variable effects. Psychol Methods. 2002;7(1):83.
36. Preacher KJ, Rucker DD, Hayes AF. Addressing moderated mediation hypotheses: theory, methods, and prescriptions. Multivar Behav Res. 2007; 42(1):185–227.
37. Hayes AF. An index and test of linear moderated mediation. Multivar Behav Res. 2015;50(1):1–22.
38. Chmura Kraemer H, Kiernan M, Essex M, Kupfer DJ. How and why criteria defining moderators and mediators differ between the Baron & Kenny and MacArthur approaches. Health Psychol. 2008;27(2S):S101.
39. von Soest T, Hagtvet KA. Mediation analysis in a latent growth curve modeling framework. Struct Equ Model. 2011;18(2):289–314.
40. Holland PW, Rubin DB. Causal inference in retrospective studies. ETS Res Rep Ser. 1987;1987(1):203–31.
41. Luo W, Lee K, Koh ICH. Do competitive performance goals and cooperative social goals conflict? A latent interaction analysis. Learn Individ Differ. 2015; 39:186–92.
42. Gardner P. The role of social engagement and identity in community mobility among older adults aging in place. Disabil Rehabil. 2014;36(15): 1249–57.
43. Pinquart M, Sorensen S. Influences on loneliness in older adults: a meta-analysis. Basic Appl Soc Psychol. 2001;23(4):245–66.
44. Stav WB, Hallenen T, Lane J, Arbesman M. Systematic review of occupational engagement and health outcomes among community-dwelling older adults. Am J Occup Ther. 2012;66(3):301–10.
45. Infurna FJ, Grimm KJ. The use of growth mixture modeling for studying resilience to major life stressors in adulthood and old age: lessons for class size and identification and model selection. J Gerontol B. 2017;73(1):148–59.
46. Kuh D, Ben-Shlomo Y. A life course approach to chronic disease epidemiology. 2nd ed. Oxford: Oxford University Press; 2004.

11

Sarcopenia as a predictor of hospitalization among older people

Xiaoming Zhang†, Wenwu Zhang†, Conghua Wang, Wuyuan Tao, Qingli Dou* and Yunzhi Yang

Abstract

Background: Previous cohort studies investigating the association between sarcopenia and the risk of hospitalization have been inconsistent. We performed a meta-analysis to determine if sarcopenia is a predictor of hospitalization.

Methods: Prospective cohort studies that evaluated the association between sarcopenia and hospitalization in older people were identified via a systematic search of four electronic databases (PubMed, EMBASE, Science Citation Index, and the Cochrane Library). A random-effect model was applied to combine the results according to the heterogeneity of the included studies.

Results: Five studies (2832 participants) were included in this meta-analysis. Pooled results demonstrated that older people with sarcopenia were at an increased risk of hospitalization (pooled hazards ratio [HR] = 1.57, 95% confidence interval [CI] = 1.26, 1.94, $I^2 = 4.5\%$, $P = 0.000$) compared to those without sarcopenia. Results of subgroup analyses showed that hospitalized patients with sarcopenia had a higher rate of hospitalization (HR = 2.01, 95% CI = 1.41, 2.88, $p = 0.000$) versus patients without sarcopenia. A similar result was also found in community-dwelling older people with sarcopenia versus those without sarcopenia (HR = 1.40, 95% CI = 1.05, 1.88, $p = 0.023$). In addition, the subgroup analysis for length of follow-up showed that studies with a follow-up period of 3 years or more (pooled HR = 1.52, 95% CI = 1.19, 1.94, $P = 0.001$) reported a significantly higher rate of hospitalization among individuals with sarcopenia compared to those without sarcopenia. However, this association was not found in the studies with a follow-up period of less than 3 years (pooled HR = 1.76, 95% CI = 0.90, 3.44, $P = 0.099$).

Conclusions: Sarcopenia is a significant predictor of hospitalization among older individuals, and the association may not be significantly affected by the characteristics of the population or the definition of sarcopenia.

Keywords: Sarcopenia, Hospitalization, Older people, Meta-analysis

Background

Sarcopenia was first described by Rosenberg [1] in 1989, who defined sarcopenia as a condition of age-related loss of muscle mass characterized by a decrease in muscle strength and physical performance. Sarcopenia is a feature of aging [2], and the prevalence of sarcopenia is reported to vary from 1 to 29% in community-dwelling older people, from 14 to 33% in long-term care, and about 10% in acute hospital care populations [3]. Currently, sarcopenia is considered a geriatric syndrome rather than a disease [4], and accumulating evidence from epidemiological studies indicates that sarcopenia may be a predictor of aging related conditions, such as functional decline and frailty [5].

The clinical relevance of sarcopenia has been extensively studied in the past few decades, and these studies have demonstrated that older people with sarcopenia have an increased risk of multiple adverse health outcomes, which include falls [6] and fractures [7], decreased mobility [8], depression [9], poor quality of life [10], hospitalization [11] and mortality [12]. In particular, hospitalization is an important outcome for older people, because even a

* Correspondence: 1149646884@qq.com
†Xiaoming Zhang and Wenwu Zhang contributed equally to this work.
Department of Emergency Medicine, the Baoan Hospital affiliated with Southern Medical University, People's Hospital of Baoan District of Shenzhen, No. 118, Longjing, Baoan District, Shenzhen 518101, China

short-term stay in a hospital for an older people is associated with a decline in functional ability [13].

Recently, Bianchi [14] and colleagues reported that sarcopenia was significantly associated with hospitalization (hazard ratio [HR] 1.57; 95% CI 1.03–2.41) among community-dwelling older adults. Furthermore, Yang [15] and Gariballa [16] reported that sarcopenia was significantly associated with re-hospitalization, with HR: 2.49; 95% CI: 1.25–4.95 and HR: 2.52; 95% CI: 1.34–4.75, respectively in hospitalized patients. However, two previous longitudinal studies did not show a significant association between sarcopenia and hospitalization in older individuals. Cawthon [17] and colleagues found that none of the summary definitions or the definition components (slowness, weakness, or low lean mass) was associated with risk of hospitalization (Rate ratio [OR] = 1.27, 95% confidence interval [CI] = 0.85, 1.90) among 1516 males with sarcopenia compared to males without sarcopenia. In addition, Henwood [18] and colleagues reported no significant association between a baseline diagnosis of sarcopenia and hospitalization among 273 male and female nursing homes residents.

In view of these inconsistencies, a meta-analysis of the associated risk is warranted. Recently, Beaudart [19] performed a meta-analysis and systematic review to assess the association between sarcopenia and various health outcomes. However, only one study was available to estimate the association between sarcopenia and hospitalization, and the author analyzed and described the outcomes without a meta-analysis. Therefore, in this meta-analysis, we aimed to include all available prospective cohort studies to summarize the current understanding of the association between sarcopenia and risk of hospitalization in older adults.

Methods

This systematic review was conducted and reported according to the Preferred Reporting Items for Systematic Reviews and Meta-Analyses (PRISMA) guidelines [20].

Data sources and search strategy

A systematic literature review was conducted via searches of PubMed, EMBASE, Science Citation Index, and the Cochrane CENTRAL Library through November 2017. The search strategy was tailored to fulfill the criteria of each database. The search terms included [Hospitalization (Medical Subject Heading (MeSH)] OR (Hospitalization*) AND [(Sarcopenia (Medical Subject Heading (MeSH)] OR (Sarcopenia*). We searched the potential gray studies through Google Scholar. Furthermore, a manual search was carried out on the references of included studies to identify potentially relevant studies. The search string is included in detail in Additional file 1.

Study selection

The studies identified by our search strategy were reviewed by two independent investigators (Zhang XM, Zhang WW) who evaluated each title and abstract of the records. In cases of disagreement about inclusion or exclusion of studies, this issue was resolved by discussion with a third investigator until consensus was reached.

Inclusion and exclusion criteria

The inclusion criteria were as follows: prospective cohort studies. Since these studies could provide a longitudinal association between sarcopenia and the risk of hospitalization with less bias, we only included prospective cohort studies, studies aiming to investigate whether sarcopenia is a predictor of hospitalization, studies clearly reporting diagnostic criteria for sarcopenia, and studies clearly reporting outcomes of hospitalization or readmission. Exclusion criteria were as follows: insufficient data, conference abstracts or review articles, no clear definition of sarcopenia, studies using only components or subdomains of sarcopenia criteria (e.g., muscle mass, Muscle Strength, Physical Performance, SARC-F Questionnaire), and studies published in other languages than English.

Data extraction

Two authors (Zhang XM, Zhang WW) independently extracted data from the included studies into a standardized Microsoft Excel spreadsheet. Any disagreement was resolved by consensus with a third investigator. The following data were extracted from the studies: year of publication, country, demographics of participants (e.g., sample size, and male proportion), follow-up period, definitions of sarcopenia, definitions of hospitalization outcome, and Newcastle–Ottawa scale scores. All data were cross-checked by the investigators. Disagreements were resolved via discussion until consensus was reached. Moreover, our meta-analysis was based on secondary data; therefore, the ethical approval or patient consent was not necessary.

Assessment of risk bias

Assessment of risk of bias was performed by two independent investigators (Zhang XM, Wang CH) according to the Newcastle Ottawa Scale (NOS) [21], which evaluates the quality of cohort studies via the following aspects: representativeness of the exposed cohort, comparability of the groups, blinding of investigators who measured outcomes, the time and completeness of follow-up, contamination bias, and other potential sources of bias. A higher score indicated better quality. A detailed description is shown in Table 3 as a supplement.

Statistical analysis

The STATA version 11.0 (Stata Corp, College Station, TX, USA) was used for all analyses. Hazard ratios (HRs), odds ratios (ORs), and 95% confidence intervals (CIs) for the incidence of hospitalization in older adults with sarcopenia were compared to those without sarcopenia. If the incidence of sarcopenia was less than 10%, we regarded ORs as RRs; otherwise, we used generic inverse variance to calculate the pooled HR. Subgroup analyses according to length of follow-up and type of participants (hospitalized, community-dwelling or nursing home residents) were implemented to analyze the association between sarcopenia and hospitalization. Statistical heterogeneity among the included studies was examined using Cochran's Q statistic using chi-square and I^2 Statistics, and I^2 value of 25%, 50% and 75% represented the cut-off values for the low, moderate, and high heterogeneity, respectively. From the perspective of research and design, there was heterogeneity because of the different evaluation methods of sarcopenia, different types of participants, and length of follow-up. Therefore, we used the random-effects model to synthesize all data, regardless of heterogeneity between the pooled studies, in statistical order to obtain more conservative results. Subgroup analyses according to different populations and length of follow-up were performed to analyze the association of sarcopenia and hospitalization.

Results

Selection processes

A total of 1083 articles were initially identified via our literature search. After eliminating duplicate articles, 935 articles were screened for potential eligibility. After screening the titles and summaries, non-related articles were removed and the remaining 24 articles were included for further investigation. Of these articles, six were removed because they were not cohort studies (e.g., review articles, cross-sectional study), three were removed because of irrelevant outcomes, eight were removed because they had no clear definition of sarcopenia, and two were same cohort studies. Figure 1 shows the flow diagram of our literature search and selection process.

Included studies

Table 1 presents the characteristics of five cohort studies [14–18] included in our meta-analysis. One studies was from America [17], one was from China [15], and the remaining three were from the UK [16], Australia [18], and Italy [14], respectively. Four studies [14–16, 18] included both male and female participants, while one study [17] included only male participants. The population included in our study included hospitalized patients [15, 16], community-dwelling older people [14, 17], and nursing home residents [18]. Sample size varied from 58 to 1516 and the mean age of the study participants was > 70 years. Moreover, all of the studies selected hospitalization [14, 17, 18] or re-hospitalization [15, 16] as the clinical outcomes. In four of the studies [14, 16–18], sarcopenia was diagnosed by the European Working Group for Sarcopenia in Older Persons (EWGSOP); in one study [15], sarcopenia was diagnosed by the Asian Working Group for Sarcopenia (AWGS). The EWGSOP [22] defined sarcopenia as ALM adjusted for height squared as ≤ 7.26 kg/m^2 in men and ≤ 5.54 kg/m^2 in women combined with low hand-grip strength (< 30 kg) and low gait speed (< 0.8 m/s), and/or low grip strength < 30 kg for men and < 20 kg for women. According to AWGS [23], participants were classified as having sarcopenia if the participants had a lower muscle mass with a low handgrip strength of < 26 kg in men and < 18 kg in women, and a lower gait speed < 0.8 m/s. Follow-up periods ranged from 0.5 to 10 years. The largest study [17] involved 1516 participants, while the minimum cohort [18] involved 58 participants. The prevalence of sarcopenia ranged from 7.5 to 40.2%. The results of each study were displayed in our studies. Table 2 shows the different tools and cut-off of muscle mass, muscle strength, and physical performance.

Quality assessment

Table 3 shows the detailed description of the methodological quality evaluation using NOS. Scores ranged from six to eight and three studies reported scores > 7.

Sarcopenia as a predictor of hospitalization

Meta-analysis of studies

Five studies [14–18] evaluated the association between sarcopenia and hospitalization. Because of the different evaluation methods of sarcopenia, different type of participants, and length of follow-up, and considering the presence of the heterogeneity of the study itself, we used the random-effects model to synthesize all data, regardless of heterogeneity between the pooled studies, in statistical order to obtain more conservative results. The data are shown in Fig. 2. The pooled results showed that older people with sarcopenia had significantly higher risk of hospitalization (pooled HR = 1.57, 95% CI = 1.26, 1.94, $P = 0.000$) versus participants without sarcopenia. No significant heterogeneity was observed in these studies (Q-value = 4.19, degree of freedom = 4, $I^2 =$ 4.5%, $P = 0.381$).

Subgroup analyses

The HR of hospitalization risk for sarcopenia in five studies [14–18] was further assessed by subgroup analyses. According to the type of the participants, the association between sarcopenia and hospitalization was consistent in studies with hospitalized patients (pooled

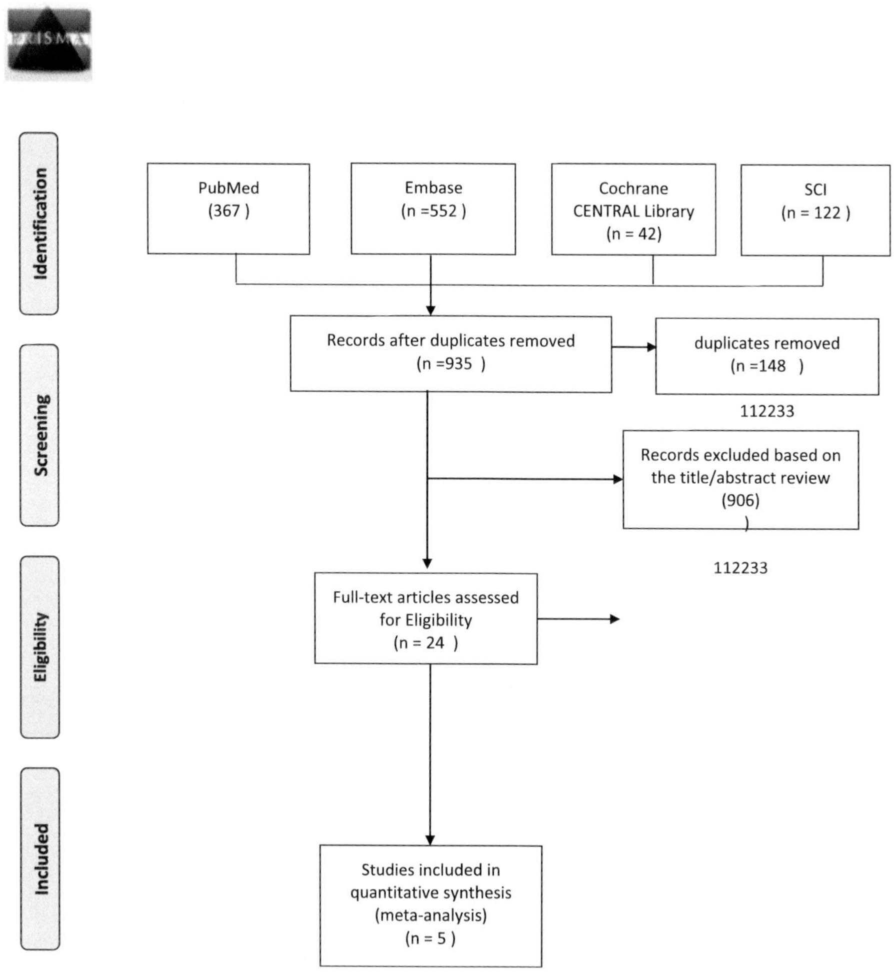

Fig. 1 The flow diagram of studies selection

HR = 2.01, 95% CI = 1.41, 2.88, $P = 0.004$) [15, 16] and studies with community-dwelling individuals (pooled HR = 1.62, 95% CI = 1.26, 2.09, $P = 0.000$) [14, 17], but not individuals living in nursing homes (pooled HR = 1.27, 95% CI = 0.73, 2.21, $P = 0.400$) [18] with a between subgroup p-value of 0.23. In addition, the subgroup analysis for length of follow-up showed that studies with a follow-up period of 3 years or more [14, 15, 17] (pooled HR = 1.52, 95% CI = 1.19, 1.94, $P = 0.001$) indicated a significantly higher rate of hospitalization in participants with sarcopenia compared to those without sarcopenia. However, this association was not

Table 1 Characteristics of included studies

First author	Year	Country	Male	Sample size	Age (years)	[b]Definitions of sarcopenia	Follow-up durations	Result of effect size	Outcome	Quality[a]
P.M Cawthon	2017	USA	100%	1516	70–80	EWGSOP	3 years	OR:1.27 (0.85, 1.90)	hospitalization	7
S.Gariballa	2013	UK	74.30%	432	70–80	EWGSOP	0.5 years	HR:2.52(1.34,4.74)	re-hospitalization	6
L.Bianchi	2016	Italy	46.80%	538	77.1	EWGSOP	10 years	HR:1.57(1.03,2.41)	hospitalization	7
T.Henwood	2017	Australia	29.30%	58	80–90	EWGSOP	1.5 years	RR:1.27(0.73,2.22)	hospitalization	6
M.Yang	2017	China	78.10%	288	81.1 ± 6.6	AWGS	3 years	HR:1.81(1.17,2.80)	re-hospitalization	8

[a]Quality of the studies were assessed with Newcastle-Ottawa Scale (NOS);
[b]EWGSOP (European Working Group for Sarcopenia in Older Persons) defines sarcopenia in men as ALM adjusted for height squared < 7.25 kg/m2 combined with low hand-grip strength (< 30 kg) and/or low gait speed (< 0.8 m/s)
Asian Working Group for Sarcopenia (AWGS): participants had a lower muscle mass with a low handgrip strength of < 26 kg in men and < 18 kg in women, and/or a lower gait speed ≦ 0.8 m/s
OR, odds ratio; RR, risk ratio; HR, hazard ratio

Table 2 Study and sarcopenia criteria

study	Sarcopenia criteria	Item,tool, Cutoff points						Prevalence (%)	Ref
		Muscle mass		Muscle strength		Physical performance			
		Tool	Cutoff points	Tool	Cutoff points	Tool	Cutoff point		
P.M Cawthon	EWFSOP	ALM/ height2	Men ALM/height^2: ≤ 7.23 kg/m^2)	Grip strength:	GS < 30 k	Gait speed	≤ 0.8 m/s	7.5	[17]
S.Gariballa	EWFSOP	MAMC	Men: MAMC <21.1 cm Women: MAMC <19.2 cm	Grip strength:	Men:GS<30 kg Women: GS<20 kg	None	None	10	[16]
L.Bianchi	EWFSOP	BIA	Men:SMI < 8.87 kg/m^2 Women:SMI < 6.42 kg/m^2	Grip strength:	Men: BMI ≤ 24 kg/m^2 GS ≤29 kg, BMI 24.1–28 kg/m^2 GS ≤30 kg, BMI > 28 kg/m^2 GS ≤ 32 kg; women: BMI ≤ 23 kg/m2 GS ≤17 kg, BMI 23.1–26 kg/m2 GS ≤17.3 kg, BMI 26.1–29 kg/m2 GS ≤18 kg, BMI > 29 kg/m^2 GS ≤21 kg)	Gait speed:4 m	≤ 0.8 m/s	10.2	[14]
T.Henwood	EWFSOP	BIA	Men:SMI < 8.87 kg/m^2 Women:SMI < 6.42 kg/m^2	Grip strength	Men:GS<30 kg Women: GS<20 kg	Gait speed: 4 m	≤ 0.8 m/s	40.2	[18]
M.Yang	AWGS	SMI	men: SMI < 6.70 kg/m^2, women: SMI < 4.75 kg/m^2	Grip strength	Men:GS<26 kg Women: GS<18 kg	Gait speed: 4 m	≤ 0.8 m/s	17	[15]

ALM appendicular lean mass, *ASM* appendicular muscle mass, *AWGS* Asian Working Group for Sarcopenia, *BIA* bioimpedance analysis, *BMI* body mass index, *DXA* dual-energy X-ray absorptiometry, *EWGSOP* the European Working Group on Sarcopenia in Older People, *GS* grip strength, *MAMC* mid-arm muscle circumference, *SMI* skeletal muscle mass index

found in the studies with a follow-up period of less than 3 years [16, 18] (pooled HR = 1.76, 95% CI = 0.90, 3.44, $P = 0.099$). All the subgroup analyses are displayed in Table 4.

Publication bias assessment

We could not conduct publication bias assessment due to the small number of the studies included.

Discussion

This meta-analysis of five available cohort studies showed that older adults with sarcopenia have an increased risk of hospitalization. Moreover, results of subgroup analyses showed that the association between sarcopenia and increased risk of hospitalization is consistent in older people from hospital- or community-based data and in studies with different diagnostic criteria of sarcopenia. Our results highlight that sarcopenia is an

Table 3 Result of the Newcastle-Ottawa Scale quality assessment

Newcastle-Ottawa scale		P.M Cawthon 2017 [17]	S.Gariballa 2013 [16]	L.Bianch 2016 [14]	T.Henwood 2017 [18]	M.Yang 2017 [15]
Selection(4)	Representativeness of the exposed cohort	1	1	1	0	1
	Selection of the non-exposed cohort	1	1	1	1	1
	Ascertainment of exposure	1	1	1	1	1
	Demonstration that outcome of interest was not present at start of study	1	1	1	1	1
Comparability(2)	Comparability of cohorts on the basis of the design or analysis	1	0	0	1	2
Outcome(3)	Assessment of outcome	1	1	1	1	1
	Was follow-up long enough for outcome to occur	1	0	1	0	0
	Adequacy of follow up of cohorts	1	1	1	1	1
Quality(9)	Total	8	6	7	6	8

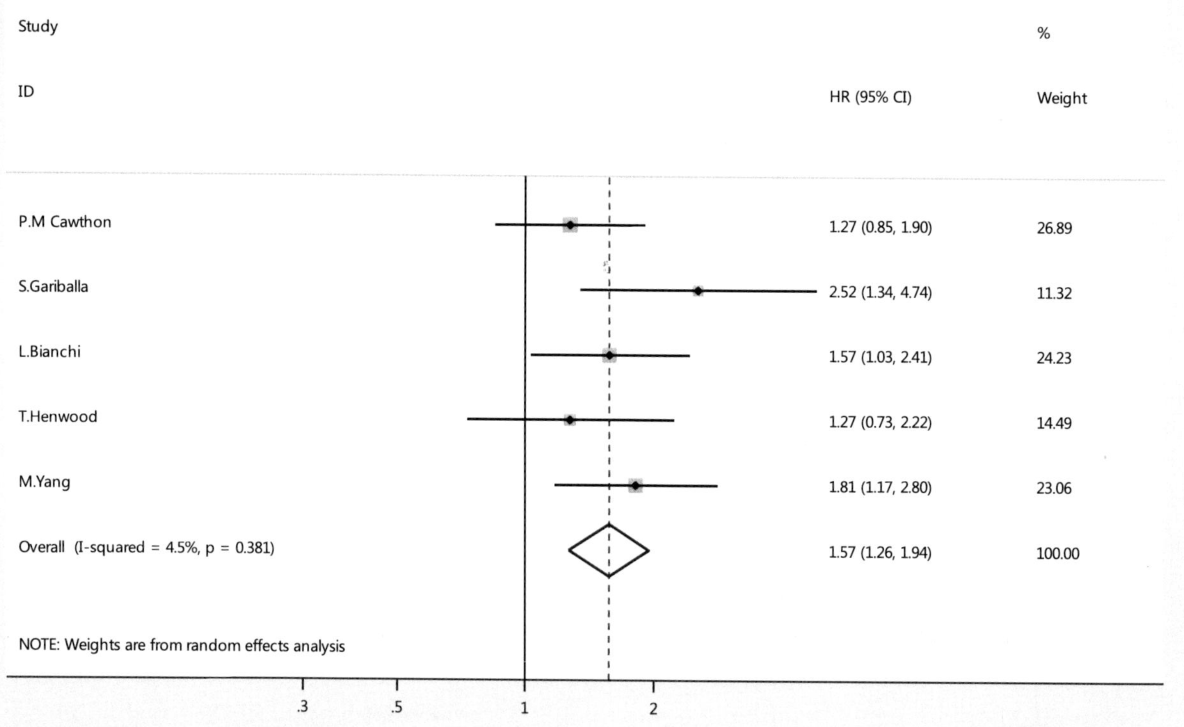

Fig. 2 Forest plots for the meta-analysis of the association between sarcopenia and hospitalization

Table 4 Subgroup analyses of the meta-analysis

Subgroup	Effect model	Number of studies	Mean difference (95% CI)	P for Heterogeneity	I-squared Value	*P* Value for effect	*P* Value Between Groups
Type of participant	Random effect						
hospitalized patients		2	2.01[1.41, 2.88]	0.40	0%	0.0001	
community-dwelling individuals		2	1.40[1.05, 1.88]	0.48	0%	0.02	
nursing homes residents		1	1.27 [0.73,2.21]			0.40	*P* = 0.23
Follow-up	Random effect						
> = 3 years		3	1.52[1.19, 1.94]	0.496	0%	0.0007	
< 3 years		2	1.76[0.90, 3.44]	0.111	60.7%	0.10	*P* = 0.69
Outcome	Random effect						
hospitalization		3	1.37[1.06, 1.78]	0.74	0%	0.02	
re-hospitalization		2	2.01[1.41, 2.88]	0.40	0%	0.0001	*P* = 0.09
NOS score	Random effect						
≥7		3	1.52[1.19, 1.94]	0.496	0%	0.0007	
<7		2	1.76[0.90, 3.44]	0.111	60.7%	0.10	*P* = 0.69

important determinant of hospitalization outcome in older people, and preventative strategies against sarcopenia may improve the outcome of hospitalization for older people [24].

Beaudart [19] assessed the association between sarcopenia and various health outcomes in 2017. However, only one study was available that estimated the association between sarcopenia and hospitalization, and the author analyzed and described the outcomes without a meta-analysis. Compared to this previous systematic review, our meta-analysis included five cohort studies and focused on all hospitalizations. To the best of our knowledge, our study is the most comprehensive review summarizing cohort studies that included all definitions of sarcopenia and hospitalization.

In our systematic review, the prevalence rates of sarcopenia varied from 7.5 to 40.2%. Diversity in our analysis was mainly due to the characteristics of the older adults and the different diagnostic methods of sarcopenia. Subgroup analyses of types of participants indicate that the association between sarcopenia and hospitalization was consistent in studies with hospitalized patients (pooled HR = 2.01, 95% CI = 1.41, 2.88, $P = 0.004$) and studies with community-dwelling individuals (pooled HR = 1.62, 95% CI = 1.26, 2.09, $P = 0.000$). Although the HR of hospitalization was more than the HR of community-dwelling individuals, there was no significant difference between the groups. Generally, community-dwelling individuals were relatively healthy and had well-preserved functional ability compared to hospitalized patients. This can be attributed to the fact that hospitalized patients [15, 16] often presenting with multiple comorbidities and activated inflammatory conditions, which can result in higher levels of inflammatory markers, such as C-reactive proteins (CRP) and cytokines. In addition, according to a recent meta-analysis, sarcopenia is associated with higher serum inflammatory parameters, particularly increased CRP levels [25]. Therefore, more prospective cohort studies are needed to compare hospitalized patients with community-dwelling older people. There was only one study [18] that addressed nursing home residents. That study included 102 older adults at baseline from 11 nursing homes; 58 of these older adults were followed-up for 18 months. The author concluded that there were no statistical significant association between sarcopenia and hospitalization in nursing home residents (pooled HR = 1.27, 95% CI = 0.73, 2.21, $P = 0.400$).

Subgroup analysis for length of follow-up indicated that a follow-up period of 3 years or more resulted in significantly higher rates of hospitalization in participants with sarcopenia compared to those without sarcopenia. However, this association was not found in the studies with a follow-up period of less than 3 years. The difference in results may be attributed to aging or sarcopenia-aggravated hospitalization [26], which may increase the rate of hospitalization. This suggests that if sarcopenia is detected early, it can potentially be managed nutritionally or with physical activity to reduce the hospitalization probability.

The underlying mechanisms driving the association of sarcopenia and risk of hospitalization were unable to draw conclusions. Some results of previous studies provide potential explanations. First, sarcopenia has been associated with poor endurance, physical disability, slow gait speed, and decreased mobility [6]. Besides disability, muscle strength is also a strong predictor of hospitalization [27, 28], and older people with sarcopenia tend to have low muscle mass or poor physical performance [29], which increases their risk of hospitalization. Secondly, multiple studies [30–33] found that sarcopenia is a significant predictor of future falls among older adults. When older people fall, they can suffer hip, spine, hand, and/or pelvic fractures, which could increase the probability of hospital admission. According to the US Centers for Disease Control and Prevention, there were 2.5 million nonfatal falls among older adults presenting to the emergency department, 734,000 hospitalizations, and a direct medical cost of $30 billion in 2013. [34] Thirdly, sarcopenia is multifactorial, in that it can be associated with a range of ages [35], multiple chronic health conditions, unhealthy lifestyle [36], deregulated hormonal factors [37], inflammation [38] and so on [39]. All of these factors are considered risk factors for hospitalization and can exacerbate sarcopenia. In addition, sarcopenia has been considered a predictor of future fracture in older adults [40–42], which raises the risk of subsequent hospitalization. As a geriatric syndrome rather than a disease, the underlying mechanisms for the pathogenesis of sarcopenia may be complex. Intensive studies are needed to clarify the potential mechanisms underlying the association between sarcopenia and hospitalization. Of the utmost importance, prevention of the multiple factors underlying sarcopenia, particularly nutrition and physical activity, may be very important. There is a growing body of literature that recognizes specific physical activity programs as the most important approach to slowing the decline of muscle mass and muscle strength associated with aging and to treat sarcopenia [43]. Adequate nutrition [44], specifically protein and micronutrients (vitamin D), has to be regarded as an essential requisite for any successful therapeutic approach for prevention and treatment of sarcopenia. By taking preventative measures to decrease the rate of sarcopenia, we can further decrease the medical expenses and resources related to hospitalization.

There are some strengths and limitations in our systematic review and meta-analysis. One of the strengths is that we performed an extensive search of electronic data-bases and evaluated the quality of each study. The primary limitation of our analysis is the limited number of longitudinal studies and the small sample sizes of the studies, which may have affected the quality of our systematic review and the results of subgroup analyses. Secondly, we only included studies published in English and, consequently, may have overlooked data from important studies published in other languages, which may have resulted in potential bias. Third, although we combined adjusted results, we could not exclude the residual confounding factors that may affect the association between sarcopenia and hospitalization risk.

Conclusion

This meta-analysis suggests that sarcopenia is associated with increased risk of hospitalization of community-dwelling and hospitalized older adults. These results indicate that we should more closely monitor older adults in hospitals and community-dwelling locations. Comprehensive diagnosis and treatment of sarcopenia should be conducted in hospitalized older people to reduce the progression of sarcopenia and improve prognosis. Early detection of sarcopenia is beneficial in community-dwelling older people, and appropriate nutrition and exercise interventions are necessary to reduce the harmful consequences of sarcopenia and ultimately reduce the risk of hospitalization of older adults.

Abbreviation

AWGS: Asian Working Group for Sarcopenia; EWGSOP: European Working Group on Sarcopenia in Older People definition; NOS: Newcastle-Ottawa scale

Acknowledgements

The authors thank the staffs in the Department of Emergency Medicine, the Affiliated Baoan Hospital of Southern Medical University, and the People Hospital of Baoan Shenzhen for their guidance and support. No sponsors had any role in the design, subject recruitment, data collection, analysis, or preparation of this manuscript.

Authors' contributions

XMZ initiated the study concept, performed the literature review, data analysis and interpretation, and was responsible for drafting, revising and finalizing the manuscript. WWZ contributed to the study design, literature search and was responsible for extracting data and drafting the manuscript. CHW was involved in the study design and literature review, and critically revised the manuscript. WYT helped perform statistical analysis and interpret the data, and critically revised the manuscript. YZY was responsible for screening the papers and quality assessment, and helped analyze and interpret the data, and critically revised the manuscript. QLD initiated and designed the study and was responsible for quality assessment, statistical analysis, and revision of the manuscript. All authors read and approved the final version of the manuscript. All authors agreed to be accountable for all aspects of the work.

Competing interests

The authors declare that they have no competing interests.

References

1. Rosenberg IH. Sarcopenia: origins and clinical relevance. J. Nutr. 1997;127(5 Suppl):990s–1s.
2. Marzetti E, Calvani R, Tosato M, Cesari M, Di Bari M, Cherubini A, Collamati A, D'Angelo E, Pahor M, Bernabei R, et al. Sarcopenia: an overview. Aging Clin Exp Res. 2017;29(1):11–7.
3. Cruz-Jentoft AJ, Landi F, Schneider SM, Zuniga C, Arai H, Boirie Y, Chen LK, Fielding RA, Martin FC, Michel JP, et al. Prevalence of and interventions for sarcopenia in ageing adults: a systematic review. Report of the international sarcopenia initiative (EWGSOP and IWGS). Age Ageing. 2014;43(6):748–59.
4. Cruz-Jentoft AJ, Landi F, Topinkova E, Michel JP. Understanding sarcopenia as a geriatric syndrome. Curr Opin Clin Nutr Metab Care. 2010;13(1):1–7.
5. Marty E, Liu Y, Samuel A, Or O, Lane J. A review of sarcopenia: enhancing awareness of an increasingly prevalent disease. Bone. 2017;105:276–86.
6. Landi F, Liperoti R, Russo A, Giovannini S, Tosato M, Capoluongo E, Bernabei R, Onder G. Sarcopenia as a risk factor for falls in elderly individuals: results from the ilSIRENTE study. Clin Nutr (Edinburgh, Scotland). 2012;31(5):652–8.
7. Yu R, Leung J, Woo J. Incremental predictive value of sarcopenia for incident fracture in an elderly Chinese cohort: results from the osteoporotic fractures in men (MrOs) study. J Am Med Dir Assoc. 2014;15(8):551–8.
8. Gale CR, Martyn CN, Cooper C, Sayer AA. Grip strength, body composition, and mortality. Int J Epidemiol. 2007;36(1):228–35.
9. Chang KV, Hsu TH, Wu WT, Huang KC, Han DS. Is sarcopenia associated with depression? A systematic review and meta-analysis of observational studies. Age Ageing. 2017;46(5):738–46.
10. Woo J. Sarcopenia. Clin Geriatr Med. 2017;33(3):305–14.
11. Wang SY, Shamliyan TA, Talley KM, Ramakrishnan R, Kane RL. Not just specific diseases: systematic review of the association of geriatric syndromes with hospitalization or nursing home admission. Arch Gerontol Geriatr. 2013;57(1):16–26.
12. Liu P, Hao Q, Hai S, Wang H, Cao L, Dong B. Sarcopenia as a predictor of all-cause mortality among community-dwelling older people: a systematic review and meta-analysis. Maturitas. 2017;103:16–22.
13. Cawthon PM, Fox KM, Gandra SR, Delmonico MJ, Chiou CF, Anthony MS, Sewall A, Goodpaster B, Satterfield S, Cummings SR, et al. Do muscle mass, muscle density, strength, and physical function similarly influence risk of hospitalization in older adults? J Am Geriatr Soc. 2009;57(8):1411–9.
14. Bianchi L, Ferrucci L, Cherubini A, Maggio M, Bandinelli S, Savino E, Brombo G, Zuliani G, Guralnik JM, Landi F, et al. The predictive value of the EWGSOP definition of sarcopenia: results from the InCHIANTI study. J Gerontol A Biol Sci Med Sci. 2016;71(2):259–64.
15. Yang M, Hu X, Wang H, Zhang L, Hao Q, Dong B. Sarcopenia predicts readmission and mortality in elderly patients in acute care wards: a prospective study. J Cachexia Sarcopenia Muscle. 2017;8(2):251–8.
16. Gariballa S, Alessa A. Sarcopenia: prevalence and prognostic significance in hospitalized patients. Clin Nutr. 2013;32(5):772–6.
17. Cawthon PM, Lui LY, Taylor BC, McCulloch CE, Cauley JA, Lapidus J, Orwoll E, Ensrud KE. Clinical definitions of sarcopenia and risk of hospitalization in community-dwelling older men: the osteoporotic fractures in men study. J Gerontol A Biol Sci Med Sci. 2017;72(10):1383–9.
18. Henwood T, Hassan B, Swinton P, Senior H, Keogh J. Consequences of sarcopenia among nursing home residents at long-term follow-up. Geriatr Nurs. 2017;38(5):406–11.
19. Beaudart C, Zaaria M, Pasleau F, Reginster JY, Bruyere O. Health outcomes of sarcopenia: a systematic review and meta-analysis. PLoS One. 2017;12(1): e0169548.
20. Moher D, Liberati A, Tetzlaff J, Altman DG. Preferred reporting items for systematic reviews and meta-analyses: the PRISMA statement. Int. J. Surg. 2010;8(5):336–41.
21. Stang A. Critical evaluation of the Newcastle-Ottawa scale for the assessment of the quality of nonrandomized studies in meta-analyses. Eur J Epidemiol. 2010;25(9):603–5.
22. Lera L, Albala C, Sanchez H, Angel B, Hormazabal MJ, Marquez C, Arroyo P. Prevalence of sarcopenia in community-dwelling Chilean elders according to an adapted version of the European working group on sarcopenia in older people (EWGSOP) criteria. J Frailty Aging. 2017;6(1):12–7.
23. Chen LK, Liu LK, Woo J, Assantachai P, Auyeung TW, Bahyah KS, Chou MY, Chen LY, Hsu PS, Krairit O, et al. Sarcopenia in Asia: consensus report of the Asian working Group for Sarcopenia. J Am Med Dir Assoc. 2014;15(2):95–101.
24. Padilla Colon CJ, Sanchez Collado P, Cuevas MJ. Benefits of strength training for the prevention and treatment of sarcopenia. Nutr Hosp. 2014;29(5):979–88.

25. Bano G, Trevisan C, Carraro S, Solmi M, Luchini C, Stubbs B, Manzato E, Sergi G, Veronese N. Inflammation and sarcopenia: a systematic review and meta-analysis. Maturitas. 2017;96:10–5.
26. Waltz TB, Fivenson EM, Morevati M, Li C, Becker KG, Bohr VA, Fang EF. Sarcopenia, aging and prospective interventional strategies. Curr Med Chem. 2017;24(1):1–8.
27. Volpato S, Cavalieri M, Sioulis F, Guerra G, Maraldi C, Zuliani G, Fellin R, Guralnik JM. Predictive value of the short physical performance battery following hospitalization in older patients. J Gerontol A Biol Sci Med Sci. 2011;66(1):89–96.
28. Legrand D, Vaes B, Mathei C, Adriaensen W, Van Pottelbergh G, Degryse JM. Muscle strength and physical performance as predictors of mortality, hospitalization, and disability in the oldest old. J Am Geriatr Soc. 2014;62(6): 1030–8.
29. Fuggle N, Shaw S, Dennison E, Cooper C. Sarcopenia. Best Pract Res Clin Rheumatol. 2017;31(2):218–42.
30. Matsumoto H, Tanimura C: Sarcopenia is a risk factor for falling in independently living Japanese older adults: a 2-year prospective cohort study of the GAINA study. 2017.
31. Bischoff-Ferrari HA, Orav JE, Kanis JA, Rizzoli R, Schlogl M, Staehelin HB, Willett WC, Dawson-Hughes B. Comparative performance of current definitions of sarcopenia against the prospective incidence of falls among community-dwelling seniors age 65 and older. Osteoporos Int. 2015;26(12): 2793–802.
32. Clynes MA, Edwards MH, Buehring B, Dennison EM, Binkley N, Cooper C. Definitions of sarcopenia: associations with previous falls and fracture in a population sample. Calcif Tissue Int. 2015;97(5):445–52.
33. Scott D, Seibel M, Cumming R, Naganathan V, Blyth F, Le Couteur DG, Handelsman DJ, Waite LM, Hirani V. Sarcopenic obesity and its temporal associations with changes in bone mineral density, incident falls, and fractures in older men: the concord health and ageing in men project. J Bone Miner Res Off J Am Soc Bone Miner Res. 2017;32(3):575–83.
34. Khow KSF, Visvanathan R. Falls in the aging population. Clin Geriatr Med. 2017;33(3):357–68.
35. Marzetti E, Lees HA, Wohlgemuth SE, Leeuwenburgh C. Sarcopenia of aging: underlying cellular mechanisms and protection by calorie restriction. BioFactors (Oxford, England). 2009;35(1):28–35.
36. Cruz-Jentoft AJ, Kiesswetter E, Drey M, Sieber CC. Nutrition, frailty, and sarcopenia. Aging Clin Exp Res. 2017;29(1):43–8.
37. Martone AM, Lattanzio F, Abbatecola AM, Carpia DL, Tosato M, Marzetti E, Calvani R, Onder G, Landi F. Treating sarcopenia in older and oldest old. Curr Pharm Des. 2015;21(13):1715–22.
38. Westbury LD, Fuggle NR, Syddall HE, Duggal NA, Shaw SC, Maslin K, Dennison EM, Lord JM, Cooper C. Relationships between markers of inflammation and muscle mass, Strength and Function: Findings from the Hertfordshire Cohort Study. Calcif Tissue Int. 2018;102(3):2872–95.
39. Malafarina V, Uriz-Otano F, Iniesta R, Gil-Guerrero L. Sarcopenia in the elderly: diagnosis, physiopathology and treatment. Maturitas. 2012;71(2): 109–14.
40. Hars M, Biver E, Chevalley T, Herrmann F, Rizzoli R, Ferrari S, Trombetti A. Low lean mass predicts incident fractures independently from FRAX: a prospective cohort study of recent retirees. J Bone Miner Res Off J Am Soc Bone Miner Res. 2016;31(11):2048–56.
41. Chalhoub D, Cawthon PM, Ensrud KE, Stefanick ML, Kado DM, Boudreau R, Greenspan S, Newman AB, Zmuda J, Orwoll ES, et al. Risk of nonspine fractures in older adults with sarcopenia, low bone mass, or both. J Am Geriatr Soc. 2015;63(9):1733–40.
42. Scott D, Chandrasekara SD, Laslett LL, Cicuttini F, Ebeling PR, Jones G. Associations of Sarcopenic obesity and Dynapenic obesity with bone mineral density and incident fractures over 5-10 years in community-dwelling older adults. Calcif Tissue Int. 2016;99(1):30–42.
43. Zembron-Lacny A, Dziubek W, Rogowski L, Skorupka E, Dabrowska G. Sarcopenia: monitoring, molecular mechanisms, and physical intervention. Physiol Res. 2014;63(6):683–91.
44. Bosaeus I, Rothenberg E. Nutrition and physical activity for the prevention and treatment of age-related sarcopenia. Proc Nutr Soc. 2016;75(2):174–80.

12

Item distribution, internal consistency, and structural validity of the German version of the DEMQOL and DEMQOL-proxy

Christian G. G. Schwab[1,2], Martin Nikolaus Dichter[1,2*] and Martin Berwig[3,1]

Abstract

Background: Accurate assessment of health-related quality of life as an endpoint in intervention studies is a major challenge in dementia research. The *DEMQOL* (29 items) and the *proxy* version (32 items), which is partly based on the *DEMQOL*, are internationally used instruments. To date, there is no information on the structural validity, item distribution, or internal consistency for the German language version of these questionnaires.

Methods: This psychometric study is based on a secondary data analysis of a sample of 201 outpatients with a mild form of Alzheimer's disease (AD) and their informal caregivers. The informal caregivers who were interviewed were involved in the care of the person with AD several times per week. The analysis for the evaluation of the structural validity was performed using Mokken scale analysis. The internal consistency was calculated using the ρ of the Molenaar Sijtsma statistic and Cronbach's α.

Results: For both versions, four subscales were identified: [A] "positive emotions", [B] "negative emotions", [C] "physical and cognitive functioning", and [D] "daily activities and social relationships". For both instruments, the internal consistency of all subscales was considered "good" ($\rho = 0.71–0.88$, $\alpha = 0.72–0.87$).

Conclusions: The results are a first indication of good construct validity of the instruments used for the German setting. We recommend further investigations of the test-retest reliability and the inter-rater reliability of the proxy instrument.

Keywords: Dementia, Quality of life, Structural validity, Internal consistency

Background

According to the World Alzheimer Report, a person was diagnosed with dementia every 3.2 s in 2015. Currently, approximately 46.8 million people worldwide are living with dementia [1]. Dementia is a neurocognitive disorder associated with a significant cognitive decline from a previous level of performance, resulting in a dependency on others to perform activities of daily living [2].

Health-related quality of life (HRQoL) reflects an important desire for persons living with dementia and is therefore used as a general endpoint in many interventional studies. Additionally, HRQoL is increasingly used for assessments of anti-dementia drugs and by the European Medicines Agency to determine the benefits of such drugs [3]. HRQoL in persons living with dementia also is also considered by regulatory authorities and administrative agencies who must judge this parameter based on a resident's degree of self-sufficiency. Furthermore, HRQoL is used in economic evaluations of persons in all stages of dementia [4–6].

HRQoL is defined by Hays and Reeve as how well a person functions in his/her life and perceives his/her well-being in the physical, mental, and social domains of health [7]. In this definition, functioning refers to the individual's ability to achieve predefined activities, and well-being refers to individual's subjective feelings [8, 9]. Based on this and similar definitions of HRQoL, Karimi and Brazier [8] conclude that HRQoL is a particular type of health description; therefore, the World Health Organization (WHO) defines *health* as "a state of complete physical, mental and social well-being, and not merely the absence of disease and infirmity" [10]. This definition indicates that HRQoL measurements reflect

* Correspondence: Martin.Dichter@dzne.de
[1]German Center for Neurodegenerative Diseases (DZNE), Stockumer Straße 12, 58453 Witten, Germany
[2]School of Nursing Science, Witten/Herdecke University, Stockumer Straße 12, 58453 Witten, Germany
Full list of author information is available at the end of the article

health in a wider sense (i.e., well-being and functioning) than solely other clinical outcomes (e.g., 5-year survival rate, rate of restenosis, death, and tumor recurrence).

According to Bakas et al. [11], three models of HRQoL are frequently used: the WHO [12] International Classification of Functioning, Disability and Health (ICF) Model of Functioning and Disability, the HRQoL Model from Wilson and Cleary [9], and, based on this model, the quality of life (QoL) measurement by Ferrans et al. [13].

Smith et al. observed the need to develop a conceptual framework that addressed the differences between the views expressed about HRQoL by people with dementia and their caregivers [14]. The results of the literature analysis and the findings from expert opinions could also be verified by data from interviews of individuals with dementia and their family caregivers [14]. Thus, an empirical justification of the conceptual framework can be assumed. Based on the five domains of the conceptual framework ("health and well-being", "cognitive functioning", "daily activities", "social relationships", and "self-concept"), they developed two interviewer-administered instruments called Dementia Quality of Life (*DEMQOL*) and its proxy version (*DEMQOL-Proxy*). The authors conducted a pretest factor analysis during the development of the instrument (*DEMQOL* $n = 130$, *DEMQOL-Proxy* $n = 126$) that covered the same four dimensions: "positive emotions", "negative emotions", "memory", and "daily activities". For the *DEMQOL-Proxy*, a two-factor solution, as given by "emotion" and "functioning", has been suggested by the results of the pretest. The factors of both the self-report and proxy version, however, did not fully support the original conceptual framework [15]. Mulhern and colleagues [4] published a factor analysis with a sample of 644 persons with mild to moderate dementia and 682 proxies. In their study, the subscales "cognition", "positive emotion" and "negative emotion" could be used on both instruments [4]. However, "social relationships" and "loneliness" were observed only in the *DEMQOL*, while the subscales "daily activities" and "appearance" only occurred in the *DEMQOL-Proxy* [4].

The *DEMQOL* consists of 28 items, while the *DEMQOL-Proxy* includes 31 items on a four-point Likert-type scale with the following responses: a lot, quite slightly, a little, and not at all. The scale includes an additional global QoL item (item 29 resp. 32). Items were scored from 1 to 4, with higher scores indicating better HRQoL. It must be noted that there are five contraindicative items in the *DEMQOL* and the *DEMQOL-Proxy* (4 = a lot, ..., 1 = not at all). The global QoL item also contraindicates the answer options of "very good", "good", "fair", and "poor". Fifteen items, in addition to the global QoL item, are similar in both versions of the *DEMQOL*; however, there are also items that are not part of the other instrument [15].

The *DEMQOL* can be used in mild to moderate dementia as a self-report form and also for severe dementia in a proxy version (*DEMQOL-Proxy*) across different types of dementia and care arrangements [15]. The utility score (*DEMQOL-U*), which is created from a subset of items from the *DEMQOL*, can also be used for economic assessments [4]. The *DEMQOL* instrument was developed and tested in the UK, which was reported in a Health Technology Assessment (HTA) report [15]. Consequently, it is used more frequently in the UK. While there is a German translation, the results of a linguistic validation have not been reported [16]. No adequate results are available for psychometric testing of the German versions, which are required for both research and applied purposes [17]. To date, the *DEMQOL* has been subjected to at least four more latent variable modeling investigations in two countries since its foundation work [15], two factor analyses [4, 18], bifactor modeling [19], and Rasch modeling [20].

This paper consequently targets the first evaluation of the item distribution, structural validity as a part of the construct validity, and internal consistency of the German version of both the *DEMQOL* and *DEMQOL-Proxy*. For this purpose, a parallel iterative Mokken scale analysis (MSA) is used as a further procedure in addition to the aforementioned methods.

Methods

The analysis for the present study was performed on a secondary data analysis using anonymous baseline data of a randomized controlled trial called the *Cognitive Rehabilitation and Cognitive Behavioral Treatment for Early Dementia in Alzheimer's Disease* (CORDIAL) study [21]. To test the structure found in terms of a sensitivity analysis, we used the data of the follow-up surveys after three (T_1) and after nine months (T_2). The CORDIAL study was performed to provide clinically meaningful benefits and to evaluate the feasibility, acceptance, efficacy, and usefulness of interventions in cognitive rehabilitation. The study was accomplished as a multicenter randomized controlled trial on persons living with Alzheimer's disease (AD) and their informal caregivers (as proxy raters). Ethical clearance was granted for the CORDIAL study by the Ethics Commission of the Faculty of Medicine of the Technical University of Munich on 12/10/2009 under the number 2113/08 S. We have refrained from re-auditing as ethical clearance is not required for analyses based on secondary data [22] or for studies using anonymous data.

Setting and participants

The baseline data of the CORDIAL study were collected from July 2008 to September 2009. The first inclusion criterion required participants to be elderly outpatients with an established ICD-10 diagnosis of AD with mild severity, as defined by a Mini-Mental State Examination (MMSE) score of 21 or above. A differential diagnosis to other forms of dementia was conducted by the recruitment centers. This process was completed to obtain a similar picture of symptoms of the participants, in which memory problems in the early stage are the focus of their everyday problems. Patients were recruited from the ten recruitment centers of the study, including memory clinics and neurological and psychotherapeutic practices throughout Germany.

The need for a designated informal caregiver who was involved in the care of the person living with AD several times a week was the second inclusion criterion for the study. Exclusion criteria were comprised of acute psychiatric or physical disorders, ongoing formal psychotherapy or cognitive training, regular visits to day care facilities, an impending hospital or nursing home admission, a poor command of the German language, alcohol or substance dependence, and participation in another interventional trial. Stable doses of cholinesterase inhibitors, memantine, nootropics, antidepressants, and antipsychotics were permissible as concomitant medications of the person living with AD [21].

Procedures

The task of the recruitment centers was to inform possible study participants in advance of the study. This process was completed through personal conversations and informational materials. Written informed consent was obtained from both, persons living with AD and their informal caregivers. Independent psychologists, serving as raters, conducted the assessments of the CORDIAL study. The raters received a one-day seminar with case studies for use during the assessments, including the *DEMQOL*-questionnaires. The two interviews with the persons living with AD and the informal caregivers were completed separately. Thus, the informal caregivers were blinded to the answers of the persons living with AD. The monitoring of the study was conducted by an interdisciplinary data monitoring and safety board.

Measurements

In addition to the previously described *DEMQOL* and *DEMQOL-Proxy*, which are the main topics of interest for our study, further instruments were used. To determine the cognitive ability of the persons living with AD, the German version of the MMSE was used [23]. It is an eleven-question assessment covering five areas of cognitive functioning: orientation, registration, attention and calculation, recall, and language. Each of the 30 tasks is evaluated using a point (range of total scores: 0 to 30). A lower MMSE score indicates a more severe cognitive impairment. To assess impairment of activities of daily living among persons living with AD, the Bayer Activities of Daily Living Scale (B-ADL) by Hindmarch et al. [24] was used. The B-ADL displays a proxy rating assessment for elderly persons with loss of cognitive performance. It is comprised of 25 items rated on a 10-point scale (1 = never, ..., 10 = always). The total scores range from 1 to 10, and higher scores indicate higher impairment. To evaluate depressive symptoms, the long form of the Geriatric Depression Scale (GDS) from Yesavage [25] was used. This assessment has 30 dichotomous items (yes or no; directed differently); thus, the total score ranges from 0 to 30 points (higher scores reflect more severe depression). Finally, the Neuropsychiatric Inventory (NPI) by Cummings [26] was used to characterize the neuropsychiatric symptoms and psychopathology of persons living with AD. The NPI covers twelve types of neuropsychiatric disturbances. The frequencies of the symptoms are rated on a 4-point scale multiplied by their severities on a 3-point scale. A higher score (0 to 144) indicates more challenging behavior.

For a description of the informal caregiver, two assessments were used. First, the Beck Depression Inventory (BDI) from Hautzinger et al. [27] is an instrument that assesses the severity of depression. For each of the 21 questions, there are four different answers that are arranged according to their intensity (e.g., item 1: 0 = I do not feel sad; ..., 3 = I am so sad or unhappy that I cannot stand it). A higher BDI score (range for total scores: 0 to 63) indicates greater severity of depressive symptoms. Second, the full Zarit Burden Interview (ZBI-22; 22 items) by Zarit et al. [28] measures the subjective burden of informal caregivers, associated with functional/behavioral impairments and the home care situation. The ZBI-22 is rated on a 5-point scale (0 = never, ..., 4 = nearly always), and higher scores (range for total scores: 0 to 88) indicates a higher burden.

The socio-demographic data collected for the informal caregiver included age in years and sex, and for the person living with AD, education in years was recorded. In addition, the informal caregiver was asked to explain his/her relationship to the person living with AD.

Statistical analysis

The descriptions of the participants, missing data, and item distribution were conducted using descriptive statistics. The analysis of the item difficulty was based on the proportion of responses endorsing the best and worst ratings (i.e., ceiling/floor effects). A corresponding effect was assumed conservatively, as long as the mean value of the item was in the lower end (upper 20%) of the respective item range.

For the analysis of the structural validity of the *DEMQOL* and *DEMQOL-Proxy*, as part of the construct validity, we used the MSA. The MSA is a useful tool for researchers who wish to construct unidimensional tests or use questionnaires that comprise multiple binary or polytomous items and enable the examination of reliability without the use of Cronbach's alpha [29]. The MSA is a method of the non-parametric item response theory originating from assumptions of the unidimensionality of tests or scales, local independency and monotonicity [30]. The method is established in the context of scale development and has been widely used in QoL research [31, 32].

The MSA provides additional information about the relationship between items. As an indicator of the internal correlation of each subscale, the MSA uses Loevinger's H coefficient (H^S). According to Sijtsma and Molenaar [33], the following interpretation of H^S scores was applied to describe the scale: > 0.5 = "strong", > 0.4 = "medium", and > 0.3 = "weak". The correlation of a single item to the other items of the scale is expressed by the value H_i. The H_i should be non-negative for the Mokken model to hold. Depending on the source, an H_i-value from 0 to 0.55 is recommended. We have fixed the H_i-value to the typically used minimum of > 0.3. Items that fall below this level have weak discrimination power and are not useful for this scale. The H_{ij} designated the coefficient of two items.

The criterion (Crit) of the MSA by Molenaar and Sijtsma [34] was used to identify items that partially satisfy the assumptions for monotonous homogeneity or double monotonicity. For each item, this diagnostic value combines the H coefficient, the frequency and size of the violations, and their significance. Every item should have a Crit value of less than 40, and optimally a Crit value of 0. A Crit value of greater than 80 displays a strong indication that an item has violated the assumption for the MSA in this subscale. The critical values were calculated separately for each of the ten imputed records (see below). As a result, individual injuries of double monotonicity should not be systematically increased by a factor of ten.

For the exploratory investigation of the instruments, a method of parallel iteration was used, which consists of two steps. In the first step, cores were determined. The cores are items in an item pool that are strongly correlated with each other (H_{ij}) and are less correlated with the other cores when examined as a dyad. This finding means that other items from the pool could improve the H^S value in a similar way that a second core could. Otherwise, the weaker second core was returned into the item pool as single items. As a strong correlation for a core, we defined a minimum H_{ij}-value of 0.45 as a reference according to Müller-Schneider [35]. Analogous to the procedure in a factor analysis, the number of subscales is thereby predefined. In the second step, an iterative MSA was performed in parallel for each core determined. All items were tested in parallel. Accordingly, all remaining items would be tested against any core, and the item with the highest H_i-value to a specific core would be chosen. In doing so, the assignment of an item should not lead to a violation of monotonicity (Crit > 40). This procedure was used with regard to content in the case of a possible allocation to two different cores (cross loader). The search procedure stopped when there were no further items that fulfilled the requirements ($H_i \geq 0.3$ or Crit > 40) or when all the items had been incorporated into a scale. This method of parallel iterative analysis allowed for the identification of smaller subscales with higher H^S values, as opposed to the Automated Item Selection Procedure (AISP) for MSA [36].

As a precondition, the MSA assumes only complete cases and integers as values. Therefore, missing values may have to be imputed. In the case of instrument testing, however, the imputation of missing data should be performed with caution. We used a two-way imputation, which is a Bayesian method for estimating missing data in tests and questionnaires [37].

The internal consistency was assessed with the coefficient rho (ρ) of the Molenaar Sijtsma statistic. The ρ coefficient is not as prone to bias as Cronbach's α and should therefore be preferentially used [38, 39]. For comparison purposes, we also calculated Cronbach's alpha (α). Values for a ρ or α between 0.70 and 0.95 indicated "good" internal consistency [40]. Finally, we conducted a part-whole-corrected item-total correlation (r_{it}) calculation. For this purpose, the coefficient for the item to be examined against the scale without this item was computed. Items with r_{it} coefficients > 0.5 reflected a "high" correlation, and those with r_{it} > 0.3 reflected a "moderate" correlation [41]. An r_{it} correlation of 0.3 and below indicated that the item did not correlate well with the scale as the item may not measuring the same construct as the other variables.

All analysis were performed using R environment for statistical computing version 3.4.1 (30.06.2017) [42]. The following packages were used for the MSA and the imputation, respectively: "mokken" version 2.8.6 [43, 44] and "miceadds" version 2.5–9 [45].

Results

Study population

A summary of participant characteristics is shown in Table 1. The total number of participants was 201 dyads (persons living with mild AD and their informal caregivers). Notably, 48% (n = 90) of informal caregivers did not specify their relationship to the person with AD (Table 1).

Missing value analysis

For the *DEMQOL*, with its 28 items and with 201 participants, there were seven missing responses (0.1%), while in the proxy version of the *DEMQOL* (31 items), there were eleven missing responses (0.2%; Table 2). The missing values corresponded to seven cases of one missing

Table 1 Participant characteristics

Characteristics	$n = 201$
Persons with dementia	
Age (years)	73.74 (±7.92)
Female	88 (43.8%)
Education level (years)	12.53 (±3.05)
General cognitive ability (MMSE)	25.06 (±2.17)
Functional ability (B-ADL, proxy rating)	3.57 (±1.88) [a]
Depression (GDS)	8.90 (±5.16)
Challenging behavior (12 types NPI)	9.72 (±9.30)
Informal caregivers (proxy raters)	
Age (years)	64.82 (±13.17)
Female	143 (71.1%)
Spouse of the person with dementia	80 (72.1%) [b]
Depression (BDI)	8.35 (±6.53) [a]
Burden (ZBI-22)	19.12 (±12.52)

Data are reported as the mean (±standard deviation) or number (%).*MMSE* Mini-Mental Status Examination, *B-ADL* Bayer Activities of Daily Living Scale;*GDS* Geriatric Depression Scale, *NPI* Neuropsychiatric Inventory;*BDI* Beck Depression Inventory, *ZBI-22* Zarit Burden Interview with 22 items
[a]Missing value in 1 case
[b]Missing values in 90 cases

item (3.6%) in the *DEMQOL*, as well as nine cases in which one item (3.2%) and one case in which two items (6.5%) were missing in the *DEMQOL-Proxy*. Ten complete datasets with two-way imputed integers for missing data were generated for the MSA.

Item distribution

Five items (20–22, 25, 26) for the *DEMQOL* and six items (21–24, 28, 29) for the *DEMQOL-Proxy* showed a ceiling effect (Table 2). The 15 identical items of the *DEMQOL* and *DEMQOL-Proxy* demonstrated that proxy ratings are typically lower than the corresponding self-ratings (Table 2).

Structural validity

Four cores were found for the *DEMQOL*: items 21/24, 7/9, 17/19, and 6/10 (all $H_{ij} \geq 0.49$). In addition, for the *DEMQOL-Proxy*, four cores were found, consisting of items 4/8, 12/14, 5/7, and 23/24 (all $H_{ij} \geq 0.65$). The results of the iterative MSA are shown in Table 3. We found four equal subscales for both instruments, i.e., [A] "positive emotions", [B] "negative emotions", [C] "physical and cognitive functioning", and [D] "daily activities and social relationships" (Table 3).

For the *DEMQOL*, the H^S coefficient showed a "medium" correlation for three subscales ($H = 0.42$–0.46) in comparison to the subscale [A], which presented only a "weak" ($H = 0.37$) correlation. The correlations of the *DEMQOL-Proxy* subscales are "strong" ([A] $H^S = 0.66$) and "medium" subscales ([C] $H^S = 0.50$; [B] $H^S = 0.46$; [D] $H^S = 0.42$). Subscale [A] differed between both instruments, with only a "weak" H^S in the *DEMQOL* but a "strong" H^S in the *DEMQOL-Proxy* version. The MSA used all items of the proxy version, while in the *DEMQOL*, two items (11: "irritable"; 15: "forgetting who people are") could not be assigned. With regard to content, item 11 could have matched to subscale [B], while item 15 would have matched to subscale [C]. However, both showed a H_i of < 0.3. Item 24 from the *DEMQOL*, "making yourself understood", and the corresponding item 20 of the *DEMQOL-Proxy* version, "making him/herself understood", are in different subscales ([C] vs. [D]). Apart from this finding and the missing item 11 in the *DEMQOL* version, the remaining 13 of the 15 identical items of the two instruments have been assigned to the same subscales. In the *DEMQOL*, the item 18 ("difficulty making decisions") presented as a cross loader, which could have assigned to subscale [C] with $H_i = 0.45$ as well as to subscale [D] with $H_i = 0.39$. For a better fit with respect to content and the conceptual framework of Smith et al. [15], we decided to move item 18 into subscale [C]. The assumption of monotonicity for the MSA has been achieved for each of the ten imputed samples for all items (Crit = 0). All items with a ceiling effect could be found in subscale [D].

Sensitivity analyses were carried out to determine the stability of the identified subscales using the data from the CORDIAL study follow-up surveys, which can be found in Additional file 1: Table A1 for time T_1 after three months and in Additional file 2: Table A2 for the nine-month survey (T_2) in the supplemental material of this article. With the exception of item 26 in the *DEMQOL* version at time T_2, the results were confirmed. The H^S values in the *DEMQOL* version are comparable to the baseline values with "medium" correlations for subscale [B] to [D] and to a "weak" correlation for subscale [A] (Additional file 1: Table A1). At T_2, the assessment on subscale [A] improved to a "medium", whereas subscale [D] marginally worsened. The subscales [B] and [C] of the *DEMQOL-Proxy* improved to "strong" for both timepoints. The same result was found for subscale [D] at T_2. Therefore, at T_2, all subscales of the *DEMQOL-Proxy* are "strong" (Additional file 2: Table A2).

Internal consistency

The subscales revealed a ρ of 0.71–0.84 ($\alpha = 0.72$–0.83) for the *DEMQOL* and a ρ of 0.79–0.88 ($\alpha = 0.81$–0.87) for the *DEMQOL-Proxy*. According to the ρ- and α-values, all subscales were considered "good" (Table 3). The internal consistency was also "good" for T_1 and T_2 for all subscales, with ρ- and α-values > 0.72 (Additional file 1: Table A1 and Additional file 2: Table A2). The r_{it} revealed only one item (item 9 from the *DEMQOL-Proxy*, "irritable") that was below 0.4, which was not scalable at all in the *DEMQOL* version. All other items had a "high" ($n = 41$) or "moderate" ($n = 15$) r_{it}-values of 0.4 or more.

Table 2 Item distribution on the German version of the *DEMQOL* and *DEMQOL-Proxy* (No. of original item order; $n = 201$)

DEMQOL									*DEMQOL-Proxy*								
No.	Item	Response options				Descriptive			No.	Item	Response options				Descriptive		
		a lot	quite a bit	a little	not at all	missing	mean	(±SD)			a lot	quite a bit	a little	not at all	missing	mean	(±SD)
Feelings In the last week, have you felt …									Feelings In the last week, would you say that *(your relative)* has felt …								
1.	…cheerful? [a]	85	90	24	2	0	3.28	(±0.71)	1.	…cheerful? [a]	67	91	41	2	0	3.11	(±0.75)
2.	…worried or anxious?	22	65	60	54	0	2.73	(±0.98)	2.	…worried or anxious?	31	90	50	29	1	2.39	(±0.92)
3.	…that you are enjoying life? [a]	110	61	27	3	0	3.38	(±0.77)									
4.	…frustrated?	14	43	75	69	0	2.99	(±0.92)	3.	…frustrated?	15	73	72	41	0	2.69	(±0.88)
5.	…confident? [a]	82	77	34	8	0	3.16	(±0.85)									
6.	…full of energy? [a]	93	75	26	6	1	3.28	(±0.80)	4.	…full of energy? [a]	42	77	62	20	0	2.70	(±0.91)
7.	…sad?	17	59	64	61	0	2.84	(±0.96)	5.	…sad?	14	86	68	33	0	2.60	(±0.84)
									6.	…content? [a]	104	72	22	2	1	3.39	(±0.72)
8.	…lonely?	12	24	51	114	0	3.33	(±0.91)									
9.	…distressed?	6	23	62	110	0	3.37	(±0.80)	7.	…distressed?	27	94	51	29	0	2.41	(±0.90)
10.	…lively? [a]	73	74	38	16	0	3.01	(±0.94)	8.	…lively? [a]	55	76	52	18	0	2.84	(±0.93)
11.	…irritable?	19	50	74	57	1	2.85	(±0.95)	9.	…irritable?	30	75	63	32	1	2.49	(±0.93)
12.	…fed-up?	4	40	54	103	0	3.27	(±0.85)	10.	…fed-up?	12	69	64	56	0	2.82	(±0.91)
									11.	…that he/she has things to look forward to? [a]	80	92	26	3	0	3.24	(±0.73)
13.	…that there are things that youwanted to do but couldn't?	8	42	68	82	1	3.12	(±0.88)									
Memory In the last week, how worried have you been about …									Memory In the last week, how worried would you say *(your relative)* has been about …								
									12.	…his/her memory in general?	89	73	26	13	0	1.82	(±0.89)
									13.	…forgetting things that happened a long time ago?	28	58	73	42	0	2.64	(±0.96)
14.	…forgetting things that happened recently?	59	79	35	28	0	2.16	(±1.00)	14.	…forgetting things that happened recently?	85	66	33	15	2	1.89	(±0.94)
15.	…forgetting who people are?	26	44	42	88	1	2.96	(±1.09)									
									15.	…forgetting people's names?	52	79	45	24	1	2.21	(±0.96)
									16.	…forgetting where he/she is?	12	24	61	104	0	3.28	(±0.90)
16.	…forgetting what day it is?	27	51	50	73	0	2.84	(±1.07)	17.	…forgetting what day it is?	36	56	50	59	0	2.66	(±1.08)
17.	…your thoughts being muddled?	32	55	56	58	0	2.70	(±1.05)	18.	…his/her thoughts being muddled?	30	68	54	48	1	2.60	(±1.01)
18.	…difficulty making decisions?	11	51	54	85	0	3.06	(±0.95)	19.	…difficulty making decisions?	29	54	66	51	1	2.70	(±1.01)

Table 2 Item distribution on the German version of the *DEMQOL* and *DEMQOL-Proxy* (No. of original item order; $n = 201$) *(Continued)*

19.	…poor concentration?	63	65	43	29	1	2.19 (±1.04)								
24.	…making yourself understood? [b]	14	31	57	99	0	3.20 (±0.94)	20.	…making him/herself understood?	12	48	56	85	0	3.06 (±0.95)
Everyday life In the last week, how worried have you been about …								Everyday life In the last week, how worried would you say *(your relative)* has been about …							
20.	…not having enough company?	4	17	51	129	0	3.52 [d] (±0.74)	28.	…not having enough company?	5	25	49	121	1	3.43 [d] (±0.81)
21.	…how you get on with people close to you?	8	19	47	126	1	3.46 [d] (±0.83)								
22.	…getting the affection that you want?	4	17	42	137	1	3.56 [d] (±0.73)								
23.	…people not listening to you?	9	25	50	117	0	3.37 (±0.87)								
25.	…getting help when you need it?	4	23	42	132	0	3.50 [d] (±0.78)								
26.	…getting to the toilet in time?	12	20	20	149	0	3.52 [d] (±0.90)								
27.	…how you feel in yourself?	14	29	45	113	0	3.28 (±0.95)								
28.	…your health overall?	28	67	49	57	0	2.67 (±1.04)								
								21.	…keeping him–/herself clean(e.g. washing and bathing)?	2	7	23	169	0	3.79 [d] (±0.55)
								22.	…keeping him–/herself looking nice?	6	18	41	136	0	3.53 [d] (±0.78)
								23.	…getting what he/she wants from the shops?	3	25	49	124	0	3.46 [d] (±0.77)
								24.	…using money to pay for things?	12	23	38	128	0	3.40 [d] (±0.91)
								25.	…looking after his/her finances?	14	38	37	112	0	3.23 (±0.99)
								26.	…things taking longer than they used to?	33	61	48	58	1	2.66 (±1.07)
								27.	…getting in touch with people?	1	31	61	108	0	3.37 (±0.76)
								29.	…not being able to help other people?	3	22	58	118	0	3.45 [d] (±0.75)
								30.	…not playing a useful part in things?	12	41	41	107	0	3.21 (±0.97)
								31.	…his/her physical health?	37	73	42	48	1	2.51 (±1.05)
Frequencies of the response options in total, n		**860**	**1316**	**1340**	**2105**	**7**		Frequencies of the response options in total, n		**978**	**1785**	**1522**	**1935**	**11**	

Table 2 Item distribution on the German version of the *DEMQOL* and *DEMQOL-Proxy* (No. of original item order; $n = 201$) *(Continued)*

Frequencies of the response options in total, %	**15.3**	**23.4**	**23.8**	**37.5**	**0.1**		Frequencies of the response options in total, %	**15.7**	**28.7**	**24.5**	**31.1**	**0.2**	
No. Item	Response options				Descriptive		No. Item	Response options				Descriptive	
	very good	good	fair	poor	missing	mean (±SD)		very good	good	fair	poor	missing	mean (±SD)
OverallThinking about all of these things in the last week, how would you rate …							OverallThinking about all of these things in the last week, how would you say *(your relative)* would rate …						
29. …your quality of life overall?[c]	23	139	37	2	0	2.91 (±0.58)	32. …his/her quality of life overall? [a]	11	125	58	7	0	2.70 (±0.63)
Frequencies of the response options, %	**11.4**	**69.2**	**18.4**	**1.0**	**0.0**		Frequencies of the response options, %	**5.5**	**62.2**	**28.9**	**3.5**	**0.0**	

[a]Contraindicative items
[b]The item corresponds to both versions, however in the original questionnaire it is part as number 24 of "Everyday life"
[c]Contraindicative items
[d]Ceiling effect, the mean is in the last 20% of the scale (≥ 3.4)

Table 3 Scale analysis and internal consistency of the *DEMQOL* and *DEMQOL-Proxy* ($n = 201$)

DEMQOL	ρ	α	H^S			*DEMQOL-Proxy*	ρ	α	H^S		
A. Positive emotions	**0.71**	**0.72**	**0.38**	H_i	r_{it}	A. Positive emotions	**0.88**	**0.86**	**0.66**	H_i	r_{it}
10. …lively?				0.41	0.52	8. …lively?				0.71	0.78
6. …full of energy?				0.39	0.50	4. …full of energy?				0.65	0.69
1. …cheerful?				0.37	0.47	11. …that he/she has things to look forward to?				0.66	0.70
3. …that you are enjoying life?				0.37	0.46	1. …cheerful?				0.66	0.69
5. …confident?				0.34	0.43	6. …content?				0.58	0.59
B. Negative emotions	**0.80**	**0.80**	**0.45**	H_i	r_{it}	B. Negative emotions	**0.79**	**0.81**	**0.46**	H_i	r_{it}
7. …sad?				0.52	0.66	7. …distressed?				0.51	0.65
9. …distressed?				0.51	0.63	5. …sad?				0.51	0.65
8. …lonely?				0.41	0.50	3. …frustrated?				0.53	0.67
4. …frustrated?				0.47	0.58	2. …worried or anxious?				0.43	0.53
12. …fed-up?				0.41	0.49	10. …fed-up?				0.46	0.55
2. …worried or anxious?				0.40	0.48	9. …irritable?				0.31	0.37
C. Physical and cognitive functioning	**0.83**	**0.82**	**0.42**	H_i	r_{it}	C. Physical and cognitive functioning	**0.88**	**0.87**	**0.50**	H_i	r_{it}
19. …poor concentration?				0.50	0.66	12. …his/her memory in general?				0.50	0.59
17. …your thoughts being muddled?				0.47	0.64	14. …forgetting things that happened recently?				0.50	0.60
14. …forgetting things that happened recently?				0.42	0.53	15. …forgetting people's names?				0.51	0.62
27. …how you feel in yourself?				0.40	0.49	18. …his/her thoughts being muddled?				0.57	0.75
18. …difficulty making decisions?				0.42	0.55	19. …difficulty making decisions?				0.52	0.66
28. …your health overall?				0.40	0.53	17. …forgetting what day it is?				0.49	0.63
16. …forgetting what day it is?				0.37	0.49	16. …forgetting where he/she is?				0.46	0.53
13. …that there are things that you wanted to do but couldn't?				0.33	0.43	20. …making him/herself understood?				0.46	0.54
						13. …forgetting things that happened a long time ago?				0.45	0.57
D. Daily activities and social relationships	**0.84**	**0.83**	**0.46**	H_i	r_{it}	D. Daily activities and social relationships	**0.86**	**0.86**	**0.42**	H_i	r_{it}
21. …how you get on with people close to you? [a]				0.49	0.65	23. …getting what he/she wants from the shops? [a]				0.48	0.67
24. …making yourself understood?				0.50	0.62	24. …using money to pay for things? [a]				0.43	0.59
23. …people not listening to you?				0.52	0.68	21. …keeping him-/herself clean (e.g. washing and bathing)? [a]				0.45	0.50
22. …getting the affection that you want? [a]				0.49	0.63	27. …getting in touch with people?				0.49	0.67
25. …getting help when you need it? [a]				0.47	0.62	22. …keeping him-/herself looking nice? [a]				0.45	0.59
20. …not having enough company? [a]				0.39	0.49	30. …not playing a useful part in things?				0.42	0.58
26. …getting to the toilet in time? [a]				0.34	0.40	29. …not being able to help other people? [a]				0.42	0.58
						26. …things taking longer than they used to?				0.40	0.51
						31. …his/her physical health?				0.38	0.45
						28. …not having enough company? [a]				0.38	0.52
						25. …looking after his/her finances?				0.36	0.48

The criterion (Crit) by Molenaar, Sijtsma, and Boer used to check the monotonicity assumption is for all items in every of the ten imputed datasets = 0
ρ = rho (Molenaar Sijtsma statistic); α = Cronbach's alpha (> 0.7 and < 0.95 = good); r_{it} = part-whole-corrected item-total correlation (> 0.50 = high, > 0.30 = moderate);
H^S = Loevinger's H coefficient of scalability of the scale (> 0.50 = strong, > 0.40 = medium, > 0.30 = weak); H_i = Loevinger's H coefficient for an item and the remaining items of the scale
[a] Item with ceiling effect (see Table 2)

Discussion

The evaluation of the German versions of the *DEMQOL* and *DEMQOL-Proxy* revealed the following major findings. First, the MSA for the *DEMQOL* and the *DEMQOL-Proxy* revealed that four subscales ([A] "positive emotions", [B] "negative emotions", [C] "physical and cognitive functioning", and [D] "daily activities and social relationships") were found with stable H^S values ≥0.38. Second, the internal consistency showed consistently "good" values. Third, the item description showed ceiling effects, as exhibited by 18% of the items on the *DEMQOL* and 19% of the items on the *DEMQOL-Proxy*. Furthermore, the results of the MSA for the German versions of the *DEMQOL* and *DEMQOL-Proxy* are largely comparable to findings from previous studies on the HRQoL of persons living with dementia [4, 15], especially to the conceptual framework of Smith and colleagues [14] as well as to their explorative factor analysis of the pretest during the development of the instrument. As such, our results can be considered to be first indications of the structural validity of the *DEMQOL* and the *DEMQOL-Proxy*.

In our data evaluation, the domain "health and well-being" of the conceptual framework is represented by subscales [A], "positive emotions", and [B], "negative emotions", except items 27 ("how you feel in yourself") and 28 ("your health overall"), which have been loaded onto subscale [C], "physical and cognitive functioning". Therefore, this subscale has been complemented by the word "physical". For the *DEMQOL-Proxy*, only item 31 ("his/her physical health") from the framework was loaded onto subscale [D], "daily activities and social relationships". Subscale [C] characterizes the domain "cognitive functioning" of the conceptual framework in our data evaluation. Herein, 100% conformity for the *DEMQOL-Proxy* could be shown. However, item 24 of the *DEMQOL* ("making yourself understood") loaded onto subscale [D]. The domains "daily activities" and "social relationships" of the framework were combined into the fourth subscale of our study, which was designated as subscale [D], "daily activities and social relationships". However, item 13 of the *DEMQOL* ("that there are things that you wanted to do but couldn't") was an exception, as it was loaded to the subscale [C], "physical and cognitive functioning". This loading may be due to the translation of the word "inability" into German. Furthermore, item 30 of the *DEMQOL-Proxy* ("not playing a useful part in things") was added to subscale [D]. This was the only item that could be assigned to the "self-concept" domain of the conceptual framework.

Compared to the findings of Mulhern and colleagues, we also found subscales for "positive emotions" and "negative emotions" in our study. In contrast, in our assessment, subscale [C], "physical and cognitive functioning", is related to what has been termed "cognition" in the HTA report by Mulhern and colleagues [4]. The subscales "social relationships" in the *DEMQOL* and "daily activities" in the *DEMQOL-Proxy* were referred to the common subscale [D], "daily activities and social relationships", for both instruments within our data evaluation. Taken together, 71% of the *DEMQOL* items and 65% of the *DEMQOL-Proxy* items coincided with the results of Mulhern et al. [4]; that is, 20 items that are equally distributed in both instruments.

Furthermore, the subscales "positive emotions" (both instruments) and "negative emotions" (*DEMQOL-Proxy* only) are completely identical, if the cross loaders of the *DEMQOL-Proxy* in the Mulhern study are not removed. Subscale [B] of the *DEMQOL*, "negative emotions", exhibits a difference, as given by the loading of items 8 and 9, while item 11 is not loaded. In contrast, the subscale "cognition" shows high consistencies with the *DEMQOL* and *DEMQOL-Proxy*. Differences in the *DEMQOL*, however, exist only in the additional loading of the items 13, 27 and 28, while item 15 was not loaded. On the *DEMQOL-Proxy*, item 26 was not loaded, while all other items were identical. Item 20 of *DEMQOL* was additionally loaded within subscale [D], "daily activities and social relationships", which was named "social relationships" by Mulhern et al. [4]. Only three items of the *DEMQOL-Proxy* could be seen in the data set of Mulhern et al. [4], while our data evaluation further loaded the items 21, 22, and 26–31.

In summary, our data demonstrated the determined subscales to be highly consistent with the conceptual framework of Smith et al. [15] and that these subscales further exhibit similarities to those of Mulhern et al. [4]. The sensitivity analysis at times T_1 and T_2 showed a stable result for assignment of the items to the subscales (Additional file 1: Table A1 and Additional file 2: Table A2). In contrast, the designation of subscale [D] was identical in the *DEMQOL* and *DEMQOL-Proxy*, while this finding differed according to Mulhern et al. [4] and was therefore presented as "social relationships" in the *DEMQOL* and "daily activities" in the *DEMQOL-Proxy*. However, if both subscales were taken together, they represent a similar construct as our subscale [D], "daily activities and social relationships".

In accordance with the HRQoL definition from Hays and Reeve [7] provided in the background, the subscales we found in our study cover the aspects of "how well a person functions in his/her life" (physical and cognitive functioning [C]) and his or her "perceived well-being in physical (daily activities), mental (positive and negative emotions [A-B]), and social domains (social relationships [D]) of health".

Limitations

The presented data of this psychometric study used datasets from the CORDIAL study by Kurz et al. [21]. Thus, since additional data could not be obtained, no statements on the inter-rater reliability of the *DEMQOL-Proxy* can be made to estimate the quality of the underlying data. Similarly, it was no longer possible to influence the number of study participants. According to a study by Straat et al. [46], a sample of more than 250 respondents should be given if the quality of the answers is high. In the present study, however, only the data of 201 persons could be used, reflecting a limitation of the results. Furthermore, the CORDIAL study included only persons with a mild severity of AD. The mild form might explain the ceiling effects of subscale [D]. Thus, the generalizability of the results is limited due to the absence of other forms of dementia.

Conclusions

In this psychometric study using the German versions of the instruments *DEMQOL* and *DEMQOL-Proxy*, four equal subscales were found in both instruments, demonstrating "good" internal consistency. The subscales reflect the conceptual framework of the instrument developers to a high degree. Thus, the results can be considered a first indication of the construct validity of the two German versions. In our opinion, *DEMQOL* subscale scores are more explanatory than a total score because HRQoL is a multidimensional concept and respective domain scores may help clarify treatment impacts. Moreover, our internal consistency results reflect the homogeneity of the subscales. However, Chua et al. [19] used bifactor models for direct comparisons between total and subscale scores and showed that the latter scores had poor reliability and should not be used. Such direct comparisons were not performed in our study due to differences in modeling decisions (parallel iterative MSA rather than bifactor modeling). The merits of MSA and bifactor modeling for clarifying multidimensionality are debatable [47, 48]. Therefore, more empirical data are needed before definitive recommendations can be made.

However, we recommend further investigations prior to or integrated in future studies using the German version of the *DEMQOL* and *DEMQOL-Proxy*. In particular, we advise the integration of the evaluation of test-retest reliability (both *DEMQOL* versions) and inter-rater reliability (*DEMQOL-Proxy*) as part of the instrument application in future studies. Continued research should also be carried out on structural validity using various latent variable models. In addition, further investigation of data from persons living with moderate dementia, or with severe dementia for the proxy version, should be performed according to the ceiling effects we found in our study. For the proxy version, it would also be important to conduct a study with professional nurses to make statements on the use of the instrument in German nursing homes. Similarly, an investigation should be conducted to analyze against external criteria for other proportions of the construct validity.

Abbreviations

AD: Alzheimer's disease; B-ADL: Bayer Activities of Daily Living Scale; BDI: Beck Depression Inventory; CORDIAL: Cognitive Rehabilitation and Cognitive Behavioral Treatment for Early Dementia in Alzheimer's Disease (study); Crit: Criterion by Molenaar, Sijtsma, and Boer; DEMQOL: Dementia Quality of Life; GDS: Geriatric Depression Scale; H_i: Loevinger's H coefficient for an item and the remaining items of the scale; HRQoL: Health-related quality of life; H^S: Loevinger's H coefficient of scalability of a scale; HTA: Health Technology Assessment; ICF: International Classification of Functioning, Disability and Health; MMSE: Mini-Mental Status Examination; MSA: Mokken scale analysis; NPI: Neuropsychiatric Inventory; QoL: Quality of life; r_{it}: Part-whole-corrected item-total correlation; SD: Standard deviation; WHO: World Health Organization; ZBI-22: Zarit Burden Interview with 22 items; α: Cronbach's alpha; ρ: rho (Molenaar Sijtsma statistic)

Acknowledgments

We would like to thank the participants and colleagues from the CORDIAL study. We would especially like to thank Professor Dr. Alexander Kurz for providing the data.

Funding

The German Federal Ministry of Health funded the CORDIAL study (2008–2010; funding code: IIA5-2508FSB105//44–034). This study was also a "lighthouse project dementia". The German Center for Neurodegenerative Diseases supported the data analysis for this article. Both funding institutions had no role in the design, conduct, analyses or reporting of this study.

Authors' contributions

Study concept: CGGS, MND, and MB. Data collection and handling: CGGS and MB. Data analysis: CGGS and MND. Manuscript preparation: CGGS, MND, and MB. All authors have read and approved the final version of the manuscript.

Competing interests

The authors declare that they have no competing interests.

Author details

[1]German Center for Neurodegenerative Diseases (DZNE), Stockumer Straße 12, 58453 Witten, Germany. [2]School of Nursing Science, Witten/Herdecke University, Stockumer Straße 12, 58453 Witten, Germany. [3]Clinic for Cognitive Neurology, Medical Faculty, Leipzig University, Liebigstraße 16, 04103 Leipzig, Germany.

References

1. Alzheimer's Disease International (ADI). World Alzheimer Report 2015: The global impact of dementia. In London; 2015.
2. American Psychiatric Association (ed.): DSM-5. Diagnostic and statistical manual of mental disorders, Fifth Edition edn. Washington/DC: American Psychiatric Publishing; 2013.
3. Guidelines on medicinal products for the treatment of Alzheimer's disease and other dementias [http://www.ema.europa.eu/docs/en_GB/document_library/Scientific_guideline/2009/09/WC500003562.pdf].
4. Mulhern B, Rowen D, Brazier J, Smith S, Romeo R, Tait R, Watchurst C, Chua KC, Loftus V, Young T et al: Development of DEMQOL-U and DEMQOL-PROXY-U: generation of preference-based indices from DEMQOL and DEMQOL-PROXY for use in economic evaluation. Health Technology Assessment 2013, 17(5):v-xv, 1–140.
5. Rowen D, Mulhern B, Banerjee S, Hout B, Young TA, Knapp M, Smith SC, Lamping DL, Brazier JE. Estimating preference-based single index measures for dementia using DEMQOL and DEMQOL-Proxy. Value Health. 2012;15. United States:346–56.
6. Rowen D, Mulhern B, Banerjee S, Tait R, Watchurst C, Smith SC, Young TA, Knapp M, Brazier JE. Comparison of general population, patient, and carer

utility values for dementia health states. Medical Decision Making. 2015;35. United States:68–80.
7. Hays RD, Reeve BB: Measurement and modeling of health-related quality of life. In: Epidemiology and demography in public health. Edited by Killewo J, Heggenhougen HK, Quah SR. San Diego CA: Academic Press; 2010: 195–205.
8. Karimi M, Brazier J. Health, health-related quality of life, and quality of life: what is the difference? PharmacoEconomics. 2016;34(7):645–9.
9. Wilson IB, Cleary PD. Linking clinical variables with health-related quality of life. A conceptual model of patient outcomes. Jama. 1995;273(1):59–65.
10. World Health Organization (WHO). Constitution of the World Health Organization. Basic documents of the Word Helath Organization. Geneva: World Health Organization; 2014.
11. Bakas T, McLennon SM, Carpenter JS, Buelow JM, Otte JL, Hanna KM, Ellett ML, Hadler KA, Welch JL. Systematic review of health-related quality of life models. Health Qual Life Outcomes. 2012;10:134.
12. World Health Organization (WHO). International Classification of Functioning, disability, and Health: Children and Youth Version: ICF-CY. Geneva: World Health Organization; 2007.
13. Ferrans CE, Zerwic JJ, Wilbur JE, Larson JL. Conceptual model of health-related quality of life. Journal of nursing scholarship : an official publication of Sigma Theta Tau International Honor Society of Nursing. 2005;37(4):336–42.
14. Smith SC, Murray J, Banerjee S, Foley B, Cook JC, Lamping DL, Prince M, Harwood RH, Levin E, Mann A. What constitutes health-related quality of life in dementia? Development of a conceptual framework for people with dementia and their carers. International journal of geriatric psychiatry. 2005;20(9):889–95.
15. Smith SC, Lamping DL, Banerjee S, Harwood R, Foley B, Smith P, Cook JC, Murray J, Prince M, Levin E, et al. Measurement of health-related quality of life for people with dementia: development of a new instrument (DEMQOL) and an evaluation of current methodology. Health Technol Assess. 2005;9(10):1–93 iii-iv.
16. Berwig M, Leicht H, Gertz HJ. Critical evaluation of self-rated quality of life in mild cognitive impairment and Alzheimer's disease - further evidence for the impact of anosognosia and global cognitive impairment. The journal of nutrition health and aging. 2009;13(3):226–30.
17. Dichter MN, Schwab CGG, Meyer G, Bartholomeyczik S, Halek M. Linguistic validation and reliability properties are weak investigated of most dementia-specific quality of life measurements - a systematic review. J Clin Epidemiol. 2016;70:233–45.
18. Lucas-Carrasco R, Lamping DL, Banerjee S, Rejas J, Smith SC, Gomez-Benito J. Validation of the Spanish version of the DEMQOL system. International psychogeriatrics / IPA. 2010;22(4):589–97.
19. Chua KC, Brown A, Little R, Matthews D, Morton L, Loftus V, Watchurst C, Tait R, Romeo R, Banerjee S. Quality-of-life assessment in dementia: the use of DEMQOL and DEMQOL-proxy total scores. Quality of life research : an international journal of quality of life aspects of treatment, care and rehabilitation. 2016;25(12):3107–18.
20. Hendriks AAJ, Smith SC, Chrysanthaki T, Cano SJ, Black N. DEMQOL and DEMQOL-proxy: a Rasch analysis. Health Qual Life Outcomes. 2017;15(1):164.
21. Kurz A, Thone-Otto A, Cramer B, Egert S, Frolich L, Gertz HJ, Kehl V, Wagenpfeil S, Werheid K. CORDIAL: cognitive rehabilitation and cognitive-behavioral treatment for early dementia in Alzheimer disease: a multicenter, randomized, controlled trial. Alzheimer Dis Assoc Disord. 2012;26(3):246–53.
22. Swart E, Gothe H, Geyer S, Jaunzeme J, Maier B, Grobe TG, Ihle P, et al. [Good Practice of Secondary Data Analysis (GPS): Guidelines and Recommendations] Gute Praxis Sekundärdatenanalyse (GPS): Leitlinien und Empfehlungen. Gesundheitswesen. 2015;77(02):120–6.
23. Kessler J, Markowitsch HJ, Denzler PE. [Mini-Mental State Examination (MMSE) - German version] Mini-Mental-Status-Test (MMSE) - Deutsche Fassung. Beltz: Weinheim; 1990.
24. Hindmarch I, Lehfeld H, de Jongh P, Erzigkeit H. The Bayer activities of daily living scale (B-ADL). Dement Geriatr Cogn Disord. 1998;9(suppl 2):20–6.
25. Yesavage JA. Geriatric depression scale. Psychopharmacol Bull. 1988;24(4): 709–11.
26. Cummings JL. The neuropsychiatric inventory: assessing psychopathology in dementia patients. Neurology. 1997;48(5 Suppl 6):10–6.
27. Hautzinger M, Bailer M, Worall H, Keller F: [Beck-depression-inventory (BDI): editing of the German version - test manual] Beck-depressions-Inventar (BDI): Bearbeitung der deutschen Ausgabe - Testhandbuch, 2. Auflage edn. Bern: Hans Huber; 1994.
28. Zarit SH, Reever KE, Bach-Peterson J. Relatives of the impaired elderly: correlates of feelings of burden. The Gerontologist. 1980;20(6):649–55.
29. Stochl J, Jones PB, Croudace TJ. Mokken scale analysis of mental health and well-being questionnaire item responses: a non-parametric IRT method in empirical research for applied health researchers. BMC Med Res Methodol. 2012;12:74.
30. Watson R, van der Ark LA, Lin LC, Fieo R, Deary IJ, Meijer RR. Item response theory: how Mokken scaling can be used in clinical practice. J Clin Nurs. 2012;21(19–20):2736–46.
31. Dichter MN, Dortmann O, Halek M, Meyer G, Holle D, Nordheim J, Bartholomeyczik S. Scalability and internal consistency of the German version of the dementia-specific quality of life instrument QUALIDEM in nursing homes -- a secondary data analysis. Health Qual Life Outcomes. 2013;11(1):91.
32. Bouman AI, Ettema TP, Wetzels RB, van Beek AP, de Lange J, Droes RM. Evaluation of Qualidem: a dementia-specific quality of life instrument for persons with dementia in residential settings; scalability and reliability of subscales in four Dutch field surveys. International journal of geriatric psychiatry. 2011;26(7):711–22.
33. Sijtsma K, Molenaar IW. Introduction to nonparametric item response theory, vol. 5. Thousand Oaks, CA: Sage Publications; 2002.
34. Molenaar IW, Sijtsma K. User's manual MSP5 for windows [software manual]. IEC ProGAMMA: Groningen, The Netherlands; 2000.
35. Müller-Schneider T. Multiple Skalierung nach dem Kristallisationsprinzip. Eine alternative zur explorativen Faktorenanalyse [multiple scaling according to the principle of crystallization. An alternative method to exploratory factor analysis]. Z Soziol. 2001;30(4):305–15.
36. Schwab CGG. [Construct validity and internal consistency of the instrument "burden in dealing with dementia" (BelaDem) in nursing homes - unpublished master thesis] Konstruktvalidität und interne Konsistenz des Instrumentes "Belastungserleben im Umgang mit Demenz" (BelaDem) in der stationären Altenhilfe - unveröffentlichte Masterarbeit. Herdecke: Witten: Universität Witten/Herdecke; 2013.
37. Van Ginkel JR, Andries van Der Ark LA, Sijtsma K, Vermunt JK. two-way imputation: a Bayesian method for estimating missing scores in tests and questionnaires, and an accurate approximation. Computational Statistics & Data Analysis. 2007;51(8):4013–27.
38. Sijtsma K, Molenaar IW. Reliability of test scores in nonparametric item response theory. Psychometrika. 1987;52.
39. van der Ark LA, van der Palm DW, Sijtsma K. A latent class approach to estimating test-score reliability. Appl Psychol Meas. 2011;35(5):380–92.
40. Terwee CB, Bot SD, de Boer MR, van der Windt DA, Knol DL, Dekker J, Bouter LM, de Vet HC. Quality criteria were proposed for measurement properties of health status questionnaires. J Clin Epidemiol. 2007;60(1):34–42.
41. Bortz J, Döring N, Bortz D. [Research methods and evaluation: for human and social sciences] Forschungsmethoden und Evaluation: für Human- und Sozialwissenschaftler, fourth revised edition edn. Heidelberg: Springer-Medizin-Verlag; 2006.
42. Core R. Team R: a language and environment for statistical computing. Vienna, Austria: R Foundation for Statistical Computing; 2017.
43. van der Ark LA. Mokken scale analysis in R. J Stat Softw. 2007;20(11):19.
44. van der Ark LA. New developments in Mokken scale analysis in R. J Stat Softw. 2012;48(5):27.
45. Robitzsch A, Grund S, Henke T: TAM: Some additional multiple imputation functions, especially for mice. R package version 2.5–9. https://CRAN.R-project.org/package=miceadds; 2017.
46. Straat JH, van der Ark LA, Klaas S. minimum sample size requirements for Mokken scale analysis. Educ Psychol Meas. 2014;74(5):809–22.
47. Reise SP, Kim DS, Mansolf M, Widaman KF. Is the Bifactor model a better model or is it just better at modeling implausible responses? Application of iteratively reweighted least squares to the Rosenberg self-esteem scale. Multivariate Behav Res. 2016;51(6):818–38.
48. Smits IAM, Timmerman ME, Meijer RR. Exploratory Mokken scale analysis as a dimensionality assessment tool: why scalability does not imply Unidimensionality. Appl Psychol Meas. 2012;36(6):516–39.

13

Health-related quality of life on tele-monitoring for users with pacemakers 6 months after implant: the NORDLAND study, a randomized trial

Antonio Lopez-Villegas[1,2,3], Daniel Catalan-Matamoros[4,5*], Remedios Lopez-Liria[6], Terje Enebakk[2], Hilde Thunhaug[2] and Knut Tore Lappegård[2,3]

Abstract

Background: With an ageing population and widening indications for pacemakers implantation, the number of persons carrying an implant is steadily increasing. The routine follow-up is thus a heavy burden for the respective NHS as well as for the patients and their relatives. Most of them of the studies have been performed in densely populated areas and nearby to the hospital. It is thus unknown whether these results could be applied also in rural areas such as Northern Norway with a more scattered population. The aim of this study was to assess the effectiveness of tele-monitoring (TM) in patients with pacemakers regarding reliability, safety and health-related quality of life, compared to traditional follow-up in outpatient clinic in a setting where geographical effects could possible influence the results.

Methods: The NORDLAND study is a controlled, randomized, non-masked clinical trial in pacemaker patients, with data collection carried out during the pre-implant stage and after 6 months. Between August of 2014 and November of 2015, 50 patients were assigned to either a tele-monitoring group ($n = 25$) or a conventional hospital monitoring (HM) group ($n = 25$). The *EuroQol-5D* (EQ-5D) utilities and visual analogue scale (VAS) and the Minnesota Living with Heart Failure Questionnaire *(MLHFQ)* were used to measure Health-Related Quality of Life. Baseline characteristics and number of hospital visits were also analyzed.

Results: The baseline characteristics of the two study groups were similar for EQ-5D utilities (TM:0.81; HM:0.76; $p = 0.47$) , EQ-5D VAS (TM: 64.00; HM:64.88; $p = 0.86$) and the *MLHFQ* (TM:20.20; HM:28.96; $p = 0.07$). At the 6 month follow-up, there were no significant differences between the groups in EQ-5D utilities (TM: 0.81; HM: 0.76; $p = 0.54$) and EQ-5D VAS scores (TM: 72.71; HM: 59.79; $p = 0.08$). The *MLHFQ* score was improved in both groups (TM: -4.40; HM: -15.13; $p < 0.001$). The number of in-office visits was similar in both groups (TM: 1.24 vs HM: 1.12; $P = 0.30$).

Conclusions: The NORDLAND trial shows that HRQoL is improved after implant in both groups. Without significant differences with regards to effectiveness and safety. In addition, provides a scientifically rigorous method to the field of HRQoL evaluations in patients with pacemakers.

Keywords: Health-related quality of life, Older adults, Pacemaker follow-up, Randomized study, Remote monitoring, Telemedicine

* Correspondence: dcatalan@ual.es
[4]Department of Journalism and Communication, Universidad Carlos III de Madrid, Calle Madrid 133, 28903 Getafe, Madrid, Spain
[5]Health Sciences CTS-451 Research Group, University of Almeria, Almería, Spain
Full list of author information is available at the end of the article

Background

International guidelines of professional practice advises that users with pacemakers (PM) must be monitored in periods between 3 and 12 months [1, 2]. Every hospital visit usually involves an assessment of pacemakers function, cardiovascular events and an analysis of patient physical status and, whether is necessary the medication is modified and/or the device is re-configured again [1, 3]. With an ageing population and widening indications for PM implantation, the number of persons carrying an implant is steadily increasing. The routine follow-up is thus a heavy burden for the respective national health services [4] as well as for the pacemakers users and their caregivers [5, 6].

Remote monitoring or tele-monitoring (TM) systems have potential advantages such as early detection of cardiovascular events and early response to technical problems of the device or changes in the patient's clinical status [7–10]. TM may be a potential alternative to help reduce the number of in-office visits to hospital, thereby optimizing medical resources [11]. Along last decade, several studies have showed that TM is as effective as traditional follow-up in hospital [2, 10–13]. In addition, the number of unscheduled visits to the hospital for assistance at the emergency services and hospitalizations can be reduced [4, 14]. In the last decade a limited number of studies have shown results on efficiency [4, 7, 15, 16] particularly based on patient-reported outcomes such as HRQoL [10–12, 15–18]. On the other part, a study published recently affirms that telemedicine is not significantly more effective than usual care on mental and physical Health-Related Quality of Life (HRQoL) [19].

However, the majority of these studies have not been randomized, but have based their allocation to mode of follow-up to patient or observer preference. Furthermore, several of them have been performed in densely populated areas with most of the patients living only a short distance to the following centre. It is thus unknown whether these results apply also in a randomized study and in rural areas such as Northern Norway with a more scattered population.

Regarding previous paragraph, there is no international standard for defining rural areas, and the existing ones may vary even within a same country [20, 21]. Previous publications indicate that the healthcare needs of patients living in rural areas usually be different from those in urban areas, and patients living in rural areas often they tend to have problem access to healthcare [22]. Nordland county (Norway) has a scattered population of 6,3 inhab/sq. km (for comparison Canada has 3,7, USA 34,8 and United Kingdom 274 inhab/sq. km) [20, 23]. Although a large fraction of the population in Nordland county (Norway) lives in cities, the cities are small and there is still a significant proportion of inhabitants living in communities with less than 2500 individuals and at distances a long way from the hospital.

The purpose of the present study was to assess the effectiveness of TM in patients with pacemakers regarding reliability, safety and health-related quality of life, compared to traditional follow-up in outpatient clinic in a setting where geographical effects could possible influence the results.

Methods

Design

Controlled, randomized, non-masked clinical trial with patient assignment to conventional follow-up in the hospital or tele-monitoring follow-up by electronic data transmission with 6 months monitoring from the date of implantation.

The randomization process was performed as follows: A person unrelated to the study prepared a total of 50 sealed envelopes, 25 which included at note reading "tele-monitoring" and 25 with a note reading "hospital monitoring". The envelopes were thoroughly mixed and numbered from 1 to 50. When a patient had accepted the invitation to participate in the study and signed the informed consent he was given a consecutive study number and allocated to follow-up in accordance with the specification included in the corresponding envelope. Thus, the investigators had no knowledge of or influence on the randomization result prior to inclusion.

Environment

The study was carried out in Nordland Hospital, Bodø, Norway, a hospital with a pacemaker center that serves a population of 170,000 inhabitants and performs around 80–90 pacemakers implants per year.

Participants and selection

All patients who were scheduled for implant with a pacemaker between August of 2014 and October of 2015 and met all the inclusion criteria (age 18 years or older, ability to give informed consent and to operate the home monitor, life expectancy > 1 year) and none of the exclusion criteria (scheduled for implantable cardioverter-defibrillator (ICD) or cardiac resynchronization therapy (CRT), participation in other trials) were invited to participate. A total of 76 patients were screened and 50 patients were included and randomized to either telemonitoring (TM, $n = 25$) or hospital monitoring (HM, $n = 25$). No changes to methods were performed after trial commencement.

Devices

According to their diagnosis, patients received either a single (VVIR) or a dual chamber pacemaker (DDDR). Patients assigned to tele-monitoring received either a Biotronik Estella SR-T/ DR-T or a Biotronik Evia SR-T/ DR-T. Patients assigned to hospital monitoring received either one of the aforementioned Biotronik pacemakers, a St Jude Medical Endurity SR/DR or a Sorin Reply 200 SR/DR.

Home monitoring was performed through the Biotronik Home Monitoring® system, an internet-based TM service for users with Biotronik implantable heart devices. Biotronik devices equipped with Home Monitoring (T-devices) have additional storage capacity and contain a small RF-antenna for wireless communication and data transmission from the implant to a wireless patient device, the CardioMessenger. Home Monitoring has no negative effects on devices' battery life [24].

Every night, the CardioMessenger automatically collects and transmits important, encrypted health information to the Biotronik service center using the global network of T-Mobile and its partners (GPRS). The transmitted patient data is collected, automatically analyzed and filtered at the Biotronik Home Monitoring Service Center, according to patients'needs as defined by their physician. Health and system-related issues are ranked and marked in order of importance. All event and trend reports can be accessed and reviewed on a protected online platform. Furthermore, according to pre-set definitions, the physician can receive automatic warnings (e.g. by e-mail or text message) concerning safety issues such as premature battery depletion, lead fracture etc.

Primary outcome measures

HRQoL of the users with pacemakers was assessed through the Norwegian version of the utility scores of the EuroQol-5D (EQ-5D) [25] from − 1 [the worst state of health] to 1 [the best state of health], and the self-rated HRQoL was analyzed through of the EQ-5D Visual Analogue Scale (EQ-5D-VAS), from 0 [worst imaginable health state or death] to 100 [perfect health]).

Secondary outcome measures

To measure the effects of symptoms, functional limitations and psychological reactions commonly associated with heart failure or its treatment on an individual's quality of life, the Norwegian validated version of the MLHFQ. It consists of 21 questions regarding patients' perception of the effects of HF on their daily lives; the score for each question ranges from 0 to 5, producing a total score of 0 to 105, with a higher score indicating a poorer HRQoL [26–29].

Other outcome measures

Differences between TM and HM groups, in regards to: 1) Cardiovascular events (AE), including exitus, percutaneous coronary intervention, angina and lead dislodgement 2) monitoring visits and transmissions from home vs. hospital and 3) changes of medication and pacemakers reprogramming.

Follow-up

Patients were given 3 interviews (on the day of the pacemakers implant, and at 1 and 6 months after the implant) in which the corresponding questionnaires were administered. These interviews were carried out in a personalized way during hospitalization or by telephone interviews after discharge.

To ensure that the sample size was representative, due to the limited capacity of patient enrolment in the hospital, the following formula was used: $n = \frac{N.Z^2.p(1-p)}{(N-1)e^2+Z^2.p(1-p)}$ Thus, from a target population of $n = 70$, assuming a standard deviation of Z = 1.96, with a margin of error e = 0.10, a proportion of $p = 0.5$, and a 10% of possible losses, we got a size sample necessary of $n = 45$. We did not have any prior information on the value that was expected to be found. For this reason, 50% has been used as the statistical power ($p = 0.5$) meaning that, if there was any effect, it would be detected at the 50% of the total events.

Statistical analysis

Continuous variables were assessed as mean ± standard deviation. Categorical data in both groups were compared using difference in proportions test (binomial method) or Chi-Square test or Fisher exact test, when was appropriated. Differences between both groups were also assessed in the pre-specified endpoints using the difference in means or proportions tests and Wilcoxon signed ranks test for *Minnesota Living with Heart Failure Questionnaire*. Results are presented, including the corresponding 95% confidence intervals (95% CI). All statistical analyses were performed with SPSS (SPSS Institute, Inc., Chicago, IL, USA) statistical software.

Results

Participants

Between August of 2014 and October of 2015, 50 patients (mean age: 75 ± 12 years, 48% women) were enrolled in the NORDLAND study, of which 25 were included in the TM group and 25 in the HM group (Fig. 1). Dizziness was the most common symptom, and the patients were most commonly referred from the hospital's own cardiology ward or from other local hospitals. The most common pacing indication was sick sinus syndrome (48%) followed by atrioventricular block (40%). In 88% of the cases, DDDR pacemakers were used. Hypertension was the most frequent comorbidity (64%). None of the baseline characteristics, including HRQoL were different between the two groups (Table 1).

Health-related quality of life basal analysis

In basal analysis patients had a mean score of 0.78 (95%CI:0.72;0.85) for EQ5D utilities and 64.83 (95%

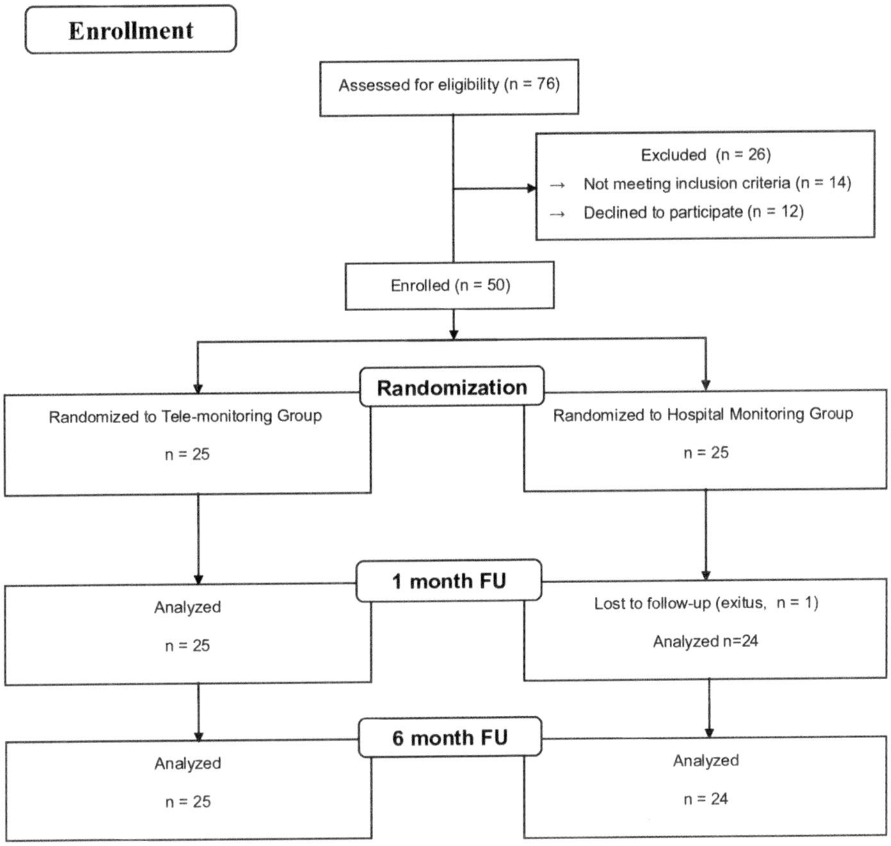

Fig. 1 Flow (CONSORT) diagram of the study

CI:56.74;70.14) for EQ5D VAS, which was increased to 0.81 (95%CI: -0.75;0.87) and 67.80 (95%CI: 62.49;73.10) respectively at 1 month after PM implantation (Table 2). Changes between baseline and 1 month EQ5D utilities and VAS were not statistically significant ($p = 0.81$ and $p = 0.20$, respectively). TM and HM groups showed no significant differences in EQ5D utilities and VAS scores between enrollment and at month (Table 2), nor at any EQ5D utilities dimensions. Regarding MLHFQ, the patients had a mean score at baseline of 24.58 (95%CI:19.30;29.86). This improved significantly to 16.55 (95%CI:11.40–21.70) at the 1 month assessment ($p < 0.05$). There were no significant differences in MLHFQ scores between TM and HM groups (20.20 vs. 28.96; $p = 0.07$) at baseline or at 1 month of follow-up (18.64 vs. 14.38, $p = 0.59$) (Table 3).

Cardiovascular adverse events and workload

After 6 months of follow-up, 6% of patients had experienced at least one AE (TM: 6%, HM: 4.2%; $p = 0.40$) (Table 4). After PM implantation, 38.2% of patients were hospitalized at least once (TM: 42%, HM: 33.4%; $p = 0.55$). The main causes of hospitalization were due to coronary problems (TM, 16% vs. HM, 20.8%) and PM dysfunction (TM, 12% vs. HM, 0%), however no significant differences between the groups were found. One patient (HM group) died for non-cardiovascular causes. As for workload, a mean of 1.20 ± 0.50 in-hospital visits per patient were registered during the follow-up period (TM:1.24 vs. HM:1.17; $p = 0.26$).

Health related quality of life results at 6 months

At 6 months, the EQ5D utilities score (Table 5) was increased to 0.79 (95%CI: 0.71;0.86; $p = 0.54$), 0.01 points more than baseline and 0.02 points less than the scores reached in month 1 (95% CI: -0.16;0.10; $p = 0.64$). On the EQ-5D VAS, the mean score reached 66.74 points, 1.91 points higher than in basal analysis (relative increase of 2.86%; $p = 0.42$) and 1.06 points less than the obtained in month 1 after implant (relative decrease of 1.59%; $p = 0.72$).

The MLHFQ scores (Table 5) revealed a significant improvement for both groups (– 9.65 points; 95% CI: 9.04–20.02), with significant differences compared to baseline scores ($p < 0.001$) and 2.02 points less than the obtained at month 1 after implant (reduction of 12.21%; $P = 0.39$). At the end of the study period, HM group experienced the better response with respect to month 0 (TM: – 4.4 vs. HM: – 15.75). At 6 months, there were no significant differences between the two groups (TM: 15.80 versus HM: 13.21; $p = 0.97$).

Table 1 Patients' demographic and clinical characteristics at baseline

	All (*n* = 50)	Groups		*P*-value
		TM (*n* = 25)	HM (*n* = 25)	
Age (mean) ± SD	74.84 ± 11.8	73.68 ± 14.2	76.00 ± 8.8	0.68
Men (mean)	26 (52.0)	13 (52.0)	13 (52.0)	1.00
MLHFQ [95CI]	24.58 [19.30;29.86]	20.20 [14.48;25.92]	28.96 [19.97–37.95]	0.07
EQ5D utilities [95CI]	0.78 [0.72;0.85]	0.81 [0.74;0.87]	0.76 [0.64;0.88]	0.47
Pacing indication *(%)*				
Sick sinus syndrome	24 (48.0)	12 (48.0)	12 (48.0)	0.65
Atrioventricular block	20 (40.0)	11 (44.0%)	9 (36.0)	
Chronic AF with Bradycardia	6 (12.0)	2 (8.0)	4 (16.0)	
Disease manifestations *(%)*				
Syncope	14 (28.0)	8 (32.0)	6 (24.0)	0.81
Dizziness	25 (50.0)	12 (48.0)	13 (52.0)	
Dyspnoea	11 (22.0)	5 (20.0)	6 (24.0)	
Service derivated (%)				
Emergency dept.	3 (6.0)	1 (4.0)	2 (8.0)	0.51
Cardiology ward	14 (28.0)	5 (20.0)	9 (36.0)	
Primary healthcare	4 (8.0)	2 (8.0)	2 (8.0)	
Other hospitals	29 (58.0)	17 (68.0)	12 (48.0)	
Stimulation (%)				
DDDR	44 (88.0)	23 (92.0)	21 (84.0)	0.33
VVIR	6 (12.0)	2 (8.0)	4 (16.0)	
Comorbidities (%)				
Dislipidemia	27 (54.0)	13 (52.0)	14 (56.0)	0.50
Obesity (BMI > 30)	1 (2.0)	0 (0.0)	1 (4.0)	0.50
Tachyarrhythmia	18 (36.0)	7 (28.0)	11 (44.0)	0.19
Hypertension	32 (64.0)	17 (68.0)	15 (60.0)	0.38
Diabetes Mellitus	6 (12.0)	0 (0.0)	6 (24.0)	0.01
Other comorbidities (%)				
None	18 (36.0)	11 (44.0)	7 (28.0)	0.39
Others	10 (20.0)	6 (24.0)	4 (16.0)	
Coronary heart diseases	22 (44.0)	8 (32.0)	14 (56.0)	
Pharmaceutical treatment (%)				
Antiaggregants	18 (36.0)	8 (32.0)	10 (40.0)	0.38
Anticoagulants	25 (50.0)	10 (40.0)	15 (60.0)	0.13
Antiarrhythmics	18 (36.0)	7 (28.0)	11 (44.0)	0.19
Antihypertensives	32 (64.0)	18 (72.0)	14 (56.0)	0.19

N = 50 (Telemonitoring group: 25; Hospital Monitoring group: 25). Values are expressed as means or proportions. 95CI: 95% confidence interval of means; *AF* atrial fibrillation, *BMI* body mass index, *EQ5D* EuroQoL-5D, *DDD* bicameral pacemaker with two electrodes placed in the atrium and in the ventricle with the ability to modulate frequency of stimulation, *MLHFQ* Minnesota Living with Heart Failure, *VVIR* unicameral pacemaker with an electrode in the ventricle with the ability to modulate frequency of stimulation

Discussion

Principal findings

Among the main results of the NORDLAND study, we found that, a) there was not significant differences in HRQoL assessed through EQ-5D utilities and VAS questionnaires administered at 1 and 6 months after implant between users included in the two groups of follow-up, b) in MLHF questionnaire were found significant differences in both groups between the enrolment and the end of follow-up period, c) safety was similar between both groups and no significant differences were found, d) that number of visits to hospital

Table 2 Health-related quality of life at 6 months of follow-up

EQ-5D Utilities		Month 0				Month 1				Month 6			
		TM n (%)	HM n (%)	Total n (%)	p	TM n (%)	HM n (%)	Total n (%)	p	TM n (%)	HM n (%)	Total n (%)	p
Mobility	No problems	15 (60.0)	12 (48.0)	*27 (54.0)*	*0.29*	16 (64.0)	*14 (58.3)*	30 (61.2)	0.46	17 (68.0)	16 (66.7)	33 (67.3)	0.58
	Some problems	10 (40.0)	13 (52.0)	*23 (46.0)*		9 (36.0)	*10 (41.7)*	19 (38.8)		8 (32.0)	8 (33.3)	16 (32.7)	
	Extreme problems	0 (0.0)	0 (0.0)	0 (0.0)		0 (.0)	0 (0.0)	0 (0.0)		0 (0.0)	0 (0)	0 (0.0)	
Self-care	No problems	22 (88.0)	22 (88.0)	*44 (88.0)*	*0.67*	23 (92.0)	*22 (91.7)*	45 (91.8)	0.68	21 (84.0)	23 (95.8)	44 (89.8)	0.19
	Some problems	22 (88.0)	22 (88.0)	*6 (12.0)*		2 (8.0)	*2 (8.3)*	4 (8.2)		4 (16.0)	1 (4.2)	5 (10.2)	
	Extreme problems	0 (0.0)	0 (0.0)	0 (0.0)		0 (0.0)	0 (0.0)	0 (0.0)		0 (0.0)	0 (0.0)	0 (0.0)	
Usual activities	No problems	16 (64.0)	14 (56.0)	*30 (60.0)*	*0.84*	13 (52.0)	*13 (54.2)*	26 (53.1)	0.55	18 (72.0)	12 (50.0)	30 (61.2)	0.22
	Some problems	8 (32.0)	10 (40.0)	18 (36.0)		12 (48.0)	*11 (45.8)*	23 (46.9)		7 (28.0)	11 (45.8)	18 (36.7)	
	Extreme problems	1 (4.0)	1 (4.0)	2 (4.0)		0 (0.0)	0 (0.0)	0 (0.0)		0 (0.0)	1 (4.2)	1 (2.0)	
Pain / discomfort	No problems	11 (44.0)	14 (56.0)	*25(50.0)*	*0.08*	13 (52.0)	*15 (62.5)*	28 (57.1)	0.71	13 (52.0)	12 (50.0)	25 (51.0)	0.87
	Some problems	14 (56.0)	8 (32.0)	*22 (44.0)*		10 (40.0)	*8 (33.3)*	18 (36.7)		9 (36.0)	10 (41.7)	19 (38.8)	
	Extreme problems	0 (0.0)	3 (12.0)	*3 (6.0)*		2 (8.0)	*1 (2.0)*	3 (6.1)		3 (12.0)	2 (8.3)	5 (10.2)	
Anxiety / depression	No problems	16 (64.0)	16 (64.0)	*32 (64.0)*	*0.62*	18 (72.0)	*19 (79.2)*	37 (75.5)	0.58	16 (64.0)	19 (79.2)	35 (71.4)	0.50
	Some problems	9 (36.0)	9 (36.0)	*18 (36.0)*		6 (24.0)	*5 (20.8)*	11 (22.4)		7 (28.0)	4 (16.7)	11 (22.4)	
	Extreme problems	0 (0.0)	0 (0.0)	0 (0.0)		1 (4.0)	*0 (0.0)*	1 (2.0)		2 (8.0)	1 (4.2)	3 (6.1)	
	TOTAL [95CI]	0.81 [0.74;0.87]	0.76 [0.64;0.88]	0.78 [0.72;0.85]	*0.47*	0.79 [0.70;0.88]	0.83 [0.74;0.92]	0.81 [0.75;0.87]	0.49	0.82 [0.69;0.93]	0.76 [0.65;0.87]	0.79 [0.71;0.86]	0.54
EQ-5D VAS													
	TOTAL [95CI]	64.00 [55.77;72.23]	64.88 [51.69;74.07]	64.83 [56.74;7C.14]	0.86	69.38 [60.82;76.38]	66.96 [59.17;74.75]	67.80 [62.49;73.10]	0.71	72.71 [65.58;79.83]	59.79 [49.44;70.14]	66.74 [60.46;73.01]	0.08

TM tele-monitoring group, *HM* hospital monitoring group; N (month 0) = 50 (TM group: 25; HM group: 25). N (month 1) =49 (TM group: 25; HM group: 24). N (month 6) =49 (TM group: 25; HM group: 24). Values are expressed as means [95CI: 95% confidence interval of means]. EQ5D: EuroQoL-5D; VAS: Visual Analog Scale

Table 3 Minnesota Living with Heart Failure Questionnaire (MLHFQ) scores at 6 months

	Month 0			Month 1			Month 6		
	TM *N* = 25	HM *N* = 25	p	TM *N* = 25	HM *N* = 24	p	TM *N* = 25	HM *N* = 24	p
Swelling in ankles, legs	0.84	1.00	0.72	0.50	0.58	0.88	0.25	0.42	0.57
Rest during the day	1.28	2.08	0.13	1.29	1.08	0.75	1.08	0.88	0.69
Walking and climbing stairs	0.96	1.92	0.09	0.96	0.54	0.41	0.63	0.63	0.96
Working around the house	1.20	2.36	0.03	0.96	1.25	0.61	0.50	1.13	0.18
Going away from home	0.28	1.44	0.01	0.92	0.21	0.06	0.79	0.83	0.92
Sleeping	0.84	1.32	0.27	0.71	0.71	0.94	0.58	0.50	0.83
Doing things with friends or family	0.88	1.96	0.04	1.04	0.71	0.42	1.04	0.83	0.68
Working to earn a living	0.40	0.72	0.23	0.50	0.08	0.14	0.00	0.04	0.32
Recreational pastimes	1.24	1.76	0.23	1.29	0.88	0.39	1.21	1.17	0.92
Sexual activities	0.32	0.68	0.31	0.25	0.42	0.52	0.71	0.67	0.96
Eat less of the food liked	0.60	1.00	0.21	0.71	0.42	0.36	0.50	0.17	0.34
Shortness of breath	2.44	2.48	0.99	1.46	1.04	0.32	1.29	1.50	0.60
Fatigue, tireness, low on energy	2.36	3.20	0.08	1.54	1.38	0.76	1.38	1.38	0.97
Stay in the hospital	1.48	1.76	0.58	1.00	1.38	0.55	0.58	0.38	0.60
Costing money for medical care	0.60	0.80	0.50	0.71	0.42	0.19	0.25	0.13	0.85
Side effects from medication	0.44	0.68	0.47	0.13	0.83	0.06	0.54	0.79	0.53
Feeling burdensome	0.32	0.76	0.19	0.46	0.08	0.12	0.21	0.21	0.71
Feeling a loss of self control	0.80	0.76	0.95	0.54	0.46	0.72	0.42	0.38	0.92
Worry	1.00	0.88	0.64	0.79	0.67	0.81	0.67	0.38	0.41
Difficulty remembering & concentrating	1.16	0.96	0.53	1.00	0.75	0.59	0.92	0.54	0.37
Feeling depressed	0.44	0.76	0.37	0.71	0.50	0.72	0.54	0.29	0.50
TOTAL [95CI]	20.20 [14.48–25.92]	28.96 [19.97–37.95]	0.07	18.64 [11.01–26.27]	14.38 [6.99–21.76]	0.59	15.80 [7.18–24.42]	13.21 [5.86–20.56]	0.97

TM: Tele-monitoring group; HM: Hospital monitoring group; N (month 0) = 50 (TM group: 25; HM group: 25). N (month 1) = 49 (TM group: 25; HM group: 24). N (month 6) = 49 (TM group: 25; HM group: 24). Items values are expressed as means. Total values are expressed as means [95CI: 95% confidence interval of means]

for both groups was similar and no significant differences were found.

Health-related quality of life

Several studies [10, 16–18, 30] have assessed HRQoL in users with pacemakers. In these clinical trials, the SF-36 [16, 17, 30] and EQ5D [10, 18] questionnaires were used to assess HRQoL. Results were improved but no significant differences between both groups in either the effectiveness or the safety of TM and HM were found.

Coinciding with previous trials [16, 17, 30] there was not found significant improvement in health-related quality of life for both groups between the enrolment and the last month of the study. In other more recent studies [17, 18], users with pacemaker implants included in both groups reported significant improvements in HRQoL assessed through the EQ-5D [10] and SF-36 [18]. On the other hand, in NORDLAND study the MLHF questionnaire score was improved in the studied groups (21.78% vs. 54.42%) and at 6 months there were statistically significant differences between the groups. These results were similar to those obtained in other studies in which HRQoL questionnaires for specific heart-diseases such as MLHFQ [30], AQUAREL [18], Duke Activity Status Index (DASI) [10] were improved. In all the studies, similar results have been found regardless their research design, either randomized or non-randomized.

Safety of tele-monitoring of pacemaker users

Previous studies [7, 10, 17, 30] showed a reduction in the percentage of in-office follow-up visits (31 to 58%). These results contrast with the obtained in the NORDLAND study where the visits to the hospital were 2% higher in TM group with respect to the other group (TM:1.24 vs. HM:1.17; $p = 0.26$). Additionally, in NORDLAND study, there were 98 transmissions scheduled for home patient (TM group) plus 10 extra ones (unscheduled transmissions).

Table 4 Follow-up information at 6 months

	Total N (%)	Tele-monitoring N (%)	Hospital Monitoring N (%)	*P*-value
Number of transmissions from consultation room				
0	0 (0.0)	0 (0.0)	0 (0.0)	0.26
1	41 (83.7)	21 (84.0)	20 (83.3)	
2	6 (12.2)	2 (8.0)	4 (16.7)	
3	2 (4.1)	2 (8.0)	0 (0.0)	
Transmissions from patients home				
0	29 (59.2)	5 (20.0)	24 (100)	< 0.001
3–5	15 (30.6)	15 (60.0)	0 (0.0)	
6–8	5 (10.2)	5 (20.0)	0 (0.0)	
Extra transmissions from patients home				
0	45 (91.8)	21 (84.0)	24 (100)	0.12
1	1 (2.0)	1 (4.0)	0 (0.0)	
3	3 (6.2)	3 (12.0)	0 (0.0)	
Cardiovascular adverse events				
None	46 (93.9)	23 (92.0)	23 (95.8)	0.40
PCI	1 (2.0)	1 (4.0)	0 (0.0)	
Angina	1 (2.0)	0 (0.0)	1 (4.2)	
Lead dislodgement ×2	1 (2.0)	1 (2.0)	0 (0.0)	
Changes of medication				
0	33 (67.3)	17 (68.0)	16 (66.7)	0.11
1	7 (14.3)	5 (20.0)	2 (8.3)	
2	3 (6.1)	1 (4.0)	2 (8.3)	
3	4 (8.2)	0 (0.0)	4 (16.7)	
4	2 (4.1)	2 (8.0)	0 (0.0)	
Changes of pacemakers reprogramming				
0	34 (69.4)	16 (64.0)	18 (75.0)	0.34
1	13 (26.5)	7 (28.0)	6 (25.0)	
2	2 (4.1)	2 (8.0)	0 (0.0)	
Hospitalizations days after implant				
0	30 (61.2)	14 (56.0)	16 (66.7)	0.55
1	14 (28.6)	7 (28.0)	7 (29.2)	
2	4 (8.2)	3 (12.0)	1 (4.2)	
5	1 (2.0)	1 (2.0)	0 (0.0)	
Days hospitalizated				
0	30 (61.2)	14 (56.0)	16 (66.7)	0.54
1–5	12 (24.5)	6 (24.0)	6 (25.1)	
6–10	4 (8.1)	2 (8.0)	2 (8.4)	
+ 10	3 (6.0)	3 (12.0)	0 (0.0)	
Reasons for hospitalization				
None	30 (61.2)	14 (56.0)	16 (66.7)	0.37
Others	6 (12.3)	3 (12.0)	3 (12.5)	
Cancer	1 (2.0)	1 (4.0)	0 (0.0)	
Coronary problems	9 (18.4)	4 (16.0)	5 (20.8)	
PM disfuction	3 (6.1)	3 (12.0)	0 (0.0)	

TM tele-monitoring group, *HM* hospital monitoring group, N (month 6) = 49 (TM group: 25; HM group: 24). Items values are expressed as N (%). *PCI* percutaneous coronary intervention, *PM* pacemakers

Table 5 Differences in Health-Related Quality of Life at 6 months of follow-up

	All				Tele-Monitoring				Hospital Monitoring			
	Month 0	Month 6	Differences	p	Month 0	Month 6	Differences	p	Month 0	Month 6	Differences	p
Health Related Quality of Life - Specific												
MLHFQ [95CI]	24.58 [19.30–29.86]	14.53 [9.04–20.02]	−9.65 [4.03;15.27]	< 0.001	20.20 [14.48–25.92]	15.80 [7.18–24.42]	−4.40 [−3.08;11.88]	0.04	28.96 [19.97–37.95]	13.21 [5.86–20.56]	−15.13 [6.73;23.52]	< 0.001
Health Related Quality of Life - General												
EQ5D VAS [95CI]	64.83 [56.74;70.14]	66.74 [60.46;73.01]	1.91 [−10.41;4.37]	0.42	64.00 [55.77;72.23]	72.71 [65.58;79.83]	8.71 [−16.79;0.54]	0.07	64.88 [51.69;74.07]	59.79 [49.44;70.14]	5.09 [−8.97;19.13]	0.46
EQ5D utilities [95CI]	0.78 [0.72;0.85]	0.79 [0.71;0.86]	0.01 [−0.08;0.12]	0.71	0.81 [0.74;0.87]	0.81 [0.69;0.93]	0.00 [−0.14;0.12]	0.92	0.76 [0.64;0.88]	0.76 [0.65;0.87]	0.00 [−0.07;0.13]	0.50

N (month 1) =49 (TM group: 25; HM group: 24). N (month 6) =49 (TM group: 25; HM group: 24). Values are expressed as means [95CI: 95% confidence interval of means]
EQ5D EuroQoL-5D, *VAS* visual analog scale, *MLHFQ* Minnesota Living with Heart Failure Questionnaire

The results on early detection of cardiovascular events and safety were similar to those obtained in previous studies [10, 16, 17, 31–35]. There were no found significant differences among the two groups with regards to cardiovascular events. The cumulative number of cardiovascular events was slightly higher in the TM (6%) than in the HM group (4.2%) although no statistically significant differences were found. This is relevant since it has been demonstrated that either a high burden of atrial fibrillation can be an important predictor of stroke and even mortality [5, 11, 13]. On the other hand, results found in previous studies showed that users included in TM group were more satisfied, the number of in-office visits to hospital was reduced, feeling safer, and being closely monitored by competent health care professionals with negligible impact of tasks to be fulfilled to comply with monitoring [5, 18, 36, 37] and although the number of studies on HRQoL and costs performed up to present on telemonitoring of pacemakers is quite reduced, preliminary studies suggest costs-saving [15]. A very reduced number of studies on effectiveness in pacemakers telemonitoring have used the HRQoL (EQ5D and SF-36) [10, 16, 17] questionnaires.

The added value of the NORDLAND study

To our knowledge, the NORDLAND study is the first randomized clinical trial (RCT) evaluating HRQoL in the tele-monitoring of users with pacemakers. The RCT is the most scientifically rigorous method of hypothesis testing available [38], and is regarded as the gold standard trial for evaluating the effectiveness of interventions [39]. Therefore, the NORDLAND study provides an important input for future systematic reviews and clinical decision-making with regards to the use of tele-monitoring of users with pacemakers. In addition, to our knowledge, the NORDLAND study is first using the Minnesota Living with Heart Failure Questionnaire, which offers an innovative approach in the field of internet-based health technologies assessments.

Strengths and limitations

Despite the relevant results obtained, the study has some limitations. First, it is a trial where patients and health staff knew the type of monitoring assigned, possibly this aspect may have influenced in their behavior. However, such influence has been decreased as much as possible since the NORDLAND study is a randomized trial. This ensures major evidence level, less chance of bias due to random selection of the groups and it might be repeatable and comparable with other studies. Second, the final size of patients included in this trial (with a limited number of pacemakers implants per year) made it difficult to detect differences between the two groups. The lack of a larger final sample size and the limited differences between groups may have reduced the real statistical power. However, the proximity between the results found in both groups in the analyses performed do not indicate significant differences. In addition, our study is a single centre study which may also be an advantage as different clinical practice among different hospitals sometimes makes it difficult to conduct multicenter studies.

Moreover, the comparison and generalization of results to other settings may be supported as participant characteristics were quite similar to those reported in previous studies [2–7, 10, 16, 17] in terms of age, gender, symptoms and indications.

Finally, it must be considered the phenomenon known as the Hawthorne effect [40, 41]. The fact that people tend to change their behavior when they are the targets of interest and attention, regardless of the specific nature of an intervention could be a limitation of our results. In such situations, patients become eager to please their physicians and make them feel successful. Additionally, patients wish to participate so that "good" results can be achieved in the study [40, 41].

Conclusions

To conclude, data obtained in the NORDLAND study show that health-related quality of life in patients with pacemakers is improved 6 months after implant in both groups. No significant differences between tele-monitoring and in-office follow-up groups were found with regards to effectiveness in terms of health-related quality of life, feasibility, reliability, safety and number of visits to hospital. Finally, this randomized clinical trial provides a scientifically rigorous method to the field of health-related quality of life evaluations in users with pacemakers.

Future research in this area should focus on interventions based on quality of life perceived by the patients and costs of multi-center studies involving a long-term follow-up of users with the telemonitoring of pacemakers and other types of cardiovascular implantable electronic devices.

Abbreviations

AE: Adverse events; AF: Atrial fibrillation; CRT: Cardiac resynchronization therapy; DDDR: Dual chamber pacemaker; EQ-5D: EuroQol-5D; HM: Hospital monitoring; HRQoL: Health-Related Quality of Life; ICD: Implantable cardioverter-defibrillator; *MLHFQ*: Minnesota Living with Heart Failure Questionnaire; PM: Pacemakers; RCT: Randomized clinical trial; TM: Tele-monitoring; VAS: Visual analogue scale; VVIR: Single chamber pacemaker

Funding

This Project, the NORDLAND study, has been funded by the European Economic Area, project reference number 008/ABELCM/2014A, under the research call "NILS Science and Sustainability Program", 2014 and by the General Secretariat for Research, Development and Innovation, Regional Government of Andalusia (Spain), project reference number PI/0256/2017, under the research call "Development and Innovation Projects in the Field of Biomedicine and Health Sciences", 2017.

Authors' contributions

ALV, DCM, KTL and RLL contributed to study conception and participated in critically appraising and revising the intellectual content of the manuscript. TE, HT and KTL participated in acquisition of data. ALV was responsible for the study analyses and the manuscript draft. All authors read and approved the final manuscript.

Competing interests

The authors declare that they have no competing interests.

Author details

[1]Social Involvement of Critical and Emergency Medicine, CTS-609 Research Group, Hospital de Poniente, Almeria, Spain. [2]Division of Medicine, Nordland Hospital, Bodø, Norway. [3]Institute of Clinical Medicine, Faculty of Health Sciences, University of Tromsø, Tromsø, Norway. [4]Department of Journalism and Communication, Universidad Carlos III de Madrid, Calle Madrid 133, 28903 Getafe, Madrid, Spain. [5]Health Sciences CTS-451 Research Group, University of Almeria, Almería, Spain. [6]Nursing Science, Physiotherapy and Medicine, Faculty of Health Sciences, University of Almeria, Almería, Spain.

References

1. Epstein AE, JP DM, Ellenbogen KA, et al. ACC/AHA/HRS 2008 Guidelines for Device-Based Therapy of Cardiac Rhythm Abnormalities: a report of the American College of Cardiology/American Heart Association Task Force on Practice Guidelines (Writing Committee to Revise the ACC/AHA/NASPE 2002 Guideline Update for Implantation of Cardiac Pacemakers and Antiarrhythmia Devices) developed in collaboration with the American Association for Thoracic Surgery and Society of Thoracic Surgeons. J Am Coll Cardiol. 2008;51(21):e1–62. https://doi.org/10.1016/j.jacc.2008.02.032.
2. Wilkoff BL, Auricchio A, Brugada J, et al. HRS/EHRA expert consensus on the monitoring of cardiovascular implantable electronic devices (CIEDs): description of techniques, indications, personnel, frequency and ethical considerations. Heart Rhythm. 2008;5(6):907–25.
3. Cronin E, Varma N. Remote monitoring of cardiovascular implanted electronic devices: a paradigm shift for the 21st century. Expert Rev Med Devices. 2012;9(4):367–76.
4. Folino AF, Breda R, Calzavara P, Migliore F, Iliceto S, Buja G. In-home controls of pacemakers in debilitated elderly patients. Geriatr Gerontol Int. 2012;12:30–5.
5. Folino A, Breda R, Calzavara P, et al. Remote follow-up of pacemakers in a selected population of debilitated elderly patients. Europace. 2013;15(3):382–7.
6. López-Villegas A, Catalán-Matamoros D, Robles-Musso E, Peiró S. Workload, time and costs of the informal cares in patients with tele-monitoring of pacemakers. The PONIENTE study. Clin Res Cardiol. 2016;105(4):307–13.
7. Perl S, Stiegler P, Rotman B, et al. Socio-economic effects and cost saving potential of remote patient monitoring (SAVE-HM trial). Int J Cardiol. 2013;169:402–7.
8. Varma N, Ricci RP. Telemedicine and cardiac implants: what is the benefit? Eur Heart J. 2013;34(25):1885–95.
9. Osca J, Sanchotello MJ, Navarro J, et al. Technical reliability and clinical safety of a remote monitoring system for antiarrhythmic cardiac devices. Rev Esp Cardiol. 2009;62(8):886–95.
10. López-Villegas A, Catalán-Matamoros D, Robles-Musso E, Peiró S. Comparative effectiveness of remote monitoring of people with cardiac pacemaker versus conventional: quality of life at the 6 months. Rev Esp Salud Pública. 2015;89:149–58.
11. Lopez-Villegas A, Catalan-Matamoros D, Robles-Musso E, Peiro S. Effectiveness of pacemaker tele-monitoring on quality of life, functional capacity, event detection and workload: the PONIENTE trial. Geriatr Gerontol Int. 2016;16(11):1188–95. https://doi.org/10.1111/ggi.12612.
12. Guédon-Moreau L, Lacroix D, Sadoul N, Clémenty J, Kouakam C, Hermida JS, et al. A randomized study of remote follow-up of implantable cardioverter defibrillators: safety and efficacy report of the ECOST trial. Eur Heart J. 2013;34(8):605–14.
13. Ricci RP, Morichelli L, Santini M. Home monitoring remote control of pacemaker and implantable cardioverter defibrillator patients in clinical practice: impact on medical management and health-care resource utilization. Europace. 2008;10:164–70.
14. Halimi F, Cantu F. Remote monitoring for active cardiovascular implantable electronic devices; a European survey. Europace. 2010;12(12):1778–80.
15. López-Villegas A, Catalán-Matamoros D, Martín-Saborido C, Villegas-Tripiana I, Robles-Musso E. A Systematic Review of Economic Evaluations of Pacemaker Telemonitoring Systems. Rev Esp Cardiol (Engl Ed). 2016;69(2):125–33. https://doi.org/10.1016/j.rec.2015.06.020 Review.
16. Halimi F, Clémenty J, Attuel P, Dessenne X, Amara W on behalf of the OEDIPE trial investigators. Optimized post-operative surveillance of permanent pacemakers by home monitoring: the OEDIPE trial. Europace. 2008;10:1392–9.
17. Mabo P, Victor F, Bazin P, et al. A randomized trial of long-term remote monitoring of pacemaker recipients (the COMPAS trial). Eur Heart J. 2012;33(9):1105–11.
18. Comoretto RI, Facchin D, Ghidina M, Proclemer A, Gregori D. Remote control improves quality of life in elderly pacemaker patients versus standard ambulatory-based follow-up. J Eval Clin Pract. 2017;23(4):681–9. https://doi.org/10.1111/jep.12691.
19. Knox L, Rahman RJ, Beedie C. Quality of life in patients receiving telemedicine enhanced chronic heart failure disease management: a meta-analysis. J Telemed Telecare. 2017;23(7):639–49. https://doi.org/10.1177/1357633X16660418.
20. United Nations Department of Economic and Social Affairs. Demographic Yearbook - 2016. https://unstats.un.org/unsd/demographic-social/products/dyb/dybsets/2016.pdf.
21. Pong RW, Pitbaldo RJ. Don't take "geography" for granted! Some methodological issues in measuring geographic distribution of physicians. Canadian J Rural Med. 2001;6:105.
22. DesMeules M, Pong R, Lagacé C, et al. How healthy are rural Canadians? An assessment of their health status and health determinants. Otawa: Canadian Institute for Health Information; 2006.
23. Ministry of Finance, Norway Government. Statistics Norway 2015. https://web.archive.org/web/20150924125714/http://www.ssb.no/en/befolkning/statistikker/folkemengde/aar/2015-02-19?fane=tabell&sort=nummer&tabell=218738
24. Telecardiology system BIOTRONIK. BIOTRONIK Home Monitoring. https://www.biotronik.com/en-de/products/home-monitoring.
25. EuroQol Group. EuroQol a new facility for the measurement of health-related quality of life. Health Policy. 1990;16:199–208.
26. Thomas S. FDA Medical Device Development Tool (MDDT) Qualification Package for the Minnesota Living with Heart Failure Questionnaire (MLHFQ). 2017. https://djhurij4nde4r.cloudfront.net/attachments/files/000/000/483/original/MLHFQ_FDA_Medical_Device_Development_Tool_(MDDT)_Qualification_Package.pdf?1516113948.
27. Hole T, Grundtvig M, Gullestad L, Flønæs B, Westheim A. Improved quality of life in Norwegian heart failure patients after follow-up in outpatient heart failure clinics: results from the Norwegian heart failure registry. Eur J Heart Fail. 2010;(11):1247–52. https://doi.org/10.1093/eurjhf/hfq156.
28. Kularatna S, Byrnes J, Chan YK, Carrington MJ, Stewart S, Scuffham PA. Comparison of contemporaneous responses for EQ-5D-3L and Minnesota living with heart failure; a case for disease specific multiattribute utility instrument in cardiovascular conditions. Int J Cardiol. 2017;227:172–6. https://doi.org/10.1016/j.ijcard.2016.11.030.
29. Austin J, Williams WR, Hutchison S. Patterns of fatigue in elderly heart failure patients measured by a quality of life scale (Minnesota living with heart failure). Eur J Cardiovasc Nurs. 2012;11(4):439–44. https://doi.org/10.1016/j.ejcnurse.2011.04.002.
30. Blum K, Gottlieb SS. The effect of a randomized trial of home telemonitoring on medical costs, 30-day readmissions, mortality, and health-related quality of life in a cohort of community-dwelling heart failure patients. J Card Fail. 2014;20(7):513–21. https://doi.org/10.1016/j.cardfail.2014.04.016.
31. Lazarus A. Remote, wireless, ambulatory monitoring of implantable pacemakers, cardioverter defibrillators, and cardiac resynchronization therapy systems: analysis of a worldwide database. Pacing Clin Electrophysiol. 2007;30:S2–12.
32. Neuzil P, Taborsky M, Holy F, Wallbrueck K. Early automatic remote detection of combined lead insulation defect and ICD damage. Europace. 2008;10:556–7.
33. Ricci RP, Morichelli L, Santini M. Remote control of implanted devices

through home monitoring technology improves detection and clinical management of atrial fibrillation. Europace. 2009;11:54–61.
34. Spencker S, Coban N, Koch L, Schirdewan A, Muller D. Potential role of home monitoring to reduce inappropriate shocks in implantable cardioverter defibrillator patients due to lead failure. Europace. 2009;11:483–8.
35. Ricci RP, Morichelli L, D'Onofrio A, et al. Effectiveness of remote monitoring of CIEDs in detection and treatment of clinical and device-related cardiovascular events in daily practice: the HomeGuide registry. Europace. 2013;15(7):970–7.
36. Schoenfeld MH, Compton SJ, Mead RH, et al. Remote monitoring of implantable cardioverter defibrillators: a prospective analysis. Pacing Clin Electrophysiol. 2004;27:757–63.
37. Joseph GK, Wilkoff BL, Dresing T, Burkhardt J, Khaykin Y. Remote interrogation and monitoring of implantable cardioverter defibrillators. J Interv Card Electrophysiol. 2004;11:161–6.
38. Last JM. A dictionary of epidemiology. New York: Oxford University Press; 2001.
39. Akobeng AK. Principles of evidence based medicine. Arch Dis Child. 2005; 90:837–40. https://doi.org/10.1136/adc.2005.071761.
40. Meneguin S, Machado César LA. Motivation and frustration in cardiology trial participation: the patient perspective. Clinics. 2012;67(6):603–7.
41. Fletcher RH, Fletcher SW. Epidemiologia clinica: elementos essenciais. Artmed. 2006;8:154–78.

14

Nordic walking training and nutritional supplementation in pre-frail older Indians: an open-labelled experimental pre-test and post-test pilot study to develop intervention model

Prasun Chatterjee[1], Prakash Kumar[1], Ramesh Kandel[2], Ruchika Madan[1], Meenakshi Tyagi[1], Deepa Anil Kumar[3], Maroof Ahmad Khan[4], Gaurav Desai[1], Preeti Chaudhary[1], Shyama Gupta[5], Kanika Grover[6] and Aparajit Ballav Dey[1*]

Abstract

Background: Identifying and treating people in a pre-frail state may be an effective way to prevent or delay frailty and preserve their functional capacity. This study aimed to assess the efficacy of, and compliance with, a 12 week individualized nutritional supplementation (INS) and Nordic walking (NW) program in pre-frail older Indians. The primary measure is physical performance, as indicated by Fried's Frailty scale. Other measures include: cognition, as indicated by the Hindi Mental Status Examination; mood, by the Geriatric Depression Scale; and nutritional status, by the Mini Nutritional Assessment.

Methods: This is an open-labeled experimental pre-test and post-test study, which took place from October 2012 to December 2014. The study was approved by Institute Ethics committee (IEC/NP-350/2012/RP-26/2012) at the All India Institute of Medical Sciences (AIIMS), New Delhi. Participants were sixty-six pre-frail elderly, who were randomly allocated into three subgroups, namely: A (NW only), B (INS only), and C (NW and INS). One-way ANOVA was used to statistically assess differences in baseline characteristics for quantitative variables, with the Chi-Square/Fischer exact test utilized for qualitative variables. Paired t-tests were used to assess pre and post intervention difference within the group for quantitative variables, with McNemar's Chi-Square test used for qualitative variables. Kruskal Wallis test was used to assess significant intervention effects among the groups. A p-value < 0.05 was considered as statistically significant.

Results: There was significant effect of intervention in gait speed in group A ($p = 0.001$) and C ($p = 0.002$), but not in group B ($p = 0.926$). While there was no significant change in grip strength in Group A ($p = 0.488$) and B ($p = 0.852$), a statistically significant increase was observed in group C ($p = 0.013$). Mood significantly improved in group B ($p = 0.025$) and C ($p = 0.021$). No significant difference was noted in cognitive status across groups. Following the interventions, a total of 18.18% of pre-frail participants were classified as non-frail.

Conclusions: Combining NW and INS provides a simple, pragmatic intervention with efficacy in the management of functionally vulnerable older adults, and allows their maintained independence. Future studies should replicate this readily applicable intervention in a larger cohort with a longer follow-up period.

(Continued on next page)

* Correspondence: abdey@hotmail.com
[1]Department of Geriatric Medicine, All India Institute of Medical Sciences, New Delhi, India
Full list of author information is available at the end of the article

(Continued from previous page)

Keywords: Frailty, Adapted indoor Nordic walk, Individualized nutritional supplementation

Background

Frailty syndrome is arguably the greatest challenge faced by an aging population. It also has obvious significance for clinicians, scientists and policy planners [1]. Frailty syndrome is a state of increased vulnerability due to poor resolution of homeostasis after a stressor event, thereby increasing the risk of adverse outcomes including falls, delirium and disability [2]. The paradigm of precision medicine may be readily applied to the concept of frailty, allowing its better management within main stream modern medicine [3]. The prevalence of frailty is variable across studies, due to differences in defining criteria and study samples. In community dwelling western population over the age of 65 years, a systematic review indicates an overall frailty prevalence of 10.7%, which increases with age, being evident in 15.7% in 80 to 84 year olds and 26% in those over 85 years of age [3].

'Fitness' and 'frailty' may be seen as forming the poles of a continuum [4], with the former indicating complete independence, and the latter indicating complete dependence. Age-associated progression along this continuum often results in stages from healthy, to a semi-robust, subclinical frailty, to a pre-frail and eventual frail state [5]. Frail populations have a substantially increased risk of falls, disability, and the need of institutional care as well as of mortality [6]. Systematic reviews indicate that the pre-frail state, an intermediate stage between non-frail and frail, to have a 41.6% prevalence in community samples, compared to the 10.7% prevalence of a frail state [7]. One study of an Indian tertiary care hospital shows a 21% frailty prevalence and a 20% pre-frailty prevalence, using Fried's phenotypic criteria [8].

Pre-frail individuals have more than twice the risk of becoming frail compared to non-frail people [9]. Identifying and treating people in the pre-frail state is an opportunity to prevent or effectively delay frailty. Further, evidence suggests that older adults in a pre-frail, compared to a frail, state respond better to more intensive interventions [10].

Frailty has a multi-faceted pathogenesis and pathophysiology, with sarcopenia proposed to play an important role [8, 11]. Sarcopenia is a syndrome that is characterized by the progressive and generalized loss of skeletal muscle mass and strength, thereby increasing the risk of many adverse outcomes, including physical disability and poor quality of life, as well as and mortality [12]. Consequently, interventions focused on improving muscle strength should have utility. However, improving muscle strength can be challenging, given its dependence on multiple factors, such as nutritional status [13], and the functional capacity of the individual [14]. Numerous multi-factorial interventions consisting of nutritional supplementation and various forms of exercise have been studied in the frail elderly, with variable results [15–17]. Unfortunately, the compliance to regular exercise in frail older adults is low, due to intrinsic weakness, lack of inertia and the perceived risks of exercise [18]. Resistance training and/or diet seem the only effective interventions to treat or prevent sarcopenia in frail or pre-frail individuals [13].

Walking is a rhythmic, dynamic, and aerobic activity with numerous benefits for the musculoskeletal system and almost no negative effects [19]. Nordic walking (NW) is a form of walking that uses muscles of the upper and lower body in a continuous and reciprocal movement [20] (Fig. 1). Due to the higher muscle mass involved, NW produces a higher cardio-respiratory workload, whilst improving endurance and flexibility as well as benefitting body balance functioning [21]. It is a whole-body aerobic or alternating aerobic/anaerobic discipline, rarely associated with physical injury and easily practiced by people of all ages, including older adults [15, 22–24]. A systematic review and meta-analysis by Bullo et al. summarizes the effectiveness of NW interventions on the physical fitness and quality of life in the elderly [25].

Inadequate dietary intake, especially of proteins and amino acids contributes to the development of sarcopenia and frailty [26–29], with a noticeable improvement in muscle strength occuring after protein and micro-nutrients supplementation [26]. Nutritional supplementation (protein and amino acid) in combination with physical training could further improve the functional status in frail populations. However, such work has focused on the combination of nutritional supplementation plus exercise for all study participants. It is important to clarify the relative contributions of exercise and diet. We hypothesized that, without pain and discomfort, an older person performing NW with individualized nutritional supplementation for 12 weeks would show a 20% greater improvement, versus either NW or INS alone. The current investigation is a pilot initiative study evaluating the efficacy of NW in functionally vulnerable older Indians, with or without INS, as well as in comparison to INS alone.

Methods

This is an open-labeled experimental pre-post study from October 2012 to December 2014. The study was

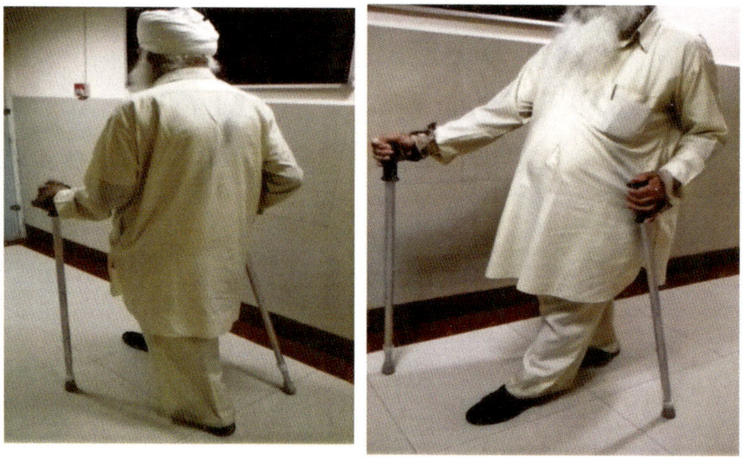

Fig. 1 Adapted indoor Nordic Walk training

conducted with the approval of the Institute Ethics committee of All India Institute of Medical Sciences (AIIMS), New Delhi (Ref. No: IEC/NP-350/2012/RP-26/2012).

Participants: Individuals aged 60 years and above were recruited from the out-patient department of Geriatrics Medicine, AIIMS. Study inclusion criteria were: Pre-frail, as assessed by a Fried's phenotypic scale [30] score of 1 or 2. Exlusion criteria: Any form of resistive training exercise or nutritional supplementation in the previous 6 months; having an acute illness, severe obstructive airway disease (Forced ExpiratoryVolume< 30%); severe systolic dysfunction (Ejection Fraction < 30% by Echocardiogram); severe depression (Geriatric Depression Scale > 11); severe, painful lower limb muscle condition; and severe cognitive impairment (Mini-Cog =0).

As per the out-patient department posting schedule of the first author (PC) and the principal investigator (ABD), three patients were randomly selected after obtaining consent to carry out frailty assessment. This was done three times a week for 18 months, giving a total of 648 patients. Of these 648 patients, 129 were found to be pre-frail as per Fried's criteria. However, 63 patients declined to participate in the study, due to a variety of reasons, including transport, mobility issues and the lack of care giver support. Consequently, the 66 patients who gave informed written consent were recruited into the study.

A standard randomization procedure for intervention allocation was generated using the n-query 2.0 software and allocation of the participants in three groups was done by sequentially numbered opaque sealed envelope. Sixty-six participants were therefore randomly allocated into three groups of twenty-two: Group A: NW; Group B: INS; and Group C: NW + INS (Fig. 2).

Demographic details including age, gender, education and income were obtained. A detailed assessment on nutritional status and physical performance was carried out by a qualified nutritionist (Masters degree in Food and Nutrition with two-years research experience in Geriatric Medicine) and an occupational therapist (Bachelors degree in Occupational Therapy with two years of clinical research experience in geriatric medicine), which provided baseline scores on these parameters.

Nutritional assessment was carried out by anthropometric measures, including weight, height, body mass index (BMI), and mid upper arm circumference (MUAC). A MUAC < 23.5 cm in males and < 22 cm in females was indicative of malnutrition. The nutritional status of the participants was assessed by Mini Nutritional Assessment (MNA®, Nestle Nutrition Institute) [31], an 18-point questionnaire with a maximum score of 24. Participants scoring < 17, 17–23.5 and 24–30 were labelled as 'Malnourished', 'At risk of malnutrition' and with 'Normal nutritional status' respectively.

To determine the concentration of serum albumin 5 ml blood was drawn from each study participant at baseline and after intervention. Serum was separated and albumin concentration was determined using standard protocols. Various functional assessments were performed. The assessment of the physical domain utilized the Modified Physical Performance Test (MPPT) and Berg Balance Scale (BBS). MPPT consists of nine components each with a minimum score of zero and maximum of 4 (total:36) [32]. Participants scoring between 0 and 16, 17–24, 25–31 and 32–36 are classified as severe, moderate, mild and non-frail, respectively. The BBS measure of balance consists of a 14-item scale designed to measure balance of the older adult in a clinical setting out of a total score of 56. Based on the scoring between 0 and 20, 21–40 and 41–56, participants were categorized into 'low risk', 'medium risk' and 'high risk' group respectively [33]. The assessment of daily living

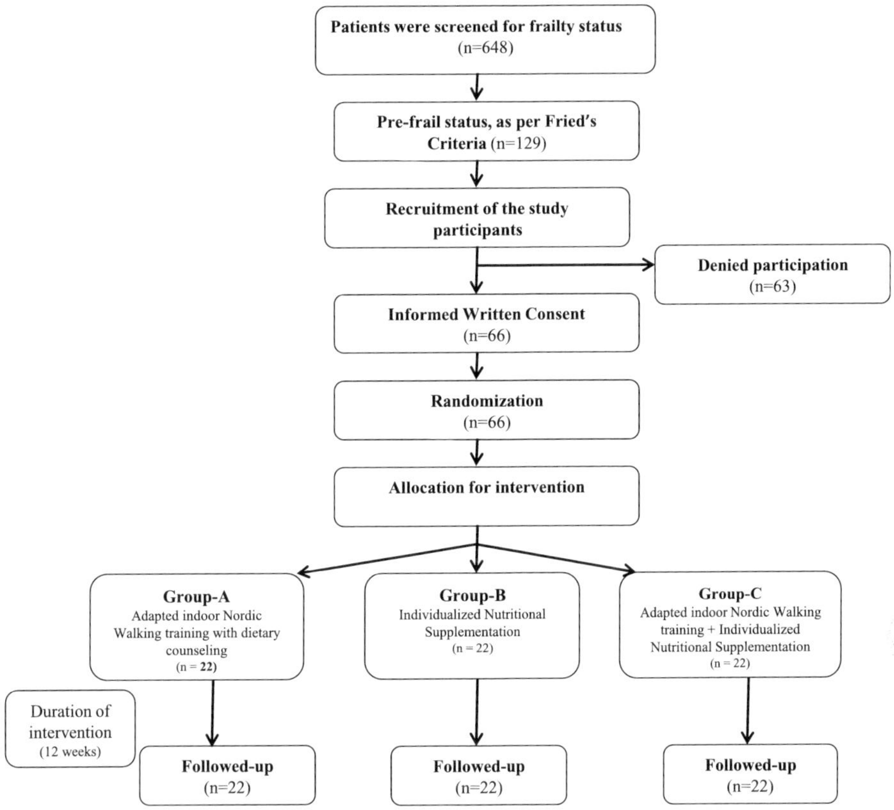

Fig. 2 Flowchart showing the sequence of the study design

functioning utilized the 'Barthel activity of daily living (BADL)' and 'Lawton and Brody instrumental activity of daily living (IADL).' The BADL is an ordinal scale with 10 components, scored either 0 or 1, giving a total scale range of 0–20 [34]. The IADL consists of eight components, scored either 0 or 1, giving a total scale range of 0–8 [35]. Mood was assessed by 15-item short form of the geriatric depression scale (GDS), with a score over 5 denoting depression [36]. The cognitive domain was assessed by the 'Hindi Mental Status Examination (HMSE)' scale. The HMSE is a 23-item questionnaire with a maximum score of 30. Patients scoring less than 24 are regarded as cognitively impaired [37].

Frailty Assessment: Frailty was assessed by Fried's phenotypical criteria [30], whereby one point is scored for each criterion met to specification. The components were: a) slow walking speed -walking 0.6 m/sec with or without a walking aid. b) Weakness (grip strength) was measured using hand dynamometer (in kg), taking the best of three attempts, with a grip strength of less than 6 kg in females and less than 15 kg in males as positive indicant of frailty. These cut-offs are also the 25th percentile of age matched control, which were taken as cut off value in previous published data from AIIMS [38]. c) An unintentional loss of weight greater than 5% of body weight or 10 lb. in the last one year was taken as positive indicant of frailty. d) Self Reported Exhaustion in the previous week, as indicated by response to being asked how often they felt that "everything they did was an effort" and "whether they could get going?". Answer indicating this to be for3–4 days in the past week were taken as positive indicants of frailty. e) Low Physical Activity (over the past three months), with positive indicants of frailty being "not performing minimum weight-bearing physical activity" or "spending more than 6 hours per day sitting or lying other than sleep time." Individuals with 3 or more of these characteristics were considered as frail, with those having 1 or 2 of these scale characteristics regarded as pre-frail.

Adapted indoor Nordic walking training

The participants were trained for 12 weeks (36 training sessions each of 60 min duration), with a frequency of three times a week. Training sessions were individualized and provided by a qualified physiotherapist having Masters in Physiotherapy, with specialization in Orthopaedics, and using the NW technique according to the guidelines of the International Nordic Walking Federation (INWA)

[39]. Each training session began with a short warm-up (5–10 min) which consisted of flexibility exercise for upper and lower extremities and spine. Training ended with stretching and breathing exercises (3–5 min). The pole length was adopted according to the participant's physique, permitting a smooth arm motion and based on the INWA formula (0.7 X height cm). NW took place in a departmental corridor. Two walking poles were used to push against the ground with each stride, actively engaging the trunk and upper limbs during walking and maintaining natural gait, whilst the hands performed an open-close cycle in an alternating manner [15] (Fig. 1). Therapist walked side by side with the participant, providing encouragement throughout the walking sessions. During this training period, participants did not engage in any other physiotherapy and occupational therapy programs. Assessment of post-intervention dependent variables was done within 1 week of the final NW session.

Nutritional Intervention: Considering the high prevalence of malnutrition in India [40] the present study carried out assessment for both calorie and protein deficiency, with supplementation given as required. Calorie and protein requirement of each participant were assessed by a nutritionist. The participants from group A were counselled at baseline about their deficiency and were asked to improve their nutritional status by improving their diet. Participants belonging to group B and C were supplemented with the deficit quantity of nutrients, as per individual need, for 12 weeks. Carbohydrates were supplemented at the rate of ≈50% of total daily calorie requirement and protein was supplemented at the rate of 1.2 g/kg body weight. The objective of the supplementation was to provide an additional 100 Kcal with 8-10 g protein per day. Participants or their care-providers were called on weekly basis to provide nutritional supplementation powder. This gave the research team an indication of participant compliance towards nutrient supplementation, as well as any issues or complications that emerged. Participants were also instructed to return with the empty container after completion of the intervention.

Statistical analysis

Qualitative variables of participant characteristics were reported as numbers or percentages, whilst quantitative data were reported as the mean ± standard deviation (SD). Normality assumption among the groups was tested using the Kolmogorov-Smirnov Test. If normality was established, one-way ANOVA was carried out to see the association among the groups for quantitative variables and Chi-Square/Fischer Exact Test for qualitative variables. Paired t-tests were used to find the pre and post intervention differences within the group for quantitative data and McNemar's Chi-Square Test for qualitative data. Kruskal Wallis Test was used to find the actual change effect among the groups. A p-value < 0.05 was considered as statistically significant.

Results

The ages of participants (mean ± SD) in groups A, B, C were 75.77 ± 6.25, 76.88 ± 5.89 and 77.41 ± 3.78 years, respectively (p = 0.607). Table. 1 shows both quantitative and qualitative data at baseline. Similar baseline demographics were noted in each group and there were no statistically significant differences in age, gait speed, grip strength, BADL, IADL, serum albumin concentration and qualitative parameters such as GDS, HMSE, MNA, MPPT, BBS and frailty score.

Participants' gait speed (mean ± SD) in groups A, B and C were 0.66 ± 0.11, 0.67 ± 0.10 and 0.67 ± 0.11 respectively. There was significant effect of intervention on gait speed in group A (p = 0.001) and C (p = 0.002), but not in group B (p = 0.926). Grip strength (mean ± SD) in groups A, B and C were 8.91 ± 2.11 kg, 9.09 ± 2.20 kg and 8.45 ± 2.32 kg, respectively. No significant change was seen in grip strength in group A (p = 0.488) and B (p = 0.852), but a statistically significant increase was observed in group C (p = 0.013). Intervention resulted in statistically significant increase in BADL and IADL scores for all three groups. While a significant effect on MPPT score was observed only in group C (p = 0.020), whilst a significant effect of intervention on the balance measure, BBS, occurred in group A (p = 0.046) and C (p = 0.024), but not in group B (p = 0.270) (Table 2).

There was statistically significant decrease in the serum albumin concentration in group A (p < 0.001), whilst groups B (p < 0.001) and C group (p < 0.001) showed significant increases. A statistically significant (p < 0.001) improvement in the nutritional status, as assessed by MNA, was also evident.

The effect of interventions on depression, as indicated by GDS score, showed significant improvement in groups B (p = 0.025) and C (p = 0.021). There was no significant impact on cognition across interventions.

Among the study groups, a significant difference was observed in gait speed between groups A and B (p = 0.003), B and C (p = 0.012) but the difference was not significant between A and C (p = 0.944). The difference in albumin concentration was significant among groups A and B (p<0.001) and groups A and C (p<0.001), but not significant among groups B and C (p = 0.603). A significant difference in BADL score was observed between group A and C (p<0.001), and groups B and C (p<0.001), but not between groups A and B (p = 0.677) (Table 3).

As shown in the Fig. 3, two participants (9.09%) in group A became non-frail, one became frail (4.55%) and the rest (86.36%) remained as prefrail. For group B these figure were 4 (18.18%), 2 (9.09%) and 16 (72.73%). In

Table 1 Baseline characteristics of the study participants

Variables	Group A ($n = 22$)	Group B ($n = 22$)	Group C ($n = 22$)	*p*- value
Sex				
Male	13	11	18	0.078
Female	9	11	4	
Age ± SD (years)	75.7 ± 6.24	76.68 ± 5.8	77.4 ± 3.78	0.607
Gait speed ± SD (metre/sec)	0.66 ± 0.1	0.67 ± 0.1	0.67 ± 0.1	0.970
Grip strength ± SD (Kg)	8.90 ± 2.1	9.09 ± 2.2	8.45 ± 2.32	0.620
BADL	3.95 ± 1.46	3.36 ± 0.90	3.77 ± 1.15	0.251
IADL	1.40 ± 0.50	1.36 ± 0.58	1.59 ± 1.00	0.555
Serum albumin (g/dl)	4.24 ± 0.48	3.97 ± 0.47	4.07 ± 0.55	0.207
GDS				
< 5	10	11	6	0.268
≥ 5	12	11	16	
HMSE				
< 24	10	9	9	0.940
≥ 24	12	13	13	
MNA				
Malnourished	9	9	12	0.518
At the risk	9	12	8	
Normal	4	1	2	
MPPT				
Severe	11	11	13	0.538
Moderate	6	9	7	
Mild	3	0	0	
Non-frail	2	2	2	
BBS				
Low - risk	5	5	5	1.000
Medium- risk	15	16	15	
High - risk	2	1	2	
Pre- frail status	22	22	22	0.676

Analysed by One-way ANOVA and Chi-square test

group C, 6 (27.27%) became non-frail whilst 16 (72.73%) remained pre-frail.

Compliance with the protocol and adverse events

All of the randomized participants completed the trial. The values for median compliance within all three groups were also 100%. Diarrhea occurred in three participants receiving the nutritional supplement but they stopped the supplement for a week, and then restarted. No cardiovascular complications occurred during any testing or training sessions.

Discussion

NW is a promising and practicable intervention for the maintenance of functionality in late life. In the present study, gait speed significantly improved with NW alone and in combination with INS. However, lone nutritional supplementation without NW did not show any impact on the gait speed of pre-frail adults. Our finding support previous report by Figueiredo et al., who observed an improvement in gait speed in older individuals following NW practice, versus an over-ground walking comparison group [20]. The combination of NW and INS also improved grip strength, although this effect was not evident for either alone. An earlier study reported a significant change in the grip strength of elderly women who practiced NW for the same duration as the present study [41]. This difference across studies may arise from variations in the levels of baseline malnutrition, 45.45% being malnourished and 43.94% at risk of malnourishment in the current study. Further, it might require a longer duration for lone nutritional supplementation to show any impact on muscle strength under variations in levels of malnourishment. The combined intervention seems to have an additive or synergistic effect in improving the strength of hand muscles.

All three groups showed improvements in functionality, indicating the utility of diet and NW on this parameter. Such data also highlights the importance of readily-modifiable nutritional deficiency in functional decline. Improvement of functional status is a primary goal for vulnerable older adults [42]. A study conducted by Persson et al. on the effects of combined nutritional treatments, in patients at risk of protein-energy malnutrition, also showed improved functionality as compared to controls [43].

NW + INS and INS alone significantly improved participants' mood. Many forms of exercise can improve mood, with some of the efficacy of exercise mediated via a lowering of the immune-inflammatory cascade that is evident in depression, as well as in pre-frail and frail older adults [44]. Previous work indicates the positive effect of NW on mood [44, 45]. However, the present study showed no mood improvement in the NW alone group. This again may arise from variations in study populations, with diet being more relevant to mood improvement in the current study. Previous studies have indicated that diet could regulate mood due to increased availability of key compounds, such as tryptophan, which is a necessary precursor or serotonin synthesis, thereby linking to the long-standing effects of serotonin in mood regulation [46]. In addition, small sample size and unmeasured factors/confounders may have contributed to the differences across studies. It is also of note, that due to the bidirectional association between depression and frailty [47], mood improvement may have a direct

Table 2 Effect of intervention on different variables within groups

Variables	Categories	Group A			Group B			Group C		
		Pre	Post	*p*-value	Pre	Post	*p*-value	Pre	Post	*p*-value
Gait Speed		0.66 ± 0.11	0.99 ± 0.41	0.001	0.67 ± 0.11	0.66 ± 0.10	0.926	0.67 ± 0.10	1.00 ± 0.45	0.002
Grip Strength		8.9 ± 2.1	8.27 ± 3.9	0.488	9.09 ± 2.2	9.22 ± 2.5	0.852	8.45 ± 2.3	9.86 ± 2.8	0.013
BADL		3.95 ± 1.46	5.27 ± 1.20	<0.001	3.36 ± 0.90	4.81 ± 0.90	<0.001	3.77 ± 1.15	6.40 ± 0.95	<0.001
IADL		1.40 ± 0.50	2.59 ± 1.00	<0.001	1.36 ± 0.58	2.22 ± 0.81	<0.001	1.59 ± 1.00	3.31 ± 1.21	<0.001
Serum Albumin		4.24 ± 0.48	3.93 ± 0.48	< 0.001	3.97 ± 0.47	4.26 ± 0.5	<0.001	4.07 ± 0.5	4.40 ± 0.49	<0.001
MNA	Malnourished	9	12	0.050	9	1	0.005	12	0	0.003
	At the risk	9	9		12	20		8	17	
	Normal	4	1		1	1		2	5	
MPPT	Severe	11	6		11	8		13	2	
	Moderate	6	11	0.226	9	12	0.072	7	4	0.020
	Mild	3	4		0	2		0	12	
	Non-frail	2	1		2	0		2	4	
BBS	Low-risk	5	3		5	4		5	3	
	Medium-risk	15	10	0.046	16	14	0.270	15	10	0.024
	High-risk	2	9		1	4		2	9	
Frailty	Non-frail	0	2		0	4		0	6	
	Pre-frail	22	19	0.035	22	16	0.01	22	16	0.001
	Frail	0	1		0	2		0	0	
GDS	<5	10	9	0.739	11	16	0.025	6	14	0.021
	≥5	12	13		11	6		16	8	
HMSE	<24	12	13	0.564	13	12	0.564	13	10	0.083
	≥24	10	9		9	10		9	12	

Paired t-test and Mc Nemar's Chi-Square test was performed to see the effect within the groups

impact on the functionality of an individual and vice versa, possibly via immune-inflammatory regulation, including as arising from alterations in the microbiome and associated intestinal permeability. Many dietary factors can also act to regulate cognition, including more directly via brain neurotransmitter pathways, synaptic transmission, membrane fluidity and signal-transduction pathways [48], whilst diet and exercise may interact at the molecular level to influence cognitive abilities [48]. However, neither solitary nor multimodal interventions in the present study had any impact on cognitive status. This may have arisen due to the relatively short duration of the current pilot study, given that increased physical activity for at least 6 months may be necessary to improve cognition in older adults [49]. The current results also highlight the role of these simple interventions in the improvement of overall physical performance, as indicated by better frailty score in 18.18% of total study participants. However, intervention for a short duration might not show any significant impact on parameters

Table 3 Intervention effects across groups

Variables	Group A	GROUP B	GROUP C	*p*-value			
	Median (Min, Max)			A Vs B Vs C	A Vs B	A Vs C	B Vs C
Grip strength (Kg)	- 1.5 (−6, 7)	0.5 (−8, 5)	1 (−2, 7)	0.10	–	–	–
BADL	1.5 (0, 2)	1.5 (0, 3)	3 (1,3)	0.001	0.677	<0.001	<0.001
Serum albumin (g/dl)	−0.3 (− 1.1, 0.09)	0.25 (0, 0.7)	0.3 (−0.29, 0.8)	< 0.001	<0.001	<0.001	0.603
Gait speed (m/s)	0.33 (−0.33, 1.71)	0 (−0.2, 0.4)	0.21 (−0.3, 1.2)	0.007	0.003	0.944	0.012
IADL	0 (0, 2)	1 (0, 2)	3.72 (0, 4)	0.013	0.258	0.055	0.005

$p < 0.016$ was considered to be significant for multiple comparison (Kruskal-Wallis test followed by Wilcoxon Rankson test)

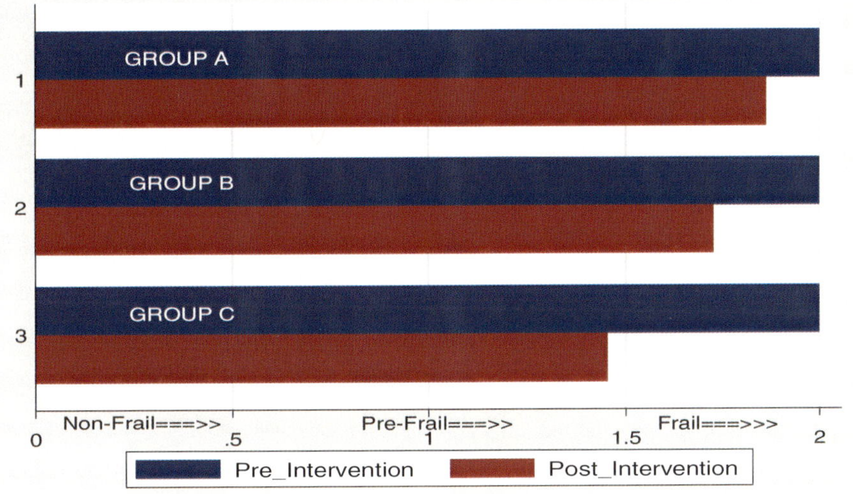

Fig. 3 Frailty status on Pre and Post intervention

such as weight loss, self reported physical exertions and physical performance (Fig. 4).

A recently published review of 17 studies of older adults (> 65 years) showed enhanced benefits of exercise training when combined with dietary supplementation [50]. This review also included studies of nutrition and exercise interventions aiming to impact on mass and/or muscle strength as indicants of improved physical performance [50].A study conducted by Rydwik et al. similarly showed a positive effect on lower-extremity muscle strength after a multi modal intervention [51]. The data of the present and previous studies are promising and of significant clinical importance, including as indicated by the comfort and high compliance with which older Indians practiced NW, coupled to no adverse events. Importantly, NW is regarded as a safe form of physical activity that helps in maintaining the body's centre of gravity, thereby decreasing the risk of falls [52]. Further, NW can be performed by individuals who have relatively low levels of endurance and requires no added supervision. It is clear that this pilot study requires replication in a larger cohort and for a longer duration.

This is the first study to have focused on a simple, yet effective intervention model in pre-frail older adults from India. With proper health awareness among various society stakeholders, NW and INS can be incorporated as a healthy life style, thereby promoting active and healthy aging in late life.

Limitation of the study

A major limitation of this study was that there was no non-treatment or control group. Further, this is a pilot study that clearly requires investigation in a larger cohort for a longer duration. Given the small sample size and the diversity of geriatric populations, the findings cannot be generalized.

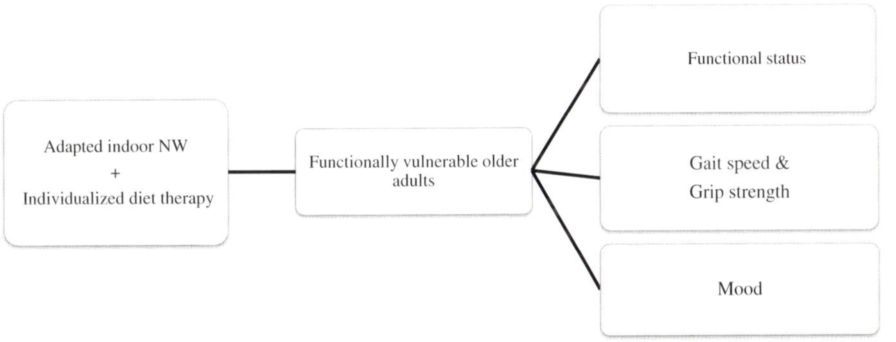

Fig. 4 Changes in various domains after multimodal intervention

Conclusions

NW and INS were a simple pragmatic interventions to better optimize the benefits of exercise and nutrition on the functionally of vulnerable, pre-frail, older adults, allowing their greater independence. Although indications of some benefits are shown from NW and INS alone, there combination seems more effective in preventing the shift from a pre-frail to frail state. The current data need to be replicated and extended in a larger cohort with a longer follow-up period.

Abbreviations

AIIMS: All India Institute of Medical Sciences; BADL: Barthel activity of daily living; BBS: Berg balance scale; BMI: Body mass index; GDS: Geriatric depression scale; HMSE: Hindi mental status examination; IADL: Instrumental activity of daily living; IEC: Institutional ethical committee; INS: Individualized nutritional supplementation; INWA: International Nordic walking federation; MNA: Mini nutritional assessment; MPPT: Modified physical performance test; MUAC: Mid upper arm circumference; NW: Nordic walking; SD: Standard deviation

Acknowledgements

The research group acknowledges, with thanks, the supports rendered by all faculties and staff of the Department of Geriatric Medicine and most importantly the study participants and care provider who proactively brought their seniors to the hospital for the intervention. The study was financially supported by the funds from National Programme for Health Care of the Elderly (NPHCE), Government of India.

Funding

National Programme for Health Care of the Elderly (NPHCE) was launched by Ministry of Health and Family Welfare, Government of India to fund Regional Geriatric Centres to carry out research. Department of Geriatric Medicine, AIIMS, New Delhi is one such centre recognized by the Government of India. The funding body did not have any role in the design of the study nor in the collection, analysis, interpretation of the data and in the writing the manuscript.

Authors' contributions

First author PC1 conceived and designed the entire study and was also involved in the conceptualization and preparation of the first draft of the manuscript. PK conceived, designed, initiated the concept of Nordic walking and reviewed and modified the manuscript. RK, RM and MT were involved in data collection. DAK assisted the first author in writing the manuscript. GD and PC2 were involved in the revision of the manuscript. MAK, KG and SG performed the statistical analysis and wrote the results. Corresponding author ABD was involved in conceptualization of the concept along with the first author and guided in writing the entire manuscript. All authors read and approved the final version of the manuscript.

Competing interest

The authors declare that they have no competing interests.

Author details

[1]Department of Geriatric Medicine, All India Institute of Medical Sciences, New Delhi, India. [2]Division of Geriatric Medicine, Patan Academy of Health Sciences, Patan, Nepal. [3]Healthy Aging India, New Delhi, India. [4]Department of Biostatistics, All India Institute of Medical Sciences, New Delhi, India. [5]Corner Office Advisors, New Delhi, India. [6]University of Manitoba, Winnipeg, Canada.

References

1. Frailty is the most problematic expression of population ageing". British Geriatrics Society. 2018. Available at: https://britishgeriatricssociety.wordpress.com/2017/04/21/frailty-is-the-most-problematic-expression-of-population-ageing/. Accessed 5 April 2018.
2. Clegg A, Young J, Iliffe S, Rikkert M, Rockwood K. Frailty in elderly people. Lancet. 2013;381(9868):752–62. https://doi.org/10.1016/s0140-6736(12)62167-9.
3. Halter J B, Ouslander JG, Studenski S, High K P, Asthana S, Supiano M A, Ritchie C. Hazzard's Geriatric Medicine and Gerontology. Seventh edition. New York, N.Y. : McGraw-Hill Education LLC., 2017.
4. Romero-Ortuno R, O'Shea D. Fitness and frailty: opposite ends of a challenging continuum! Will the end of age discrimination make frailty assessments an imperative? Age Ageing. 2013;42(3):279–80. https://doi.org/10.1093/ageing/afs189.
5. Sergi G, Veronese N, Fontana L, De Rui M, Bolzetta F, Zambon S. Pre-frailty and risk of cardio vascular disease in elderly men and women. J Am Coll Cardiol. 2015;65(10):976–83. https://doi.org/10.1016/j.jacc.2014.12.040.
6. Bagshaw SM, Stelfox HT, McDermid RC, et al. Association between frailty and short- and long-term outcomes among critically ill patients: a multicentre prospective cohort study. CMAJ : Canadian Medical Association Journal. 2014;186(2):E95–E102. https://doi.org/10.1503/cmaj.130639.
7. Collard RM, Boter H, Schoevers RA, et al. Prevalence of frailty in community-dwelling older persons: a systematic review. J Am Geriatr Soc. 2012;60(8): 1487–92. https://doi.org/10.1111/j.1532-5415.2012.04054.x.
8. Chatterjee P, Krishnaswamy B. Prevalence and predisposing factors of frailty syndrome in elderly (> 75 YEARS) Indian population in subacute care setup. J Aging Res Clin practice. 2012;1(1):3–5.
9. Fairhall N, Kurrle SE, Sherrington C, Lord SR, Lockwood K, John B, et al. Effectiveness of a multifactorial intervention on preventing development of frailty in pre-frail older people: study protocol for a randomized controlled trial BMJ Open. 2015;5:e007091. https://doi.org/10.1136/bmjopen-2014-007091.
10. Cameron I D, Fairhall N, Gill L, et al. Developing Interventions for Frailty. Advances in Geriatrics 2015, Article ID 845356, 7 pages, 2015. doi:https://doi.org/10.1155/2015/845356.
11. Morley JE, Baumgartner RN, Roubenoff R, Mayer J, Nair KS. Sarcopenia. J Lab Clin Med. 2001;137(4):231–43. https://doi.org/10.1067/mlc.2001.113504.
12. Santilli V, Bernetti A, Mangone M, Paoloni M. Clinical definition of sarcopenia. Clinical Cases in Mineral and Bone Metabolism. 2014;11(3): 177–80.
13. Michel J-P, Cruz-Jentoft AJ, Cederholm T. Frailty, exercise and nutrition. Clin Geriatr Med. 2015;31:375–87. https://doi.org/10.1016/j.cger.2015.04.006.
14. Tomás MT, Galán-Mercant A, Carnero EA, Fernandes B. Functional capacity and levels of physical activity in aging: a 3-year follow-up. Front Med. 2018; 4:244. https://doi.org/10.3389/fmed.2017.00244.
15. Ossowski ZM, Skrobot W, Aschenbrenner P, Cesnaitiene VJ, Smaruj M. Effects of short-term Nordic walking training on sarcopenia-related parameters in women with low bone mass: a preliminary study. Clin Interv Aging. 2016;11:1763–71. https://doi.org/10.2147/CIA.S118995.
16. Tieland M, van de Rest O, Dirks ML, van der Zwaluw N, Mensink M, van Loon LJ, de Groot LC. Protein supplementation improves physical performance in frail elderly people: a randomized, double-blind, placebo-controlled trial. J Am Med Dir Assoc. 2012;13(8):720–6. https://doi.org/10.1016/j.jamda.2012.07.005.
17. Morgulec-Adamowicz N, Marszałek J, Jagustyn P. Nordic walking—a new form of adapted physical activity (a literature review). Human Movement. 2011;12(2):124–32. https://doi.org/10.2478/v10038-011-0009-7.
18. AAHF. Articles: aging. Aahfinfo: Exercise and Motivation; 2018. http://aahf.info/sec_news/section/aging-motivation_petersen_012407.htm. Accessed 5 April 2018
19. Notthoff N, Carstensen LL. Positive messaging promotes walking in older adults. Psychol Aging. 2014;29(2):329–41. https://doi.org/10.1037/a0036748.
20. Figueiredo S, Finch L, Mai J, Ahmed S, Huang A, Mayo NE. Nordic walking for geriatric rehabilitation: a randomized pilot trial. Disabil Rehabil. 2013; 35(12):968–75. https://doi.org/10.3109/09638288.2012.717580.
21. Tschentscher M, Niederseer D, Niebauer J. Health benefits of Nordic walking. Am J Prev Med. 2013;44(1):76–84. https://doi.org/10.1016/j.amepre.2012.09.043.
22. Schiffer T, Knicker A, Hoffman U, Harwig B, Hollmann W, Strüder HK. Physiological responses to Nordic walking, walking and jogging. Eur J Appl Physiol. 2006;98:56–61. https://doi.org/10.1007/s00421-006-0242-5.
23. British Nordic Walking | Instructor Training | Nordic Walking Events. British Nordic Walking. 2018. Available at: https://britishnordicwalking.org.uk/. Accessed 5 April 2018.

24. Morsø L, Hartvigsen J, Puggaard L, Manniche C. Nordic walking and chronic low back pain: design of a randomized clinical trial. BMC Musculoskelet Disord. 2006;7(77):21e26. https://doi.org/10.1186/1471-2474-7-77.
25. Bullo V, Gobbo S, Vendramin B, Cugusi L, Di BA, et al. Nordic walking can be incorporated in the exercise prescription to increase aerobic capacity, strength, and quality of life for elderly: a systematic review and meta-analysis. Rejuvenation Res. 2017; https://doi.org/10.1089/rej.2017.1921.
26. Fukagawa NK, Young VR. Protein and amino acid metabolism and requirements in older persons. Clin Geriatr Med. 1987;3(2):329–41.
27. Morais JA, Chevalier S, Gougeon R. Protein turnover and requirements in the healthy and frail elderly. J Nutr Health Aging. 2006;10(4):272–83.
28. Baum JI, Kim I-Y, Wolfe RR. Protein consumption and the elderly: what is the optimal level of intake? Nutrients. 2016;8(6):359. https://doi.org/10.3390/nu8060359.
29. Fujita S, Volpi E. Amino acids and muscle loss with aging. J Nutr. 2006;136(1 Suppl):277S–80S.
30. Fried LP, Tangen CM, Walston J. Frailty in older adults: evidence for a phenotype. J Gerontol A BiolSci Med Sci. 2001;56(3):M146–56.
31. Guigoz Y, Vellas B, Garry PJ. Mini Nutritional Assessment: a practical assessment tool for grading the nutritional state of elderly patients. Facts Res Gerontol. 1994;4(suppl 2):15.
32. Reuben DB, Siu AL. An objective measure of physical function of elderly outpatients. The physical performance test. J Am Geriatr Soc. 1990;38(10): 1105–12. https://doi.org/10.1111/j.1532-5415.1990.tb01373.x
33. Berg K, Wood-Dauphinee S, Williams J, et al. Measuring balance in the elderly: preliminary development of an instrument. Physiother Can. 1989; 41(6):304–11. https://doi.org/10.3138/ptc.41.6.304
34. Wade DT, Collin C. The Barthel ADL index: a standard measure of physical disability? Int Disabil Stud. 1988;10(2):64–7.
35. Lawton M.P, Brody E.M. Assessment of older people: self-maintaining and instrumental activities of daily living. Gerontologist 1969;9: 179–186.
36. Greenberg SA. How to try this: the geriatric depression scale: short form. Am J Nurs. 2007;107(10):60–9. https://doi.org/10.1097/01.NAJ.0000292204.52313.f3.
37. Ganguli M, Ratcliff G, Chandra V, Sharma S, Gilby J, Pandav R, et al. A Hindi version of the MMSE: the development of a cognitive screening instrument for a largely illiterate rural elderly population in India. International Journal of Geriatric Psychiatry. 1995;10(5):367–77.
38. Gunasekaran V, Banerjee J, Dwivedi SN, Upadhyay AD, Chatterjee P, Dey AB. Normal gait speed, grip strength and thirty seconds chair stand test among older Indians. Arch Gerontol Geriatr. 2016;67:171–8.
39. Homepage - INWA. INWA. 2018. Available at: http://www.inwa-nordicwalking.com/. Accessed 5 April 2018.
40. Pai MK. Comparative study of nutritional status of elderly population living in the home for aged Vs those living in the community. Biomedical Research. 2011;22(1):120–6.
41. Song MS, Yoo YK, Choi CH, Kim NC. Effects of nordic walking on body composition, muscle strength, and lipid profile in elderly women. Asian Nurs Res (Korean Soc Nurs Sci). 2013;7(1):1–7. https://doi.org/10.1016/j.anr.2012.11.001.
42. Bierman AS. Functional status: the sixth vital sign. J Gen Intern Med. 2001; 16(11):785–6. https://doi.org/10.1111/j.1525-1497.2001.10918.x.
43. Persson M, Hytter-Landahl Å, Brismar K, Cederholm T. Nutritional supplementation and dietary advice in geriatric patients at risk of malnutrition. Clin Nutr. 2007;26(2):216–24. https://doi.org/10.1016/j.clnu.2006.12.002.
44. Suija K, Pechter Ü, Kalda R, Tähepöld H, Maaroos J, Maaroos H. Physical activity of depressed patients and their motivation to exercise: Nordic walking in family practice. Int J Rehabil Res. 2009;32(2):132–8. https://doi.org/10.1097/mrr.0b013e32831e44ef.
45. Lee HS, Park JN. Effects of Nordic walking on physical functions and depression in frail people aged 70 years and above. J Phys Ther Sci. 2015; 27(8):2453–6. https://doi.org/10.1589/jpts.27.2453.
46. Rao TSS, Asha MR, Ramesh BN, Rao KSJ. Understanding nutrition, depression and mental illnesses. Indian J Psychiatry. 2008;50(2):77–82. https://doi.org/10.4103/0019-5545.42391.
47. Soysal P, Nicola V, Thompson T, Kahl KG, Fernandes BS, Prina AM. Solmi M et al. Relationship between depression and frailty in older adults: A systematic review and meta-analysis Ageing Research Reviews. 2017;36:78–87. https://doi.org/10.1016/j.arr.2017.03.005.
48. Gómez-Pinilla F. Brain foods: the effects of nutrients on brain function. Nat Rev Neurosci. 2008;9(7):568–78. https://doi.org/10.1038/nrn2421.
49. Lautenschlager N, Cox K. Can participation in mental and physical activity protect cognition in old age? JAMA Intern Med. 2013;173(9):805. https://doi.org/10.1001/jamainternmed.2013.206.
50. Denison HJ, Cooper C, Sayer AA, Robinson SM. Prevention and optimal management of sarcopenia: a review of combined exercise and nutrition interventions to improve muscle outcomes in older people. Clin Interv Ageing. 2015;11(10):859–69. https://doi.org/10.2147/CIA.S55842.
51. Rydwik E, Lammes E, Frändin K, Akner G. Effects of a physical and nutritional intervention program for frail elderly people over age 75. A randomized controlled pilot treatment trial. Aging Clin Exp Res. 2008;20(2):159–70. https://doi.org/10.1007/bf03324763.
52. Dalton C. Effect of Nordic Walking on Older Adult Gait and Posture Available at https://ruor.uottawa.ca/bitstream/10393/34091/5/Dalton_Christopher_2016_Thesis.pdf.Accessed June 3, 2018.

15

Association among handgrip strength, body mass index and decline in cognitive function among the elderly women

Su-min Jeong†, Seulggie Choi†, Kyuwoong Kim[2], Sung Min Kim[2], Sujin Kim[3] and Sang Min Park[1,2*]

Abstract

Background: The association between handgrip strength combined with body mass index (BMI) and cognitive impairment has not been thoroughly examined. We aimed to investigate whether the relationship between handgrip strength and risk of cognitive impairment is altered by the presence of obesity in older women.

Methods: A total of 544 older women aged over 65 years without cognitive impairment from the Korean Longitudinal Study of Aging (KLoSA) were included in the study. Handgrip strength was classified in a binary manner (weak or strong) or in tertiles and obesity was defined as a BMI ≥ 25 kg/m^2, in accordance with the Asia-Pacific World Health Organization criteria. Incident cognitive impairment was defined as a Korean Mini-mental State Examination (K-MMSE) score of less than 24 after eight years of follow-up.

Results: Strong handgrip strength was associated with reduced likelihood of developing cognitive impairment compared to weak handgrip strength in obese women (adjusted odds ratio, aOR 0.23, 95% confidence interval, CI 0.08–0.66). The highest tertile of handgrip strength was associated with reduced risk of incident cognitive impairment (aOR 0.16, 95% CI 0.04–0.70), compared to the lowest tertile of handgrip strength in obese women, with a significant linear trend (p for trend = 0.016). Furthermore, the highest tertile of handgrip strength was significantly associated with smaller decline in K-MMSE scores compared to the lowest tertile of handgrip strength in obese women (p value = 0.009). There was no association between handgrip strength and incident cognitive impairment in non-obese women.

Conclusions: Strong handgrip strength was associated with reduced risk of cognitive impairment among obese women, but not in non-obese women. Handgrip strength may be a simple and useful marker for predicting future cognitive impairment among obese women.

Keywords: Handgrip strength, Obesity, Cognitive function

Background

Cognitive decline may lead to mild cognitive impairment or dementia among older adults. A recent study has shown that the conversion rate to cognitive impairment is 6% per person-year among healthy adults [1]. Therefore, identifying and managing modifiable risk factors for cognitive decline are imperative. Previously, body mass index (BMI) and weight change has been shown to be associated with cognitive decline [2, 3]. A recent meta-analysis reported that being underweight, overweight, and obese in mid-life were associated with increased risk of dementia [4]. However, in other studies, overweight in late-life was associated with lower risk of dementia [5]. In addition, decline in BMI was associated with reduced memory function.

The protective effect of high BMI on the risk of dementia may be affected by handgrip strength, a surrogate marker for muscle strength. Handgrip strength, which is positively correlated with BMI, is a valid and representative measure of muscle strength that reflects total power from the upper limb muscles [6]. Previous studies have shown that handgrip strength is associated with mortality

* Correspondence: smpark.snuh@gmail.com
†Su-min Jeong and Seulggie Choi contributed equally to this work.
[1]Department of Family Medicine, Seoul National University Hospital, 101 Daehak-ro, Jongno-gu, Seoul, South Korea
[2]Department of Biomedical Sciences, Seoul National University Graduate School, 101 Daehak-ro, Jongno-gu, Seoul, South Korea
Full list of author information is available at the end of the article

[7, 8], cardiovascular disease [9, 10] and cognitive function [11–13]. In terms of the temporal relationship between handgrip strength and cognitive function, many studies reported that cognitive decline preceded handgrip strength weakness [11, 14]. Moreover, handgrip strength could be a predictive value for cognitive decline [15]. Strong handgrip strength may imply that the intact neuromuscular integrity is associated with reduced risk of dementia and cognitive decline. Although handgrip strength differs according to BMI [16], most previous studies have simply adjusted for height, weight [11] or BMI [12, 13].

Therefore, we hypothesized that different associations may exist between handgrip strength and cognitive strength according to obesity. This study aimed to investigate whether the relationship between handgrip strength and risk of cognitive impairment is altered by the presence of obesity in older women.

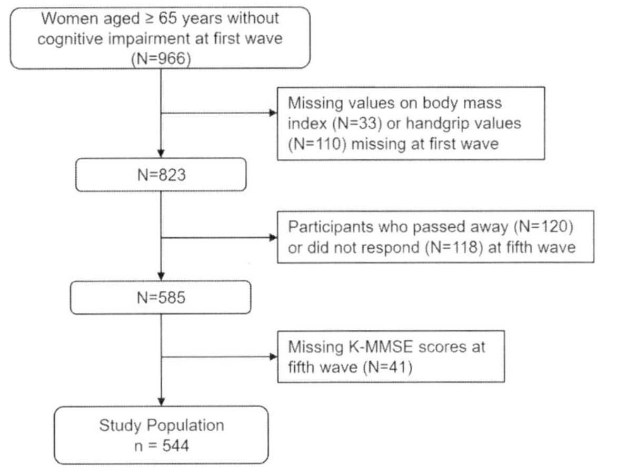

Fig. 1 Flow diagram of the study population. Acronyms: K-MMSE, Korea Mini-mental State Examination

Methods

Study population

The study population was derived from a nationwide panel survey on individuals over the age of 45 years, called the Korean Longitudinal Study of Aging (KLoSA) [17]. The Korea Labor Institute sampled 6171 households from 1000 enumeration districts since 2006 and obtained data on demographics, health status, family structure, income and employment status, and medical history via interviews with follow-up interviews every two years. Five waves are publicly available (2006, 2008, 2010, 2012, and 2014), among which we used the first (2006) and fifth (2014) waves. A total of 966 older women without cognitive impairment (24 points or more of the Korea Mini-mental State Examination, K-MMSE) aged 65 years or older were initially included during the first wave. Individuals without information on BMI or handgrip strength values ($n = 143$) at first wave, who passed away ($n = 120$) and did not respond at the fifth wave ($n = 118$) were excluded. After excluding individuals who lack K-MMSE scores during the fifth wave ($n = 41$), the final study population consisted 544 respondents (Fig. 1).

Measurement of handgrip strength

Two primary exposure variables were used in this study: handgrip strength and BMI from the first wave. Handgrip strength was measured by using a dynamometer (Model number: NO6103, Manufacturer: TANITA, Japan), which measures handgrip strength in units of 0.1 kgF and has been used in multiple previous studies that determined handgrip strength [18, 19]. Upon measurement, the participant was in a seated or standing position, her elbow at a right angle, and the wrist in neutral position. Two measurements for each hand were taken, with the maximum value from each hand were averaged to determine the final handgrip strength. Handgrip strength was either classified in a binary manner as weak (lower half of handgrip strength, ≤18.5 kgF) or strong (upper half of handgrip strength, > 18.5 kgF), or into tertiles (4.5–17.5 kgF, 18.0–20.5 kgF, and 20.8–27.5 kgF).

Classification of handgrip strength and BMI

The other primary exposure variable, BMI, was calculated by self-reported data on weight and height during the first wave. As the revised Asia-Pacific BMI criteria by the Western Pacific Region of the World Health Organization classified those with BMI of 25 kg/m^2 or greater as obese [20], we divided the study population into non-obese (BMI of less than 25 kg/m^2) and obese (BMI of 25 kg/m^2 or greater). A previous study investigating the association between BMI calculated by self-reported weight and height data from KLoSA and BMI calculated by measured weight and height on the same study sample (from a sub-sample of 510 individuals from KLoSA) revealed acceptable Pearson's correlation coefficients (0.865) and specificity (98.0%), but low sensitivity (60.1%) for obesity diagnosis among women [21].

We combined handgrip strength and BMI by first dividing the population into non-obese and obese individuals. Then, the population was further divided according to handgrip strength (lower half and upper half). The population was ultimately divided into: 1) non-obese and weak (lower half) handgrip strength, 2) non-obese and strong (upper half) handgrip strength, 3) obese and weak handgrip strength, and 4) obese and strong handgrip strength.

Assessment of cognitive impairment and cognitive decline

Incident cognitive impairment was determined by the K-MMSE score on the fifth wave. K-MMSE is used to determine cognitive function by questions designed to assess various categories of cognitive function, such as time and place, orientation, registration, attention and calculation, memory recall, language, and visual construction [22, 23]. The validity of K-MMSE scores has been verified in a previous study [22], in which decreasing scores from a perfect score of 30 indicate declining cognitive function. As K-MMSE scores of 24 or greater are considered normal [22, 23], we defined cognitive impairment as a change of K-MMSE score into 23 or less. Furthermore, we calculated the degree of cognitive function decline by subtracting the K-MMSE scores in 2014 by those in 2006 for each individual.

Covariates

The covariates considered in this study are age, marital status (married and unmarried), education (elementary, middle school, high school, and college or higher), income (divided into quartiles), insurance (Medicaid and National Health Insurance), area of residence (urban and rural), smoking status (never smoker, ex-smoker, and current smoker), drinking (no and yes), physical activity (self-reported questionnaire of none and at least once per week of exercise), weight change determined by the change in BMI between the fifth and first waves (loss of less than 1 kg/m^2, no change, and gain of more than 1 kg/m^2), activities of daily living (0 and 1 or more), depression (the Depression 10-item Scale of 4 or less and more than 4, the Center for Epidemiologic Studies), comorbidity (none among cardiovascular disease, stroke, hypertension, and diabetes, and at least one), and baseline K-MMSE score from the first wave.

Statistical analysis

The analysis of variance (ANOVA) method for continuous variables and χ^2 test for categorical variables were performed to compare differences in baseline variables according to BMI and handgrip strength. We first determined the association between baseline handgrip strength and BMI values in the first wave (2006) and cognitive decline in the fifth wave (2014), resulting in an eight-year follow-up period. This was carried out in two ways. We performed logistic regression analyses between the four groups categorized according to BMI and handgrip strength and cognitive decline. Then, the study population was divided into tertiles of increasing handgrip strength and logistic regression analyses was conducted in non-obese and obese groups. The *P* for interaction was calculated to determine whether obesity was a significant factor in the association between handgrip strength and cognitive impairment. Furthermore, the association between baseline handgrip strength and BMI values and degree of cognitive function decline was investigated by linear regression analyses between handgrip strength tertiles and change in K-MMSE scores. Finally, the association between change in handgrip strength and cognitive impairment among those with strong handgrip strength during the first wave was determined by logistic regression analysis to confirm the causality. Among those with strong handgrip strength in the first wave, those with strong handgrip strength (maintained handgrip strength) and weak handgrip strength (weakened handgrip strength) during the fifth wave were compared for development of cognitive decline.

For logistic and linear regression analyses, covariates were adjusted for in a sequential manner: model 1 (age), model 2 (additionally marital status, education, income, insurance, and area of residence), model 3 (additionally smoking status, drinking, and physical activity), and model 4 (additionally activities of daily living, depression, comorbidity, and baseline K-MMSE score). Statistical significance was defined as a p value of less than 0.05 in a two-sided manner. All statistical analyses were conducted via Stata version 13.0 (College Station, TX; StataCorp LP).

Results

Baseline characteristics

The descriptive characteristics of the study population during the first wave in 2006 are presented in Table 1. The distribution of individuals according to BMI and handgrip strength was 33.1% for non-obese with weak handgrip strength, 39.3% for non-obese with strong handgrip strength, 12.5% for obese with weak handgrip strength and 15.1% for obese with strong handgrip strength. Among the four groups divided by BMI and handgrip strength, those with strong handgrip strength were younger compared to those with weak handgrip strength. Non-obese and obese women with strong handgrip were younger than those with weak handgrip strength. Mean ages were 68.7 and 68.8 years in non-obese and obese women with strong handgrip strength, while 71.4 and 70.6 years in non-obese and obese women with weak handgrip strength, respectively. Obese women with strong handgrip strength were likely to be less depressive and more physically active than obese women with weak handgrip strength. There was no significant difference in baseline K-MMSE score at baseline according to the handgrip strength and obesity. Furthermore, a sensitivity analysis of the characteristics between study participants and non-participants are shown in (Additional file 1: Table S1) There was a significance difference in age, area of residence, activities of daily living, and baseline K-MMSE score among participants and non-participants (all p values < 0.05).

Association between handgrip strength with BMI and development of cognitive impairment

The association between handgrip strength with BMI and cognitive decline is depicted in Table 2. There was a significant interaction between obesity and handgrip strength

Table 1 Descriptive characteristics of study participants divided by BMI and handgrip strength

BMI	Non-obese [a]		Obese [a]		*p* value
Handgrip Strength [b]	Weak	Strong	Weak	Strong	
Number of people	180	214	68	82	
Proportion, %	33.1	39.3	12.5	15.1	
Age, years					
Mean	71.4	68.7	70.6	68.8	< 0.001
SD	4.8	3.9	4.3	3.6	
Marital status, %					
Married	31.1	44.0	10.4	14.5	0.209
Unmarried	34.7	35.6	14.2	15.5	
Education, %					
Elementary	32.0	40.7	12.9	14.4	0.351
Middle	37.3	30.5	10.2	22.0	
High	40.7	32.2	11.9	15.3	
College or higher	18.8	62.5	12.5	6.3	
Income, %					
1st quartile	34.7	33.3	16.9	15.1	0.060
2nd quartile	34.7	45.2	8.1	12.1	
3rd quartile	34.9	45.8	4.8	14.5	
4th quartile	27.1	41.7	10.4	20.8	
Insurance, %					
Medicaid	50.0	18.4	21.1	10.5	0.012
NHI	31.8	40.9	11.9	15.4	
Area of residence, %					
Urban	32.7	37.1	13.7	16.6	0.087
Rural	34.3	46.3	9.0	10.5	
Smoking status, %					
Never smoker	35.0	39.5	12.8	14.7	0.561
Ex-smoker	25.0	25.0	0.0	50.0	
Current smoker	37.5	37.5	6.3	18.8	
Drinking, %					
No	34.8	36.6	12.8	15.8	0.002
Yes	19.0	62.1	10.3	8.6	
Physical activity, %					
None	31.1	39.0	14.6	15.2	0.258
1 or more/week.	36.1	39.8	9.3	14.8	
Weight change, %					
Loss	49.1	34.0	11.3	5.7	0.025
No change	31.0	40.2	12.2	16.6	
Gain	43.8	31.3	25.0	0.0	
ADL, %					
0	33.0	39.3	12.6	15.1	0.938
1 or more	35.7	42.9	7.1	14.3	

Table 1 Descriptive characteristics of study participants divided by BMI and handgrip strength *(Continued)*

BMI	Non-obese [a]		Obese [a]		*p* value
Depression, %					
No	28.0	43.7	10.5	17.8	0.001
Yes	41.4	32.3	15.2	11.0	
Comorbidity, %					
0	31.3	43.5	11.8	13.4	0.273
1 or more	34.8	35.5	13.1	16.7	
Baseline K-MMSE					
Mean	26.3	26.7	26.5	26.8	0.072
SD	1.7	1.7	1.6	1.6	

[a]non-obese, BMI < 25 kg/m^2; obese, BMI ≥ 25 kg/m^2
[b]Handgrip strength: weak, lower half, < 18.5 kgF; strong, upper half, ≥18.5 kgF
Acronyms: *BMI* body mass index, *K-MMSE* Korea Mini-mental state examination, *SD* standard deviation, *NHI* National Health Insurance, *ADL* activities of daily living

(*p* value = 0.013 in model 4) (see Additional file 2). Strong handgrip strength was associated with reduced likelihood of developing cognitive decline compared to weak handgrip strength in obese women (adjusted odds ratio, aOR 0.23, 95% confidence interval, CI 0.08–0.66) (Table 2). Strong handgrip strength in non-obese women did not show the significant association with cognitive decline (aOR 1.26, 95% CI 0.75–2.13).

Association between handgrip tertiles according to BMI and cognitive impairment

The risk for cognitive impairment was not significantly different according to tertiles of handgrip strength in the total study population (Table 3). However, among obese women, those with the highest tertile of handgrip strength had reduced likelihood of developing cognitive impairment compared to the lowest tertile of handgrip strength (aOR 0.16, 95% CI 0.04–0.70). Furthermore, there was a significant linear trend between handgrip strength and the risk of cognitive decline among obese women (*p* for trend 0.016). Such associations were not observed in non-obese women.

Association between handgrip strength with BMI and change in K-MMSE score

The association between handgrip strength with BMI and the degree of cognitive function decline calculated by difference in K-MMSE scores were presented in Fig. 2. The highest tertile handgrip strength was significantly associated with smaller declines in K-MMSE scores compared to the lowest tertile handgrip strength in obese women (*p* value 0.009), while the highest tertile of handgrip strength did not in non-obese women. Furthermore, there was a notable linear trend between the degree of cognitive function decline and handgrip strength among obese women (*p* for trend 0.048).

Table 2 Associations between handgrip strength with BMI and cognitive decline

BMI [a]	Non-obese		Obese		$P_{interaction}$
Handgrip Strength [b]	Weak	Strong	Weak	Strong	
Number of cases	94	105	39	32	
Model 1	1.00 (reference)	1.15 (0.71–1.84)	1.00 (reference)	0.66 (0.32–1.38)	0.065
Model 2	1.00 (reference)	1.04 (0.63–1.73)	1.00 (reference)	0.39 (0.17–0.92)	0.029
Model 3	1.00 (reference)	1.13 (0.67–1.88)	1.00 (reference)	0.28 (0.11–0.72)	0.025
Model 4	1.00 (reference)	1.26 (0.75–2.13)	1.00 (reference)	0.23 (0.08–0.66)	0.013

[a]non-obese, BMI < 25 kg/m^2; obese, BMI ≥ 25 kg/m^2
[b]Handgrip strength: weak, lower half, < 18.5 kgF; strong, upper half, ≥18.5 kgF
Model 1: odds ratio by logistic regression analysis adjusted for age (95% confidence interval)
Model 2: additionally adjusted for marital status, education, income, insurance, and area of residence
Model 3: additionally adjusted for smoking status, drinking, physical activity, and weight change
Model 4: additionally adjusted for activities of daily living, depression, comorbidity, and baseline K-MMSE score
P for interaction of BMI and handgrip strength for cognitive impairment
Acronyms: BMI, body mass index

Change in handgrip strength and cognitive impairment

We evaluated the association weakened handgrip strength and cognitive impairment at fifth wave among those who had strong handgrip strength at first wave ($n = 137$) regardless of obesity (Table 4). Weakened handgrip strength was associated with increased risk of cognitive impairment (aOR 2.28, 95% CI 1.23–4.24) compared to maintained handgrip strength.

Discussion

In this longitudinal study, we have demonstrated that strong handgrip strength was associated with lower risk of cognitive impairment compared to weak handgrip strength among obese women. Meanwhile, strong handgrip strength was not associated with lower risk of cognitive impairment in non-obese women. Moreover, decline in handgrip strength was significantly associated with cognitive impairment.

Table 3 Associations between handgrip strength with BMI and cognitive decline according to handgrip strength tertiles and obesity

Handgrip Strength [a]	1st tertile	2nd tertile	3rd tertile	*p* for trend
BMI combined				
Number of cases	104	93	73	
Model 1	1.00 (reference)	1.04 (0.67–1.61)	0.90 (0.55–1.47)	0.684
Model 2	1.00 (reference)	1.05 (0.64–1.71)	0.75 (0.44–1.28)	0.303
Model 3	1.00 (reference)	1.08 (0.66–1.77)	0.77 (0.45–1.33)	0.361
Model 4	1.00 (reference)	1.12 (0.67–1.87)	0.88 (0.50–1.53)	0.649
Non-obese [b]				
Number of cases	70	75	53	
Model 1	1.00 (reference)	1.31 (0.77–2.23)	1.13 (0.61–2.07)	0.669
Model 2	1.00 (reference)	1.27 (0.70–2.30)	1.09 (0.57–2.11)	0.752
Model 3	1.00 (reference)	1.30 (0.71–2.39)	1.16 (0.59–2.26)	0.633
Model 4	1.00 (reference)	1.45 (0.77–2.72)	1.42 (0.72–2.79)	0.296
Obese [b]				
Number of cases	34	18	20	
Model 1	1.00 (reference)	0.53 (0.23–1.23)	0.56 (0.23–1.34)	0.205
Model 2	1.00 (reference)	0.51 (0.18–1.40)	0.29 (0.10–0.86)	0.027
Model 3	1.00 (reference)	0.42 (0.14–1.28)	0.19 (0.05–0.68)	0.011
Model 4	1.00 (reference)	0.35 (0.10–1.17)	0.16 (0.04–0.70)	0.016

[a]Handgrip strength: 1st tertile (≤17.5 kgF), 2nd tertile (18.0 to 20.5 kgF), and 3rd tertile (≥20.8 kgF)
[b]non-obese, BMI < 25 kg/m^2; obese, BMI ≥ 25 kg/m^2
Model 1: odds ratio by logistic regression analysis adjusted for age (95% confidence interval)
Model 2: additionally adjusted for marital status, education, income, insurance, and area of residence
Model 3: additionally adjusted for smoking status, drinking, physical activity, and weight change
Model 4: additionally adjusted for activities of daily living, depression, comorbidity, and baseline K-MMSE score
Acronyms: BMI, body mass index

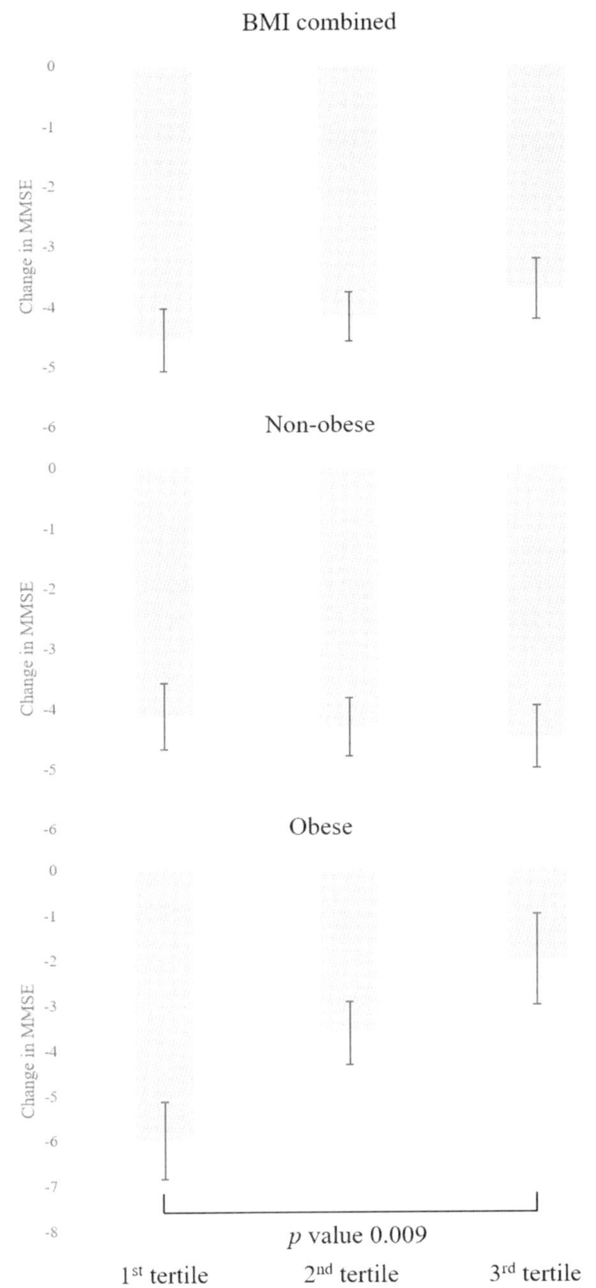

Fig. 2 Adjusted means of change in K-MMSE scores according to handgrip tertiles and obesity. Non-obese, BMI < 25 kg/m^2; obese, BMI ≥ 25 kg/m^2. Handgrip strength: 1st tertile (≤17.5 kgF), 2nd tertile (18.0 to 20.5 kgF), and 3rd tertile (≥20.8 kgF). Adjusted mean values adjusted for age, marital status, education, income, insurance, area of residence smoking status, drinking, physical activity, activities of daily living, depression, comorbidity, and baseline K-MMSE score, *p*-value calculated by linear regression analysis. Black bar indicates standard error. Acronyms: BMI, body mass index

Our results are in agreement with previous studies that have shown that strong handgrip strength was protectively associated with cognitive decline [12, 13]. In a cross-sectional study, mild cognitive impairment was associated with weak handgrip strength [12]. A longitudinal study among 2160 Mexican Americans aged over 65 years have also shown that the highest handgrip strength quartile was associated with better cognitive function over 7 years [13]. A study from the Rush Memory and Aging Project has also reported that strong muscle strength was associated with decreased risk of Alzheimer's disease and mild cognitive impairment [24]. The Rush Memory and Aging Project assessed comprehensive muscle strength with measurement of nine muscle groups including handgrip strength. However, both longitudinal studies adjusted for BMI as a covariate and did not stratify the subjects according to obesity.

Table 4 Associations between change in handgrip strength and cognitive decline among those with strong handgrip strength

Change in Handgrip Strength [a]	Maintained	Weakened
Number of cases	68	69
Model 1	1.00 (reference)	2.15 (1.29–3.61)
Model 2	1.00 (reference)	2.13 (1.19–3.81)
Model 3	1.00 (reference)	2.07 (1.13–3.79)
Model 4	1.00 (reference)	2.28 (1.23–4.24)

[a]Change in handgrip strength: maintained, strong handgrip strength in fifth wave; weakened, weak handgrip strength in fifth wave
Model 1: odds ratio by logistic regression analysis adjusted for age (95% confidence interval)
Model 2: additionally adjusted for marital status, education, income, insurance, and area of residence
Model 3: additionally adjusted for smoking status, drinking, physical activity, and weight change
Model 4: additionally adjusted for activities of daily living, depression, comorbidity, and baseline K-MMSE score

Several possible mechanisms may explain the association between handgrip strength and cognitive function. First, weak handgrip strength may be an early sign of cognitive impairment, as handgrip strength could be reflected by change of nervous system activity or white matter integrity [25]. A prospective study among 555 subjects aged 85 years at baseline revealed that better cognitive performance for attention and processing speed was significantly associated with both stronger and slower decline in handgrip strength [11]. The authors suggested that cognitive function may precede muscle weakness, which could be explained by the fact that strong handgrip strength needs better neuromuscular coordination under well-operated executive functions, especially in the frontal lobe [25]. In our study, weakened handgrip strength was associated with cognitive impairment compared to sustained strong handgrip strength, suggesting that weakened handgrip strength could precede cognitive impairment. Therefore, handgrip strength could be a simple and useful marker in predicting future cognitive impairment.

Second, weak muscle strength and cognitive impairment may share common pathophysiological pathways such as systemic inflammation, insulin resistance and oxidative stress, all of which may contribute to both weak muscle strength and cognitive impairment [26, 27]. Furthermore, factor related to sociodemographics [28], depressive symptoms, health behavior or nutritional state may also affect the risk of cognitive impairment according to muscle strength. Specifically, increased physical activity is highly associated with handgrip strength [29], while also attenuating cognitive decline by the promotion of increased neuroplasty and cerebral blood flow [30]. Previous studies have shown that under-nutrition is associated with weak handgrip strength as well as cognitive impairment in older adults [31].

Our study showed that strong handgrip strength was associated with lower risk of cognitive impairment in obese women, but not in non-obese women. This discrepancy in association of handgrip strength and cognitive impairment according to obesity could be explained by differences of body composition [32]. Participants with high BMI who have strong handgrip strength may have greater muscle mass and less fat mass compared to those with weak handgrip strength. On the other hand, obese participants with weak handgrip strength may have low muscle mass and high fat mass, a state referred to sarcopenic obesity. Excess body fat has previously been shown to be associated with brain atrophy [33] and reduction of hippocampal function through alteration in deoxyribonucleic acid methylation of memory-associated genes [34]. Sarcopenia may also aggravate the risk of cognitive impairment via decreased secretion of cytokines such as insulin-like growth factors [35].

Several limitations must be considered upon interpreting out results. First, the number of subjects was relatively small and may thus lack sufficient statistical power. Our results cannot be generalized to men as the study population was limited to women. Second, selection bias of the study population may exist considering of different baseline characteristics between participants and non-participants. People with poor health conditions are more likely to have passed away or not respond during the fifth wave. Third, BMI was measured using self-reported height and weight. Particularly, as obesity determined by self-reported values yielded high specificity but low sensitivity, there may have been an underestimation of obese individuals. In a previous study using the National Health and Nutrition Examination Survey, there was an average – 0.67 (SD, 0.04) kg/m2 in difference between self-reported and measured BMI values in women. However, there were no difference in the association between self-reported BMI-defined obesity and obesity-related markers compared to association between measured BMI-defined obesity and obesity-related markers, suggesting that self-reported BMI is sufficiently acceptable for epidemiological studies [36]. In addition, we could consider applying high BMI threshold for obesity in older adults because of the low risk of cognitive decline [24] and mortality [37] in overweight groups or due to height reduction [38]. Moreover, other measures of body composition, particularly the proportions of fat and muscle mass, would be useful in further investigating the association between obesity and cognitive function.

Fourth, although the modality of exercise may be an important factor in the association between handgrip strength and cognitive function, we could not adjust for this potential confounder due to the lack of information. Fifth, while MMSE is a widely used cognitive test, it is insensitive detecting early stages of cognitive decline [39], and thus other measurements of cognitive impairment in future studies would be beneficial. Sixth, although measurement of handgrip strength is a useful and simple method to assess upper extremity muscle strength, we could not reflect other aspects of muscle strength, such as quadriceps strength [40] due to the lack of data. Seventh, confounding factors that affect handgrip strength over time such as nutritional state or presence of arthritis in hand could not be considered [41]. Finally, handgrip strength was determined by the maximum value of two measurements rather than three. Future studies using handgrip strength measured by the best of three measurements are needed.

Despite these limitations, to our knowledge, this is first study to elucidate the association between handgrip strength and cognitive function stratified by obesity. In addition, we used a national representative survey. KLoSA is conducted by the Ministry of Labor of Korea from 2006 enrolled participants who randomly selected by a multistage, stratified probability sampling among of community-dwelling Koreans aged ≥45 years after consideration of age, sex, and geographic area [42].

Conclusions

In conclusion, strong handgrip strength in obese women was associated with reduced risk of cognitive impairment. Handgrip strength may be a simple and useful marker for predicting future cognitive impairment among obese women. Further research is needed to determine why the relationship between grip strength and cognitive function was more prominent in obese groups.

Additional files

Additional file 1: Table S1. Sensitivity analysis of the descriptive characteristics between study participants with non-participants.

Additional file 2: Figure S1. Predictive margins for cognitive impairment according to handgrip strength and obesity. Predictive margins calculated by logistic regression analysis after adjustments for age, marital status, education, income, insurance, area of residence, smoking status, drinking, physical activity, weight change, activities of daily living, depression, comorbidity, and baseline K-MMSE score. Obesity: non-obese, BMI < 25 kg/m^2; obese, BMI ≥ 25 kg/m^2. Handgrip strength: weak, lower half, < 18.5 kgF; strong, upper half, ≥18.5 kgF.

Abbreviations
BMI: Body mass index; KLoSA: Korean Longitudinal Study of Aging; K-MMSE: Korean Mini-Mental State Examination

Authors' contributions
SM-J and SG-C contributed study concept and design, analysis and interpretation, drafting and critical revision of the manuscript. SM-J and SG-C designed statistical analysis. SJ-K, KW-K and SM-K critically revised and approved the manuscript. SM-P had full access to all of the data in the study and takes responsibility for this study. All authors read and approved the final manuscript.

Competing interests
The authors declare that they have no competing interests.

Author details
[1]Department of Family Medicine, Seoul National University Hospital, 101 Daehak-ro, Jongno-gu, Seoul, South Korea. [2]Department of Biomedical Sciences, Seoul National University Graduate School, 101 Daehak-ro, Jongno-gu, Seoul, South Korea. [3]Korea Institute for Health and Social Affairs, Sejong, South Korea.

References
1. Chen Y, Denny KG, Harvey D, Farias ST, Mungas D, DeCarli C, et al. Progression from normal cognition to mild cognitive impairment in a diverse clinic-based and community-based elderly cohort. Alzheimers Dement. 2017;13:399–405.
2. Kim S, Kim Y, Park SM. Body mass index and decline of cognitive function. PLoS One. 2016;11(2):e0148908. https://doi.org/10.1371/journal.pone.0148908.
3. Tolppanen AM, Ngandu T, Kareholt I, Laatikainen T, Rusanen M, Soininen H, Kivipelto M. Midlife and late-life body mass index and late-life dementia: results from a prospective population-based cohort. J Alzheimers Dis. 2014;38(1):201–9. https://doi.org/10.3233/JAD-130698.
4. Anstey KJ, Cherbuin N, Budge M, Young J. Body mass index in midlife and late-life as a risk factor for dementia: a meta-analysis of prospective studies. Obes Rev. 2011;12(5):e426–37. https://doi.org/10.1111/j.1467-789X.2010.00825.x
5. Suemoto CK, Gilsanz P, Mayeda ER, Glymour MM. Body mass index and cognitive function: the potential for reverse causation. Int J Obes. 2015;39(9):1383–9. https://doi.org/10.1038/ijo.2015.83.
6. Roberts HC, Denison HJ, Martin HJ, Patel HP, Syddall H, Cooper C, Sayer AA. A review of the measurement of grip strength in clinical and epidemiological studies: towards a standardised approach. Age Ageing. 2011;40(4):423–9. https://doi.org/10.1093/ageing/afr051.
7. Leong DP, Teo KK, Rangarajan S, Lopez-Jaramillo P, Avezum A, Orlandini A, Seron P, Ahmed SH, Rosengren A, Kelishadi R, et al. Prognostic value of grip strength: findings from the prospective urban rural epidemiology (PURE) study. Lancet. 2015;386(9990):266–73. https://doi.org/10.1016/S0140-6736(14)62000-6.
8. Ling CH, Taekema D, de Craen AJ, Gussekloo J, Westendorp RG, Maier AB: Handgrip strength and mortality in the oldest old population: the Leiden 85-plus study. CMAJ 2010, 182(5):429–435.
9. Xu L, Hao YT. Effect of handgrip on coronary artery disease and myocardial infarction: a Mendelian randomization study. Sci Rep. 2017;7(1):954.
10. Lawman HG, Troiano RP, Perna FM, Wang CY, Fryar CD, Ogden CL. Associations of relative handgrip strength and cardiovascular disease biomarkers in U.S. adults, 2011-2012. Am J Prev Med. 2016;50(6):677–83. https://doi.org/10.1016/j.amepre.2015.10.022.
11. Taekema DG, Ling CH, Kurrle SE, Cameron ID, Meskers CG, Blauw GJ, Westendorp RG, de Craen AJ, Maier AB. Temporal relationship between handgrip strength and cognitive performance in oldest old people. Age Ageing. 2012;41(4):506–12. https://doi.org/10.1093/ageing/afs013.
12. Jang JY, Kim J. Association between handgrip strength and cognitive impairment in elderly Koreans: a population-based cross-sectional study. J Phys Ther Sci. 2015;27(12):3911–5. https://doi.org/10.1589/jpts.27.3911.
13. Alfaro-Acha A, Snih SA, Raji MA, Kuo Y-F, Markides KS, Ottenbacher KJ. Handgrip strength and cognitive decline in older Mexican Americans. J Gerontol A Biol Sci Med Sci. 2006;61(8):859–65. https://doi.org/10.1093/gerona/61.8.859.
14. Fritz NE, McCarthy CJ, Adamo DE. Handgrip strength as a means of monitoring progression of cognitive decline - a scoping review. Ageing Res Rev. 2017;35:112–23. https://doi.org/10.1016/j.arr.2017.01.004.
15. Rijk JM, Roos PR, Deckx L, van den Akker M, Buntinx F. Prognostic value of handgrip strength in people aged 60 years and older: a systematic review and meta-analysis. Geriatr Gerontol Int. 2016;16(1):5–20. https://doi.org/10.1111/ggi.12508.
16. Liao K-H. Hand grip strength in low, medium, and high body mass index males and females. Middle East J Rehabil Health. 2016;3(1). https://doi.org/10.17795/mejrh-33860.
17. Korea Labor Institute. User Guide for. KLoSA. In: 2007; 2007.
18. Kim K-N, Lee M-R, Choi Y-H, Hwang H, Oh S-Y, Park C, Hong Y-C. Association between phthalate exposure and lower handgrip strength in an elderly population: a repeated-measures study. Environ Health. 2016;15(1):93.
19. Iinuma T, Arai Y, Fukumoto M, et al. Maximum occlusal force and physical performance in the oldest old: the Tokyo oldest old survey on Total health. J Am Geriatr Soc. 2012;60(1):68–76. https://doi.org/10.1111/j.1532-5415.2011.03780.x.
20. Consultation WHOE. Appropriate body-mass index for Asian populations and its implications for policy and intervention strategies. Lancet. 2004;363(9403):157–63. https://doi.org/10.1016/S0140-6736(03)15268-3.
21. Yoon K, Jang SN, Chun H, Cho SI. Self-reported anthropometric information cannot vouch for the accurate assessment of obesity prevalence in populations of middle-aged and older Korean individuals. Arch Gerontol Geriatr. 2014;59(3):584–92. https://doi.org/10.1016/j.archger.2014.08.008.
22. Kang YND, Hahn S. A validity study on the Korean mini-mental state examination (K-MMSE) in dementia patients. J Korean Neurol Assoc. 1997;15(2):300–8.
23. Thomas F, Bean K, Pannier B, Oppert JM, Guize L, Benetos A. Cardiovascular mortality in overweight subjects: the key role of associated risk factors. Hypertension. 2005;46(4):654–9. https://doi.org/10.1161/01.HYP.0000184282.51550.00.
24. Boyle PA, Buchman AS, Wilson RS, Leurgans SE, Bennett DA. Association of muscle strength with the risk of Alzheimer disease and the rate of cognitive decline in community-dwelling older persons. Arch Neurol. 2009;66(11):1339–44. https://doi.org/10.1001/archneurol.2009.240.
25. Choudhary AK, Jiwane R, Alam T, Kishanrao SS. Grip strength and impact on cognitive function in healthy kitchen workers. Achiev Life Sci. 2016;10(2):168–74.
26. Weaver JD, Huang MH, Albert M, Harris T, Rowe JW, Seeman TE. Interleukin-6 and risk of cognitive decline: MacArthur studies of successful aging. Neurology. 2002;59(3):371–8. https://doi.org/10.1212/WNL.59.3.371.
27. Mangialasche F, Polidori MC, Monastero R, Ercolani S, Camarda C, Cecchetti R, Mecocci P. Biomarkers of oxidative and nitrosative damage in Alzheimer's disease and mild cognitive impairment. Ageing Res Rev. 2009;8(4):285–305. https://doi.org/10.1016/j.arr.2009.04.002.
28. Wu F, Guo Y, Zheng Y, Ma W, Kowal P, Chatterji S, Wang L. Social-economic status and cognitive performance among Chinese aged 50 years and older. PLoS One. 2016;11(11):e0166986. https://doi.org/10.1371/journal.pone.0166986.
29. Dodds R, Kuh D, Aihie Sayer A, Cooper R. Physical activity levels across adult life and grip strength in early old age: updating findings from a British birth cohort. Age Ageing. 2013;42(6):794–8. https://doi.org/10.1093/ageing/aft124.
30. Carvalho A, Rea IM, Parimon T, Cusack BJ. Physical activity and cognitive function in individuals over 60 years of age: a systematic review. Clin Interv Aging. 2014;9:661–82. https://doi.org/10.2147/CIA.S55520.
31. Shawky Khater M, Fawzy Abouelezz N. Nutritional status in older adults with mild cognitive impairment living in elderly homes in Cairo, Egypt. J Nutr Health Aging. 2011;15(2):104–8. https://doi.org/10.1007/s12603-011-0021-9.
32. Levine ME, Crimmins EM. Sarcopenic obesity and cognitive functioning: the mediating roles of insulin resistance and inflammation? Current Gerontology and Geriatrics Research. 2012;2012:7.

33. Gustafson D, Lissner L, Bengtsson C, Bjorkelund C, Skoog I. A 24-year follow-up of body mass index and cerebral atrophy. Neurology. 2004;63(10):1876–81. https://doi.org/10.1212/01.WNL.0000141850.47773.5F.
34. Heyward FD, Gilliam D, Coleman MA, Gavin CF, Wang J, Kaas G, Trieu R, Lewis J, Moulden J, Sweatt JD. Obesity weighs down memory through a mechanism involving the Neuroepigenetic dysregulation of Sirt1. J Neurosci. 2016;36(4): 1324–35. https://doi.org/10.1523/JNEUROSCI.1934-15.2016.
35. Ashpole NM, Sanders JE, Hodges EL, Yan H, Sonntag WE. Growth hormone, insulin-like growth factor-1 and the aging brain. Exp Gerontol. 2015;68:76–81. https://doi.org/10.1016/j.exger.2014.10.002.
36. A. MM, M. DR, B. HF: Comparison of self-reported and measured BMI as correlates of disease markers in U.S. adults. Obesity 2007, 15(1):188–188.
37. Flicker L, McCaul KA, Hankey GJ, Jamrozik K, Brown WJ, Byles JE, Almeida OP. Body mass index and survival in men and women aged 70 to 75. J Am Geriatr Soc. 2010;58(2):234–41.
38. Han TS, Tajar A, Lean MEJ. Obesity and weight management in the elderly. Br Med Bull. 2011;97(1):169–96. https://doi.org/10.1093/bmb/ldr002.
39. Tombaugh TN, McIntyre NJ. The mini-mental state examination: a comprehensive review. J Am Geriatr Soc. 1992;40(9):922–35.
40. Chen W-L, Peng T-C, Sun Y-S, Yang H-F, Liaw F-Y, Wu L-W, Chang Y-W, Kao T-W. Examining the association between quadriceps strength and cognitive performance in the elderly. Medicine. 2015;94(32):e1335. https://doi.org/10.1097/MD.0000000000001335.
41. Granic A, Davies K, Jagger C, Kirkwood TB, Syddall HE, Sayer AA. Grip strength decline and its determinants in the very old: longitudinal findings from the Newcastle 85+ study. PLoS One. 2016;11(9):e0163183. https://doi.org/10.1371/journal.pone.0163183.
42. Jang SN, Kawachi I, Chang J, Boo K, Shin HG, Lee H, Cho SI. Marital status, gender, and depression: analysis of the baseline survey of the Korean longitudinal study of ageing (KLoSA). Soc Sci Med. 2009;69(11):1608–15. https://doi.org/10.1016/j.socscimed.2009.09.007.

16

Prevalence of malnutrition and associated factors among community-dwelling older persons

H. D. W. T. Damayanthi[1,2*], F. M. Moy[3], K. L. Abdullah[1] and S. D. Dharmaratne[4,5,6]

Abstract

Background: Malnutrition in older persons is a public health concern. This study aimed to estimate the prevalence of malnutrition and its associated factors among community-dwelling older persons in Sri Lanka.

Methods: A cross-sectional study was conducted in the Kandy district, Sri Lanka. The nutritional status of older persons was assessed using the Mini Nutritional Assessment –Short Form (MNASF). A standardised questionnaire was used to record factors associated with malnutrition: demographic characteristics, financial characteristics, food and appetite, lifestyle, psychological characteristics, physical characteristics, disease and care, oral health, and social factors. Complex sample multinomial logistic regression analysis was performed.

Results: Among the 999 participants included in the study, 748 (69.3%) were females and 251 (25.1%) were males. The mean age was 70.80 years (95% CI: 70.13, 71.47). The prevalence of malnutrition, risk of malnutrition and well-nutrition was 12.5%, 52.4% and 35.1% respectively. In the multivariate model, hypertension (adjusted OR = 1.71; 95% CI: 1.02, 2.89), alcohol consumption (aOR = 4.06; 95% CI: 1.17, 14.07), and increased age (aOR = 1.06; 95% CI: 1.01, 1.11) were positively associated with malnutrition. An increased number of people living with the older person (aOR: 0.91; 95% CI: 0.85, 0.97) was a protective factor among those at risk for malnutrition.

Conclusion: Both the prevalence of malnutrition and risk of malnutrition were commonly observed among community-dwelling older persons in Sri Lanka. The associated factors identified in this study might help public health professionals to implement necessary interventions that improve the nutritional status of this population.

Keywords: Elderly persons, Malnutrition, Mini nutritional assessment, Prevalence, Sri Lanka

Background

Sri Lanka is experiencing rapid growth of its older population due to the improvement of health care facilities. In the South Asian region, Sri Lanka has the fastest-growing ageing population [1]. By year 2041, one out of every four persons in Sri Lanka is expected to be an older person aged 60 years and older [2, 3]. Changes in physiological, pathological, social, and psychological conditions can be observed among older persons as they go through the process of aging [4]. Malnutrition among older persons is a key determinant of their mortality, health care and quality of life [5–8].

Malnutrition is often defined as 'a faulty or inadequate nutrition status' [9]. Malnutrition causes adverse effects on health as well as the quality of life of older persons. Further, it presents high costs to health care systems [10, 11]. Hence, malnutrition has become an important component of geriatric care that warrants monitoring.

The prevalence of malnutrition among older persons varies according to the setting in which they reside. In Sri Lanka, the prevalence of malnutrition among older persons who resided in nursing homes was 30% [12]. It ranged from 21 to 67% in the hospital setting [13]. However, there is a lack of literature on malnutrition among community-dwelling older persons in Sri Lanka.

* Correspondence: trbaasu@yahoo.com
[1]Department of Nursing Sciences, Faculty of Medicine, University of Malaya, Kuala Lumpur, Malaysia
[2]Department of Nursing, Faculty of Allied Health Sciences, University of Peradeniya, Peradeniya, Sri Lanka
Full list of author information is available at the end of the article

Malnutrition among older persons is a multifactorial condition. A recent systematic review identified several domains of malnutrition: demographic characteristics, financial characteristics, food and appetite, lifestyle, psychological characteristics, physical functioning, disease and care, oral health, and social factors [14]. Previous studies have identified additional potential risk factors of malnutrition related to the above domains: advanced age, female and single/widowed/divorced [15, 16], low education level [17], poverty [17, 18], loss of appetite, food allergies and eating/swallowing/tasting difficulties, [12, 19, 20], cigarette smoking and alcohol consumption [21, 22], betel nut chewing [23], lack of interest, low mood, frequent negative thoughts, loneliness, depression, dementia and low cognition [17, 24], physical inactivity [12], diseases [11], tooth loss and not wearing dentures [25] and social factors such as living alone [26].

As most studies were conducted in high-income countries, where lifestyles and foods differ from that in Sri Lanka [5, 6, 17], research studies need to be conducted in Sri Lanka to reflect the nutrition status of the population. In addition, the magnitude of malnutrition among older persons in community settings in Sri Lanka has been under-reported thus far. Factors associated with malnutrition among community-dwelling older persons in Sri Lanka need to be identified in order to determine suitable interventions that can improve their nutritional status [12]. Therefore, this study was conducted to determine the prevalence and associated factors of malnutrition among community-dwelling older persons in Sri Lanka.

Methods

Study design and sample

This cross-sectional study was conducted to determine the prevalence and associated factors of malnutrition among community-dwelling older persons in Sri Lanka. A total of 1267 respondents were recruited and 1015 of them completed the questionnaires (response rate of 80.1%). Sixteen cases were subsequently excluded because of missing data. The final sample used for analysis was 999.

This study was conducted in Kandy district, Sri Lanka from July 2015 to May 2016. The Open Source Epidemiologic Statistics for Public Health software (version 3.01) was used to calculate the sample size. Sample size was calculated using the odds ratios of selected factors associated with malnutrition among older persons in previous studies and the largest sample size was taken for the present study. Nazemi and colleagues (2015) reported that older persons with diabetes mellitus were twice more likely [(OR): 1.67; 95% confidence interval (CI): 1.1–2.4] to have malnutrition compared to older persons without diabetes. The estimated sample size was 1056. Considering the 20% non-response rate, 1267 older persons were needed for the sample size of the study. Participants were included in the study if they were aged 60 years and older, stayed in the community and consented to participate in the study. Exclusion criteria included being physically frail and/or mentally unable to answer the questionnaire. Participants were selected using multistage sampling from twenty-six Grama Niladari (GN) divisions, among seven randomly-selected Divisional Secretariats in Kandy district. At the GN level, a list of older persons was obtained from the 2012 electoral registers utilizing the simple random sample approach.

Data collection and procedures

The selected participants completed the questionnaires at a community centre. All participants were informed about the aim and content of the study and each participant signed an informed consent form prior to data collection. Anthropometric measurements (height and weight) were recorded using standardized procedures.

The nutritional status was assessed using the Sinhala version of the Mini Nutritional Assessment – short form (MNA-SF), which is an instrument specifically designed for elderly people; it has been validated in many settings including hospitals, nursing homes and communities [27, 28]. The MNA-SF is simple, non-invasive, inexpensive, and easy to use. The questionnaire consists of six items: food intake, weight loss, mobility, psychological stress or acute disease, neuropsychological problems and body mass index (BMI) [27]. The following cut-off values were used: 0 to 7 for malnourished, 8 to 11 for risk of malnutrition, and 12 to 14 for well-nutrition [29].

Body mass index (BMI) was calculated to assess the nutritional status of participants. BMI is calculated as weight in kilograms (kg) divided by height in square meters (m^2). The World Health Organization classifies BMI < 18.5 as underweight, BMI 18.5–24.9 as normal weight, BMI ≥ 25 as overweight [30]. Reliable measurements of height of older persons, however, can be difficult due to vertebral compression, loss of muscle tone and postural changes. Hence, BMI was considered only for the assessment of nutritional status [31].

Interviewer-administered questionnaires were used to collect data on all explanatory variables, including demographic characteristics, financial characteristics, food and appetite, lifestyle, psychological characteristics, physical functioning, disease and care, oral health, and social factors. Demographic factors were age, sex, marital status and level of education. Selected older persons were categorized into three groups by age: the young old (60 to 69 years), the middle old (70 to 79 years), and the very old (80 years and older) [32]. With respect to marital status, participants were categorised as married, single, or divorced/widowed. Based on level of education, participants were also classified into three groups: no formal education, primary education and secondary/tertiary education.

Participants' financial status was determined by whether their last monthly income was below or above the poverty level, which was Rs. 3999 (Sri Lankan rupees). Living arrangements and the number of people living with the older person were considered as social factors. Participants were divided into three groups based on social factors: alone, living with children/spouse or living with relatives/friends.

Loss of appetite, eating/swallowing difficulties, food allergies and vegetarian diet were included under food and appetite. Lifestyle factors included alcohol consumption, cigarette smoking and betel chewing. Disease and care included suffering from chronic illnesses, usage of medicines, and chronic conditions such as diabetes mellitus, hypertension and hypercholesterolemia. Tooth loss and use of dentures were considered oral factors. For these four explanatory variables – food and appetite, lifestyle, disease and care, and oral factors, participants were classified based on self-reported responses of 'yes' or 'no'.

Physical characteristics included physical activity, which was measured using the Sinhala version of the International Physical Activity Questionnaire (IPAQ) short form validated for Sri Lankans [33]. All participants were asked to answer the IPAQ, which consisted of four parts: the frequency and time spent on vigorous intensity activity, moderate intensity activity, walking for at least 10 min at one time, and sitting and/or lying down (excluding sleeping) [34]. Physical activity value was obtained in Metabolic Equivalent of Task (MET) minutes per week; values were obtained by multiplying the value of energy expenditure for the given physical activity in MET by the weekly frequency (days per week) and the time (minutes per day). MET values for vigorous physical activity, moderate physical activity and walking were 8.0, 4.0 and 3.3 respectively. For the purpose of the current study, participants were grouped into three categories based on physical activity; 'inactive/low', 'moderately active' and 'highly active'. Participants with scores of < 600 MET minutes per week were considered low in physical activity; those with scores of 600–2999 MET minutes per week were moderately active; and those with scores of ≥3000 MET minutes per week were highly active. The validly and reliability of this questionnaire for elderly people also has been ensured [35].

The depression level of the participants was considered as a psychological factor. It was measured using the Sinhala version of the geriatric depression scale (GDS) [36]. The GDS-short form contains 15 items with a 'yes' or 'no' answer format. It has been tested for psychometric properties [37, 38]. Participants were considered depressed if they had scores of more than 8 on the GDS [39].

Statistical analysis

Data analysis was performed using the IBM Statistical Program for Social Sciences (SPSS) version 21. This sampling utilized multistage sampling of Divisional Secretariats (DS), Grama Niladari (GN) Divisions and households. Households within clusters are more similar than households randomly sampled from the population as a whole [40]. Complex sample analysis with weighting was carried out. The weights were determined by the proportion of the respective stratum in the population divided by the proportion of that stratum in the sample (the inverse of the probability of selection). Weights were applied to correct for unequal selection probabilities of multistage sampling. We computed the weights for each person based on DS, GN and household levels.

Initially, descriptive analyses was conducted to describe socio-demographic characteristics. The mean and 95% confidence interval (CI) were calculated for continuous variables. Unweighted counts and weighted percentages for categorical variables were reported. Then the independent variables were compared between nutritional categories (malnourished, at risk of malnutrition and well-nourished) using one way analysis of variance for continuous variables and Chi-square tests for categorical study variables. Then, complex samples multinomial logistic regression analyses, in the form of univariate and multivariate, were used to examine the associations between malnutrition and risk of malnutrition and study variables. Well-nutrition was used as the reference category. Variables entered into the multivariate model were those found to have significant associations ($p < .05$) with malnutrition and risk of malnutrition in the univariate analysis, while those with $p > .25$ in the univariate analysis were excluded from the multivariate model [41]. The multivariate analysis was adjusted for gender and all other variables in the model. Crude odds ratios (OR) and adjusted odds ratios (aOR) with 95% confidence intervals (CI) were reported in univariate and multivariate analysis respectively. Significant level was pre-set at 0.05.

Results

The participants' mean age was 70.80 years (CI: 70.13, 71.47). Almost half of the participants (48.1%) were young old, 42.3% were middle old and 9.5% were very old. Two-thirds (71.9%) were females. The majority were Sinhalese (94.0%). About half of them (55.6%) had completed secondary or tertiary education, while 10.2% had no formal education. The majority (73.9%) of the participants earned an income below the poverty line and lived with family members (88.8%) (Table 1).

The mean MNA score was 10.45 (CI: 10.24, 10.67). Based on the MNA scores, 12.5% of the participants were malnourished, about half (52.4%) were at risk of malnutrition and one-third (35.1%) were well-nourished. Table 1 further shows the results of comparison of different nutritional status (malnourished, risk of malnutrition and well-nourished) across various factors. Alcohol consumption, betel chewing and BMI categories showed statistically significant differences with the nutritional status. With reference to BMI,

Table 1 Nutritional status of older persons according to demographic, social, financial, food and appetite, lifestyle, psychological, physical, disease & care, oral characteristics and BMI categories ($N = 999$)

Variable	Total $n = 999$ (n, weighted %)	Malnutrition, $n = 151$ (n, weighted %)	At risk of malnutrition, $n = 485$ (n, weighted %)	Well nutrition, $n = 363$ (n, weighted %)	*p* value
Demographic characteristics					
Age categories					0.104
Young old	542(48.1)	52(8.0)	267(50.5)	223(41.4)	
Middle old	375(42.3)	81(15.4)	178(53.5)	116(31.2)	
Old old	81(9.5)	18(12.5)	39(55.1)	24(27.9)	
Sex					0.256
Male	251(28.1)	42(12.7)	128(58.0)	81(29.3)	
Female	748(71.9)	109(12.3)	357(50.0)	282(37.7)	
Marital status					0.095
Married	840(79.4)	135 (13.8)	407(50.6)	298(35.7)	
Single	15(2.2)	0	10(90.7)	5(9.3)	
Divorced/widowed	144(18.4)	16(9.8)	68(53.7)	60(36.5)	
Level of education					0.435
No formal	76(10.2)	13(13.9)	44(60.8)	19(25.3)	
Primary	270(34.2)	40(12.3)	141(54.6)	89(33.0)	
Secondary/tertiary	653(55.6)	98(12.2)	300(48.2)	255(39.6)	
Financial characteristic					
Income					0.276
Below poverty line	678(73.9)	104(13.1)	321(50.6)	253(36.3)	
Above poverty line	321(26.1)	47(9.8)	164(59.4)	110(30.7)	
Social characteristics					
Living arrangements					0.256
Alone	89(10.4)	17(11.8)	47(53.3)	25(35.0)	
With family members	900(88.8)	133(12.6)	434(52.2)	333(35.1)	
With friends/relatives	10(0.8)	1(2.3)	4(61.1)	5(36.6)	
Food & appetite characteristics					
Loss of appetite					0.659
Yes	140(11.0)	26(11.2)	70(58.0)	44(30.7)	
No	859(89.0)	125(12.6)	415(51.7)	319(35.7)	
Eating/swallowing difficulties					0.935
Yes	125(10.7)	19(13.4)	63(49.9)	43(36.7)	
No	874(89.3)	132(12.3)	422(52.7)	32(34.9)	
Food allergies					0.521
Yes	73(6.7)	10(19.4)	31(48.9)	32(31.4)	
No	926(93.3)	141(11.9)	454(52.7)	331(35.4)	
Vegetarian					0.587
Yes	328(34.7)	52(13.3)	155(48.8)	121(37.8)	
No	671(65.3)	99(12.0)	330(54.3)	242(33.7)	
Lifestyle characteristics					
Alcohol consumption					0.016*
Yes	36(5.2)	9(31.4)	17(55.9)	10(12.7)	
No	963(94.8)	142(11.4)	468(52.2)	353(36.4)	

Table 1 Nutritional status of older persons according to demographic, social, financial, food and appetite, lifestyle, psychological, physical, disease & care, oral characteristics and BMI categories (*N* = 999) *(Continued)*

Variable	Total *n* = 999 (n, weighted %)	Malnutrition, *n* = 151 (n, weighted %)	At risk of malnutrition, *n* = 485 (n, weighted %)	Well nutrition, *n* = 363 (n, weighted %)	*p* value
Cigarette smoking					0.069
Yes	28(3.5)	6(32.4)	15(52.8)	7(14.8)	
No	971(96.5)	145(11.7)	470(52.4)	356(35.9)	
Betel chewing					0.027*
Yes	269(46.3)	46(17.1)	131(49.7)	92(33.1)	
No	730(53.7)	105(8.4)	354(54.7)	271(36.8)	
Psychological characteristics					
Depression					0.378
Normal	413(36.7)	61(12.4)	203(51.8)	149(35.8)	
Depression	586(63.3)	90(12.5)	282(52.8)	214(34.7)	
Physical characteristics					
Physical activity					0.991
Low	164(15.4)	24(11.1)	80(52.9)	60(36.0)	
Moderate	729(68.4)	111(12.4)	349(52.6)	269(35.1)	
High	106(16.2)	16(14.2)	56(51.3)	34(34.5)	
Disease & care characteristics					
Chronic illness					0.325
Yes	503(55.0)	69(10.4)	248(56.1)	186(33.5)	
No	496(45.0)	82(14.1)	237(49.4)	177(36.5)	
Usage of medicines					0.110
Yes	568(60.1)	92(15.2)	275(50.1)	201(34.7)	
No	431(39.9)	59(8.4)	210(55.9)	162(35.7)	
Medical conditions					
DM					0.385
Yes	62(3.9)	8(7.6)	31(64.2)	23(28.2)	
No	937(96.1)	143(12.6)	454(51.9)	340(35.4)	
HPT					0.320
Yes	203(23.5)	28(8.5)	101(57.8)	74(33.7)	
No	796(76.5)	123(13.7)	384(50.8)	289(35.6)	
HCH					0.728
Yes	14(0.5)	3(15.3)	7(41.3)	4(43.4)	
No	985(99.5)	148(12.4)	478(52.5)	359(35.1)	
Oral characteristics					
Tooth loss					0.503
Yes	881(89.5)	137(13.1)	430(52.3)	314(34.7)	
No	118(10.5)	14(7.3)	55(53.7)	49(39.1)	
Use dentures					0.877
Yes	270(15.1)	46(12.0)	129(50.3)	95(37.7)	
No	729(84.9)	105(12.5)	356(52.8)	268(34.7)	
BMI categories					< 0.001*
Underweight	127(13.7)	78(44.7)	49(55.3)	0	
Normal	541(58.1)	71(10.9)	297(58.3)	173(30.8)	

Table 1 Nutritional status of older persons according to demographic, social, financial, food and appetite, lifestyle, psychological, physical, disease & care, oral characteristics and BMI categories ($N = 999$) *(Continued)*

Variable	Total $n = 999$ (n, weighted %)	Malnutrition, $n = 151$ (n, weighted %)	At risk of malnutrition, $n = 485$ (n, weighted %)	Well nutrition, $n = 363$ (n, weighted %)	*p* value
Over weight	323(28.3)	2(0.4)	135(37.9)	186(61.7)	
Age, mean(CI)	70.80(70.13,71.47)	72.3(70.6,74.0)	70.90(69.9,71.7)	70.2(69.0,71.4)	0.140
Number of people living with (CI)	3.60(3.42,3.77)	3.4(3.1,3.8)	3.5(3.3,3.8)	3.8(3.5,4.1)	0.256

Data are presented as number & weighted percentage (%) or as mean & 95% confidence interval (CI)
Significance between groups was determined using chi-square test for categorical variables and one way ANOVA for continuous variables
DM diabetes mellitus, *HPT* hypertension, *HCH* hypercholesterolemia, *BMI* body mass index
Poverty line-Kandy district poverty line July 2015 Rs.3909
$^*p < 0.05$ is significant

44.7% of the malnourished older persons were categorized as being underweight compared to 0% of the well-nourished.

In the univariate analyses, age, hypertension, cigarette smoking and alcohol consumption were significantly associated with malnutrition. The number of people living with the older person was statistically significant for risk of malnutrition (Table 2).

Factors associated with malnutrition and at risk of malnutrition in the multinomial logistic regression analysis after adjusting for age, number of people living with, alcohol use, smoking, betel chewing, usage of medication and gender are shown in Table 3. Participants who consumed alcohol were found to be four times more likely (aOR = 4.06, 95% CI: 1.17, 14.07) to have malnutrition. In addition, older persons with hypertension had approximately 71% more chance of being malnourished (aOR = 1.71, 95% CI: 1.02, 2.89). Age remained independently associated with an increased risk of malnutrition with OR of 1.06 (95% CI: 1.01, 1.11). The number of people living with was a protective factor for being at risk of malnutrition (aOR: 0.91, 95% CI: 0.85, 0.97).

Discussion

This study was conducted among community-dwelling older persons in the Kandy district in Sri Lanka. About half of the participants were young old, while a small proportion consisted of very old participants. This pattern is similar to the age structure of the Sri Lankan population and represents the Sri Lankan older population [42]. The majority of the participants were of the Sinhala ethnic group and is comparable with the findings of other community based studies conducted in Sri Lanka [43, 44]. The education level of the participants also was consistent with the national levels reported, in that the larger proportion of the participants had secondary/tertiary education [45].

We found that the prevalence of malnutrition among community-dwelling older persons was 12.5%, with more than half of the population being at risk of malnutrition; this corroborates the findings of other studies in India which used MNA [46, 47]. Several studies conducted in South Africa, Portugal, and Korea using MNA as the measurement tool, reported prevalence of malnutrition among community-dwelling older persons as 10.4%, 5.6% and 10.5% respectively [5, 20, 48]. In comparison to these studies, the present study found a higher prevalence of malnutrition. A possible reason for this discrepancy may be the low economic conditions faced by Sri Lankans, which may be closely intertwined with the household food security of the older population. However, we feel that further detailed studies could propose more evidence based explanation for this finding.

In comparison to studies conducted among older persons in other care settings of Sri Lanka, the community-dwelling older persons of the current study were less likely to be malnourished [12, 13]. This may be due to the extended family support involved in their nutritional care. Older persons living in other settings, especially institutions, often lack family support; most institutions have set menus for three meals, which may be lacking in essential nutrients [12]. Another possible reason for the low prevalence of malnutrition in our study might be because the definitions and tools used to assess malnutrition are different from those used in other studies [12]. For instance, malnutrition among older persons who stayed in nursing homes was assessed using BMI [5].

In the multivariate analysis, age was associated with malnutrition. The physiological changes of aging directly affect the metabolism of nutrients. Also, physiological conditions of aging, such as sarcopenia and osteoporosis, might progressively limit the mobility of older individuals, further limiting their ability in shopping, preparing foods and even consuming foods [49]. This finding is similar to that reported in another study [4]. Our participants with hypertension were 70% more likely to be malnourished. The reason behind this may be the pathophysiological effects of diseases which lead to loss of appetite and decreased digestion, absorption and metabolism [50].

Alcohol consumption was also found to contribute to the prevalence of malnutrition. Alcohol and malnutrition may be linked to impaired liver function which directly affects protein metabolism [51]. Further, vitamin and mineral

Table 2 Crude odds ratio (95% CI) of nutritional status according to associated factors in multinomial logistic regression

Variable	Risk of malnutrition, $n = 485$		Malnutrition, $n = 151$	*p* value
	OR (95% CI)	*p* value	OR (95% CI)	
Age	1.02(0.99, 1.05)	0.291	1.06(1.02,1.10)	0.008*
Gender	1.49(0.91,2.45)	0.110	1.32(0.65,2.68)	0.437
Male				
Level of education				
No formal	1.79(0.58,5.50)	0.311	1.98(0.90,4.34)	0.288
Primary	1.21(0.61,2.41)	0.581	1.36(0.85, 2.17)	0.297
Secondary/tertiary	Reference			
Income (Below poverty line)	1.29(0.69,2.41)	0.400	1.05(0.45,2.44)	0.909
Living arrangement				
Alone	1.17(0.48,2.83)	0.714	1.25(0.24,6.42)	0.782
With family members	5.56(0.63,53.0)	0.926	5.38(0.48,60.67)	0.273
With relatives/friends	Reference			
No of people living with	0.91(0.86,0.97)	0.006*	0.90(0.76,1.70)	0.216
Loss of appetite	1.28(0.80,2.05)	0.290	1.28(0.65,2.54)	0.456
Eating/swallowing difficulties	1.02(0.58,1.80)	0.931	1.06(0.51,2.24)	0.866
Food allergies	0.84(0.34,2.70)	0.685	1.14(0.45,2.88)	0.777
Vegetarian	0.88(0.45,1.70)	0.680	1.03(0.72,1.47)	0.843
Alcohol consumption	2.04(0.73,5.71)	0.167	4.60(2.35,8.98)	< 0.001*
Cigarette smoking	2.20(0.75–6.45)	0.141	4.70(2.21,9.99)	< 0.001*
Betel chewing	1.09(0.71,1.69)	0.669	1.65(0.93,2.92)	0.082
Depression				
Depression	1.05(0.68, 1.64)	0.823	1.04(0.54, 2.02)	0.906
Normal	Reference			
Physical activity				
Low	0.75(0.23,2.44)	0.631	0.99(0.45, 2.20)	0.983
Moderate	0.86(0.35,2.09)	0.737	1.01(0.54,1.90)	0.638
High	Reference			
Chronic illness	1.11(0.87,1.42)	0.385	0.81(0.40,1.64)	0.546
Usage of medicines	0.98(0.75,1.28)	0.901	1.47(0.87,2.49)	0.142
DM	0.87(0.36,2.07)	0.731	0.80(0.27,2.44)	0.686
HPT	1.02(0.81,1.29)	0.859	1.89(1.15,3.09)	0.014*
HCH	0.99(0.19,5.06)	0.992	0.64(0.16,2.58)	0.526
Tooth loss	1.17(0.47,2.87)	0.727	1.85(0.43,8.02)	0.390
Use dentures	0.96(0.65,--1.43)	0.840	1.16(0.64,2.13)	0.596

DM diabetes mellitus, *HPT* hypertension, *HCH* hypercholesterolemia, *BMI* body mass index, *OR* odds ratio, *CI* 95% confidence interval
Poverty line-Kandy district poverty line July 2015 Rs.3909
*$p < 0.05$ is significant
Reference category is well nutrition ($n = 363$); reference category for loss of appetite, eating/swallowing difficulties, food allergies, vegetarian, alcohol consumption, cigarette smoking, betel chewing, chronic illness, usage of medicine, DM, HPT, HCH, tooth loss, use dentures is 'no'; reference for gender is female

deficiencies associated with heavy alcohol consumption deteriorate the nutritional status of older persons [52]. However, there were contradictory findings on the association between alcohol consumption and malnutrition reported in other studies [22]. Tian et al. (2017) reported that moderate alcohol consumption had beneficial effects on malnutrition [53] whereas Mathew et al. (2016) found no association between alcohol consumption and malnutrition among older persons in their study [16]. Therefore, further investigations on patterns of

Table 3 Factors associated with risk of malnutrition and malnutrition after adjusted for confounders using multinomial logistic regression

Variable	Risk of malnutrition, $n = 485$ aOR (95% CI)	p value	Malnutrition, $n = 151$ aOR (95% CI)	p value
Age	1.02 (0.99,1.05)	0.268	1.06 (1.01,1.11)	0.020*
Gender (Male)	1.26(0.59,2.72)	0.533	0.95(0.33,2.68)	0.912
No of people living with	0.91 (0.85,0.97)	0.006*	0.89(0.74,1.09)	0.277
Usage of medication	0.97 (0.74,1.28)	0.827	1.47(0.82,2.66)	0.186
Alcohol consumption	1.63 (0.65,4.08)	0.281	4.06(1.17,14.07)	0.029*
Cigarette smoking	1.57 (0.75,3.29)	0.222	2.28(0.88,5.93)	0.087
Betel chewing	0.99 (0.66–1.50)	0.986	1.30(0.77,2.19)	0.304
HPT	0.99 (0.79,1.27)	0.994	1.71 (1.02,2.89)	0.044*

HPT hypertension; The reference category is well-nutrition ($n = 363$); Reference category for alcohol consumption, cigarette smoking, betel chewing, usage of medicine, HPT is 'no'; Reference for Gender is female
Multinomial regression was used, with a removal probability of 0.25
Adjusted for gender and for all other variables in the model. * $p < 0.05$ is significant
Model Fit: $R^2 = 0.048$ (Cox and Snell); 0.056 (Nagelkerke); 0.025 (McFadden)

alcohol consumption among this population is required to postulate a final conclusion.

Traditionally, Sri Lankan society holds older persons in reverence and provides social and financial support for them [54]. The majority of our participants were married and stayed with their family. In Sri Lanka, provision of older person care is considered to be the responsibility of family members; in large families, care responsibilities might be shared by family members, with each contributing a smaller effort than would be observed in a smaller family [1]. Our results showed that the number of people living with the older person was a protective factor of being at risk of malnutrition. Living with more family members might help older persons to prevent loneliness and social isolation which are common reasons why older persons eat more poorly [55]. Therefore, support from family members may be crucial in nutritional interventions that aim to improve the nutritional status of older persons in the community.

While previous studies have suggested that marital status, level of education, income, tooth loss, use of dentures, chronic illnesses, diabetes, dyslipidaemia, depression, physical activity, eating difficulty, food allergy, loss of appetite and vegetarianism are associated with malnutrition among older persons, our study did not find these factors to be associated with malnutrition [16–19]. A reason for this may be the effect of multiple unidentified confounders which distort or mask actual associations. Although the identified confounders could be controlled, unidentified confounders could not be controlled using statistical analysis [56, 57]. Similarly, a recent systematic review on determinants of malnutrition among community-dwelling older persons highlighted strong evidence that there is no association between various factors and malnutrition. The same review identified poor appetite as the single factor which had a strong association with malnutrition among older persons [14]. Although poor appetite is probably a major cause of malnutrition, it is mediated by a variety of factors such as age, several peptide hormones released by the gut including; ghrelin, CCK, peptide-YY, glucagon-like peptide 1, oxyntomodulin, and pancreatic polypeptide and many neurotransmitters [58–61]. A possible reason for not finding a strong association for loss of appetite with malnutrition in our study might be a result of interactions among the risk factors on appetite among our participants.

Strengths and limitations

There were a few limitations which warrant consideration in the present study. First, this was a cross-sectional study, which limits the establishment of causality. Second, as the majority of the participants were Sinhalese, our sample may not be representative of the community-dwelling older persons in the country. Third, recall bias may be another limitation. However, the questionnaire was interviewer-administered and probing was used to ensure that the participants recalled information as well as they could. Fourth, non-respondents are likely to be malnourished or at risk of malnutrition [62]. Excluding disabled and mentally-ill older persons may also have affected findings on the prevalence of malnutrition and risk of malnutrition. Fifth, this study did not assess dietary intake which may directly affect the nutritional status of the participants.

On the other hand, to the best of our knowledge, this is the first study on malnutrition conducted among community-dwelling older persons in Sri Lanka. The use of validated and internationally-accepted questionnaires is a strength of the current study. Finally, the use of multistage sampling ensured that a representative sample was recruited from the community.

Conclusion

Prevalence of risk of malnutrition is high among older persons in the community-dwelling setting. Age, having hypertension and alcohol consumption were significantly associated with malnutrition among the participants. Moreover, the number of people living with the older persons decreased the probability of being at risk of malnutrition. Public health professionals should be encouraged to develop screening strategies according to the identified factors to improve the nutritional status of this vulnerable population.

Abbreviations

BMI: Body mass indexCIConfidence intervalMNA-SFMini nutritional assessment tool – short formOROdds ratio

Acknowledgments

The authors would like to thank all the participants for their cooperation.

Funding

This research received no specific grant from any funding agency in the public, commercial, or not-for-profit sectors.

Authors' contributions

HDWTD, FMM, KLA and SDD participated in the design of the study. HDWTD collected data under supervision of SDD, FMM and KLA. HDWTD, FMM and KLA performed the data analysis. HDWTD drafted the manuscript. FMM, KLA, SDD revised the manuscript critically for important intellectual content. All authors read and approved the final version of the manuscript.

Competing interests

The authors declare that they have no competing interests.

Author details

[1]Department of Nursing Sciences, Faculty of Medicine, University of Malaya, Kuala Lumpur, Malaysia. [2]Department of Nursing, Faculty of Allied Health Sciences, University of Peradeniya, Peradeniya, Sri Lanka. [3]Julius Centre University of Malaya, Department of Social and Preventive Medicine, Faculty of Medicine, University of Malaya, Kuala Lumpur, Malaysia. [4]Department of Community Medicine, Faculty of Medicine, University of Peradeniya, Peradeniya, Sri Lanka. [5]Department of Family and Community Medicine, College of Medicine, University of Kentucky, Kentucky, USA. [6]Department of Health Metric Sciences, School of Medicine, University of Washington, Seattle, USA.

References

1. Watt MH, Perera B, Østbye T, Ranabahu S, Rajapakse H, Maselko J. Caregiving expectations and challenges among elders and their adult children in southern Sri Lanka. Aging Soc. 2014;34(5):838–58. https://doi.org/10.1017/S0144686X12001365
2. DeSilva WI. A population projection of Sri Lanka for the new millennium. 2001–2101 trends and implications. Institute for Health Policy: Colombo; 2007.
3. Gallo JJ, Rebok GW, Lesikar SE. The driving habits of adults aged 60 years and older. J Am Geriatr Soc. 1999;47(3):335–41.
4. Amarya S, Singh K, Sabharwal M. Changes during aging and their association with malnutrition. Journal of Clinical Gerontology and Geriatrics. 2015;6(3):78–84. https://doi.org/10.1016/j.jcgg.2015.05.003.
5. Santos ALM, Amaral TMSPF, Borges NPGFB. Undernutrition and associated factors in a Portuguese older adult community. Rev Nutr. 2015;28:231–40.
6. Boulos C, Salameh P, Barberger-Gateau P. Factors associated with poor nutritional status among community dwelling Lebanese elderly subjects living in rural areas: results of the AMEL study. J Nutr Health Aging. 2014; 18(5):487–94. https://doi.org/10.1007/s12603-014-0463-y.
7. Kvamme J-M, Olsen JA, Florholmen J, Jacobsen BK. Risk of malnutrition and health-related quality of life in community-living elderly men and women: the Tromsø study. Qual Life Res. 2011;20(4): 575–82. https://doi.org/10.1007/s11136-010-9788-0.
8. de Hollander EL, Van Zutphen M, Bogers RP, Bemelmans WJ, De Groot LC. The impact of body mass index in old age on cause-specific mortality. J Nutr Health Aging. 2012;16(1):100–6.
9. Chen CC, Schilling LS, Lyder CH. A concept analysis of malnutrition in the elderly. J Adv Nursing. 2001;36 https://doi.org/10.1046/j.1365-2648.2001.01950.x.
10. Rasheed S, Woods RT. An investigation into the association between nutritional status and quality of life in older people admitted to hospital. J Hum Nutr Diet. 2014;27(2):142–51. https://doi.org/10.1111/jhn.12072.
11. Leslie W, Hankey C. Aging, nutritional status and health. Healthcare. 2015; 3(3):648–58. https://doi.org/10.3390/healthcare3030648.
12. Rathnayake KM, Wimalathunga M, Weech M, Jackson KG, Lovegrove JA. High prevalence of undernutrition and low dietary diversity in institutionalised elderly living in Sri Lanka. Public Health Nutr. 2015;18(15): 2874–80. https://doi.org/10.1017/s1368980015000749.
13. Jayalath WATA, Kumara SKGPH. Assessment of Nutritional Status of Elderly Hospitalised Patients According to Their Co-Morbid Conditions and Educational Levels Using Mini Nutrition Assessment Tool. Sri Lanka: Peradeniya University Research Sessions; 2011.
14. van der Pols-Vijlbrief R, Wijnhoven HA, Schaap LA, Terwee CB, Visser M. Determinants of protein-energy malnutrition in community-dwelling older adults: a systematic review of observational studies. Ageing Res Rev. 2014; 18:112–31. https://doi.org/10.1016/j.arr.2014.09.001.
15. Montejano Lozoya AR, Ferrer Diego RM, Clemente Marín G, Martínez-Alzamora N, Sanjuan Quiles Á, Ferrer Ferrándiz E. Factores asociados al riesgo nutricional en adultos mayores autónomos no institucionalizados. Nutr Hosp. 2014;30:858–69.
16. Mathew AC, Das D, Sampath S, Vijayakumar M, Ramakrishnan N, Ravishankar SL. Prevalence and correlates of malnutrition among elderly in an urban area in Coimbatore. Indian J Public Health. 2016; 60(2):112–7. https://doi.org/10.4103/0019-557x.184542.
17. Torres MJ, Dorigny B, Kuhn M, Berr C, Barberger-Gateau P, Letenneur L. Nutritional status in community-dwelling elderly in France in urban and rural areas. PLoS One. 2014;9(8):e105137. https://doi.org/10.1371/journal.pone.0105137.
18. Donini LM, Scardella P, Piombo L, Neri B, Asprino R, Proietti AR, et al. Malnutrition in elderly: social and economic determinants. J Nutr Health Aging. 2013;17(1):9–15. https://doi.org/10.1007/s12603-012-0374-8.
19. Vanderwee K, Clays E, Bocquaert I, Gobert M, Folens B, Defloor T. Malnutrition and associated factors in elderly hospital patients: a Belgian cross-sectional, multi-Centre study. Clin Nutr. 2010;29(4):469–76. https://doi.org/10.1016/j.clnu.2009.12.013.
20. Hyun HS, Lee I. Nutritional status and risk factors for malnutrition in low-income urban elders. J Korean Acad Nurs. 2014;44(6):708–16. https://doi.org/10.4040/jkan.2014.44.6.708.
21. Barcelo M, Torres O, Mascaro J, Francia E, Cardona D, Ruiz D. Assessing nutritional status in the elderly evaluation of Chumlea equations for weight. Nutr Hosp. 2013;28(2):314–8. https://doi.org/10.3305/nh.2013.28.2.6320.

22. Fares D, Barbosa AR, Borgatto AF, Coqueiro RS, Fernandes MH. Fatores associados ao estado nutricional de idosos de duas regiões do Brasil. Rev Assoc Med Bras. 2012;58:434–41.
23. Tsai AC, Chang TL. Association of dental prosthetic condition with food consumption and the risk of malnutrition and follow-up 4-year mortality risk in elderly Taiwanese. J Nutr Health Aging. 2011;15(4):265–70.
24. Akın S, Mucuk S, Öztürk A, Mazıcıoğlu M, Göçer Ş, Arguvanlı S, et al. Muscle function-dependent sarcopenia and cut-off values of possible predictors in community-dwelling Turkish elderly: calf circumference, midarm muscle circumference and walking speed. Eur J Clin Nutr. 2015;69(10):1087–90. https://doi.org/10.1038/ejcn.2015.42
25. Kazemi S, Savabi G, Khazaei S, Savabi O, Esmaillzadeh A, Keshteli AH, et al. Association between food intake and oral health in elderly: SEPAHAN systematic review no. 8. Dent Res J. 2011;8(Suppl1):S15–20.
26. Westergren A, Hagell P, Sjodahl Hammarlund C. Malnutrition and risk of falling among elderly without home-help service--a cross sectional study. J Nutr Health Aging. 2014;18(10):905–11. https://doi.org/10.1007/s12603-014-0469-5.
27. Guigoz Y, Vellas B, Garry PJ. Assessing the nutritional status of the elderly: the mini nutritional assessment as part of the geriatric evaluation. Nutr Rev. 1996;54
28. Vellas B, Villars H, Abellan G, Soto ME, Rolland Y, Guigoz Y, et al. Overview of the MNA--its history and challenges. J Nutr Health Aging. 2006;10(6):456–63. discussion 63-5
29. Rubenstein LZ, Harker JO, Salva A, Guigoz Y, Vellas B. Screening for undernutrition in geriatric practice: developing the short-form mini-nutritional assessment (MNA-SF). J Gerontol A Biol Sci Med Sci. 2001;56(6):M366–72.
30. WHO Expert Consultation. Appropriate body-mass index for Asian populations and its implications for policy and intervention strategies. Lancet. 2004; 363(9403):157–63. https://doi.org/10.1016/s0140-6736(03)15268-3.
31. Balcombe NR, Ferry PG, Saweirs WM. Nutritional status and well being. Is there a relationship between body mass index and the well-being of older people? Curr Med Res Opin. 2001;17(1):1–7.
32. Forman DE, Berman AD, McCabe CH, Baim DS, Wei JY. PTCA in the elderly: the "young-old" versus the "old-old". J Am Geriatr Soc. 1992;40(1):19–22.
33. Arambepola C. Abdominal obesity and its association with selected risk factors of coronary heart disease in an adult population in the district of Colombo. Colombo: Postgraduate Institute of Medicine, University of Colombo; 2004.
34. Ibrahim S, Karim NA, Oon NL, Ngah WZW. Perceived physical activity barriers related to body weight status and sociodemographic factors among Malaysian men in Klang Valley. BMC Public Health. 2013; 13(1):275. https://doi.org/10.1186/1471-2458-13-275.
35. Tomioka K, Iwamoto J, Saeki K, Okamoto N. Reliability and validity of the international physical activity questionnaire (IPAQ) in elderly adults: the Fujiwara-kyo study. J Epidemiol. 2011;21(6):459–65. https://doi.org/10.2188/jeaJE20110003.
36. Kulathunga M, Umayal S, Somaratne S, Srikanth S, Kathriarachchi S, De Silva K. Validation of the geriatric depression scale for an elderly Sri Lankan clinic population. Indian J Psychiatry. 2010;52(3):254–6. https://doi.org/10.4103/0019-5545.70979.
37. Friedman B, Heisel MJ, Delavan RL. Psychometric properties of the 15-item geriatric depression scale in functionally impaired, cognitively intact, community-dwelling elderly primary care patients. J Am Geriatr Soc. 2005; 53(9):1570–6. https://doi.org/10.1111/j.1532-5415.2005.53461.x.
38. Burns A, Lawlor B, Craig S. Rating scales in old age psychiatry. Br J Psychiatry. 2002;180:161–7.
39. Wong SY, Mercer SW, Woo J, Leung J. The influence of multi-morbidity and self-reported socio-economic standing on the prevalence of depression in an elderly Hong Kong population. BMC Public Health. 2008;8(1):119. https://doi.org/10.1186/1471-2458-8-119.
40. Woyessa A, Deressa W, Ali A, Lindtjørn B. Ownership and use of long-lasting insecticidal nets for malaria prevention in Butajira area, south-Central Ethiopia: complex samples data analysis. BMC Public Health. 2014;14(1):99. https://doi.org/10.1186/1471-2458-14-99.
41. Bursac Z, Gauss CH, Williams DK, Hosmer DW. Purposeful selection of variables in logistic regression. Source Code Biol Med. 2008;3:17. https://doi.org/10.1186/1751-0473-3-17.
42. Department of Census & Statistics SL. Vital statistics. 2013. http://www.statistics.gov.lk/PopHouSat/VitalStatistics/Tables.asp?Year=2013.
43. Malhotra R, Chan A, Ostbye T. Prevalence and correlates of clinically significant depressive symptoms among elderly people in Sri Lanka: findings from a national survey. Int Psychogeriatr. 2010;22(2):227–36. https://doi.org/10.1017/s1041610209990871.
44. Katulanda P, Ranasinghe P, Jayawardana R, Sheriff R, Matthews DR. Metabolic syndrome among Sri Lankan adults: prevalence, patterns and correlates. Diabetol Metab Syndr. 2012;4(1):24. https://doi.org/10.1186/1758-5996-4-24.
45. Census of Population and Housing Sri Lanka 2012. http://www.statistics.gov.lk/PopHouSat/CPH2011/Pages/Activities/Reports/CPH_2012_5Per_Rpt.pdf.
46. Agarwalla R, Saikia AM, Baruah R. Assessment of the nutritional status of the elderly and its correlates. J Family Community Med. 2015;22(1):39–43. https://doi.org/10.4103/2230-8229.149588.
47. Lahiri S, Biswas A, Santra S, Lahiri SK. Assessment of nutritional status among elderly population in a rural area of West Bengal, India. Int J Med Sci Public Health. 2015;4(4):569–72.
48. Naidoo I, Charlton KE, Esterhuizen T, Cassim B. High risk of malnutrition associated with depressive symptoms in older south Africans living in KwaZulu-Natal, South Africa: a cross-sectional survey. J Health Popul Nutr. 2015;33(1):19. https://doi.org/10.1186/s41043-015-0030-0.
49. Alzahrani SH, Alamri SH. Prevalence of malnutrition and associated factors among hospitalized elderly patients in king Abdulaziz University hospital, Jeddah, Saudi Arabia. BMC Geriatr. 2017;17(1):136. https://doi.org/10.1186/s12877-017-0527-z
50. Zhu Z, Xiong S, Liu D. The gastrointestinal tract: an initial organ of metabolic hypertension? Cell Physiol Biochem. 2016;38(5):1681–94. https://doi.org/10.1159/000443107
51. Stickel F, Hoehn B, Schuppan D, Seitz HK. Review article: nutritional therapy in alcoholic liver disease. Aliment Pharmacol Ther. 2003;18(4):357–73.
52. Ijaz S, Jackson J, Thorley H, Porter K, Fleming C, Richards A, et al. Nutritional deficiencies in homeless persons with problematic drinking: a systematic review. Int J Equity Health. 2017;16(1):71. https://doi.org/10.1186/s12939-017-0564-4.
53. Tian HY, Qiu R, Jing LP, Chen ZY, Chen GD, Chen YM. Alternate Mediterranean diet score is positively associated with skeletal muscle mass index in middle-aged adults. Br J Nutr. 2017;117:1181–8. https://doi.org/10.1017/s0007114517001118.
54. Kaluthanthri KDMS. Aging and the changing role of the family in Sri Lanka (PhD Thesis). The University of Adelaide; 2014. https://digital.library.adelaide.edu.au/dspace/bitstream/2440/93498/3/02whole.pdf.
55. Ramic E, Pranjic N, Batic-Mujanovic O, Karic E, Alibasic E, Alic A. The effect of loneliness on malnutrition in elderly population. Med Arh. 2011;65(2):92–5.
56. Pannucci CJ, Wilkins EG. Identifying and avoiding Bias in research. Plast Reconstr Surg Glob Open. 2010;126(2):619–25. https://doi.org/10.1097/PRS.0b013e3181de24bc.
57. Skelly AC, Dettori JR, Brodt ED. Assessing bias: the importance of considering confounding. Evid Based Spine Care J. 2012;3(1):9–12. https://doi.org/10.1055/s-0031-1298595.
58. de Groot CP, van Staveren WA, de Graaf C. Determinants of macronutrient intake in elderly people. Eur J Clin Nutr. 2000;54(Suppl 3):S70–6.
59. Das SK, Moriguti JC, McCrory MA, Saltzman E, Mosunic C, Greenberg AS, et al. An underfeeding study in healthy men and women provides further evidence of impaired regulation of energy expenditure in old age. J Nutr. 2001;131(6):1833–8.
60. Morley JE. Decreased food intake with aging. J Gerontol Ser A J Gerontol A Biol Sci Med Sci. 2001;56(Spec No 2):81–8.
61. Clarkston WK, Pantano MM, Morley JE, Horowitz M, Littlefield JM, Burton FR. Evidence for the anorexia of aging: gastrointestinal transit and hunger in healthy elderly vs. young adults. Am J Phys. 1997;272(1 Pt 2):R243–8.
62. Cheung KL, ten Klooster PM, Smit C, de Vries H, Pieterse ME. The impact of non-response bias due to sampling in public health studies: a comparison of voluntary versus mandatory recruitment in a Dutch national survey on adolescent health. BMC Public Health. 2017;17(1):276.

17

Challenges of conducting research in long-term care facilities

Helen R Lam[1], Selina Chow[1,2], Kate Taylor[1], Ronald Chow[1], Henry Lam[1], Katija Bonin[1], Leigha Rowbottom[1] and Nathan Herrmann[1,2*]

Abstract

Background: The aim of this review is to describe the challenges and barriers to conducting research in long-term care facilities.

Methods: A literature search was conducted in Ovid MEDLINE, Embase, Cochrane Central, PsycINFO and CINAHL. Keywords used included "long term care", "nursing home", "research", "trial", "challenge" and "barrier", etc. Resulting references were screened in order to identify relevant studies that reported on challenges derived from first-hand experience of empirical research studies. Challenges were summarized and synthesized.

Results: Of 1723 references, 39 articles were selected for inclusion. To facilitate understanding we proposed a classification framework of 8 main themes to categorize the research challenges presented in the 39 studies, relating to the characteristics of facility/owner/administrator, resident, staff caregiver, family caregiver, investigator, ethical or legal concerns, methodology, and budgetary considerations.

Conclusions: Conducting research in long-term care facilities is full of challenges which can be categorized into 8 main themes. Investigators should be aware of all these challenges and specifically address them when planning their studies. Stakeholders should be involved from an early stage and flexibility should be built into both the methodology and research budget.

Keywords: Research, Clinical trials, Challenges, Barriers, Nursing homes, Long-term care, Long term care hospitals, Chronic care, Skilled-nursing facilities, Residences for senior citizens

Background

As human life expectancy continues to increase, particularly in developed countries, more people will be living longer lives while being afflicted with chronic illnesses, multiple co-morbidities, and functional deficits [1–4]. As a result of the aging population, many individuals will require placement in long-term care (LTC) facilities [5, 6]. In the USA as of 2010, 1.2 million people or 3.1% of those aged 65 and over lived in a skilled-nursing facility, while in Canada as of 2011, 4.5% of those in the same demographic, yielding a total of 224,000 people lived in a 'nursing home' or 'LTC hospital' (LTC may be called skilled-nursing facilities, nursing homes, LTC hospitals, chronic care or residencies for senior citizens) [7, 8]. Thus, research aimed at improving geriatric medicine and the quality of care in LTC has become increasingly important. Despite this need, research in LTC settings, considered by some authors as a 'highly unstable environment' due to high attrition and turnover of staff or residents, as well as unpredictable external regulatory changes, remains challenging for various reasons [5, 9].

The challenges of conducting research in LTC facilities and/or on older adults have been described in a small number of reviews. Some of these focused on older adults as research subjects, but were not necessarily in LTC settings. For example, a Canadian guideline by Slaughter et al. reported on consent and assent of dementia patients as research subjects but this was not limited to LTC settings [2]. Another study discussed issues pertaining to intervention research in LTC, schools and critical care [9]. McMurdo et al. suggested potential

* Correspondence: nathan.herrmann@sunnybrook.ca
[1]Sunnybrook Health Sciences Centre, University of Toronto, 2075 Bayview Avenue, Toronto, ON M4N 3M5, Canada
[2]Division of Geriatric Psychiatry, Sunnybrook Health Sciences Centre, University of Toronto, 2075 Bayview Avenue, Room FG19, Toronto, ON M4N 3M5, Canada

improvements to recruitment of the elderly for research [10], and an article by Schulz discussed barriers to caregiver intervention research in various settings [11].

There have also been reviews focused on research challenges in LTC settings. A number of studies summarized ethical challenges [12–14], while others discussed the difficulties of studying a particular condition in LTC, such as falls, delirium and incontinence [15–17]. Ruckdeschel et al. targeted issues on gaining LTC staff support [18], while Reed et al. discussed the issue of research governance in LTC [19]. An article by Maas et al. in 2002 was a more extensive review, covering various challenges of nursing research in LTC, but it was not a systematic review and did not use a comprehensive literature search strategy [3]. We searched the PROSPERO website to check for existing systematic review protocols on this topic and found none [20]. The purpose of this study was to provide an updated and comprehensive systematic review of the challenges of conducting research in LTC facilities as reported in empirical research studies. By organizing these challenges into themes, we hope to provide investigators with a framework for anticipating and dealing with these challenges in order to facilitate research in LTC.

Methods

A literature search was conducted in Ovid MEDLINE (1946 to June 2017, week 4), Embase Classic & Embase (1947 to 2017, week 27), Cochrane Central Register of Controlled Trials (May 2017), PsycINFO (1806 to June 2017, week 4) and Ebsco CINAHL (1981 to Jul 5 2017). Keywords such as 'long-term care', 'nursing home', 'research', 'trial', 'challenge', 'barrier', 'issue', 'recruitment', and 'difficulty', etc., were used to retrieve relevant studies which explicitly reported on challenges or barriers encountered during LTC research (see Additional file 1 for complete database search strategies). The searches were limited to English language and human subjects only. The PRISMA checklist was used to validate the research process [21]. (Additional file 2: PRISMA Checklist).

The titles and abstracts of the search results were screened independently by two authors (HRL, KT) with discrepancies discussed and resolved. Articles were eligible for full-text screening if the title and/or abstract mentioned research and challenges, in addition to "long-term care", "LTC", "nursing home" or "care home". Full-texts were screened for inclusion by 3 authors (HRL, SC, KT) with disagreements resolved by discussion. Articles were included in this systematic review if they reported on challenges or barriers experienced during empirical research studies in LTC or a nursing home setting. Research studies that made use of previously collected or administrative data were also acceptable if they satisfied other criteria. Studies were excluded if they were secondary studies such as narrative reviews, systematic reviews, guidelines, expert commentaries, or were editorials, letters, conference abstracts, unfinished studies, research protocols, about patients living at home or receiving home care, or non-English (Fig. 1).

The primary information of interest was the challenges and barriers experienced by the investigators conducting research in a LTC setting. A text-tagging software QDA Miner Lite and a thematic synthesis approach was employed to assist in summarizing the main challenges that were discussed in the studies [22, 23]. We imported the full texts of all 39 included studies into the software. Three authors (HRL, SC, HL) carefully read through the full texts and performed line-by-line tagging of the sections within the studies where authors described actual research challenges they had experienced in LTC research. Patterns were recognized and initial categories (descriptive themes) of challenges were identified and established by the same group after discussion to resolve disagreements. The texts were re-coded according to the descriptive themes. We then revised and consolidated the descriptive themes into a final hierarchy of analytical themes which were approved by all co-authors. Coding of texts was re-done once again according to the final categorization.

Results

The literature search yielded 1723 references, of which 80 articles were selected for full-text screening as specified by the inclusion criteria, and ultimately 39 were included in this review (Fig. 1). They were all reports derived from actual experience of empirical research such as clinical trials, observational studies, surveys or epidemiological studies.

Of the 39 papers included in this review, 20 were based on studies conducted in the United States [24–43], 15 were based on those from the United Kingdom [44–58], and 1 study from each of Australia [59], New Zealand [60], France [61] and Norway [62]. Most of the 39 papers reported on challenges experienced in research with LTC residents as research subjects. A smaller number (4) of papers noted challenges encountered while studying subjects such as LTC facilities, LTC staff, or family members (see Table 1).

With the help of a thematic synthesis approach we created a framework of 8 main themes to categorize the challenges reported in the 39 studies: facility/owner/administrator factors, resident factors, staff caregiver factors, family caregiver factors, investigator factors, ethical/legal factors, methodological factors and budgetary factors (Table 1). We then described what the 8 main themes represent, and which and how many studies noted challenges that fall under a particular theme.

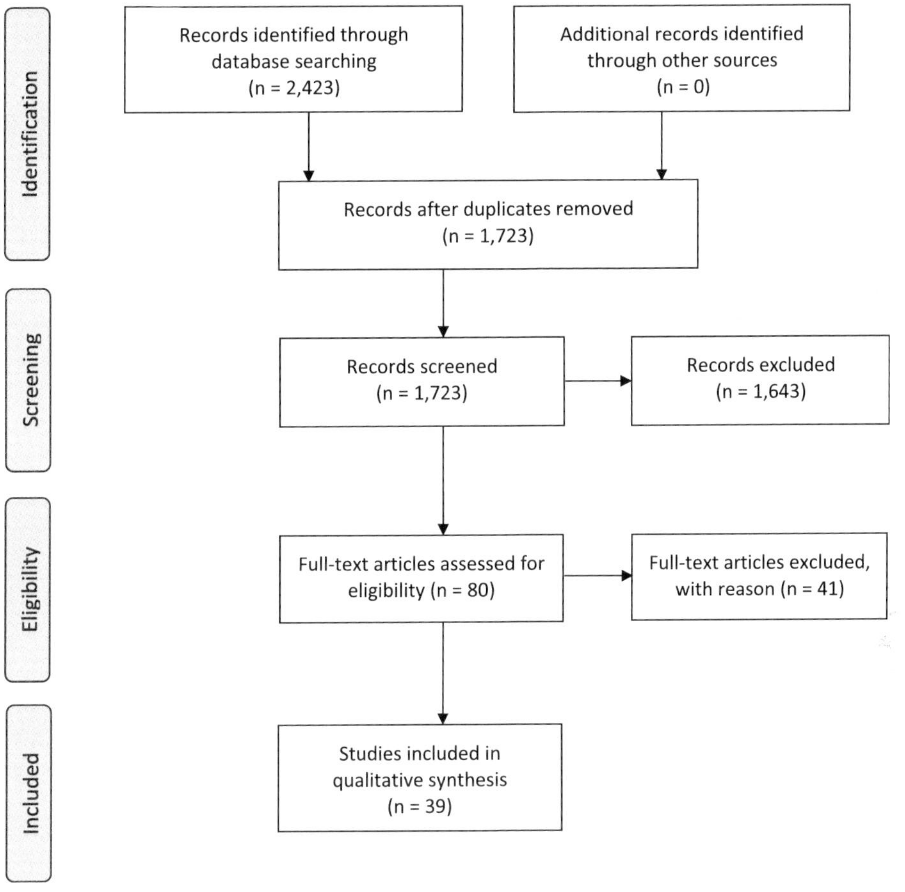

Fig. 1 PRISMA Research Process Flow Diagram

We summarized below the findings of the 39 studies under each of the eight themes.

Facility/owner/administrator factors

A total of 18 studies reported challenges that could be categorized under this theme [24–30, 32, 37, 43, 45–49, 52, 55, 59]. Some of the major issues included within this theme were: recruitment and retention of LTC facilities, owners or administrators unfamiliar with research, not interested or feel threatened.

A major challenge reported by authors was the recruitment and retention of LTC facilities to participate in clinical research, as many facilities were reluctant to do so [27, 46]. Participation in research was not a common experience for most LTC facilities [30]. Hickman et al. reported that just over half (53%) of the facilities they surveyed had previously participated in research, with experiences ranging from a single resident enrolled in an off-site study to larger scale studies involving modifications to the physical environment [30]. Some LTC owners and/or administrators refused to allow research to be conducted in their facilities, while others were prohibited from participating due to corporate policies [24, 49]. Additionally, some were reluctant to take part because their facilities would be subjected to more government inspection as a result [24]. In general, large, privately-owned LTC chains have less flexibility when there is a corporate-wide policy that prohibits research, whereas small independent non-profit facilities may be restricted from participating in research due to their limited resources [29]. In fact, Gismondi et al. reported a low participation rate of 20% from large corporations, and an even lower rate of 14% from independent facilities [32]. Moreover, recruitment of LTC facilities can be time consuming, ranging from 8 to 13 months [48, 49].

Changes in ownership posed another challenge to conducting research in LTC facilities [25, 46]. In a study conducted by Sherrell et al., 80% of nursing homes had changed their names by the time the follow-up study was administered [37]. Retention and attrition of LTC facilities was a problem, especially in longitudinal studies and among facilities with logistical deficiencies and high personnel turnover [26].

Administrators' personal views regarding the value of research were often mixed [30]. They had varied experiences and education backgrounds and many

Table 1 Research Challenges in LTC Noted by Included Studies

References	Subjects of Primary Research (F: Facilities, FM: Family members, R: Residents, S: Staff)	Type of Challenge						Methodological	Budgetary
		Facility/ Owner/ Administrator	Resident	Staff Caregiver	Family Caregiver	Investigator	Ethical/ Legal		
Zapka J et al., 2014 [24]	R	✓		✓	✓		✓		
Garcia C et al., 2013 [25]	R	✓		✓		✓	✓		✓
Tilden VP et al., 2013 [26]	F, S	✓							
Ersek M et al., 2012 [27]	R	✓	✓					✓	
Greenspan S et al., 2012 [28]	R	✓	✓	✓			✓		
Van Ness PH et al., 2012 [29]	R	✓	✓					✓	
Hickman SE et al., 2008 [30]	R	✓					✓		
Quinn CC et al., 2008 [31]	R		✓	✓					
Gismondi PM et al., 2005 [32]	R	✓	✓	✓	✓		✓		✓
Decker CL et al., 2004 [33]	R		✓		✓		✓	✓	
Mentes JC et al., 2002 [34]	R			✓					
Snyder M et al., 2001 [35]	R		✓	✓					
Cohen-Mansfield J et al., 2002 [36]	R		✓						
Sherrell K et al., 1997 [37]	R	✓	✓			✓		✓	
Phillips LR et al., 1995 [38]	R			✓					
Williams SG et al., 1993 [39]	R		✓		✓		✓		
Cassel CK et al., 1988 [40]	R		✓				✓	✓	
Cohen-Mansfield J et al., 1988 [41]	R		✓						
Lipsitz LA et al., 1987 [42]	R		✓	✓			✓		
Palumbo FB et al., 1987 [43]	R	✓					✓		
Simpson P et al., 2017 [44]	FM, R		✓		✓				
Froggatt K et al., 2016 [45]	R	✓							
Jenkins C et al., 2016 [46]	S	✓		✓			✓	✓	
Tzouvara V et al., 2016 [47]	R	✓		✓					
Shepherd V et al., 2015 [48]	R	✓		✓		✓	✓	✓	
Davies SL et al., 2014 [49]	F, S	✓		✓					✓
Whelan PJ et al., 2013 [50]	R		✓						
Wood F et al., 2013 [51]	R		✓	✓	✓				
Goodman C et al., 2011 [52]	R	✓	✓	✓			✓		✓
Lasseter G et al., 2011 [53]	R		✓						✓
Hall S et al., 2009 [54]	R		✓						
Zermansky AG et al., 2007 [55]	R	✓	✓	✓				✓	✓
Hart E et al., 2005 [56]	R							✓	
Hubbard G et al., 2003 [57]	R		✓			✓			
Shah A, 1998 [58]	R			✓			✓		
Murfield J et al., 2011 [59]	R	✓	✓			✓		✓	
Peri K et al., 2008 [60]	R			✓				✓	
Bloch F et al., 2014 [61]	R		✓						
Heggestad AKT et al., 2013 [62]	R		✓	✓	✓		✓		

were suspicious of the investigators' motives for entering the facility [37, 52]. Some might have felt threatened by an outsider investigating their service, or felt that research was uninteresting and that the results would not be applicable to their facilities [30]. There were also concerns that research might not reflect a true picture of the facility, with the potential risk of resident abuse being observed and reported to the licensing agency [25, 30]. Some administrators claimed to be too busy to return calls or messages from investigators, or simply declined without any explanation [25, 43, 47]. In contrast, some LTC facility owners only consented to research studies to prevent jeopardizing government funding [37].

Investigators also face logistical challenges. In the experiences of several investigators, experimental treatments or placebos were not always administered according to plan during the investigators' absence [24, 49, 59]. Medical and hospitalization records might not be easily accessible, due to little uniformity in the collection of health records [28, 55]. Additionally, if confidential interviews are held as part of a research study, an appropriate environment may not be available in a LTC facility due to space constraints [45, 59].

Resident factors

There were 24 studies which reported challenges that fall under this theme [27–29, 31–33, 35–37, 39–42, 44, 50–55, 57, 59, 61, 62]. Some major issues included in this theme were: recruitment, consent, residents prefer treatment over placebo, and attrition.

LTC residents are a highly heterogeneous group with different backgrounds and health conditions. As a result, their recruitment, retention, and ability to consent and participate are all potentially problematic. Some authors reported the resident recruitment phase to be the most difficult part of research in LTC, especially among residents with dementia, with a success rate of 0% to 46% in one study [53]. In another study, Bloch et al. reported that only 44% of LTC residents were willing to participate in trials, in hopes that it would provide personal benefit [61].

Participants often preferred to receive the treatment rather than the placebo, creating bias and making randomization difficult [40, 59]. On the other hand, many residents were not even willing to participate, as they did not trust the motives of the investigators and disliked the interruption to their daily routine [28, 54]. On average, low-risk observational studies experienced higher recruitment rates, whereas pharmacologic studies involving residents with frail conditions had much lower rates [36, 42, 51]. Residents often stated the following reasons for refusal: "I am too old for this type of experiment"; "I am afraid of taking an ineffective drug"; "I am already using a lot of drugs"; "I don't want to be a guinea pig" [61]. Some residents were afraid of invasive interventions, such as venipuncture or urethral catheterization [42]. Finally, recruitment within minority groups was even less successful due to cultures that might not value research participation, and the additional cost of hiring interpreters, resulting in minorities being under-represented in LTC research [24, 32, 33].

Many residents did not consent to participate in research, as they did not see how they could personally benefit from the study within their lifetime [28, 33, 36, 42, 61]. Others perceived research as an invasion of privacy, afraid that confidentiality would not be maintained [39–41, 54, 62]. The concern of lack of confidentiality was attributed to the fact that some residents shared a room with other residents, and the doors were likely kept open during the process [33, 54]. Many also felt uncomfortable with certain research topics, including sexuality, dementia and death [44, 52].

Many residents who were sick or cognitively impaired may not have had the capacity to give consent or to effectively communicate verbally [37, 44, 57]. Despite this, investigators included cognitively impaired residents, because most residents in LTC facilities typically have some degree of cognitive impairment [27, 55]. As such, recruitment requirements needed to be adjusted according to the level of disability in each facility [42].

Obtaining informed consent from LTC residents, including cognitively impaired and emotionally unstable candidates, was described as difficult and time consuming [28, 40, 50, 54, 59]. Residents' ability to consent could change during the research period, and some were excluded unnecessarily due to incorrect evaluations of their ability to consent [40, 51, 62]. Some residents lost interest during the lengthy consent process and others felt pressured by the investigators [28, 32]. Obtaining consent for research on short-stay subjects in LTC facilities was problematic due to the time constraints [31]. (The challenge of obtaining consent from residents with cognitive impairment is also listed and elaborated under Ethical/Legal Factors).

Even when investigators successfully recruited enough participants in a study, retention and attrition is a common issue, due to study withdrawal, high mortality, comorbidity, hospitalizations and transfers to another facility [29, 33, 51, 55]. In particular, some residents could not complete the study because of mood or behavioral problems [35]. For example, participants could become aggressive or agitated, or could refuse to take part because they wish to avoid disruptions to their daily routine [35]. Even if they continue to participate despite being in an agitated state, the data obtained may not be accurate [57]. (Attrition is also noted as an issue under the Methodological Factors theme).

Staff caregiver factors

There were 19 studies which reported challenges that could be categorized under this theme [24, 25, 28, 31, 32, 34–36, 38, 42, 46–49, 51, 52, 55, 58, 60, 62]. Some major issues included in this theme were: time constraint, turnover, low education level, and uncooperative attending physicians.

Staff time constraint was a major obstacle in arranging for training and execution of research [28, 31, 34, 35, 42, 46, 47, 49, 58]. In order to participate in research, LTC staff are often required to attend meetings, accompany investigators to see residents, help contact families, assist in obtaining consent, and take part in the intervention, all in addition to their regular responsibilities [24, 25, 28, 34, 52]. Initial staff enthusiasm might wear out quickly once they realize the amount of time commitment required [34, 51]. Peri et al. found that staff willingness was the main factor affecting recruitment rates [60]. If the nurses do agree to participate in a study, their assessments of residents may not necessarily be reliable, as not all nurses may be aware of the details of residents' conditions nor do they correctly recommend appropriate candidates for research [32, 62].

Another concern is high staff turnover, making it harder to carry out studies [24, 28, 34, 46]. In our experience this is a particular concern when nursing assessments are primary outcome measures, and changes in the main rater may compromise validity.

According to Phillips et al., power dynamics in LTC facilities could be complex and consequently, non-professional staff caregivers might have unexpected influences on research [38]. For instance, interventions may not have been carried out as planned when investigators were not on-site [38]. As well, the education levels among non-professional caregivers can be low and some may be hesitant to serve as witnesses to the consent process [32, 38].

Medical staff can pose other challenges. Attending physicians at a facility might be concerned about 'outsider' physicians being involved with 'their residents' [24]. There may also be billing or compensation issues [24, 31, 51]. Private physicians might not have returned calls or met with the investigators, or refused to co-operate in providing medical records [31, 48, 55].

Family caregiver factors

A total of 7 studies noted challenges that fall under this theme [24, 32, 33, 39, 44, 51, 62]. Some major issues included in this theme were: constraint of their own physical condition, schedule and education level; see no benefits to the residents, view research as invasion of privacy.

Seeking consent and assent from family members was challenging due to their own physical conditions, work schedules, visit times or education levels [24, 32, 33, 51]. While many family members believed that elderly residents should take part in studies, their opinions changed when the subjects had dementia or when they felt that there was an invasion of privacy [39]. Some believed that residents should receive financial compensation for participating in research [39]. Others had reservations about relatives participating in clinical studies, even if the latter had agreed, as they felt that there was nothing for the residents to gain or that the topic of study (e.g. sexuality) was inappropriate [24, 44, 51, 62]. It was also difficult to have family caregivers attend regular meetings during the research period [33].

Investigator factors

A total of 5 studies reported challenges that fall under this theme [25, 37, 48, 57, 59]. Some major issues included in this theme were: principal investigators (PIs) perceived as threat or outsiders, and high turnover of research assistants (RAs).

In certain countries including the United Kingdom, a PI is required to be available on-site during the intervention(s) [48]. PIs from outside the institutions can be seen as 'outsiders' or threats to the LTC facilities [25, 37]. For PIs and RAs who work primarily in other institutions, travel to the facility and communication with staff in the LTC can be significant potential barriers. Examples of communication problems included phone calls or letters from external PIs/RAs being ignored by LTC staff [25]. PIs and RAs also need to have special verbal and non-verbal communication skills to collect data from subjects with cognitive impairments, which can add to the cost due to the additional training required [57].

The cost to hire enough RAs and their high turnover are other barriers to research in LTC facilities, especially since RAs are essential in overseeing the logistics of the research process, in order to avoid over-dependence on the facilities' manpower [59].

Ethical/legal factors

A total of 15 studies reported challenges that fall under this theme [24, 25, 28, 30, 32, 33, 39, 40, 42, 43, 46, 48, 52, 58, 62]. Some major issues included in this theme were: obtaining consent legally and ethically, withholding of likely effective treatments, and lack of IRB or REB familiar with LTC.

Ethical issues were significant challenges noted by many investigators. Consenting individuals who lack the physical and mental capacity to participate in a study, especially when discomfort, pain, psychological distress or physical risk are potential side-effects, was seen as potentially problematic by some investigators [30, 42, 46, 48]. It was also an ethical dilemma when investigators incidentally discovered any sub-standard or inadequate treatment of residents in the LTC facilities during the research process [25, 33, 40, 58]. Furthermore, having a placebo group was another ethical issue when patients were knowingly withheld from a treatment that was known to improve outcomes [28]. Finally, research on subjects with dementia posed several issues, as many patients may have been unaware of their diagnosis and the concern that LTC administration might use the study's findings as a reason to raise fees for those individual patients [52, 62]. (Obtaining consent from cognitively impaired residents is also listed as a challenge under Resident Factors).

In addition to ethical challenges, researchers also encountered legal concerns when conducting their studies in LTC facilities [30, 52]. For instance while ethics committees or institutional review boards (IRBs) are required for approval of research projects, many LTC facilities lack such an oversight body [28, 30, 39, 40, 43, 62]. Since many LTC facilities do not have internal IRBs, they have to rely on external ones, which can be time consuming and troublesome, as the members of external boards may lack first-hand knowledge about LTC facilities [24, 25, 30, 32, 48, 58]. These regulatory challenges have been shown to affect LTC facilities' decision to participate in research [52].

Methodological factors

There were 11 studies which described challenges that can be categorized under this theme [27, 29, 33, 37, 40, 46, 48, 55, 56, 59, 60]. Some major issues included in this theme were: randomization and finding suitable outcome measures.

Clinical trials were described as being more complex and time consuming to set up than observational studies in LTC settings [48]. Attrition due to resident turnover and mortality posed a challenge to study design [27, 29, 37]. (Attrition is also discussed as an issue under the theme Resident Factors). Randomization of individual residents was also troublesome in clinical trials, as some residents did not understand the importance of randomization and preferred to be subjects in the active treatment groups rather than controls [40].

Some investigators tried to overcome the problem of randomization with cluster randomization, where entire institutions were randomized to either the treatment or placebo group [27, 46]. However, a larger sample size is required to achieve adequate statistical power for cluster randomization, in order to account for the correlation among subjects within a cluster [29, 46]. As a result, several studies attempted to stratify multiple LTC facilities by type, size, and quality of care, which required more resources and complicated the standardization of study protocols [27, 29, 33, 55].

Another challenge of conducting research in LTC facilities was in selecting a suitable outcome measure customized for the LTC environment and its specific population [27, 33, 56, 59, 60]. While there are increasing numbers of rating scales that have been developed specifically with LTC environment in mind (e.g. the Neuropsychiatric Inventory- Nursing Home version [63]), due to the residents' varying cognitive and functional abilities as well as their ability to communicate, many instruments and scales designed for non-LTC populations needed to be adapted before usage [27, 33].

Budgetary factors

A total of 6 studies reported challenges related to this theme [25, 32, 49, 52, 53, 55] . The major issue of this theme was high costs.

The cost of conducting research in LTC facilities could be over three times higher than studies conducted in community settings [55]. The high cost of research was primarily attributed to the lengthy recruitment process of facilities, residents and staff [25, 32, 49, 52, 53]. Other incidental costs might need to be considered including approval costs from an external REB, travel expenses to and from the LTC for investigator and RAs, and specific training of LTC staff [32, 49, 52]. Other budgetary barriers not mentioned in the included studies but were known to us from our own research experience included costs for transportation of drugs and for use of the LTC pharmacy, as well as equipment and storage costs in the LTC. Finally, the research costs are even higher when interpreters are needed in LTC facilities with large non-English speaking populations [32].

Discussion

Though lacking the attention that research in the acute care setting receives, research in LTC is important because the setting houses a population that suffers disproportionately from chronic diseases and functional deficits, consumes more medication, and has more complex health care needs than many groups [25, 40, 48, 61]. In the UK, for example, one third of the people with dementia live in LTC and approximately 80% of LTC residents have dementia, making LTC a logical location for dementia research [46]. Apart from benefits to the general population, research results from LTC are potentially more beneficial to LTC residents as they as a group are unique for their frailty and multiple-morbidity, and research results from other settings may not always be generalizable to them [55].

We think more education to residents and families about the unique advantages of LTC research in order to foster a culture of research study participation is needed. Immediate, direct benefits to participants may not frequently be obtainable, but numerous indirect benefits such as diversion from daily routine, opportunity to meet and interact with people, greater access to professional care, and to be able to feel useful and meaningful by making altruistic contribution, are not necessarily trivial to residents' well-being [2]. While LTC facilities appear to be perfect 'clinical laboratories' with 24-h on-site staff, a controlled environment and long-staying residents, there are in fact many challenges that investigators face when conducting research in these institutions [38]. We have summarized the challenges and potential solutions in Table 2.

Table 2 Suggested Solutions to Research Challenges

Challenges	Specific Issues	Suggested Solutions
Facility/owner/administrator factors	Recruitment & retention of facilities	- PI develop long-standing relationship with LTC facility [24, 47] - Establish LTC research network [49] - Target facilities with history of research participation [47] - Provide continuing education opportunities to staff
	- Unfamiliar with research - Not interested - Feel threatened	- Improve education for owners and administrators [25, 26, 49] - Share research ownership [24, 47] - Include administration in study design and development
Resident factors	- Recruitment - Consent - Lack of trust - No personal benefit - Invasion of privacy	- Carefully designed, concise, and easy to understand recruitment materials [24, 43] - Assure privacy despite difficulties [43] - Emphasize to residents that their decision will not affect relationship with staff [42] - Offer financial compensation [42] - Develop flexible recruitment criteria [28] - Have trained home staff members do the initial approach for participation
	Prefer treatment over placebo	- Double-blinded, cluster randomization [27, 46] - Educate residents about the benefits of participation e.g. more intense monitoring
	Attrition	- Consider possibility of high attrition when calculating sample size
Staff caregiver factors	Time constraint & disruption to schedule	- Careful planning to minimize disruption - Offer financial compensation
	Turnover	- Recruitment of residents and study assessment carried out by investigators or RAs to reduce burden on LTC staff [28]
	Low education level	- Improve training on staff caregivers [49]
	Uncooperative attending physicians	- Offer a contract or letter of agreement [48] - Provide continuing education and online training [48]
Family caregiver factors	Constraint of their own physical condition, schedule, education level	- Carefully designed, concise, and easy to understand recruitment materials [24, 43] - Reduce travel/meeting time of family caregivers
	Sees no benefits to the resident	- Offer financial compensation [42] - Educate families about the benefits of participation e.g. more intense monitoring
	Invasion of privacy	- Assure privacy despite difficulties [43]
Investigator factors	Seen as a threat or an outsider	- PI develop long-standing relationship with LTC facility [24, 47] - Share research ownership [24, 47]
	High turnover of RAs	- Prioritize selection, training and support for RAs [34]
Ethical/legal factors	Obtaining consent legally and ethically	- Investigators should educate themselves about relevant regulations [32]

Table 2 Suggested Solutions to Research Challenges *(Continued)*

Challenges	Specific Issues	Suggested Solutions
		- Establish standard procedures for obtaining consent
	Lack of internal REB that is familiar with LTC	- Collaborate with the LTC administration to determine which REB will be consulted
Methodological factors	Resident randomization	- Consider cluster randomization [3, 9] - Consider quasi-experimental design [3, 9]
	Outcome measures	- Use outcome measures designed specifically for LTC - Adapt outcome measures not specific to LTC if necessary [27, 33]
Budgetary factors	High cost	- Good planning and coordination to reduce costs - Budget cautiously with travel costs and site specific factors in mind

Since recruitment of facilities, staff, and residents, along with obtaining resident consent are major concerns, some authors suggest that these challenges can be reduced if PIs develop long-standing, respectful relationships with LTC facilities and share ownership of the studies [24, 47]. Other methods to increase recruitment include establishing LTC research networks, providing better research training for LTC staff, and inviting the administrator(s) to take an active role in research studies, including participation in study design and share research ownership [24–26, 47, 49]. It is also recommended that PIs target institutions with a history of successful research participation [47]. PIs should pay extra attention to the selection, retention, training and support of RAs, as they are crucial to the success of a research project [34]. Attending physicians' participation can be encouraged by offering a formal contract, continuing education sessions and online training in preparation for the project [48], while better training should also be arranged for staff caregivers with lower education levels [49]. Disruption to the daily schedule of LTC facilities should be minimized with careful planning, or financial compensation can be offered to the staff affected.

In order to encourage resident and family consent, recruitment materials must be carefully designed, concise and easy to understand [24, 43]. Benefits of participation should be communicated to family caregivers. Travel and meeting times may be reduced to facilitate participation of family caregivers who might be constraint by their own physical condition, schedule and education level. Financial compensation to family caregiver may be another incentive to encourage participation [42]. Resident privacy must also be assured, although this may be difficult to maintain given the layout of certain facilities [43]. Likewise, residents and families should be informed that their decision to participate in a study will not affect their relationship with staff caregivers [42]. Trust of residents may also be improved by having trained staff caregivers with whom the residents are familiar do the initial approach for recruitment. As well, it is essential that recruitment requirements are flexible to the degree of disability in each facility, and some authors have suggested that monetary incentives can help increase resident recruitment [28, 42]. In order to counter some residents' preference to be in the treatment rather than placebo group, cluster randomization where a whole institution or ward is assigned to the same group, and/or double-blinding where caregivers do not know which group residents are assigned, may be used [27, 46]. High attrition rate should be considered when calculating sample size.

Legal and ethical challenges are relatively universal across LTC facilities and investigators must educate themselves about all relevant local and national regulations before conducting research in LTC facilities [32]. Determining what body will act as the IRB for the study should be done in consultation with the LTC administration. Having standard operating procedures for obtaining informed consent is also highly recommended.

In regard to the methodology of research studies, while investigators should aim for rigorous designs using control groups, randomization and concurrent data collection, compromises such as quasi-experimental designs and cluster randomization can also be considered [3, 9]. Sample size calculations should include consideration of attrition due to withdrawals, death and transfers. Pre-specified rules can be designed for dealing with caregiver changes. Whenever possible, utilizing rating scales and outcome measures designed for LTC is preferable to adapting measures designed for community dwelling individuals. Finally, considering special budgetary considerations for performing the study in a LTC environment is highly recommended.

Many of the challenges and barriers to research described above would be similar to studying a frail elderly patient population in acute care or community samples. For example, in terms of recruiting sites from an acute hospital setting, in two recent larger scale clinical trials on subjects of variable age groups, 31% and 43% of hospitals contacted eventually participated [64, 65], and while higher than the LTC site recruitment figures quoted above, these are still low. In terms of under-recruitment and attrition of elderly subjects in clinical studies, this factor is certainly not unique to LTC and is evident in many health care settings [10, 66, 67]. For instance, recruitment rates for clinical studies involving the in community and hospital settings vary greatly, with examples ranging from figures as low as 3.4%, and as high as 89.9% [67–72]. Staff time constraint or staff non-cooperation as a barrier to research participation is also not exclusive to LTC. For example, they are common reasons for non-participation in research in hospitals or palliative care facilities as well [65, 73]. Methodological challenges are not limited to research in LTC. Setting up of clinical trials, achievement of proper randomization, and selection or development of suitable outcome measures are all common challenges found in health care research in various settings [74, 75]. Finally, funding or budgetary factors is a commonly reported challenge for health care research in any setting, though some authors believe it is particularly challenging in LTC [40, 76, 77]. Having noted these similarities, we still believe the LTC setting is unique. As stated above, the patient population in LTC is generally older and frailer cognitively and physically, with greater medical comorbidity and medication polypharmacy. LTC residents are "residents" and not "patients" – the LTC facility is their home, changing the context of the relationship between subject and investigator likely affecting recruitment. The LTC facilities are generally not connected with general hospitals and universities, and are therefore unfamiliar with a research culture. Administrators may see research participation as a way to raise the profile of their LTC, or alternatively, an inconvenient and disruptive distraction from the business of caring for their elderly residents. These differences are more than sufficient to require investigators' attention if successful research is to be conducted in these unique settings.

There are some limitations to our study. We restricted our search to English language materials only, which may have led to bias against non-English papers which may be smaller scale studies, or studies with less remarkable results [78]. With our search strategies, we searched for explicit reports of challenges that contain any of the keywords such as 'challenge', 'barrier', 'issue', 'factor', 'recruit', 'problem', 'attrition', 'difficult', 'dropout', 'retention', etc. in the titles or abstracts (see Additional file 1 for complete search strategy). We did not scan through all empirical studies in LTC without these keywords to look for mention of challenges or possible solutions. While we believe the chance of missing papers focused on challenges or barriers without these keywords is low, this remains a potential limitation of our study. Finally, the thematic synthesis approach we used, as with any qualitative research method, involves a certain level of subjective judgement of the reviewers involved [22]. But despite all these limitations, we believe we are able to present a summary of the literature based on the actual experience of researchers who have conducted researches in LTC.

Conclusions

This systematic review searched and summarized studies reporting challenges of conducting research in LTC facilities. With a thematic synthesis approach, we were able to categorize the challenges noted in the 39 studies into 8 main themes: facility/owner/administrator factors, resident factors, staff caregiver factors, family caregiver factors, investigator factors, ethical/legal factors, methodological factors and budgetary factors. We think this integrative framework of 8 main themes can assist readers in understanding the challenges reported in the literature to date.

Investigators should familiarize themselves with these challenges and attempt to address each barrier in advance through careful planning. Stakeholders including IRBs, LTC owners, administrators, staff representatives and physicians should be consulted at an early stage and have input into study design. Ideally, residents and family caregivers should also provide input and/or feedback. In this way, research in LTC becomes a partnership in which quality of care and quality of life can ultimately benefit.

Abbreviations

IRB: Institutional review board; LTC: Long-term care; PI: Principal investigator; RA: Research assistant; REB: Research ethics board

Funding

Dr. Nathan Herrmann is funded in part by the Canadian Consortium on Neurodegeneration in Aging, supported by the Canadian Institute of Health Research and its partners. The funding source played no role in study design; in the collection, analysis and interpretation of data; in the writing of the report; and in the decision to submit the article for publication.

Authors' contributions

NH, SC, HRL: conception and design; NH: administrative support; HRL, HL, RC, LR: provision of study materials; HRL, SC, KT, KB: collection and assembly of data; All authors: data analysis and interpretation; All authors: manuscript writing and editing; All authors: final approval of manuscript.

Competing interests

Unrelated to the current study, Dr. Herrmann has received research funding from Lundbeck, Roche and Axovant and consultation fees from Merck, Lilly, Astellas and Mediti. None of the other authors have disclosures.

References

1. Andersen F, Engstad TA, Straume B, Viitanen M, Halvorsen DS, Hykkerud S, et al. Recruitment methods in Alzheimer's disease research: general practice versus population based screening by mail. BMC Med Res Methodol. 2010;10:35.
2. Slaughter S, Cole D, Jennings E, Reimer MA. Consent and assent to participate in research from people with dementia. Nurs Ethics. 2007;14(1):27–40.
3. Maas ML, Kelley LS, Park M, Specht JP. Issues in conducting research in nursing homes. West J Nurs Res. 2002;24(4):373–89.
4. Kontis V, Bennett JE, Mathers CD, Li G, Foreman K, Ezzati M. Future life expectancy in 35 industrialised countries: projections with a Bayesian model ensemble. Lancet. 2017;389(10076):1323–35.
5. Challenges in Research and Practice in Residential Long-Term Care. J Nurs Scholarsh. 2017;49(1):3–5.
6. Birnbaum AK, Rarick JO, Pettus TK, Mielke JW, McCarthy TC, Leppik IE. Recruiting elderly nursing home subjects for antiepileptic drug studies. Epilepsy Curr. 2013;13:437–8.
7. Statistics Canada. Census in brief: living arrangement of seniors. Ottawa: Statistics Canada; 2011. http://www12.statcan.gc.ca/census-recensement/2011/as-sa/98-312-x/98-312-x2011003_4-eng.pdf. Accessed on 15 Aug 2017
8. Werner CA. 2010 Census briefs: the older population. Washington, DC: U.S. Census Bureau; 2011. https://www.census.gov/prod/cen2010/briefs/c2010br-09.pdf. Accessed on 15 Aug 2017
9. Buckwalter KC, Grey M, Bowers B, McCarthy AM, Gross D, Funk M, et al. Intervention research in highly unstable environments. Res Nurs Health. 2009;32(1):110–21.
10. McMurdo ME, Roberts H, Parker S, Wyatt N, May H, Goodman C, et al. Improving recruitment of older people to research through good practice. Age Ageing. 2011;40(6):659–65.
11. Schulz R. Some critical issues in caregiver intervention research. Aging Ment Health. 2001;5(Suppl 1):S112–5.
12. Allen S, Francis K, O'Connor M, Chapman Y. Gaining human ethics approval: a strategy for refining research studies. Monash Bioeth Rev. 2008;27(3):54–60.
13. Cassel CK. Research in nursing homes. Ethical issues. J Am Geriatr Soc. 1985; 33(11):795–9.
14. Suhonen R, Stolt M, Leino-Kilpi H. Older people in long-term care settings as research informants: ethical challenges. Nurs Ethics. 2013;20(5):551–67.
15. Eeles E, Rockwood K. Delirium in the long-term care setting: clinical and research challenges. J Am Med Dir Assoc. 2008;9(3):157–61.
16. Igou J. Incontinence in nursing homes. Research and treatment issues from the nursing perspective. Clin Geriatr Med. 1986;2(4):873–85.
17. Kehinde JO, Pope C, Amella EJ. Methodological issues in fall prevention research involving older adults in long-term care facilities. Res Gerontol Nurs. 2011;4(4):294–304.
18. Ruckdeschel K, Van Haitsma K. Research with nursing home staff: challenges and solutions. J Ment Health Aging. 1997;3(2):209–19.
19. Reed J, Cook G, Focus CM. Research governance issues in the care home sector. NT Res. 2004;9(6):430–9.
20. University of York Centre of Reviews and Dissemination. PROSPERO - international prospective register of systematic reviews. UK: NHS; 2017. https://www.crd.york.ac.uk/PROSPERO/. Accessed on 28 Oct 2017
21. Moher D, Liberati A, Tetzlaff J, Altman DG, the Prisma group. Preferred reporting items for systematic reviews and meta-analyses: the PRISMA statement. Ann Intern Med. 2009;151(4):264–9.
22. Thomas J, Harden A. Methods for the thematic synthesis of qualitative research in systematic reviews. BMC Med Res Methodol. 2008;8(1):45.
23. Provalis. QDA Miner Lite QC: Montreal, 2016; https://provalisresearch.com/products/qualitative-data-analysis-software/freeware/. Accessed on 15 Aug 2017.
24. Zapka J, Amella E, Magwood G, Madisetti M, Garrow D, Batchelor-Aselage M. Challenges in efficacy research: the case of feeding alternatives in patients with dementia. J Adv Nurs. 2014;70(9):2072–85.
25. Garcia C, Kelley CM, Dyck MJ. Nursing home recruitment: trials, tribulations, and successes. Appl Nurs Res. 2013;26(3):136–8.
26. Tilden VP, Thompson SA, Gajewski BJ, Buescher CM, Bott MJ. Sampling challenges in nursing home research. J Am Med Dir Assoc. 2013;14(1):25–8.
27. Ersek M, Polissar N, Pen AD, Jablonski A, Herr K, Neradilek MB. Addressing methodological challenges in implementing the nursing home pain management algorithm randomized controlled trial. Clin Trials. 2012;9(5):634–44.
28. Greenspan S, Nace D, Perera S, Ferchak M, Fiorito G, Medich D, et al. Lessons learned from an osteoporosis clinical trial in frail long-term care residents. Clin Trials. 2012;9(2):247–56.
29. Van Ness PH, Peduzzi PN, Quagliarello VJ. Efficacy and effectiveness as aspects of cluster randomized trials with nursing home residents: methodological insights from a pneumonia prevention trial. Contemp Clin Trials. 2012;33(6):1124–31.
30. Hickman SE, Cartwright JC, Young HM. Administrators' perspectives on ethical issues in long-term care research. J Empir Res Hum Res Ethics. 2008; 3(1):69–78.
31. Quinn CC, Port CL, Zimmerman S, Gruber-Baldini AL, Kasper JD, Fleshner I, et al. Short-stay nursing home rehabilitation patients: transitional care problems pose research challenges. J Am Geriatr Soc. 2008;56(10):1940–5.
32. Gismondi PM, Hamer DH, Leka LS, Dallal G, Fiatarone Singh MA, Meydani SN. Strategies, time, and costs associated with the recruitment and enrollment of nursing home residents for a micronutrient supplementation clinical trial. J Gerontol A-Biol Sci Med Sci. 2005;60(11):1469–74.
33. Decker CL, Adamek ME. Meeting the challenges of social work research in long-term care. Soc Work Health Care. 2004;38(3):47–65.
34. Mentes JC, Tripp-Reimer T. Barriers and facilitators in nursing home intervention research. West J Nurs Res. 2002;24(8):918–36.
35. Snyder M, Tseng Y, Brandt C, Croghan C, Hanson S, Constantine R, et al. Challenges of implementing intervention research in persons with dementia: example of a glider swing intervention. Am J Alzheimers Dis Other Demen. 2001;16(1):51–6.
36. Cohen-Mansfield J. Recruitment rates in gerontological research: the situation for drug trials in dementia may be worse than previously reported. Alzheimer Dis Assoc Disord. 2002;16(4):279–82.

37. Sherrell K, Buckwalter KC. Geropsychiatry. Barriers to follow-up studies with the chronically mentally ill elderly in long-term care settings. J Gerontol Nurs. 1997;23(8):37–40.
38. Phillips LR, Van Ort S. Issues in conducting intervention research in long-term care settings. Nurs Outlook. 1995;43(6):249–53.
39. Williams SG. How do the elderly and their families feel about research participation? Geriatr Nurs. 1993;14(1):11–14.
40. Cassel CK. Ethical issues in the conduct of research in long term care. The Gerontologist. 1988;28(3 Suppl):90–6.
41. Cohen-Mansfield J, Kerin P, Pawlson G, Lipson S, Holdridge K. Informed consent for research in a nursing home: processes and issues. The Gerontologist. 1988;28(3):355–9.
42. Lipsitz LA, Pluchino FC, Wright SM. Biomedical research in the nursing home: methodological issues and subject recruitment results. J Am Geriatr Soc. 1987;35(7):629–34.
43. Palumbo FB, Magaziner JS, Tenney JH. Recruitment of long-term care facilities for research. J Am Geriatr Soc. 1987;35(2):154–8.
44. Simpson P, Wilson CB, Brown LJ, Dickinson T, Horne M. The challenges and opportunities in researching intimacy and sexuality in care homes accommodating older people: a feasibility study. J Adv Nurs. 2017;73(1):127–37.
45. Froggatt K, Goodman C, Morbey H, Davies SL, Masey H, Dickinson A, et al. Public involvement in research within care homes: benefits and challenges in the APPROACH study. Health Expect. 2016;19(6):1336–45.
46. Jenkins C, Smythe A, Galant-Miecznikowska M, Bentham P, Oyebode J. Overcoming challenges of conducting research in nursing homes. Nurs Older People. 2016;28(5):16–23.
47. Tzouvara V, Papadopoulos C, Randhawa G. Lessons learned from recruiting nursing homes to a quantitative cross-sectional pilot study. Nurse Res. 2016; 23(4):35–9.
48. Shepherd V, Nuttall J, Hood K, Butler CC. Setting up a clinical trial in care homes: challenges encountered and recommendations for future research practice. BMC Res Notes. 2015;8:306.
49. Davies SL, Goodman C, Manthorpe J, Smith A, Carrick N, Iliffe S. Enabling research in care homes: an evaluation of a national network of research ready care homes. BMC Med Res Methodol. 2014;14:47.
50. Whelan PJ, Walwyn R, Gaughran F, Macdonald A. Impact of the demand for 'proxy assent' on recruitment to a randomised controlled trial of vaccination testing in care homes. J Med Ethics. 2013;39(1):36–40.
51. Wood F, Prout H, Bayer A, Duncan D, Nuttall J, Hood K, et al. Consent, including advanced consent, of older adults to research in care homes: a qualitative study of stakeholders' views in South Wales. Trials. 2013;14(1):247 (no pagination).
52. Goodman C, Baron NL, Machen I, Stevenson E, Evans C, Davies SL, et al. Culture, consent, costs and care homes: enabling older people with dementia to participate in research. Aging Ment Health. 2011;15(4):475–81.
53. Lasseter G, Donald I, Hapeshi J, McNulty C. Is the mental capacity act reducing generalizable research in care homes? Public Health. 2011;125(9):604–8.
54. Hall S, Longhurst S, Higginson IJ. Challenges to conducting research with older people living in nursing homes. BMC Geriatr. 2009;9(1):38 (no pagination).
55. Zermansky AG, Alldred DP, Petty DR, Raynor DK. Striving to recruit: the difficulties of conducting clinical research on elderly care home residents. J R Soc Med. 2007;100(6):258–61.
56. Hart E, Lymbery M, Gladman J. Methodological understandings and misunderstandings in interprofessional research: experiences of researching transitional rehabilitation for older people. J Interprof Care. 2005;19(6):614–23.
57. Hubbard G, Downs MG, Tester S. Including older people with dementia in research: challenges and strategies. Aging Ment Health. 2003;7(5):351–62.
58. Shah A. Difficulties with psychiatric research in nursing homes in Melbourne. Australas J Ageing. 1998;17(3):148–50.
59. Murfield J, Cooke M, Moyle W, Shum D, Harrison S. Conducting randomized controlled trials with older people with dementia in long-term care: challenges and lessons learnt. Int J Nurs Pract. 2011;17(1):52–9.
60. Peri K, Kerse N, Kiata L, Wilkinson T, Robinson E, Parsons J, et al. Promoting Independence in residential care: successful recruitment for a randomized controlled trial. J Am Med Dir Assoc. 2008;9(4):251–6.
61. Bloch F, Charasz N. Attitudes of older adults to their participation in clinical trials: a pilot study. Drugs Aging. 2014;31(5):373–7.
62. Heggestad AKT, Nortvedt P, Slettebo A. The importance of moral sensitivity when including persons with dementia in qualitative research. Nurs Ethics. 2013;20(1):30–40.
63. Cummings JL, Mega M, Gray K, Rosenberg-Thompson S, Carusi DA, Gornbein J. The neuropsychiatric inventory: comprehensive assessment of psychopathology in dementia. Neurol. 1994;44(12):2308–14.
64. Ellery F, Borschmann K, Bernhardt J, Morrison R, Langhorne P. Trials, tribulations and the truth: recruiting hospitals to a very early rehabilitation trial (AVERT-international). Neurorehabil Neural Repair. 2012;26(6):742–3.
65. Johnson AM, Jones SB, Duncan PW, Bushnell CD, Coleman SW, Mettam LH, et al. Hospital recruitment for a pragmatic cluster-randomized clinical trial: lessons learned from the COMPASS study. Trials. 2018;19(1):74.
66. Clegg A, Relton C, Young J, Witham M. Improving recruitment of older people to clinical trials: use of the cohort multiple randomised controlled trial design. Age Ageing. 2015;44(4):547–50.
67. McHenry JC, Insel KC, Einstein GO, Vidrine AN, Koerner KM, Morrow DG. Recruitment of older adults: success may be in the details. The Gerontologist. 2015;55(5):845–53.
68. Boustani MA, Campbell NL, Khan BA, Abernathy G, Zawahiri M, Campbell T, et al. Enhancing care for hospitalized older adults with cognitive impairment: a randomized controlled trial. J Gen Intern Med. 2012;27(5):561–7.
69. Gill TM, McGloin JM, Gahbauer EA, Shepard DM, Bianco LM. Two recruitment strategies for a clinical trial of physically frail community-living older persons. J Am Geriatr Soc. 2001;49(8):1039–45.
70. Kerr J, Rosenberg D, Millstein RA, Bolling K, Crist K, Takemoto M, et al. Cluster randomized controlled trial of a multilevel physical activity intervention for older adults. Int J Behav Nutr Phys Act. 2018;15(1):32 no pagination.
71. Piantadosi C, Chapman IM, Naganathan V, Hunter P, Cameron ID, Visvanathan R. Recruiting older people at nutritional risk for clinical trials: what have we learned? BMC Res Notes. 2015;8:151.
72. Sanson G, Bertocchi L, Dal Bo E, Di Pasquale CL, Zanetti M. Identifying reliable predictors of protein-energy malnutrition in hospitalized frail older adults: a prospective longitudinal study. Int J Nurs Stud. 2018;82:40–8.
73. Blum D, Inauen R, Binswanger J, Strasser F. Barriers to research in palliative care: a systematic literature review. Prog Palliat Care. 2015;23(2):75–84.
74. Li T, Jones CMC, Shah MN, Cushman JT, Jusko TA. Methodological challenges in studies comparing prehospital advanced life support with basic life support. Prehosp Disaster Med. 2017;32(4):444–50.
75. Weinberger M, Oddone EZ, Henderson WG, Smith DM, Huey J, Giobbie-Hurder A, et al. Multisite randomized controlled trials in health services research: scientific challenges and operational issues. Med Care. 2001;39(6):627–34.
76. Eichler HG, Sweeney F. The evolution of clinical trials: can we address the challenges of the future? Clin Trials. 2018;15(1_suppl):27–32.
77. Shore BJ, Nasreddine AY, Kocher MS. Overcoming the funding challenge: the cost of randomized controlled trials in the next decade. J Bone Joint Surg - Ser A. 2012;94(SUPPL. 1):101–6.
78. McDonagh M, Peterson K, Raina P, Chang S, Shekelle P. Avoiding bias in selecting studies. In: Methods Guide for Effectiveness and Comparative Effectiveness Reviews AHRQ Publication No 10(14)-EHC063-EF. Rockville: Agency for Healthcare Research and Quality; 2008. p. 9.

18

The prevalence and characteristics of frailty by frailty phenotype in rural Tanzania

Emma Grace Lewis[1,2,6*], Selina Coles[3], Kate Howorth[2], John Kissima[4], William Gray[2], Sarah Urasa[5], Richard Walker[1,2] and Catherine Dotchin[1,2]

Abstract

Background: The frailty phenotype is defined by the presence of three from the following five clinical features: weakness, slow walking speed, unintentional weight loss, exhaustion, and low physical activity. It has been widely applied in different research and clinical contexts, including across many low and middle-income countries. However, there is evidence that the operationalisation of each component of the frailty phenotype significantly alters its characteristics and predictive validity, and care is needed when applying the phenotype across settings. The study's objective was to operationalise the frailty phenotype in a rural Tanzanian population of older community-dwelling adults.

Methods: Consenting adults aged ≥60 years, and resident in five randomly selected villages of Hai district Demographic Surveillance Site, were eligible to participate in this cross-sectional study. From a screened sample of 1207 older adults, 235 were randomised and consented to an assessment of their frailty status by the frailty phenotype. Trained research fieldworkers (Tanzanian medical doctors and nurses) carried out measurements and questionnaires at local village centres or at participants' homes.

Results: The prevalence of the frailty phenotype, calculated from complete data for 196 participants, was 9.25% (95% CI 4.39–14.12) When missing data were counted as meeting frailty criterion (i.e. missing due to inability to perform an assessment), the prevalence increased to 11.22% (95% CI 7.11–15.32). Frailty by phenotype criteria was more common in older age groups, and was associated with self-assessed poor health and depression symptoms.

Conclusions: Frailty can be successfully estimated using the frailty phenotype, however there are challenges in its operationalisation cross-culturally. Further work is needed to explore the potential clinical application of the frailty phenotype in such settings.

Keywords: Prevalence, Frailty, Frailty phenotype, Older adults, Sub-Saharan Africa

Background

Frailty was described in 2001, as being a syndromic condition, distinct from, but overlapping with, disability and comorbidity [1]. The syndromic approach to frailty asserts that frailty can be described through the measurement of five physical features, and that frailty is present when three of these features are present, and pre-frailty when 1–2 features are present. The five physical features are: unintentional weight loss, weakness (low hand grip-strength), exhaustion, slow walking speed and low physical activity [1, 2]. The phenotype model is based on a proposed theoretical "cycle of frailty" which hypothesises that clinical features measurable in frailty, and its reduced physiologic reserve, are due to a cycle of factors including disease, chronic undernutrition, sarcopenia, and a reduced resting metabolic rate [1, 3]. Since the original Frailty Phenotype (FP) described by Fried et al. as part of the Cardiovascular Health Study [1], the phenotype model has been adapted and operationalised according to differing study designs, methodologies and settings.

In low and middle-income countries (LMIC), a recent systematic review found thirty six studies had used the FP to research frailty [4]. The need for cultural adaption

* Correspondence: grace.lewis@ncl.ac.uk
[1]Institute of Health and Society, Faculty of Medical Sciences, Newcastle University, Newcastle upon Tyne, UK
[2]Northumbria Healthcare NHS Foundation Trust, North Tyneside General Hospital, North Shields, UK
Full list of author information is available at the end of the article

of the phenotype model in LMIC settings, such as Tanzania, is particularly important due to issues such as resource constraints, lower background education levels and societal health and functional norms. How the FP is operationalised impacts on the prevalence of frailty, and its predictive ability [5]. A recent study has demonstrated this phenomenon when estimating the prevalence of frailty among older adults in rural Agincourt, South Africa, where each of the nine iterations of the FP constructed, gave corresponding estimates of prevalence varying between 3.0 and 13.2% [6]. However, the benefits of the FP include its relative ease of application, making it a potential tool for screening. The FP could be applied prior to any clinical assessment serving to highlight major problems or identify those most in need [7, 8]. Another benefit to the phenotype approach is the minimal amount of data required for its calculation, particularly when compared with the deficit accumulation approach to frailty (frailty index), which requires a minimum of 20 deficits to be counted in order to produce stable estimates [9, 10]. Therefore, the study's aim was to operationalise and measure the prevalence of the FP in a rural Tanzanian population of older community-dwelling adults.

Methods

A total sample of 1207 adults, living in five randomly selected villages in Hai district Demographic Surveillance Site (DSS), and aged ≥60 years were screened using the Brief Frailty Instrument for Tanzania (B-FIT) tool [11]. This short questionnaire, previously developed by our research team, was used to categorise participants into non-frail, pre-frail or frail [11]. A random selection of 79 (8.9%) of non-frail, 120 (42.1%) of pre-frail and 37 (94.7%) of frail formed a frailty-weighted cohort of 236 who underwent Comprehensive Geriatric Assessments (CGA), following the recommendations of the British Geriatrics Society [12]. One case was excluded due to large amounts of missing data, leaving 235 older adults, who were assessed for frailty according to the FP, in their homes or at a convenient local centre. Our construction of the Hai district DSS FP, is compared with Fried's FP in Table 1. In constructing a FP in our setting, we aimed to keep as close as possible to Fried's FP, so the five measured components of frailty were operationalised thus:

Weakness: Hand grip strength (HGS) was measured with participants sitting upright with the arm in flexion at 90 degrees. Three measurements were averaged from the participant's dominant hand using a JAMAR Hydraulic Hand Dynamometer (Model J000105, Lafayette Instruments, Lafayette, IN, USA).

Walking speed: Participants were asked to walk in a straight line, a distance of 4.5 m (15 ft). The distance was measured out on a flat floor surface using a rigid tape measure. The type of floor surface varied, for example participants who were assessed at their homes were often assessed walking outside due to limited space indoors. However, if the surface was slippery due to recent rain, or uneven, a surface indoors was found. At the local assessment centres (church buildings, dispensaries and local schools) smooth concrete floors were available. Walking speed was not adjusted for height or sex. Participants walked in their usual footwear and were permitted to use any walking aids.

Exhaustion: A positive response was counted, to either of the two Centre for Epidemiological Studies Depression scale (CES-D) statements [13]: "I felt that everything I did was an effort" or "I could not get going". These questions were translated verbatim to Swahili, and participants were asked to grade how often in the past week they had felt this way.

Weight loss: Participants were asked "Have you lost weight during the last 3 months?" with the option of answering "Weight loss greater than 3kg", "weight loss between 1 and 3kg", "no weight loss" or "does not know". This variable was turned from a categorical to a binary variable for analysis as described in Table 1. BMI was calculated from weight measured using Microlife Diagnostic WS 80 digital weighing scales and height using the Marsden Leicester Height Measure. Given that no serial measurements were possible, self-reported weight loss was preferred as a measure of unintentional weight loss.

Low physical activity: The International Physical Activity Questionnaire (IPAQ), [14] was used to record participants' estimations of their physical activity over the preceding 7 days. The IPAQ has been used widely, and in similar studies of older adults, for example the Ibadan study of ageing, from Nigeria [15]. Those who reported not being able to carry out tasks of moderate physical activity on any day of the previous week scored positively on this parameter. This was felt to be appropriate, given that carrying out "small works" in the home (such as using a winnowing basket or sharpening knives) was identified as a common norm for older adults in this context when developing a culturally adapted instrumental activities of daily living (IADLs) screening tool [16].

Frailty phenotype

Other recorded parameters: A questionnaire was conducted asking participants or responding close relatives about socio-demographic characteristics as well as self-reported diagnoses, including HIV-infection. The IDEA cognitive [17], and EURO-D [18], screening tools were used to screen for cognitive function and depression respectively. A short culturally specific Instrumental Activities of Daily Living (IADL) tool was used [16], where difficulty with any one of eleven

Table 1 Comparing operationalisation of the Hai DSS frailty phenotype with fried's frailty phenotype

Component measured in both	Hai DSS frailty phenotype	Fried's frailty phenotype
Weakness (low HGS): Average of three measurements in the dominant hand using the JAMAR hand-held dynamometer.	Frail criterion met if average HGS in the dominant hand <21Kg in males or < 10Kg in females based on the median HGS in African adults aged 61–70: 18 (10–25) women, 30 (21–38) men [21].	Stratified by gender and body mass index (BMI) quartiles: Men Cut-off for grip strength (Kg) criterion for frailty BMI ≤ 24 ≤ 29 BMI 24.1–26 ≤ 30 BMI 26.1–28 ≤ 30 BMI > 28 ≤ 32 Women BMI ≤ 23 ≤ 17 BMI 23.1–26 ≤ 17.3 BMI 26.1–29 ≤ 18 BMI > 29 ≤ 21
Slow walking speed: Walking at usual pace, 4.5 m (15 ft) use of walking aid is permitted.	The slowest quintile of the sample's walking speed was taken as cut-off: ≥11.12 s to walk 4.5 m distance (not stratified by gender or height).	Slowest quintile stratified by gender and height Men Height ≤ 173 cm ≥7 s Height > 173 cm ≥6 s Women Height ≤ 159 cm ≥7 s Height > 159 cm ≥6 s
Self-reported exhaustion: CES–D Depression Scale questions were used. Frailty criterion if either was felt to be present a "moderate amount of the time" or "most of the time" over the past week.	The CES-D questions were verbatim translated into Swahili by a Tanzanian doctor and statements read aloud and scored in the same manner as the Fried FP.	CES–D Depression Scale questions, the following two statements are read. (a) I felt that everything I did was an effort; (b) I could not get going. Frailty criterion if either was felt to be present a "moderate amount of the time" or "most of the time" over the past week.
Unintentional weight loss:	Has the participant/older person lost weight during the last 3 months? Frailty criterion were met if the participant answered either "yes, more than 3 kg", or "yes, between 1 and 3 kg".	"In the last year, have you lost more than 10 pounds unintentionally (i.e., not due to dieting or exercise)?" If yes, then frail for weight loss criterion, OR ≥5% of body weight lost in the past year unintentionally.
Low physical activity	Taken from the IPAQ: "During the last 7 days, on how many days did you do moderate physical activities like gardening, cleaning, bicycling at a regular pace, swimming or other fitness activities?" Those who answered "0", were categorised as meeting frailty criterion.	Based on the short version of the Minnesota Leisure Time Activity questionnaire Kcals per week expended are calculated using standardized algorithm. This variable is stratified by gender, with frailty criterion met if less than the lowest quintile of energy expended. *Men*: < 383 Kcals/week *Women*: < 270 Kcals/week.

instrumental activities, (e.g. carrying out small works in the home, giving advice and presiding over ceremonies) was classified as IADL disability.

Setting

The study was carried out across five villages in Hai DSS of rural Northern Tanzania between 24th February and 9th of August 2017. The five villages were stratified according to high-, middle-, and low-land locations, due to differing climate, ethnic background and agricultural practices across these strata.

The majority of the background population were subsistence farmers reliant on non-mechanised farming practises and on seasonal rains. There are two rainy seasons per year in this region, the long rains of February–April and short rains of November–December. The short rains which were expected in November 2016 were disappointing, meaning that the second harvest of the year was poor. The data collection period took place during the long rainy season of 2017, and into the first harvest season.

Data analysis

Data were collected by hand-held tablet devices using Open Data Kit (ODK) open source software [19]. Completed forms were uploaded to a secure ODK 0.2 aggregate online database. Downloaded data were cleaned in Microsoft Excel 2016 workbooks and imported to Stata/SE 15.0 for analysis. Simple descriptive statistics were calculated and unadjusted Chi-squared values are presented for frailty by variables of interest (Table 3). The alpha value was set at 0.05. When calculating the prevalence of frailty, the weighted stratification was taken into account, using inverse proportions. To calculate confidence intervals (CI), bootstrapping (Stata command 'svyset') was used to control for clustering by village and to adjust for the stratified weighting [12]. In primary analysis, cases with missing data necessary for calculating the FP were excluded from the analysis, and thus, were assumed missing completely at random and non-informative. In secondary analysis, values for missing data were imputed under the assumption that they were not missing completely at random and informative.

Results

Prevalence of frailty

The total study cohort of 235 people comprised 136 females (57.9%) and the average age was 74.8 years. The prevalence of frailty by Hai DSS FP, calculated from complete data for 196 participants, was 9.25% (95% CI 4.39–14.12).

Impact of missing data on estimated frailty prevalence

The number of assessments of walking speed and grip strength which were missing were 37 and 18, respectively. Interestingly, 11 of the 37 missing walking speed assessments were due to immobility following a stroke, suggesting that such data were not missing completely at random, and that these data were informative. Overall, of the 39 participants missing data for calculation of their FP, 36 (92.3%) were deemed frail by CGA [12]. In secondary analyses, except for two erroneous walking speed recordings which were deleted, all other missing data were presumed missing due to being unable to complete the assessment (i.e. due to frailty rather than missing at random), and thus categorised as meeting the frailty criterion. The CGA-derived frailty diagnoses for participants with missing data have been provided as supplementary online data in Additional file 1: Table S1. When the Hai DSS FP was calculated using this approach the prevalence of frailty increased to 11.22% (95% CI 7.11–15.32).

Correlates of frailty by phenotype

The mean walking speed was 0.65 m/s (std. dev 0.40, range 0.04–4.29 m/s), 0.72 m/s in men and 0.60 m/s in women. The mean dominant HGS was 21.9Kg (Std. dev 8.5, range 4.3–51.3), 18.92 Kg in women and 26.02 Kg in men. The mean BMI in women was 25.01 (std. dev 5.2, range 13.9–47.2), and in men was 21.21 (std. dev 5.5, range 13.4–53.3). Table 2 reports the frequencies and percentages of frailty components by sex. Around one third of participants had no frailty components ($n = 63$, 32.1%), while roughly one third had one frailty component ($n = 67$, 34.2%), and two participants fulfilled all five components of the FP criteria.

Frailty by Hai DSS FP was associated with older age groups, self-assessed poor health, self-reported chronic diseases and with self-assessed frailty status (Table 3). It is important to note that four individuals from 196, disclosed their HIV-infected status. Being assessed at home, rather than at a local centre was strongly associated with frailty by univariate analysis. Almost half of participants were married ($n = 97$, 49.5%), however frailty was significantly associated with being widowed, separated/divorced or single. Low levels of schooling, and low literacy levels, were also significant associations with frailty with 53 participants, (27.0%) having received no formal education. High numbers considered themselves to be ill ($n = 119$, 60.7%), or living with frailty ($n = 116$, 59.1%). Depression symptoms, as reported by the EURO-D screening tool [18], were significantly associated with frailty, as was a score indicative of cognitive impairment, according to the IDEA cognitive screening tool [17]. Around a fifth of participants were found to be underweight, according to BMI, while almost two fifths were either overweight or obese (Table 3), yet BMI was not found to be associated with frailty on univariate analysis.

Table 2 The Frequencies and percentages of Hai DSS frailty phenotype components

Frequency (%) of frailty components	Total $n = 196$	Males $n = 82$	Females $n = 114$
Exhaustion	82 (41.82)	32 (39.02)	50 (43.86)
Weight loss	53 (27.04)	23 (28.05)	30 (26.32)
Low physical activity	48 (24.49)	15 (18.29)	33 (28.95)
Slow walking	39 (19.90)	10 (12.20)	29 (25.44)
Weakness (Hand-grip strength)	29 (14.80)	22 (26.83)	7 (6.14)
Number of frailty components			
0	63 (32.14)	31 (37.80)	32 (28.07)
1	67 (34.18)	23 (28.05)	44 (38.60)
2	32 (16.33)	15 (18.29)	17 (14.91)
3	18 (9.18)	4 (4.88)	14 (12.28)
4	14 (7.14)	8 (9.76)	6 (5.26)
5	2 (1.02)	1 (1.22)	1 (0.88)

Table 3 Demographic and clinical characteristics of the study sample according to Hai DSS frailty phenotype status

Demographic characteristic	Total sample $n = 196$	FP not-frail $n = 63$	FP pre-frail $n = 99$	FP frail $n = 34$	Pearson Chi^2 (*P* value) for FP frailty vs FP not-frail/FP pre-frail
Age group					
60–69	85	37 (43.53)	43 (50.59)	5 (5.88)	
70–79	61	20 (32.79)	31 (50.82)	10 (16.39)	
≥80	50	6 (12.00)	25 (50.00)	19 (38.00)	**22.705 (< 0.0001)**
Sex					
Male	82	31 (37.80)	38 (46.34)	13 (15.85)	
Female	114	32 (28.07)	61 (53.51)	21 (18.42)	0.219 (0.640)
Location where assessed					
Elsewhere	139	52 (37.41)	76 (54.68)	11 (7.91)	
Home	57	11 (19.30)	23 (40.35)	23 (40.35)	**29.664 (< 0.0001)**
Tribe					
Mchagga	176	59 (33.52)	88 (50.00)	29 (16.48)	
Others	20	4 (20.00)	11 (55.00)	5 (25.00)	0.909 (0.340)
Living arrangements					
Lives with others	174	56 (32.18)	86 (49.43)	32 (18.39)	
Lives alone	21	7 (33.33)	12 (57.14)	2 (9.52)	1.023 (0.312)
Marital status					
Married	97	39 (40.21)	48 (49.48)	10 (10.31)	
Widowed, Separated/divorced or Single	99	24 (24.24)	51 (50.52)	24 (24.24)	**6.633 (0.010)**
Education					
Secondary and higher education	16	11 (68.75)	3 (18.75)	2 (12.50)	
Primary completed	56	21 (37.50)	31 (55.36)	4 (7.14)	
Some primary	71	21 (29.58)	37 (52.11)	13 (18.31)	
No school	53	10 (18.87)	28 (52.83)	15 (28.30)	**8.811 (0.032)**
Literacy "Do you know how to read and write? (Yes if able/was able to read or write)"					
Able to read/write well	89	41 (46.07)	39 (43.82)	9 (10.11)	
Read/write with difficulty	52	13 (25.00)	30 (57.69)	9 (17.31)	
Unable to read/write	55	9 (16.36)	30 (54.55)	16 (29.09)	**8.539 (0.014)**
EURO-D score					
Depression symptoms ≤3/12	105	43 (40.95)	49 (46.67)	13 (12.38)	
Depression symptoms ≥4/12	91	20 (21.98)	50 (54.95)	21 (23.38)	**3.889 (0.049)**
IDEA cognitive test score					
0–4 (poor cognitive function)	20	2 (10.00)	9 (45.00)	9 (45.00)	
5–7 (moderate cognitive function)	37	6 (16.22)	22 (59.46)	9 (24.32)	
8–12 (good cognitive function)	139	55 (39.57)	68 (48.92)	16 (11.51)	**15.225 (< 0.0001)**
Functional ability					
≥1 ADL disability	47	5 (10.64)	20 (42.55)	22 (46.81)	**37.428 (< 0.0001)**
≥1 IADL disability	60	8 (13.33)	24 (40.00)	28 (46.67)	**51.845 (< 0.0001)**
Healthcare provision					
Health insurance	51	19 (37.25)	22 (43.14)	10 (19.61)	
No health insurance	144	43 (29.86)	77 (53.47)	24 (16.67)	0.226 (0.634)
Ability to earn money or produce food					
Working	59	27 (45.76)	31 (52.54)	1 (1.69)	

Table 3 Demographic and clinical characteristics of the study sample according to Hai DSS frailty phenotype status *(Continued)*

Demographic characteristic	Total sample *n* = 196	FP not-frail *n* = 63	FP pre-frail *n* = 99	FP frail *n* = 34	Pearson Chi^2 (*P* value) for FP frailty vs FP not-frail/FP pre-frail
Not currently working	137	36 (26.28)	68 (49.64)	33 (24.09)	**14.422 (< 0.0001)**
Household facilities					
Electricity	89	31 (34.83)	38 (42.70)	20 (22.47)	
No electricity	107	32 (29.91)	61 (57.01)	14 (13.08)	2.986 (0.084)
Provision for old age					
Pension	14	8 (57.14)	5 (35.71)	1 (7.14)	
No pension	182	55 (30.22)	94 (51.65)	33 (18.13)	1.094 (0.295)
"Do you consider yourself currently ill?"					
Yes (Ill)	119	17 (14.29)	69 (57.98)	33 (27.73)	
No (not ill)	77	46 (59.74)	30 (38.96)	1 (1.30)	**22.781 (< 0.0001)**
"Do you consider yourself to be living with frailty currently?"					
Yes (Frail)	116	22 (18.97)	65 (56.03)	29 (25.00)	
No (not frail)	80	41 (51.25)	34 (42.50)	5 (6.25)	**11.609 (0.001)**
Self-assessed health: "How is your health?"					
Good/Very good	42	24 (57.14)	16 (38.10)	2 (4.76)	
Neither good nor poor	99	35 (35.35)	51 (51.52)	13 (13.13)	
Poor/Very poor	54	4 (7.41)	31 (57.41)	19 (35.19)	**17.778 (< 0.0001)**
Self-reported medical diagnoses: "Have you ever been told you have a diagnosis of any of the following?"					
Diabetes	19	7 (36.84)	8 (42.11)	4 (21.05)	0.201 (0.654)
Hypertension	58	18 (31.03)	27 (46.55)	13 (22.41)	1.475 (0.225)
Cataracts	15	3 (20.00)	6 (40.00)	6 (40.00)	**5.747 (0.017)**
Stroke	8	1 (12.50)	3 (37.50)	4 (50.00)	**6.145 (0.013)**
Heart disease	11	4 (36.36)	4 (36.36)	3 (27.27)	0.800 (0.371)
Arthritis	44	7 (15.91)	24 (54.55)	13 (29.55)	**5.788 (0.016)**
Depression	12	2 (16.67)	8 (66.67)	2 (16.67)	0.004 (0.949)
Chronic respiratory condition (asthma/COPD)	13	4 (30.77)	6 (46.15)	3 (23.08)	0.318 (0.572)
Number of self-reported chronic diseases					
0	70	27 (38.57)	40 (57.14)	3 (4.29)	
1	67	24 (35.82)	30 (44.78)	13 (19.40)	
≥2	59	12 (20.34)	29 (49.15)	18 (30.51)	**15.654 (< 0.0001)**
BMI kg/m^2					
Underweight (< 18.49)	40	11 (27.50)	24 (60.00)	5 (12.50)	
Normal weight (18.5–24.99)	79	21 (26.58)	41 (51.90)	17 (21.52)	
Overweight (25.00–29.99)	54	22 (40.74)	24 (44.44)	8 (14.81)	
Obese (≥30.00)	21	9 (42.86)	9 (42.86)	3 (14.29)	2.008 (0.571)

Pearson Chi^2 and *P* values in bold were significant (significance level $\alpha = 0.05$)
The number of chronic diseases was derived from self-reported diagnoses of any of the following; (diabetes, hypertension, stroke, cataracts, arthritis, heart disease, respiratory disease, HIV, TB, anaemia, depression, dementia, other mental health conditions, gastro-intestinal conditions, prostatic/urinary conditions, renal failure, or cancer)

Frailty, comorbidity and ADL disability were found to be distinct, but overlapping entities. The frequencies and percentages are shown in Fig. 1. Notably, almost a fifth overlapped in having all three ($n = 36$, 18.4%). Twenty (10.2%) overlapped in having both disability and frailty, while 12 (6.1%) overlapped in having dual diagnoses of comorbidity and frailty.

Discussion

The prevalence of frailty by frailty phenotype

The prevalence of frailty according to the Hai DSS FP is lower than was found by the CGA, which found a frailty prevalence of 19.1% within the same study population [12]. One major reason for this is the fact that the FP requires participants to have a certain level of functioning

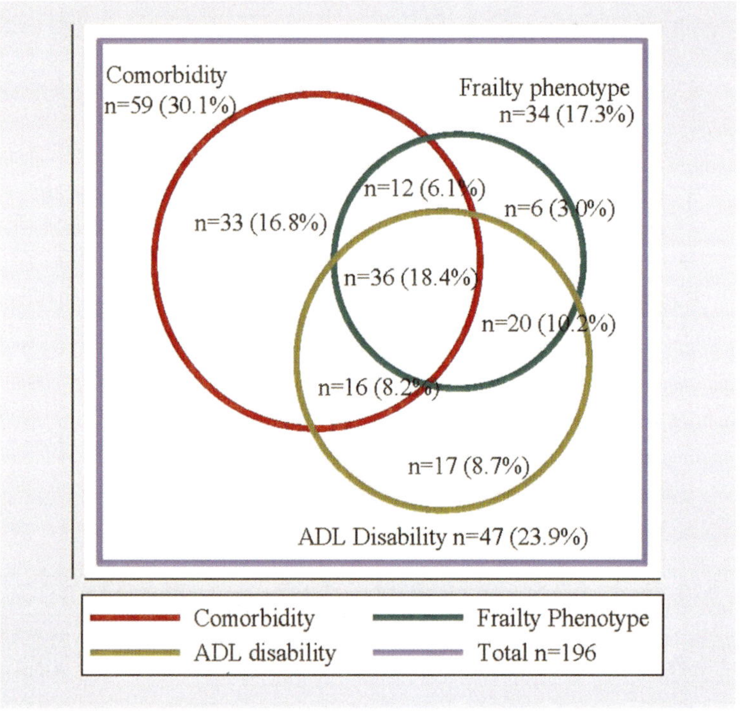

Fig. 1 Proportional Venn Diagram Illustrating the Frequencies and Percentages of Comorbidity, Disability and Frailty by Hai DSS Frailty Phenotype. Legend: Frequencies and percentages from the total sample ($n = 196$) are described. Comorbidity $n = 59$, was categorised as anyone self-reporting ≥2 diagnoses from the following (diabetes, hypertension, stroke, cataracts, arthritis, heart disease, respiratory disease, HIV, TB, anaemia, depression, dementia, other mental health conditions, gastro-intestinal conditions, prostatic/urinary conditions, renal failure, or cancer). ADL Disability $n = 47$ was categorised as being unable to do any of the Barthel Index [37] activities of daily living

in order to be assessed. They should be mobile and able to walk (walking aids are permitted), they should be able to comprehend and follow commands well enough to undertake HGS testing. The majority of missing data for assessment of FP were from patients who were immobile and/or cognitively impaired, for example due to stroke or dementia [12].

In the original Fried paper, older adults with certain clinical characteristics were excluded because their diagnoses may confound the results, by mimicking frailty [1]. For example, those with a history of Parkinson's disease, stroke, and poor cognitive function. Those taking medications for depression, Parkinson's disease or dementia were also excluded. In our rural sub-Saharan Africa (SSA) setting, excluding these participants was not possible, due to low levels of formal diagnosis, limited medication availability and poor access to healthcare. Additionally, we feel that their exclusion may significantly under-represent the true burden of frailty. This is important, given that in Europe and South Africa it has been shown that older community-dwelling adults who could not be assessed fully using the FP had higher mortality rates than those who could be assessed [6, 20]. Longitudinal assessment of this cohort would reveal whether this finding is the case in our setting.

Weakness by hand grip strength

HGS varies by ethnicity and world region, thus we have appropriately adjusted our normal values in keeping with the most up-to-date values for HGS norms in older Africans [21]. A comprehensive review of normative HGS values found that developing world regions had significantly lower HGS compared with developed regions [22], and taking a life-course approach to ageing, postulate that factors such as early growth and nutrition may be important factors accounting for this disparity. The difference in grip strength (of 14.7 Kg in males and 5.7 Kg in females) between a rural older Ghanaian study population and a comparative Dutch population disappeared when the authors standardised the Ghanaian study population against the age- group and sex- specific height and BMI of the Dutch study population [23]. Therefore, regional and ethnic variations found in HGS may, to some extent be accounted for by height and BMI [23]. The most important determinants of HGS variation globally is a complex question. Undoubtedly genetic factors contribute, however there is an increasing body of evidence for the influence of environmental factors such as early life socio-economic status on HGS variation in old age [24].

The cycle of frailty hypothesis, states that chronic undernutrition (protein, energy and micronutrient deficiencies) is integral in the development and progression of frailty [1, 3]. Indeed, dietary protein intake has been shown to be protective against loss of HGS [25]. We hypothesise that nutritional factors, including a low protein and low micronutrient diet, may be important in the development of frailty in rural SSA, supporting findings from Malawi [26]. However, more detailed assessments of dietary intake and outcomes are required in order to make comparisons with older adults in high income country (HIC) settings.

Slow walking speed

Given that there are no published norms of walking speed across SSA, we opted to use the slowest quintile as a cut-off. Stratifying by sex and height did not significantly influence our findings, but added to the complexity. The WHO Study of AGEing and Adult Health (SAGE) found a range of walking speeds between the slowest, (Russia at 0.61 m/s) and the fastest, (China, at 0.88 m/s) [27]. Our mean walking speed was slow, (0.65 m/s) when compared with the SAGE countries, and with walking speeds of HICs. For example a meta-analysis of nine cohort studies predicted a life expectancy above the median for older adults walking faster than 0.8 m/s [28]. As discussed in the methods, participants' footwear, unadjusted visual impairments, uneven ground surfaces and lack of appropriate walking aids may have led to slower walking speeds.

The concept of exhaustion

Exhaustion is a subjective and culturally dependent variable. In order to remain as close as possible to the original Fried FP, the same questions taken from the CES-D depression screening questionnaire were used, with a direct translation into Swahili. However, qualitative exploration of the meaning of "exhaustion" is needed, to ensure that this is a valid measure in this setting. For example the CES-D question; "How often in the last week did you feel you could not get going?" could have been interpreted literally as not having access to a means of transport. The fact that the majority of our study participants self-identified as living with frailty (see Table 3), is interesting in itself, suggesting that the translated term for frailty; *"udhaifu wa wazee"* or literally "weakness of the older people" doesn't hold the same negative connotations as it does in "westernised" cultures [29]. The Agincourt frailty study faced similar translation and interpretation challenges in using the CES-D questions, and substituted a question on self-reported health status [6].

Unintentional weight loss

We recorded any recent self-reported weight loss as being significant, and presumed unintentional. In the context of the HIV/AIDS epidemic, weight loss and a slim body habitus may be associated with HIV [30], which may have influenced our respondents' willingness to admit to weight loss, given that it might imply infection. Cultural views on body habitus are often counter to "western" ideas, whereby being overweight may be associated with health, wealth and social status [31]. Indeed, it would be very unusual for someone in this setting to lose weight intentionally. Given that subsistence farming is the main source of food and household income, the fact that the last short rainy season had led to a poor harvest may have influenced some of the survey responses, particularly in relation to food intake and weight loss. Very few studies of nutritional status of older adults in SSA have been conducted rurally and very few are longitudinal [32]. However, in rural Gabon a cross-sectional study showed a 25.6% prevalence of underweight by BMI among older adults, which increased to 28.2% in the rainy season [33]. In our sample the mean BMI was 25.0 for women and 21.2 for men, with 20.4% ($n = 40$) categorised as underweight. Despite a global increase in obesity it may be that in such settings, older people are at an increased risk from undernutrition, due to food and income insecurity. A cross-sectional study conducted in urban Kenya, Uganda and Tanzania described the majority of older adults as being "nutritionally vulnerable" due to problems accessing food [34]. As a consequence, the relationship between frailty and chronic undernutrition is likely to be stronger in rural SSA than might be seen in HICs and warrants further investigation.

Low physical activity

We took inability to conduct moderately difficult physical activity on any day of the week as a criterion marker for frailty. Strengths of this method are that older adults in this setting are frequently expected to take part in activities such as sweeping and gardening on a daily basis [16]. However, the measure is confounded by cognitive impairment, in a similar manner to the Minnesotta Leisure Time Physical Activity Questionnaire, in that activities such as tennis require high levels of cognitive functioning, as are required for common IADLs [8]. Given that we did not exclude older adults with cognitive impairment from our study sample, there is the possibility that this component may have been measuring their ability to perform IADLs, as assessed by the IDEA-IADL questionnaire [16]. Taking a broader multidimensional approach to frailty assessment however, this is academic, if what matters is the older adult's functional capacity.

Study limitations

The two parameters where these data's objectivity could be improved are in the measurement of weight loss and calculation of low energy expenditure. An objective measurement of weight loss would have been beneficial in providing a more accurate estimate of this component of the Hai DSS FP, but would have involved repeated home visits to remote rural areas across difficult terrain, particularly in the rainy season. One main weakness of this study is that we were unable to measure an estimated energy expenditure based on data from the IPAQ due to technical difficulties recording these data. However, the IPAQ is thought to have better reliability in urban as compared to rural samples, and it may have limited validity in rural and low literacy settings such as ours [14]. There is a need for more research into the physical activity of older adults in rural SSA (e.g. using accelerometers) in order to better assess low physical activity in this setting, where it is presumed that older adults remain more physically active than might be seen in HICs, where retirement from work is the norm.

More data on the dietary intake of older adults in this setting would help justify the use of the FP as a conceptual model. Many studies use food diaries to monitor nutritional status, but this would be difficult in this setting, given the low literacy of our studied population. Frailty is considered an important non-AIDS condition in HIV-infected individuals [35]. One weakness of this study is that HIV status was not tested, rather we relied on self-disclosure. Consequently, we may have underestimated the prevalence of HIV infection as only four participants disclosed their HIV-infection status. HIV prevalence in our background population is unknown but likely to be low based on anonymised testing conducted for a stroke risk factors study in Hai district between 2003 and 6 [36], yet this may limit the generalisability of our findings to other regions of SSA with a higher background prevalence of HIV infection. For example the recent Agincourt frailty study, reported that 21% aged ≥40 years were known to be HIV-infected [6].

A limitation of using the FP to identify frailty in this context, is its focus on physical frailty, excluding other domains of assessment, such as social and economic domains. Particularly in this rural SSA setting, older adults' frailty status, as well as the outcomes of frailty, may be closely associated with their social and economic resources. Further study is required in order to investigate the impact of these domains.

Study strengths

This study adds substantially to the limited existing body of knowledge on frailty in older rural-dwelling Africans. The FP has been successfully applied across language and cultural barriers to produce a meaningful measure close to the original phenotypic model. One significant strength of this study is in its hypothesis generation. As a result of our findings of high levels of self-reported weight loss and underweight, we propose that chronic undernutrition due to food insecurity and socio-economic factors may be important in the cyclical deterioration of energy and physiological reserve described by the "cycle of frailty" framework, and deserves further investigation in this setting.

Conclusion

The study demonstrates that the FP can be successfully operationalised in rural Tanzania to estimate frailty prevalence. The clinical application of the FP in rural SSA is unclear. JAMAR dynamometers are expensive and such technical specialist equipment is unlikely to be available for use routinely as a screening tool. Additionally, if the FP were to be applied clinically, referral for further specialist care would not be possible given the regional lack of human resources for geriatric medicine [37]. Further work assessing the nutritional status of older adults in rural SSA would help to characterise the association between chronic undernutrition and frailty in this setting. Additionally, future research should explore the optimal practical application of the FP, particularly whether a task-shifting approach to its delivery could be employed in order to reach the most vulnerable rural-dwelling older Africans.

Abbreviations

B-FIT: Brief Frailty Instrument for Tanzania; BMI: Body Mass Index; CES-D: Centre for Epidemiological Studies Depression Scale; CGA: Comprehensive Geriatric Assessment; DSS: Demographic Surveillance Site; FP: Frailty Phenotype; HGS: Hand-grip strength; HICs: High-income countries; IADL: Instrumental Activities of Daily Living; IDEA: Identification and Intervention for Dementia in Elderly Africans; IPAQ: International Physical Activity Questionnaire; ODK: Open Data Kit; SSA: sub-Saharan Africa; WHO SAGE: World Health Organization Study of AGEing and adult health

Acknowledgements

We gratefully acknowledge the Newcastle University Mres students who assisted with data collection: Greta Wood, Louise Whitton and Harry Collin. We would like to thank the Tanzanian data collection team: Aloyce Kisoli, Antusa John Kissima, Paulina Elias Tukay, Dr. Joyce Mkodo, Dr. Deborah Mdegella, Dr. Ali Mohammed Ali, Dr. Francis Zerd and Dr. Ally Mohamed Imani. Thanks to Jane Rogathi, Leila Mwakipunda and Lucy Mariki for their excellent translation work. We are grateful for the technical support of Kilimanjaro Clinical Research Institute, Kilimanjaro Christian Medical Centre, and Hai District Hospital. We would like to acknowledge the important role of the village chairmen, enumerators and ten-cell leaders. Thanks of course, go to all of the older adults and their relatives who participated.

Funding

Northumbria Healthcare NHS Foundation Trust provided the first author's salary through a Teaching and Research Fellow Grant. The sponsor had no role in the design, methods, subject enrolment, data collection, analysis or preparation of this paper.

Authors' contributions

EGL, KH, SC, WG, CD, RW and SU were involved in study concept and design. Authors EGL, KH, SC, and JK assisted in the enrolment and assessment of participants. EGL, KH, WG, CD and RW were involved in the analysis and interpretation of data, and all authors assisted in the preparation and approval of the manuscript.

Competing interests

The authors declare that they have no competing interests.

Author details

[1]Institute of Health and Society, Faculty of Medical Sciences, Newcastle University, Newcastle upon Tyne, UK. [2]Northumbria Healthcare NHS Foundation Trust, North Tyneside General Hospital, North Shields, UK. [3]The Medical school, Faculty of Medical Sciences, Newcastle University, Newcastle upon Tyne, UK. [4]Hai District Hospital, Boma Ng'ombe, Hai, Kilimanjaro, Tanzania. [5]Kilimanjaro Christian Medical Centre, Moshi, Kilimanjaro, Tanzania. [6]Education centre, North Tyneside General Hospital, Rake Lane, North Shields NE29 8NH, UK.

References

1. Fried LP, Tangen CM, Walston J, Newman AB, Hirsch C, Gottdiener J, Seeman T, Tracy R, Kop WJ, Burke G, et al. Frailty in older adults: evidence for a phenotype. J Gerontol A Biol Sci Med Sci. 2001;56(3):M146–56.
2. Fried LP, Ferrucci L, Darer J, Williamson JD, Anderson G. Untangling the concepts of disability, frailty, and comorbidity: implications for improved targeting and care. J Gerontol A Biol Sci Med Sci. 2004;59(3):255–63.
3. Fried LP, Walston J: Frailty and failure to thrive in: *Geriatric Medicine and Gerontology*. Edited by Hazzard WR, Blass JP, Ettinger WH Jr, Halter JB, Ouslander J, 5 edition (1 July 2003) edn New York: McGraw-Hill Medical; 2003: 1487–1502.
4. Gray WKRJ, McGuire J, Dewhurst F, Elder V, Weeks J, Walker RW, Dotchin CL. Frailty screening in low- and middle-income countries: a systematic review. J Am Geriatr Soc. 2016;64(4):806–23.
5. Theou O, Cann L, Blodgett J, Wallace LM, Brothers TD, Rockwood K. Modifications to the frailty phenotype criteria: systematic review of the current literature and investigation of 262 frailty phenotypes in the survey of health, ageing, and retirement in Europe. Ageing Res Rev. 2015;21:78–94.
6. Payne CF, Wade A, Kabudula CW, Davies JI, Chang AY, Gomez-Olive FX, Kahn K, Berkman LF, Tollman SM, Salomon JA, et al. Prevalence and correlates of frailty in an older rural African population: findings from the HAALSI cohort study. BMC Geriatr. 2017;17(1):293.
7. Cesari M, Gambassi G, van Kan GA, Vellas B. The frailty phenotype and the frailty index: different instruments for different purposes. Age Ageing. 2014; 43(1):10–2.
8. Theou O, Rockwood K. Comparison and clinical applications of the frailty phenotype and frailty index approaches. In: Theou O, Rockwood K, editors. Frailty in Aging Biological, Clinical and Social Implications., vol. 41. Basel: Karger; 2015. p. 74–84.
9. Rockwood K, Mitnitski A. Frailty in relation to the accumulation of deficits. J Gerontol A Biol Sci Med Sci. 2007;62(7):722–7.
10. Searle SD, Mitnitski A, Gahbauer EA, Gill TM, Rockwood K. A standard procedure for creating a frailty index. BMC Geriatr. 2008;8:24.
11. Gray WK, Orega G, Kisoli A, Rogathi J, Paddick SM, Longdon AR, Walker RW, Dewhurst F, Dewhurst M, Chaote P, et al. Identifying frailty and its outcomes in older people in rural Tanzania. Exp Aging Res. 2017;43(3):257–73.
12. Lewis EG, Wood G, Howorth K, Shah B, Mulligan L, Kissima J, Dotchin C, Gray W, Urasa S, Walker R. Prevalence of frailty in older community-dwelling Tanzanians according to comprehensive geriatric assessment. J Am Geriatr Soc. 2018.
13. Orme JG, Reis J, Herz EJ. Factorial and discriminant validity of the Center for Epidemiological Studies Depression (CES-D) scale. J Clin Psychol. 1986;42(1):28–33.
14. Craig CL, Marshall AL, Sjostrom M, Bauman AE, Booth ML, Ainsworth BE, Pratt M, Ekelund U, Yngve A, Sallis JF, et al. International physical activity questionnaire: 12-country reliability and validity. Med Sci Sports Exerc. 2003; 35(8):1381–95.
15. Gureje O, Oladeji BD, Abiona T, Chatterji S. Profile and determinants of successful aging in the Ibadan study of ageing. J Am Geriatr Soc. 2014;62(5): 836–42.
16. Collingwood CPS-M, Kisoli A, Dotchin CL, Gray WK, Mbowe G, Mkenda S, Urasa S, Mushi D, Chaote P, et al. Development and community-based validation of the IDEA study instrumental activities of daily living (IDEA-IADL) questionnaire. Glob Health Action. 2014;7(1):25988.
17. Paddick SM, Gray WK, Ogunjimi L, Lwezuala B, Olakehinde O, Kisoli A, Kissima J, Mbowe G, Mkenda S, Dotchin CL, et al. Validation of the identification and intervention for dementia in elderly Africans (IDEA) cognitive screen in Nigeria and Tanzania. BMC Geriatr. 2015;15:53.
18. Guerra M, Ferri C, Llibre J, Prina AM, Prince M. Psychometric properties of EURO-D, a geriatric depression scale: a cross-cultural validation study. BMC Psychiatry. 2015;15:12.
19. Brunette W, Sundt M, Dell N, Chaudhri R, Breit N, Borriello G. Open data kit 2.0: expanding and refining information Services for Developing Regions. In: ACM HotMobile'13; 2013. http://www.hotmobile.org/2013/papers/full/2.pdf.
20. Ravindrarajah R, Lee DM, Pye SR, Gielen E, Boonen S, Vanderschueren D, Pendleton N, Finn JD, Tajar A, O'Connell MD, et al. The ability of three different models of frailty to predict all-cause mortality: results from the European male aging study (EMAS). Arch Gerontol Geriatr. 2013;57(3):360–8.
21. Leong DP, Teo KK, Rangarajan S, Kutty VR, Lanas F, Hui C, Quanyong X, Zhenzhen Q, Jinhua T, Noorhassim I, et al. Reference ranges of handgrip strength from 125,462 healthy adults in 21 countries: a prospective urban rural epidemiologic (PURE) study. J Cachexia Sarcopenia Muscle. 2016;7(5):535–46.
22. Dodds RM, Syddall HE, Cooper R, Kuh D, Cooper C, Sayer AA. Global variation in grip strength: a systematic review and meta-analysis of normative data. Age Ageing. 2016;45(2):209–16.
23. Koopman JJ, van Bodegom D, van Heemst D, Westendorp RG. Handgrip strength, ageing and mortality in rural Africa. Age Ageing. 2015;44(3):465–70.
24. Hurst L, Stafford M, Cooper R, Hardy R, Richards M, Kuh D. Lifetime socioeconomic inequalities in physical and cognitive aging. Am J Public Health. 2013;103(9):1641–8.
25. McLean RR, Mangano KM, Hannan MT, Kiel DP, Sahni S. Dietary protein intake is protective against loss of grip strength among older adults in the Framingham offspring cohort. J Gerontol A Biol Sci Med Sci. 2016;71(3):356–61.
26. Chilima DM, Ismail SJ. Nutrition and handgrip strength of older adults in rural Malawi. Public Health Nutr. 2001;4(1):11–7.
27. Capistrant BD, Glymour MM, Berkman LF. Assessing mobility difficulties for cross-national comparisons: results from the World Health Organization study on global AGEing and adult health. J Am Geriatr Soc. 2014;62(2):329–35.
28. Studenski S, Perera S, Patel K, Rosano C, Faulkner K, Inzitari M, Brach J, Chandler J, Cawthon P, Connor EB, et al. Gait speed and survival in older adults. JAMA. 2011;305(1):50–8.
29. Britainthinks: Frailty: Language and Perceptions A report prepared by BritainThinks on behalf of Age UK and the British Geriatrics Society In.; 2015.
30. Matoti-Mvalo T, Puoane T. Perceptions of body size and its association with HIV/AIDS. S Afr J Clin Nutr. 2011;24(1):40–45 2011.
31. Renzaho AMN. Fat, rich and beautiful: changing socio-cultural paradigms associated with obesity risk, nutritional status and refugee children from sub-Saharan Africa. Health & Place. 2004;10(1):105–13.
32. Jésus P, Guerchet M, Pilleron S, Fayemendy P, Maxime Mouanga A, Mbelesso P, Preux PM, Desport JC. Undernutrition and obesity among elderly people living in two cities of developing countries: prevalence and associated factors in the EDAC study. Clin Nutri ESPEN. 2017;21:40–50.
33. Blaney S, Beaudry M, Latham M, Thibault M. Nutritional status and dietary adequacy in rural communities of a protected area in Gabon. Public Health Nutr. 2009;12(10):1946–59.
34. Cheserek MJ, Waudo JN, Tuitoek PJ, Msuya JM, Kikafunda JK. Nutritional vulnerability of older persons living in urban areas of Lake Victoria Basin in East Africa: a cross sectional survey. J Nutr Gerontol Geriatr. 2012;31(1):86–96.
35. Brothers TD, Kirkland S, Guaraldi G, Falutz J, Theou O, Johnston BL, Rockwood K. Frailty in people aging with human immunodeficiency virus (HIV) infection. J Infect Dis. 2014;210(8):1170–9.
36. Walker RW, Jusabani A, Aris E, Gray WK, Unwin N, Swai M, Alberti G, Mugusi F. Stroke risk factors in an incident population in urban and rural Tanzania: a prospective, community-based, case-control study. Lancet Glob Health. 2013;1(5):e282–8.
37. Dotchin CL, Akinyemi RO, Gray WK, Walker RW. Geriatric medicine: services and training in Africa. Age Ageing. 2013;42(1):124–8.

19

HIV testing and counselling experiences: a qualitative study of older adults living with HIV in western Kenya

Jepchirchir Kiplagat[1,2,3*] and Susann Huschke[4,5]

Abstract

Background: Finding HIV infected persons and engaging them in care is crucial in achieving UNAIDS 90–90-90 targets; diagnosing 90% of those infected with HIV, initiating 90% of the diagnosed on ART and achieving viral suppression in 90% of those on ART. To achieve the first target, no person should be left behind in their access to HIV testing services. In Kenya, HIV prevention and testing services give less emphasis on older adults. This article describes HIV testing experiences of older adults living with HIV and how their age shaped their interaction and treatment received during HIV testing and diagnosis.

Methods: We conducted a qualitative study in two HIV clinics (rural and urban) in western Kenya, and recruited 57 HIV infected persons aged ≥50 years. We conducted in depth interviews (IDIs) with 25 participants and 4 focus group discussions (FGDs) with a total of 32 participants and audio recorded all the sessions. Participants recruited were aged between 54 and 79 years with 43% being females. We transcribed audio records and analyzed the data using thematic content analysis method.

Results: Older persons' experiences with HIV testing depended on where they tested (hospital or community setting); whether they actively sought the testing or not; and the age and gender of the healthcare provider who conducted the test. Participants expressed concerns with ageist discrimination when actively seeking HIV care testing services in hospital settings, characterized by providers' reluctance or refusal to test. The testing and counseling sessions were described as short and hurried within the hospital settings, whereas the interactions with service providers in home-based testing were experienced as appropriate and supportive. Participants in this study expressed preference for healthcare providers who were older and of similar gender.

Conclusion: HIV testing services are still not tailored to target older adults' needs in our setting resulting in late diagnosis among older persons. We argue that a scale-up of community level testing services that provide adequate testing and counselling time and actively reach out to older adults is key to attaining the UNAIDS targets of having 90% of PLWH know their status.

Keywords: Older adults, Kenya, HIV testing, Ageism, Subjective experiences

* Correspondence: chiri2809@gmail.com
[1]Moi University, College of Health Sciences, School of Medicine, Nandi Road, Eldoret, Kenya
[2]Academic Model Providing Access to Healthcare (AMPATH) Program, Moi Teaching and Referral Hospital Campus, Nandi Road, Eldoret, Kenya
Full list of author information is available at the end of the article

Background

UNAIDS and WHO estimate that over 36.7 million people are currently living with HIV worldwide [1], with more than two thirds of this population residing in sub-Saharan Africa (SSA) [2]. According to UNAIDS [3], Kenya ranks the 4th largest HIV epidemic globally with about 1.6 million people living with HIV and an adult prevalence of 5.4%. Older people, that is ≥50 years, represent a growing share of the HIV population, making up 12% of the total people living with HIV (PLWH) globally [1]. In Kenya, the prevalence among older adults is estimated to be slightly higher than the country's prevalence – about 5.6%. This number is expected to rise in the coming years due to the wide access of antiretroviral treatment (ART) where people infected with HIV at a younger age are growing older as well as new infections occurring among the older adults.

Among those living with HIV in sub-Saharan Africa approximately 40%, and in Kenya 53%, do not know their status [4]. Though the Kenyan Government has adopted various testing strategies including voluntary counselling and testing (VCT), provider-initiated testing and counselling (PITC), diagnostic testing and counselling (DTC), home-based counselling and testing (HBCT), and recently self-testing, older adults still lag behind in accessing HIV testing services compared to other age groups. There are several reasons for this: first, very little HIV prevention education is targeted at older people [5], second, health care providers may not test older people for HIV [6], and third, older people may lack awareness of the risk factors for getting HIV [7]. As a result, older adults are deprived of the benefits of early diagnosis of HIV infection including timely initiation of HIV treatment.

The literature indicates that adults continue to be sexually active into their old age, including sexual practices often associated with younger people such as inconsistent condom use, sex with multiple sexual partners and casual sex [8–12]. Such sexual behaviors put older adults at risk of acquiring HIV from infected partners or transmitting HIV to an uninfected partner. Despite these risk factors, adults aged 50 years and above are less likely to be tested for HIV than younger adults testing [7, 8, 13]. As a consequence, older adults get diagnosed late into the HIV infection, likely after developing symptoms [14], and only when visiting the hospital for health complications. Despite these specific risks and concerns, there is limited literature that has explored older adults' experiences with HIV testing services. To address this gap in literature, we draw on qualitative interviews with older HIV-infected adults in western Kenya and analyze their experiences in HIV testing, including explorations on access of testing services and how they perceived their interactions with healthcare providers during testing.

Methods

Study setting and participants

The study was conducted at two facilities under the Academic Model providing Access to Healthcare (AMPATH) program [15]. The program provides comprehensive HIV care in 135 Ministry of Health (MOH) facilities spread throughout western part of Kenya and is currently the largest program providing free HIV care and treatment in the country [16].

Participants aged 50 years and above at the time of HIV care enrollment were selected from one urban and one rural facility to allow for a comparison of these settings, with a note that prevalence of HIV in Kenya is higher in urban than in rural settings [17]. Both of the selected sites served a large number of older persons when compared to other facilities.

Study design

Qualitative research methods were used to generate detailed descriptions of experiences of the participants living with HIV. In-depth interviews (IDI) and focus group discussions were employed in this study. The interviews were conducted in Kiswahili, the Kenyan national language, and lasted between 60 and 90 min each. We interviewed 25 participants; 16 (9 males and 7 females) participants from urban facility and 9 (5 males and 4 females) from rural facility. We also conducted four focus group discussions (FGD) with a total of 32 participants; two FGDs (one for male and one for female participants) were conducted in a rural and another two FGDs (also one for male and one for female participants) in the urban facility. Both IDIs and FGDs were used to triangulate information obtained from the participants.

Study procedures

Research ethics

The study was approved by the University of Witwatersrand Heath Research Ethics Committee (Clearance Certificate No: *M160449*) and the Moi University and Moi Teaching and Referral Hospital Institutional Research Ethics Committee (Formal Approval No. *FAN: IREC 1664*). Permission was granted from the AMPATH research program office to recruit participants from its clinical care sites. Prior to the interview, participants were informed about the nature of the study and the methods including the audio recording of the interviews. Participants were assured that the information obtained was going to be kept anonymous and confidentiality was going to be maintained. Participants were also informed that during reporting of the results of the study, quotes were going to be used with no link to their names. All participants who agreed and gave consent to participate in the study and to be audio recorded were interviewed.

Inclusion and exclusion criteria

HIV infected men and women aged ≥50 years at the time of HIV care enrollment and receiving care at AMPATH were targeted. For the purpose of this study a cut off age of 50 years for older persons was adopted from the WHO definition [18] for those infected with HIV.

Participants who were currently in care at the two participating outpatient HIV clinics, had been followed up for at least 1 year, and were aged 50 or older at enrolling into HIV care were included in our study. The eligible participants who did not consent to participation and audio-recording were excluded.

Of the total 65 approached participants who consented to participate in our study, we interviewed 57. The other 8 participants invited for the FGD did not turn up due to other commitments during the interview date.

Data collection

Two research assistants (RAs), recruited from the staff at the social behavioral department within the AMPATH program, were trained by the first author to conduct the data collection. We purposefully selected older research assistants, one female (52 years) and one male (55 years), and each was responsible for interviewing females and males respectively. The choice of older RAs was informed by references in other studies [19] with older adults. The chosen RAs have an educational background in social science and regularly support researchers at AMPATH by collecting qualitative data. We pilot tested the in-depth interview tool (in English) in a peri-urban HIV care clinic to ensure the clarity of the interview questions. After necessary modifications such as deleting redundant questions and including a number of new questions that arose from the pilot testing, the IDI guide (Additional file 1) was then translated from English to Kiswahili.

For FGDs, we recruited four (2 males and 2 females) research assistants, who were not affiliated with the AMPATH program. The RAs, who were all aged above 45 years, with skills in facilitating FGDs, were referred to this study by researchers at the Department of Anthropology, Moi University. The RAs were trained to use the data collection tool (FGD guide – Additional file 2) by the first author. The FGD guide provided similar questions as those of the IDI's with probes focusing on identified themes or sub themes from IDI transcripts.

Participant identification

During the clinic days, research assistants reviewed the list of persons attending the clinic on that day. The records of persons aged 50 years and above were reviewed to determine the age at first engagement in HIV care. The research assistant would then provide the clinician with the list of eligible participants (clinicians had been informed about the study). The clinician would inform the research assistant as soon as the participant completed the clinic visit. The research assistant would then approach and explain the purpose of the study to the participants. If they agreed to participate, a meeting date and time was scheduled at a venue of participant's convenience to allow privacy and comfort during the interview. All except one participant asked to do the interview on the same day they were in the clinic and wanted it done at the health facility in which they were seeking care at. Contact details were requested for one participant for the purpose of reminder and communication before the meeting time that was scheduled.

FGD participants were identified during the clinic visit, through an outreach worker stationed at the facility. Outreach workers review files of all new patients attending HIV facility and draw the patient tracer card, including patient information and their place of residence, for future follow up if patients fail to attend clinic visits. In the morning of the clinic day, patient files of the expected patients are pulled out. If a patient was 50 years and above at the time of initial enrolment, the file would be flagged with a yellow sticker. After the clinic visit, the clinician would inform the research assistant who would approach the participant and explain the purpose of the study. The consent process would be done and if the participant agreed to take part, contact information was requested for further communication regarding the date, time and venue of the FGD.

Interview process

During the in-depth interviews, the research assistant explained the purpose of the study and obtained written informed consent from the participant. There was a total of eight participants who were unable to read and write and a thumb print indicating their consent was obtained. The research assistant also asked whether the participant needed someone they trust to be present during the interview. None of them indicated the need for a companion. The interviews were conducted in one of the two enclosed research rooms within the clinical care space. The room provided privacy for the participants and a quiet environment for audio-recording. The participants' demographics were captured and they were asked a question to gauge their HIV knowledge. Participants were then invited to narrate their experiences during HIV testing and counseling.

The FGDs were conducted in a room reserved for research outside of the HIV clinic facilities but within the MTRH campus and in a teaching room at a nearby medical training college in Mosoriot. As 'neutral' spaces away from the treatment rooms of the clinic, these spaces provided a convenient environment to discuss health facility related factors that were deemed negative. The

FGD room was set with an oval table that provided seats for all participants facing each other, with the facilitators sitting among them. This set up provided an opportunity for each participant to contribute to the discussion. Two RAs participated in each FGD (female RAs conducted the female-only FGD while male RAs conducted male-only FGD). One of the RAs facilitated the discussion while the other took notes. Prior to the interviews, participants were informed of the purpose of the study and oral consent was obtained. All FGDs were conducted in Kiswahili and audio-recorded. The FGDs lasted between 90 and 135 min.

Data management and analysis

Data obtained from in-depth interviews and focus group discussions were transcribed verbatim, and translated from Kiswahili to English. All the transcripts were then uploaded to NVIVO version 10 for coding. A pre-developed codebook based on the literature on facilitators and barriers for seeking HIV testing services and accessing care was used during coding. The two RAs who conducted the IDIs and the first author coded the first three transcripts, which allowed the team to revise the codebook based on the analysis of these transcripts. The first author then shared the revised codes with the second author (SH) who made some recommendations to further clarify the structure of the codebook. The final codebook was agreed upon by the authors and the RAs. Thematic content analysis [20] was used to describe emerging patterns from in-depth interviews and FGDs. Recurrent themes identified and patterns established from the two data sources were summarized. Information obtained from the FGDs was used to complement the IDIs and to seek data saturation. Mapping and interpretation was done by searching for associations of concepts and explanations in the data. We summarize the findings according to predeveloped themes and the subthemes that emerged during the coding process.

Results

Participants' characteristics

We interviewed a total of 57 participants (25 in-depth interviews and 32 in focus group discussions) with their ages ranging from 54 to 79 years. Participant characteristics are summarized in Table 1.

In the sections below, we describe older adults' experiences with HIV testing and encounters with healthcare providers and how their age shaped their interaction and the treatment they received during their HIV testing and diagnosis.

Table 1 Participant characteristics

Variable	n (%)
Age Category (years)	
50–59	19 (33.3)
60–69	28 (49.2)
70–79	10 (17.5)
Sex	
Female	27 (47.4)
Male	30 (52.6)
Clinic Location	
Urban	31 (54.4)
Rural	26 (45.6)
Marital status	
Married	30 (54.4)
Widowed, separated, divorced	27 (45.6)
Level of Education	
No formal education	24 (42.1)
Formal education – Primary	19 (33.3)
Formal education – Secondary	10 (17.5)
Formal education – Tertiary	4 (7.1)

Experiences with HIV testing

We found that older persons' experiences with HIV testing depended on where they tested (hospital or community setting); whether they actively sought the testing or not. Participants expressed concerns with ageist discrimination when actively seeking HIV care testing services in hospital settings, characterized by providers' reluctance or refusal to test. The testing and counseling sessions were described as short and hurried within the hospital settings, whereas the interactions with service providers in home-based testing were experienced as appropriate and supportive. Age and gender of the healthcare provider also mattered to older adults in seeking HIV testing services. We did not find significant variations in experiences of older adults in urban and rural facilities hence we jointly describe their experiences.

Testing during hospital visit or during hospitalization

The majority of the participants indicated visits to the hospital as a main avenue to be tested for HIV. Participants described periods when they were sick and sought out-patient services or when they were admitted in hospital for other health conditions. Within the hospital setting, there are two approaches for HIV testing; i) opt-out HIV testing known as provider-initiated testing and counseling (PITC) and ii) opt-in HIV testing approach known as diagnostic testing and counseling (DTC) implemented as part of disease diagnosis. These two strategies of HIV testing and counseling are implemented in all healthcare facilities providing inpatient and outpatient services in Kenya. Some participants tested at the hospital setting received the HIV positive test results with shock, as the following quote exemplifies:

"I was sick with TB. I was really coughing and when I came to the hospital, I was admitted. They took an x-ray and they told me I have TB. I was also tested for HIV and that is when I found out that I had this disease [HIV]. It was shocking for me. I could never explain where I got it. It has never occurred to me that I could ever get it. At the time, I had lost so much weight".

IDI, female, 67 years, rural

Unlike the participant above, another participant tested in the hospital setting was relieved that she finally knew the condition that she had been suffering from. She had been in and out of hospital without proper diagnosis which had increased her health care seeking costs and progressed the condition. Further probing in the interview revealed that the service providers had missed two important opportunities to test this older person earlier on.

"I began coughing for some time. I went to the hospital and was given drugs for TB. I took the drugs but nothing changed. I grew so thin. I went back to the hospital because I was not improving. I was asked to take an x-ray and was told that the TB was really bad and had eaten all my chest. I was given more medicines and was told to come back after two weeks. Before the two weeks lapsed, I began to have diarrhea and also started vomiting. My face even started dying from one side [paralysis]. I went back to the hospital and I was admitted. A sister came and counseled me for HIV testing and I agreed to test. I tested positive. At this point I now knew what the problem with my body was."

FGD, female, 67 years, urban

Home based counseling and testing

Bringing HIV testing services to the older people (rather than waiting for people to actively seek out testing) proved to be critical for early diagnosis among those infected. Kenya introduced the door-to-door testing campaign after the AMPATH program showed that this strategy yielded results - with 98% of people tested [21]. During the door-to-door HIV testing, also known as home based counseling and testing (HBCT), a certified counsellor trained for HIV counseling and testing was assigned a catchment area of about 500 households. The counselor resided in the assigned area and provided perpetual testing services to his/her catchment site. The counselor went from house to house with the help of community health volunteers, and provided HIV testing services to all persons aged 13 years and above, including the elderly in the household. For all those that tested positive, the counselor worked with the patients to link them to care near them. He/she went back to the household after 3 month to offer testing services to all those who originally tested negative. Because the counselors resided in the assigned catchment area for more than a year, they spent as much time as possible with the residents in counseling before providing HIV testing services. This likely resulted in trust by the residents and acceptability of the tests.

Some of the participants we interviewed got to know their HIV status during the testing services that were provided at their homes. Participants appreciated HBCT services that were led by the AMPATH program. They perceived them as a welcome attempt to reach older persons who would otherwise not visit the hospital settings where HIV testing services are often provided.

"They came to my home (...) and I was praying to God not to be positive and when I read the results I was shocked, I didn't know where to start from. I just assumed my husband had infected me or they injected me with a used syringe in the hospital. But at least I got to know [my status] before I became too sick. Can you imagine what would have happened if I was not tested then? I probably would be dead now. Maybe, I would have grown so thin and by the time I got medication it would not work on my body anymore."

IDI, female, 69 years, urban

Just like the above mentioned participant, another participant also tested during HBCT and attributes their source of infection to their husband.

"When my husband died I didn't know what killed him so there was a time health workers were walking door to door, they counselled people before testing them. I was tested and I accepted my status, maybe I was infected by my husband"

IDI, female, 69 years, urban

Yet another participant, also tested during the door to door testing shared her testing experience. She believed she was HIV negative and agreed to be tested, and was deeply shocked when she received positive test results.

"My husband was really sick in 2008. He became so sick that he had to be admitted in the hospital. He could not eat because he had wounds in his mouth. He was transferred to the district hospital where he continued with medication. He grew so thin and died after two months. No one informed me about the condition he had. After we buried him, we continued with our normal activities. Then doctors who were

going from house to house to do HIV testing came to my house. My children were around and the doctor asked if we could be tested. My son was outside and he was sometimes helping the doctors with testing when they moved from house to house. I agreed to test because I knew I was 'clean'. I was so sure I did not have HIV. Then after the test the doctor told me the results. I was so scared and did not believe it was true. My world came crushing on me. I looked around and knew I was gone [was going to die]."

FGD, female, 64 years, rural

Proactive seeking of HIV test

A small number ($n = 4$) of participants proactively sought out an HIV test because they perceived themselves to be at risk of being infected. HIV risk perceptions were informed by condom bursts during sexual intercourse with partners they suspected could be HIV infected, having multiple partners, having taken care of HIV infected person or having signs and symptoms similar to those of HIV infected persons.

One of the female participants intimated on her engagement with multiple sexual partners and described situation of unprotected sex under the influence of alcohol. She visited a rural health facility to seek HIV testing services and was first rejected because she did not have anyone accompanying her, despite that fact that there are no existing policies in Kenya requiring that during HIV testing, one must be accompanied by another person. Her testing experience with the healthcare provider indicates likely ageism in provision of testing services to older persons:

"For me, I just went to the hospital myself. I had heard about HIV and wanted to test and get to know my status. When I got to the hospital, I found the nurse. I told her that I had come to be tested and she asked if I had come with someone. I told her that I was alone. She asked me to go home and come back the next day with a companion. I insisted that since I had made the choice to be tested I needed to [do it now]. She agreed to test. She pricked my hand and put blood in a small white stick. I could see blood move through the stick. She said that the test is incorrect and probably it can be done some other time. I told the nurse that (...) I still have a lot of blood in my body and we can do another test. We did another test and it came out positive. The nurse told me that the initial test had turned out positive but she was scared to tell me."

IDI, female, 56 years, rural

Other participants proactively sought out an HIV test following the death of a partner or a close relative or after an HIV-positive test result of a partner. Participants felt the urge to test out of curiosity, fear of being infected or fear of dying, too. The experiences with healthcare providers in these cases similarly suggest ageism and discrimination. A male participant who visited a local health facility during the early times of the HIV pandemic, when testing services were mainly provided for pregnant women as part of the national antenatal care policy, described his experience. The interaction with the healthcare provider indicates that the provider was neither used to nor comfortable with testing an older man:

"After [my wife's] demise, I became sick (...). I had bad dreams to the extent that I was communicating to the dead, and became very weak that I couldn't walk; I thought I was dying. I decided to go for a test because in my community people believe in witchcraft so I wanted to confirm so that I could tell them it wasn't witchcraft. I went home to our nearby Health Center and it took time because the doctor was hesitant to test me until I had to threaten him that I would write a letter stating that in case I die, it is my doctor who has killed me. When he heard so, he asked me whether I had made a decision and I told him I was an adult and I had decided. That I had lost my wife and I wanted to know whether it was due to HIV so it took three hours before he agreed to test me".

IDI, male, 65 years, urban

Another participant who had lost a husband to AIDS narrated her long process of seeking care for her ailing husband in several hospitals. He was only tested and diagnosed with HIV at a very late stage and died a few months after his diagnosis. She was never offered an HIV test when taking care of her husband at the hospital. After she buried the husband, she decided to get tested for HIV.

"Since I had heard that it [HIV] is transmitted sexually, I decided to go back to the hospital to get tested. When my turn came, the sister inside the room asked me if I was ready for the results in the likely event that they turn out positive. I told her any results were ok with me. When the results came out, it was positive. I was not shocked because my husband had died of HIV so I knew I could likely have [it but] of course I was praying to God for the results to come out negative".

FGD, female, 69 years, rural

Another female participant who had lost a daughter she had cared for to HIV went to seek an HIV test. She had heard that one could get infected if they cleaned an infected person's wounds without wearing gloves. Her description suggests ageist discrimination by other patients (young people) and healthcare providers:

> *"I came to the hospital and found two people, young ones, I think they were lovers, seated outside the office waiting for their turn. I sat next to them, and they stopped conversing and kept sneaking a look at me. When they went in, I stayed alone. Then another doctor passed by and asked if I was 'lost' and needed help. He went ahead to explain that the place was for HIV testing, and I say yes, I was waiting in line. He said ok and left, but I could see the shock in his face. I got tested and found with the virus. It was devastating but God has been with me now for 5 years and I am still strong."*
>
> IDI, female, 67 years, urban

Limited time spent with providers

Participants intimated that during the testing in hospital settings, it would be beneficial to spend more time with healthcare providers after testing, and to be able to discuss life after an HIV positive result. Older persons are, however, treated in a hurry during the clinic encounter with the clinician. Participants noted that the clinicians were overwhelmed by the number of patients on the queue, hence spend limited time with patients. This was perceived as an issue particularly by the older adults who may need more time to gain trust, ask questions and feel comfortable to discuss sexual matters.

> *"After the doctor counseled me, I thought I was prepared to take any results that came. I think I was convinced that I was not infected. Then during the test the doctor and I were there but we were so silent. When the results became positive, the doctor told me to go to AMPATH and ushered in the next person on the queue."*
>
> IDI, male, 54 years, urban

Unlike the above mentioned participant, a participant tested at her home expressed satisfaction with the time she spent with the doctor who provided HIV testing services and with the subsequent visits thereafter.

> *"She even took time to educate me. I asked a lot of questions and she was patient with me. She answered everything until I said I was ready. She then tested me. After the results were out, I could not remember whether one line was positive or not, she again taught me. Until I could see that my results were positive. I wanted to run outside and scream but she held me and calmed me down, she counselled me again. She stayed in my home until noon [i.e. she spent about 4 hours with the patient] and left but she visited me again the next day."*
>
> IDI, female, 65 years, urban

Age and gender matter

The age of a care provider was noted to be an important factor for HIV infected older adults during testing. Discussing sex-related issues with a healthcare provider of the same age as your child or grandchild was viewed as a 'taboo'. During an FGD, male participants unanimously expressed the need to have a male provider who can discuss male-related sexual issues which were considered 'private', including erection difficulties and sexually transmitted diseases among others. A participant shared his satisfaction after being attended to by a male provider:

> *"He is male. You know, you can talk comfortably to your fellow male and tell him everything about your private life and he would understand. There are things you cannot share with a female doctor, especially if you have private related stuff."*
>
> IDI, male, 60 years, urban

Female participants also shared similar views and prefer to be attended to by a female health care provider. Additionally, age was considered important and participants explained that an older provider would be ideal to care for older persons. Some of the participants' views are exemplified below:

> *"I wish women who are older, like us grandmothers, can be given our own doctor who would attend to us. That way, we don't have to push each other with those aged like our children on the queue".*
>
> FGD, female, 70 years, rural

> *"If also we could be given an older female doctor that understands what women go through, it would be easier to tell them even issues that are private and we would not feel embarrassed."*
>
> FGD, female, 66 years, urban

> *"I would prefer if it was a female doctor and a bit older. You cannot talk to young girls or even male [doctors] about issues down there [issues related to sexuality]."*
>
> IDI, female 54 years, rural

Discussion

This article highlights the experiences of HIV infected older adults with HIV testing services. The varied testing experiences have implications for how older people subsequently engage in HIV care services. As HIV medication continues to be widely accessible, finding the HIV infected, especially older persons, will require strategies that extend beyond facility-based HIV testing services [21–23]. This is important as countries work towards achieving the UNAIDS strategy of ending HIV transmission in 2030 by targeting to find at least 90% of those who are HIV infected, initiating them on ART and attaining viral load suppression.

Findings of our study demonstrate varied experiences of HIV testing among older adults depending on the setting of HIV test provision - whether in a hospital setting or home setting. The findings revealed that older adults are likely to be tested at the hospital in relation to another illness or when very sick and admitted to the hospital. When they test positive for HIV, older patients were shocked and devastated, likely indicating that older adults perceive themselves not to be at risk of HIV infection. These results support previous research work in similar settings [5, 24, 25] which showed that because HIV prevention messaging targets younger adults and other key populations, older adults continue to lack knowledge about HIV prevention [19]. The few older adults that actively seek HIV testing services do so amidst fear of discrimination.

The concept of ageism, 'prejudice and discrimination against older people', has been well described in literature in relation to HIV and co-morbidities with issues that include older age and sexuality [26–28]. Ageism has been associated with problems in access to HIV services, resulting in diagnosis late into HIV infection among older adults [5, 25, 28]. Healthcare providers on the other hand incorrectly assume that older adults are no longer sexually active and are more likely to misdiagnose or not diagnose an HIV infected older person presenting with flu-like symptoms [7, 8], or, as our findings show, with comorbid infections such as TB. Our findings also indicated that older adults viewed VCT services to be discriminating against older persons. The signage and directions to the VCT service station were often written in English, which older adults might not speak, or staffed with young providers who are unwilling or uncomfortable in providing services to older persons. HIV testing services were seen to target women, but focused on women at the reproductive age group (15–49 years). Once a woman is no longer in the reproductive age group, they seemed to no longer count [29]. These negative attitudes result in a lack of investments in HIV prevention education, testing and HIV care responses specifically targeting older adults. HIV policies on testing and prevention services in Kenya, and likely most parts of sub-Saharan Africa, should target older adults as a special group at risk of HIV infection.

This study also found a striking difference in experience between those who accessed the home-based testing and the hospital-based testing. Interviewees expressed a high level of satisfaction with home-based testing in terms of their interactions with the service providers. Our findings also support the view that home-based testing effectively targets subpopulations that are less likely to be tested otherwise. Globally, HBTC in many resource-limited settings appear to be acceptable and have been shown to reach as high as two-thirds of the population that did not know their HIV status [21, 30, 31]. The experiences of interviewees with hospital-based testing on the other hand were predominantly negative. Provision of HIV testing services at healthcare facilities can be challenging. Healthcare providers faced with high workloads [32–34] and the general atmosphere at the hospital setting that requires healthcare providers to spend shorter times with patients in order to provide services to a large number creates a setting that is perceived as off-putting by older patients. Our results suggests that provision of HIV testing services in a home setting (instead of hospital-based testing) would be cost effective [35] and would make an impact in finding older adults who do not have varied opportunities to test or may avoid hospital-based testing due to the unsupportive environment and/or fear of ageist discrimination [36].

Although this study observed an unsupportive environment in hospital settings compared to that of the home setting, participants who tested in hospital settings were more likely to accept the diagnosis. Unlike patients in the hospital, who were usually experiencing a range of HIV-related symptoms, those tested in home settings were likely to be asymptomatic at the time of testing. They were less likely to accept their positive result. This might indicate that pre-testing counseling in the community setting is insufficient, possibly due to ageist beliefs both by healthcare providers and older adults themselves. Beliefs by healthcare providers that older adults are no longer sexually active and are not at risk of HIV infection [27, 37, 38] may lead to presumptions of negative HIV test results when providing testing services for older adults. Additionally, older adults' beliefs that HIV is a disease of the 'young' [28, 38] may make them less likely to comprehend or ask questions during the pre-testing and counseling sessions. This study, therefore, cannot overemphasize the need for training of healthcare workers in offering counseling and testing services to older adults. HIV prevention messaging and awareness targeted towards older persons will also be key in changing older adults' attitudes towards HIV.

In provision of HIV care, patient-centered care is key to achieving better health outcomes for the HIV-infected [39, 40]. Older adults in our setting would prefer service providers of the same gender and a similar age because they felt that older healthcare providers would be more understanding of their needs. However, in Kenyan public care setting providing HIV services, patients are not able to choose healthcare providers, and there are currently no efforts made to employ particular service providers to cater to the needs of older people. Our results support studies from other settings that have shown that older people are likely to feel comfortable and discuss sexual matters with care provider of the same gender [41]. HIV care programming at facility level and possibly community level should be structured to focus on these needs of older people seeking HIV testing and care services.

While this study has highlighted potential areas for improvement in providing HIV testing services to older persons, the study had some limitations. We interviewed older adults who were still engaged in HIV care services and did not include persons who were lost to follow-up. Experiences of those who were lost to follow-up may likely be different from those of participants we interviewed. In addition, our study did not interview the healthcare providers who would shed light on their interactions with older adults. Despite this, we believe that these results are important in informing HIV care programming for HIV testing service provision in an attempt to meet Kenya's testing targets of 80% and ultimately the UNAIDS 90–90-90 targets [42].

Conclusion

This study explored HIV testing experiences among HIV infected older adults. HIV testing services in health care facilities are not tailored to target older adults in our setting resulting in late diagnosis among older persons. Community level testing services, including home-based counseling and testing, on the other hand, provide adequate testing and counselling time which is key for older persons understanding of HIV positive results. Finding HIV infected older persons by targeting testing services to them is a step in attaining the first 90 of the UNAIDS targets of having 90% of HIV infected getting to know their HIV status.

Abbreviations

AMPATH: Academic Model Providing Access to Healthcare; ART: Antiretroviral treatment; DTC: Diagnostic testing and counseling; FGD: Focus group discussion; HBCT: Home-based counseling and testing; HIV: Human immunodeficiency virus; IDI: In depth interview; MTRH: Moi Teaching and Referral Hospital; PITC: Provider Initiated testing and counseling; UNAIDS: Joint United Nations Programme on HIV/AIDS; WHO: World Health Organization

Acknowledgements

We are grateful to all older people who participated in our study. In addition, we wish to thank the research assistants Jackline Akinyi, Eunice Gift Walumbe, Julius Cheruiyot, Mark Omolo and Yvone Owino who helped a great deal in data collection and transcription. We say a big thank you to all for making this study a success.

Funding

This research was supported by the Consortium for Advanced Research Training in Africa (CARTA). CARTA is jointly led by the African Population and Health Research Center and the University of the Witwatersrand and funded by the Carnegie Corporation of New York (Grant No--B 8606.R02), SIDA (Grant No:54100029), the DELTAS Africa Initiative (Grant No: 107768/Z/15/Z). The DELTAS Africa Initiative is an independent funding scheme of the African Academy of Sciences (AAS)'s Alliance for Accelerating Excellence in Science in Africa (AESA) and supported by the New Partnership for Africa's Development Planning and Coordinating Agency (NEPAD Agency) with funding from the Wellcome Trust (UK) (Grant No: 107768/Z/15/Z) and the UK government. This study was also supported in part by the President's Emergency Plan for AIDS Relief (PEPFAR) through USAID under the terms of Cooperative Agreement No. AID-623-A-12-0001. It is made possible through joint support of the United States Agency for International Development (USAID). The contents of this study are the sole responsibility of the authors and do not necessarily reflect the views of CARTA Program, USAID or the United States Government.

Author's contribution

The study was designed by JK and SH. JK wrote the first draft of the article, SH provided guidance on the revisions of the manuscript. Both authors read and approved the final manuscript.

Competing interests

The authors declare that they have no competing interests.

Author details

[1]Moi University, College of Health Sciences, School of Medicine, Nandi Road, Eldoret, Kenya. [2]Academic Model Providing Access to Healthcare (AMPATH) Program, Moi Teaching and Referral Hospital Campus, Nandi Road, Eldoret, Kenya. [3]The University of Witwatersrand, School of Public Health, 27 St Andrews Road, Parktown, Johannesburg 2193, South Africa. [4]Graduate Entry Medical School, University of Limerick, Castletroy, Limerick V94 T9PX, Ireland. [5]School of History, Anthropology, Philosophy and Politics, Queen's University Belfast, 25 University Square, Belfast BT7 1NN, UK.

References

1. UNAIDS. Get on the Fast-Track, The life-cycle approach to HIV, Finding solutions for everyone at every stage of life. Geneva: UNAIDS; 2016.
2. UNAIDS. Global AIDS Update 2016. Geneva: UNAIDS; 2016.
3. Joint United Nations Programme on HIV/AIDS, Joint United Nations Programme on HIV/Aids: UNAIDS data 2017. UNAIDS: Geneva, Switzerland 2017.
4. World Health Organization. Progress report 2016: prevent HIV. In: Test and treat all: WHO support for country impact; 2016.
5. Negin J, Nemser B, Cumming R, Lelerai E, Amor YB, Pronyk P. HIV attitudes, awareness and testing among older adults in Africa. AIDS Behav. 2012;16(1):63–8.
6. Johnson LF, Rehle TM, Jooste S, Bekker L-G. Rates of HIV testing and diagnosis in South Africa: successes and challenges. Aids. 2015;29(11):1401–9.
7. Negin J, Cumming RG. HIV infection in older adults in sub-Saharan Africa: extrapolating prevalence from existing data. Bull World Health Organ. 2010; 88(11):847–53.
8. Mutevedzi PC, Newell M-L. A missing piece in the puzzle: HIV in mature adults in sub-Saharan Africa. Futur Virol. 2011;6(6):755–67.
9. Negin J, Geddes L, Brennan-Ing M, Kuteesa M, Karpiak S, Seeley J. Sexual behavior of older adults living with HIV in Uganda. Arch Sex Behav. 2016; 45(2):441–9.
10. Freeman E: Attitudes towards sexual health and sex behaviour among older adults with HIV in rural southern Malawi. 2016.
11. Pilowsky DJ, Wu L-T. Sexual risk behaviors and Hiv risk among Americans aged 50 years or older: a review. Subst Abus Rehabil. 2015;6:51.
12. Rosenberg MS, Gómez-Olivé FX, Rohr JK, Houle BC, Kabudula CW, Wagner RG, Salomon JA, Kahn K, Berkman LF, Tollman SM, et al. Sexual behaviors and HIV status: a population-based study among older adults in rural South Africa. J Acquir Immune Defic Syndr. 2017;74(1):e9–e17.
13. Gebo KA: Epidemiology of HIV and response to antiretroviral therapy in the middle aged and elderly. 2008.

14. Lekas H-M, Schrimshaw EW, Siegel K. Pathways to HIV testing among adults aged fifty and older with HIV/AIDS. AIDS Care. 2005;17(6):674–87.
15. Einterz RM, Kimaiyo S, Mengech HN, Khwa-Otsyula BO, Esamai F, Quigley F, Mamlin JJ. Responding to the HIV pandemic: the power of an academic medical partnership. Acad Med. 2007;82(8):812–8.
16. USAID Kenya: Academic Model Providing Access to Healthcare. 2014.
17. National AIDS and STI Control Programme (NASCOP). Kenya AIDS indicator survey 2012: Preliminary Report. Nairobi: NASCOP; 2013.
18. World Health Organization: Definition of an older or elderly person: proposed working definition of an older person in Africa for the MDS Project. http://www.who.int/healthinfo/survey/ageingdefnolder/en/. Accessed 14 Oct 2018.
19. Kuteesa MO, Seeley J, Cumming RG, Negin J. Older people living with HIV in Uganda: understanding their experience and needs. Afr J AIDS Res. 2012; 11(4):295–305.
20. Creswell JW: Qualitative, Quantitative, and mixed methods approaches. 2008.
21. Kimaiyo S, Were M, Shen C, Ndege S, Braitstein P, Sidle J, Mamlin J. Home-based HIV counselling and testing in western Kenya. East Afr Med J. 2010;87(3):100–8.
22. Osoti AO, John-Stewart G, Kiarie JN, Barbra R, Kinuthia J, Krakowiak D, Farquhar C. Home-based HIV testing for men preferred over clinic-based testing by pregnant women and their male partners, a nested cross-sectional study. BMC Infect Dis. 2015;15(1):298.
23. Krakowiak D, Kinuthia J, Osoti AO, Asila V, Gone MA, Mark J, Betz B, Parikh S, Sharma M, Barnabas R, et al. Home-based HIV testing among pregnant couples increases partner testing and identification of Serodiscordant partnerships. J Acquir Immune Defic Syndr. 2016;72(Suppl 2):S167–73.
24. Adekeye OA, Heiman HJ, Onyeabor OS, Hyacinth HI. The new invincibles: HIV screening among older adults in the US. PLoS One. 2012;7(8):e43618.
25. Kuteesa MO, Wright S, Seeley J, Mugisha J, Kinyanda E, Kakembo F, Mwesigwa R, Scholten F. Experiences of HIV-related stigma among HIV-positive older persons in Uganda–a mixed methods analysis. SAHARA-J. 2014;11(1):126–37.
26. Emlet CA, Brennan DJ, Brennenstuhl S, Rueda S, Hart TA, Rourke SB. The impact of HIV-related stigma on older and younger adults living with HIV disease: does age matter? AIDS Care. 2015;27(4):520–8.
27. Chepngeno-Langat G, Hosegood V. Older people and sexuality: double jeopardy of ageism and sexism in youth-dominated societies. Agenda. 2012;26(4):93–9.
28. DeMarco RF, Brennan-Ing M, Sprague C, Brown SM. Ageism, aging and HIV: community responses to prevention, treatment, care and support. InHIV and Aging. Karger Publishers. 2017;42:234–9.
29. Emlet CA, Poindexter CC. Unserved, unseen, and unheard: integrating programs for HIV-infected and HIV-affected older adults. Health Soc Work. 2004;29(2):86–96.
30. Dalal W, Feikin DR, Amolloh M, Ransom R, Burke H, Lugalia F, Ouma A, Laserson KF, Mermin J, Breiman RF. Home-based HIV testing and counseling in rural and urban Kenyan communities. J Acquir Immune Defic Syndr. 2013;62(2):e47–54.
31. Waruiru W, Ngare C, Ssempijja V, Gachuki T, Njoroge I, Oluoch P, Kimanga DO, Maina WK, Mpazanje R, Kim AA. The status of HIV testing and counseling in Kenya: results from a nationally representative population-based survey. J Acquir Immune Defic Syndr. 2014;66(Suppl 1):S27.
32. Burmen B, Owuor N, Mitei P. An assessment of staffing needs at a HIV clinic in a Western Kenya using the WHO workload indicators of staffing need WISN, 2011. Hum Resour Health. 2017;15(1):9.
33. Abdurahman S, Seyoum B, Oljira L, Weldegebreal F. Factors affecting acceptance of provider-initiated HIV testing and counseling services among outpatient clients in selected health facilities in Harar town, eastern Ethiopia. HIV/AIDS (Auckl). 2015;7:157.
34. Ahmed S, Bärnighausen T, Daniels N, Marlink R, Roberts MJ. How providers influence the implementation of provider-initiated HIV testing and counseling in Botswana: a qualitative study. Implement Sci. 2015;11(1):18.
35. Sharma M, Farquhar C, Ying R, Krakowiak D, Kinuthia J, Osoti A, Asila V, Gone M, Mark J, Barnabas RV. Modeling the cost-effectiveness of home-based HIV testing and education (HOPE) for pregnant women and their male Partners in Nyanza Province, Kenya. J Acquir Immune Defic Syndr. 2016;72(Suppl 2):S174–80.
36. Labhardt ND, Motlomelo M, Cerutti B, Pfeiffer K, Kamele M, Hobbins MA, Ehmer J. Home-based versus mobile clinic HIV testing and counseling in rural Lesotho: a cluster-randomized trial. PLoS Med. 2014;11(12):e1001768.
37. Eymard AS, Douglas DH. Ageism among health care providers and interventions to improve their attitudes toward older adults: an integrative review. J Gerontol Nurs. 2012;38(5):26–35.
38. Emlet CA. "You're awfully old to have this disease": Experiences of stigma and ageism in adults 50 years and older living with HIV/AIDS. Gerontologist. 2006;46(6):781–90.
39. Darin K, Bush C, Eschmann A, Moncus T, Scarsi K, DeMayo M, Whitfield C, Shankle M, Delpino A, Weidle P: Implementation of a patient-centered HIV care model to optimize outcomes. 2015.
40. Jaiswal J, Griffin-Tomas M, Singer SN, Lekas H-M. Desire for patient-centered HIV care among inconsistently engaged racial and ethnic minority people living with HIV. J Assoc Nurses AIDS Care. 2018.
41. Pascoal EL, Slater M, Guiang C. Discussing sexual health with aging patients in primary care: exploratory findings at a Canadian urban academic hospital. Can J Hum Sex. 2017;26(3):226–37.
42. Joint United Nations Programme on HIV/AIDS, Joint United Nations Programme on HIV/Aids. 90-90-90: an ambitious treatment target to help end the AIDS epidemic. Geneva: UNAIDS; 2014.

Octo- and nonagenarians' outlook on life and death when living with an implantable cardioverter defibrillator

Ingela Thylén[1*], Debra K. Moser[2] and Anna Strömberg[1,3]

Abstract

Background: Elderly individuals are increasingly represented among patients with implantable cardioverter defibrillators (ICD), but data describing life with an ICD are scarse among octo- and nonagenarians. Moreover, few studies have reported those elderly patients' perspective on timly discussions concerning what shock deactivation involves, preferences on battery replacement, and their attitudes about turning off the ICD nearing end-of-life. Consequently, the aim of the study was to describe outlooks on life and death in octo- and nonagenarian ICD-recipients.

Methods: Participants were identified via the Swedish Pacemaker- and ICD-registry, with 229 octo- and nonagenarians (82.0 ± 2.2 years, 12% female) completing the survey on one occasion. The survey involved questions on health and psychological measures, as well as on experiences, attitudes and knowledge of end-of-life issues in relation to the ICD.

Results: The majority (53%) reported their existing health as being good/very good and rated their health status as 67 ± 18 on the EuroQol Visual Analog Scale. A total of 34% had experienced shock(s), 11% suffered from symptoms of depression, 15% had anxiety, and 26% reported concerns related to their ICD. About one third (34%) had discussed their illness trajectory with their physician, with those octo- and nonagenarians being more decisive about a future deactivation (67% vs. 43%, $p < .01$). A minority (13%) had discussed what turning off shocks would involve with their physician, and just 7% had told their family their wishes about a possible deactivation in the future. The majority desired battery replacement even if they had reached a very advanced age when one was needed (69%), or were seriously ill with a life-threatening disease (55%). When asked about deactivation in an anticipated terminal illness, about one third (34%) stated that they wanted to keep the shocks in the ICD during these circumstances. About one-fourth of the octo- and nonagenarians had insufficient knowledge regarding the ethical aspects, function of the ICD, and practical consequences of withdrawing the ICD treatment in the end-of-life.

Conclusions: Increasing numbers of elderly persons receive an ICD and geriatric care must involve assessments of life expectancy as well as the patient's knowledge and attitudes in relation to generator changes and deactivation.

Keywords: Attitudes, Deactivation, End-of-life, Implantable cardioverter defibrillator, Knowledge, Nonagenarians, Octogenarians, Psychosocial distress, Quality-of-life, Shock

* Correspondence: ingela.thylen@liu.se
[1]Department of Cardiology and Department of Medical and Health Sciences, Division of Nursing Sciences, Linköping University, S-581 83 Linköping, Sweden
Full list of author information is available at the end of the article

Background

For over 20 years, implantable cardioverter defibrillators (ICDs) have been the treatment of choice for individuals at risk for - or with a history of - sudden cardiac death attributable to ventricular arrhythmias [1]. When ICDs are combined with cardiac resynchronisation therapy (CRT) in heart failure patients, symptom burden and survival are improved [1]. Therefore today, elderly individuals are increasingly represented among patients with ICDs and studies have shown that > 40% of ICDs and CRT devices are inserted in individuals ≥ 70 years of age [2]. About 12% of those deemed eligible for ICD implantation by conventional criteria are ≥ 80 years of age (i.e., octogenarians) [2]. Although guidelines state that ICD implantation is "rarely appropriate" in nonagenarians (i.e., ≥ 90 years of age) [3], they do not refer to any specific age limits, but rather to 1-year life expectancy as a mandatory criterion.

As the population ages, many are at greater risk of developing progressive multimorbidity, and therefore are likely to die of causes other than sudden cardiac death [4]. Under these circumstances, shocks may only cause a prolongation of the dying process [5]. During the first years after implantation, the risks of receiving at least one ICD shock can range from one third in primary preventive patients [6, 7] to up to 50% in patients with a secondary indication [8]. Even among those without shocks during the ICD's first battery life, the incidence of shocks at 5 years following generator exchange is > 25% [6] which can negatively affect quality-of-life (QOL) [9]. A recent systematic review that assessed > 5000 ICD-recipients reported that approximately 20% have clinically significant psychological distress with anxiety and/or depression the first year(s) post-implantation [10]. Furthermore, 31% receive a shock(s) in the last 24 h of their lives, decreasing their quality-of-death [5].

An ICD deactivation should be considered when a patient's clinical status worsens and death is near. Deactivating an ICD can be achieved in the following ways, which are ethically and legally equivalent: planned ICD deactivation through reprogramming, urgent temporary ICD deactivation using a magnet which temporarily stops the ICD delivering shocks whilst in position over the ICD, or not replacing the ICD when the device has reached the end-of-service indicator [11].

Effective communication between clinician and patient includes determining the patients' goals of care, helping patients to weigh the benefits and burdens of device therapy as their clinical situation changes, clarifying the consequences of deactivation, and discussing potential alternative treatments [12]. Therefore, in order to improve QOL for patients at the end of their lives, and to provide direction for clinicians, it is adviced that clinicians raise the question about elective ICD deactivation before implantation of the device and then recurrently during the illness trajectory [11, 13], yet few patients or families discuss the option of device deactivation with their physicians [14]. Many do not know that device deactivation is an available option, [15] which may result in a potentially painful end-of-life situation with the ICD not being deactivated [16]. There are several obstacles to effective communication and patient education regarding this issue. Firstly, many professionals still feel uncomfortable discussing end-of-life with their patients [17] and lack the competence and skills to communicate about end-of life issues [18, 19]. Secondly, professionals may feel uncertain about if and/or when patients prefer to discuss generator replacement and deactivation, which could result in a delayed end-of-life discussion [20]. Thirdly, patients might not want to discuss this topic at all [14, 21, 22].

Despite the increasingly high rate of ICD implantation in elderly patients, data describing their life-situation, experiences and perspectives on the timing of ICD deactivation discussions, and preferences on deactivation as the patient nears end-of-life, are scarse. Therefore, the overall purpose of this study was to describe outlook on life and death in octo- and nonagenarian ICD-recipients. The specific aims are as follows, using a cross-sectional design: 1) to describe self-rated perceived health and psychological distress; and 2) to describe experiences, attitudes and knowledge of end-of-life issues.

Methods

In 2012, we used the Swedish ICD- and Pacemaker registry to identify and invite all eligible ICD- and CRT-D (cardiac resynchronization therapy with defibrillator) recipients ($n = 5535$) at the time to complete standardized self-reported questionnaires, on one occasion. The survey involved questions on health and psychological measures, as well as on experiences, attitudes and knowledge of end-of-life issues in relation the the ICD/CRT-D. The inclusion criteria were being eligible for the registry (i.e., having a valid postal mail address), being ≥ 18 years old, having had the device for at least 1 year, and willingness to participate. The study was approved by the Regional Ethics Committee for Human Research at the University of Linköping, Sweden (Dnr 2011/434–31). The results from the main study are reported elsewhere [14, 23–25]. In this sub-study we have analysed data from those ≥ 80 years old.

Measures

Demographic and clinical data

Demographic data, co-morbidity and previous shock experience were obtained through purpose-designed questions whereas clinical variables such as primary vs. secondary indication and time since implantation were obtained from the Swedish ICD- and Pacemaker registry.

Quality-of-life and psychological measures

Quality-of-life was measured using the *EuroQol-5D* (EQ-5D) [26], an instrument with well-established reliability and validity. Symptoms of anxiety and depression was measured using the *Hospital Anxiety and Depression Scale* (HADS) [27], which has been used extensively in both hospitalized and non-hospitalized patients. The literaure supports the use of ≥8 as a cut-off, as it yields an optimal balance between sensitivity and specificity for the presence of symptoms of anxiety and depressive symptoms [28]. *ICD-related concerns* was measured using the 8-item Patient ICD Concerns (ICDC) questionnaire, which is a brief instrument that can be used to identify patients at risk for adverse outcomes in clinical practice. [29]. As there is no standardized cut-off for the ICDC, the instrument constructors [30] suggest dividing patients into a high vs. low concern group, using the highest tertile in the sample to indicate a high level of concerns. Perceived social support from family, friends, and significant others was measured using the *Multidimensional Scale of Perceived Social Support* (MSPSS) [31]. The higher total score, the higher the perceived social support. In addition, separate subscales can be used by summing the responses from the items in each of the three dimensions. The 4-item, *Control Attitudes Scale* (CAS) was used to measure perceived control [32]. Higher scores indicate greater perceptions of control. As recommended from the literature, we used the median in the sample as a cut-off for low vs. high perceived control [33].

End-of-life concerns

Data on experiences, attitudes and knowledge of end-of-life concerns was measured using the *EOL-ICD Questionnaire* [34]. The EOL-ICDQ is a self-rated questionnaire containing three domains that measure experiences (10 items), attitudes (18 items) and knowledge (11 items) of end-of-life in ICD-recipients. Participants list their answer as "yes/no" or "no opinion", "agree/don't agree", "true/false", or "don't know". The experiences domain includes items about patients' actual discussion experiences. Example items in this domain are "I have discussed what a battery replacement involves with my ICD doctor or nurse", and "I have told my next of kin (either in writing or orally) my wishes regarding the shocks in my ICD, if I become seriously ill with some fatal disease". The attitudes domain includes items about patients' attitudes towards potential future discussions and future events. Examples of items are "I want to have the battery in my ICD replaced even if I am seriously ill suffering from another disease" and "I want to have the shocks in my ICD even if dying of cancer or another serious disease". The knowledge domain involves 3 statements on ethical aspects, 2 statements on the fuction of the ICD, and 6 statements on practical consequences associated with ICD deactivation, such as "Deactivating the shocks is the same as active euthanasia" (i.e., false) and "When the shocks are turned off, the heart stops beating" (i.e., false).

Statistical analysis

All analyses were conducted using SPSS software, version 22 (SPSS, Chicago, Illinois). We used frequencies and proportions to describe the sample, their self-rated perceived health and psychological distress, as well as their experiences, attitudes and knowledge of end-of-life issues. Mann-Withney U-tests and chi-square tests were used to determine bivariate associations of socio-demographic, clinical, and psychological measures with positive and negative outlook on life and death (i.e., self-rated perceived health, willingness to discuss deactivation, attitudes on elective generator replacement at end-of-service indicator, and attitudes about maintaining ICD therapy in the context of terminal illness). As recommended in the literature [16], the 25th percentile in the sample (i.e., ≤3) was used as a cut-off for insufficient knowledge in the knowledge domain in the EOL-ICDQ. Probability values of $p < .05$ were considered significant.

Results

Background characteristics

Of the 5535 patients who were mailed the survey, 12% were > 80 years of age. A total of 3067 patients completed the survey, covering 55% of all Swedish ICD-recipients at the time for the study. Of these, 229 (7,5%) were octo- and nonagenarians and included in this analysis. The mean age of this sub-sample was 82.0 ± 2.2 years with a range of 80 to 94 years, with the majority being male (88%). Time since implantation ranged from one to 23 years with a mean of 5.5 ± 4.2 years, 25% had a CRT-D implanted and 32% had previously undergone an elective battery replacement. The majority (72%) had received their ICD as secondary prevention treatment, while the remainder had received their ICD for primary prevention, usually in the context of heart failure. The number of co-morbid conditions in total varied from 0 to 11, with 57% of the patients having ≥3 co-morbid conditions (mean 3.1 ± 1.9) (Table 1).

Outlook on life

The vast majority rated their general experiences as ICD-recipients as "good" or "very good" (97%). The corresponding percentage for their perceived general health experience was 53%, with a EuroQol VAS score ranging from 10 to 100 (67 ± 18) and a mean index of 0.783. The lowest proportion of reported health problems was seen in the self-care dimension (8%) whereas the highest proportion of problems were seen in the mobility dimension (52%) (Fig. 1). A worse health condition (i.e., EQ-VAS) was described by patients with a history of

Table 1 Background characteristics, $N = 229$

Characteristic[a]	Value[b]
Demographics	
Age (years)	82.0 (2.2)
Gender (male)	201 (87.8%)
Education (lower)[c]	102 (44.5%)
Living alone (yes)	55 (24.3%)
Clinical factors	
Time since implantation (years)	5.5 (4.2%)
ICD-indication (primary prevention)	65 (28.4%)
Resynchronization therapy (CRT-D, yes)	57 (24.9%)
Shock experience (yes)	76 (33.9%)
Generator replacement (yes)	73 (31.9%)
Co-morbidity	
Myocardial infarction	92 (40.2%)
Atrial fibrillation	125 (54.6%)
Heart failure	131 (57.2%)
Chronic obstructive pulmonary disease	32 (14.0%)
Diabetes mellitus	33 (14.4%)
Stroke	27 (11.8%)
Cancer	29 (12.7%)

[a]Self-reported by subjects
[b]Data are presented as mean (SD) or n (%)
[c]Compulsory secondary school, with a total education time ≤ 9 years

myocardial infarction (64 vs. 70, $p < .05$), heart failure (64 vs. 71, $p < .01$), kidney disease (57 vs. 69, $p < .01$), or intermittent claudiocation (60 vs. 69, $p < .001$) compared to their counterparts. Also patients with symptoms of depression and anxiety, and ICD-related concerns reported a worse health condition (EQ-VAS 44 vs. 70, 47 vs. 71 and 61 vs. 70, respectively, $p < .000$).

In total, 11% reported symptoms of depression, 15% anxiety, 26% had ICD-related concerns, and 32% described a low perceived control in life (Table 2). Those with symptoms of anxiety also perceived a lower control compared to them without anxiety (52% vs. 28%, respectively, $p < .01$). This was also true for the patients with high ICD-related concerns; 45% described a low control in this group compared to 26% in the group without any concerns ($p < .01$).

About one third of the patients (34%) had received at least one shock and that experience was also correlated with a higher percentage of symptoms of anxiety compared to those without any shock experience in the past (24% vs. 10%, respectively, $p < .01$). In connection with the latest shock, they rated their pain and their anxiety experience as 4.1 and 3.6 on a 10 point numeric rating scale, respectively. The ICD-recipients were least concerned about not being able to prevent the ICD from firing, with 46% being concerned for this reason. ICD-recipients were most concerned that working too hard/overdoing things might cause the ICD to fire, with 65% sharing this concern (Fig. 2). A minority (27%) stated that they had a religious faith or outlook on life helping them in their daily life as an ICD-recipient.

Outlook on death

Nearly one forth (24%) of the octo- and nonagenarians stated that they often thought about death, and one third (34%) had discussed their illness trajectory with their physician. About 40% had at some time discussed what a forthcoming generator replacement would involve for them, and 30% had discussed the topic with a family member. The vast majority (87%) had not discussed with their physician about what turning off the shocks would involve if their health deteriorates, and just 7% had told

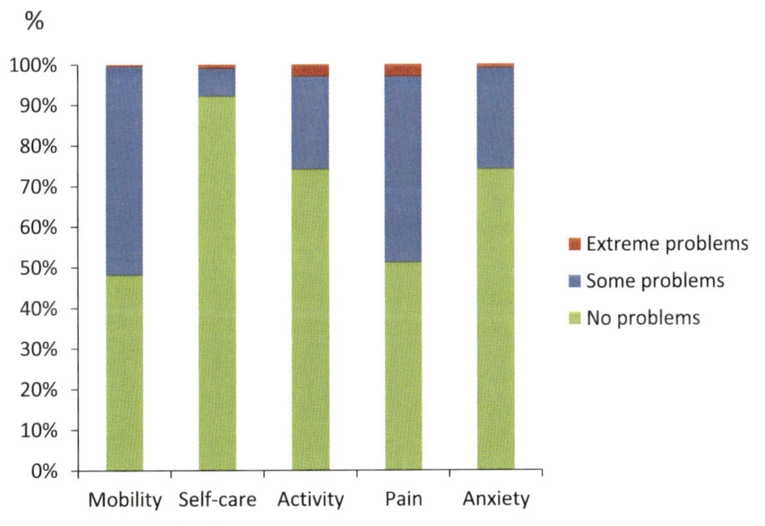

Fig. 1 ICD-recipients perceived health, measured with EQ-5D

Table 2 Psychological characteristics, N = 229

Characteristic[a]	Value[b]
Perceived ICD experience	
Experiences of the ICD-treatment ("good/very good")	213 (96.8%)
Pain experience with the latest shock, numeric rating scale (score 0–10)	4.1 (3.2)
Anxiety experience with the latest shock, numeric rating scale (score 0–10)	3.6 (2.9)
Quality-of-life (EQ-5D)	
Quality-of-life index, mean	783 (.212)
Quality-of-life, visual analogue scale, total (score 0–100)	67.4 (18.4)
Poor quality-of-life, visual analogue scale, 0–65	71 (34.1%)
Moderate quality-of-life, visual analogue scale, 66–79	74 (35.6%)
Good quality-of-life, visual analogue scale, 80–100	63 (30.3%)
Psychological distress	
Symptoms of anxiety (HADS-A)	32 (14.6%)
Symptoms of depression (HADS-D)	25 (11.2%)
ICD-related concerns (ICDC)	57 (26.1%)
Low perceived control (CAS)	71 (32.0%)
Percieved social support (MSPSS), (score 12–84)	71.4 (15.1)

[a]Self-reported by subjects
[b]Data are presented as mean (SD) or *n* (%)

their family their stance about deactivation when nearing end-of-life. Among those who had discussed their wishes, 93% perceived a high control in life compared to 65% among those that had not discussed this issue with their family ($p < .05$). Six participants had considered deactivation in the future. Many of the participants (40%) stated that they under no circumstances wanted to discuss deactivation. Among those who wanted to discuss deactivation, 51% found it appropriate to have the discussion at implantation, while 61% wanted to discuss deactivation if suffering from a poor prognosis, and 67% towards the end-of-life (Fig. 3).

When being faced with three different scenarios at the time for the end-of-service indicator in the ICD, most of the participants stated that they would like to replace the ICD even if no shock therapy had been delivered (76%), if had reached a very advanced age (69%), or if being seriously ill in a life-threatening disease at that time (55%). When asked about deactivation in an anticipated terminal illness, about one third of patients (34%) stated that they wanted to keep the shocks in the ICD during these circumstances, and 15% wanted to keep the shocks even if having shocks daily (Fig. 4). Those with a CRT-D implanted were more able to take a stand about deactivation (yes or no) if falling ill in a terminal illness compared to those without a CRT-D (77% vs. 62%, respectively, $p < .05$). This was also true for participants with a history of myocardial infarction when compared to their counterparts (76% vs. 60%, respectively, $p < .01$). Furthermore, those who had discussed deactivation with their family were more able to take a stand about deactivation in an anticipated

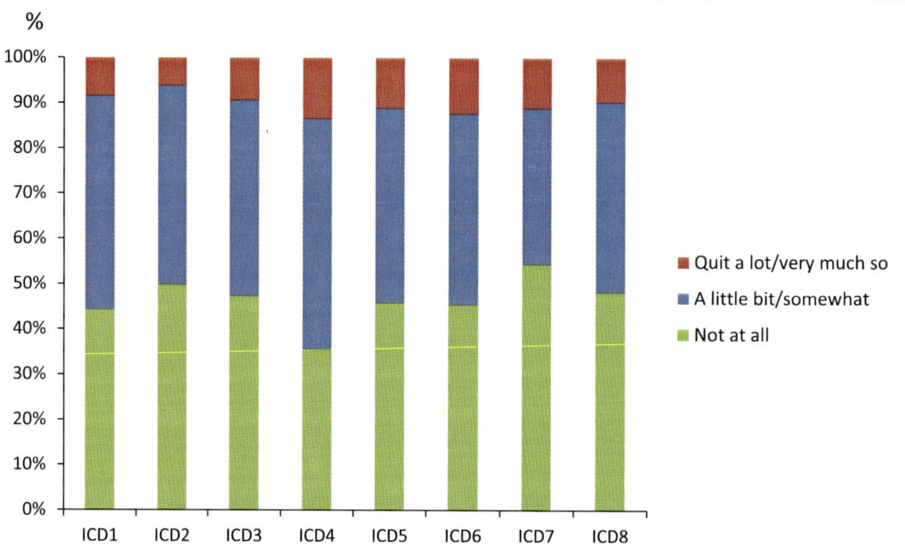

Fig. 2 ICD-related concerns, measured with ICD-C. 1) My ICD firing; 2) Doing activities/hobbies that may cause my ICD to fire; 3) Time spent thinking about my ICD firing; 4) Working too hard/overdoing things causing my ICD to fire; 5) Having no warning my ICD will fire; 6) The symptoms/pain associated with my ICD firing; 7) Not being able to prevent my ICD from firing; 8) Getting too stressed in case my ICD fires

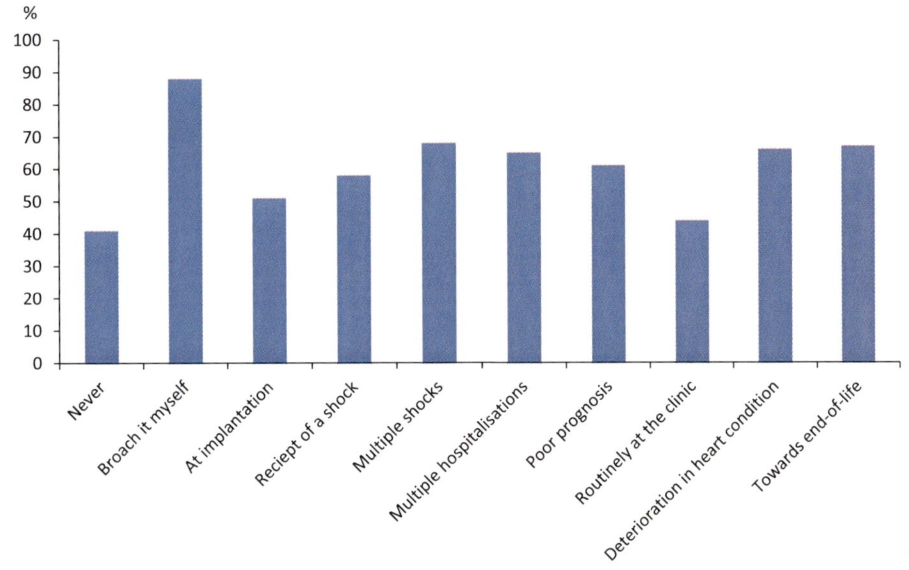

Fig. 3 Octo-nonagenarians preferences about the timing to discuss what deactivation involves

terminal illness (86% vs. 65%, respectively, $p < .05$). When it came to an anticipated situation with daily shocks, again those with a history of myocardial infarction were more able to take a stand (yes or no) about deactivation compared to those without myocardial infarction (60% vs. 45%, respectively, $p < .05$). Those who hade discussed their illness trajectory with their physician were also more decisive about this situation with 67% being able to take a stand about deactivation compared to 43% among those who had not discussed their illness trajectory with their physician, $p < .01$. Finally, those who were willing to discuss deactivation with their physician had less often had a battery replacement (44% vs. 66%, $p < .01$), more often a history of atrial fibrillation (68% vs. 49%, $p < .01$) or

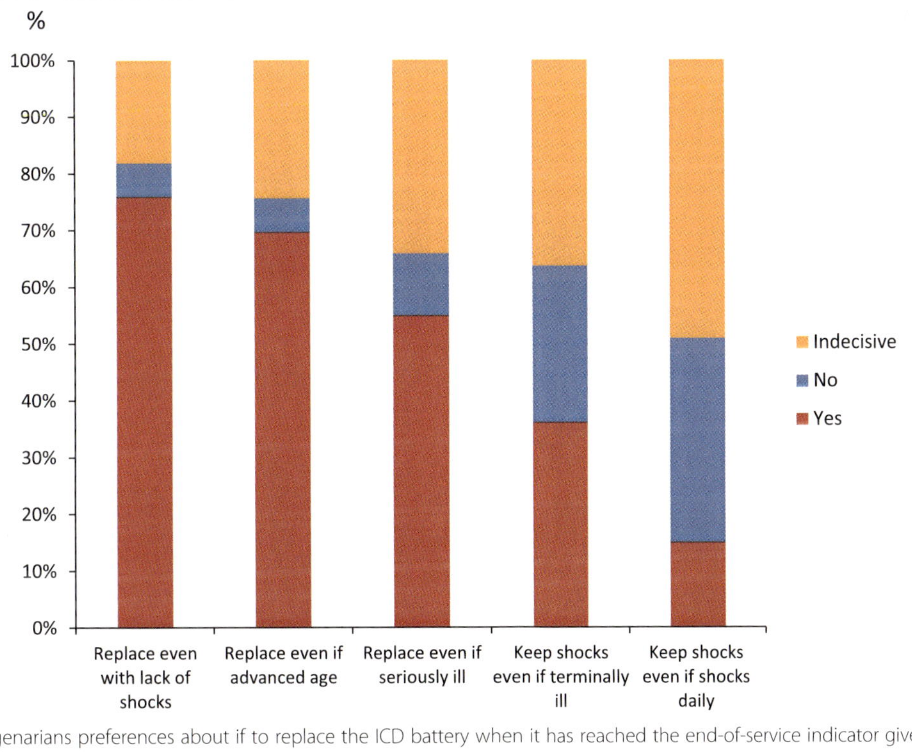

Fig. 4 Octo-nonagenarians preferences about if to replace the ICD battery when it has reached the end-of-service indicator given three different scenarios, and if keep shocks in an anticipated future with worsening of the health

diabetes (75% vs. 57%, $p < .05$). There were no other significant differences in the bivariate analyses between different socio-demographic, clinical, or psychological measures and those who were willing to discuss deactivation of the ICD, or were able to take a stand about deactivation (yes or no) or were indecisive about their standpoint in case of terminal illness or having shocks daily.

Only two participants (1%) recieved the highest possible points on the knowledge questionnaire, whereas 17 participants (8%) did not know or scored incorrectly on all statements. The mean score in the sample was 5.6 ± 3.0 out of 11 possible scores, with 54 participants (26%) having insufficient knowledge. In the ethical domain, the statement "When an ICD's defibrillating shocks are turned off, the heart stops beating," (i.e., false) resulted in the highest score with 74% responding correctly. Approximately one third (36%) in-correctly believed that deactivation was the same as active euthanasia. The two statements in the domain covering the function of the ICD, i.e., "When the battery voltage is beginning to wear, the ICD's functioning worsens" and "When the shocks are turned off, the pacemaker function in the ICD is also turned off," were correctly responded to as false by 23% and 30%, respectively. In the last domain about practical consequences of drawing the ICD treatment at the end-of-life, only 24% scored correct (i.e., false) to the statement "An ICD always delivers defibrillating shocks in connection with end-of-life". Additionally, approximately one third of the octo- and nonagenarians (37%) incorrectly believed that the ICD must be removed by surgery in order to be turned off, and 44% believed that when the ICD has been deactivated, it cannot be activated again.

Discussion

Our study, conducted in a national sample of octo- and nonagenarian ICD-recipients, demonstrated that nearly one-third of the participants experienced a good QOL and their overall ICD experience was considered good or very good in almost all the participants. Further, they reported similar prevalence of symptoms of anxiety and depression as in a Swedish norm population in this age group [35]. As many as 26% had ICD-related concerns and were most concerned about that working too hard/overdoing things may cause the ICD to fire. This is noteworthy since fear may influence and decrease activity levels in daily life [36, 37] which in turn has been found to strongly correlate with survival following ICD-implantation [38].

We found that only a minority had discussed the implications of generator replacement at battery-end-of-service or had discussed potential ICD deactivation at the end-of-life. Moreover, many participants were unable to foresee what they might prefer to do with their ICD in an end-of-life situation. Two thirds of the participants in our study wanted to replace their battery irrespectable of age and half of them wanted this done also when being seriously ill. As many as one third required to keep the ICD active until they died. These findings suggest that many patients with an ICD are at risk of not dying peacefully, painlessly and with dignity. It is the reality that many dying ICD-recipients receive shocks in their last days of life. A recent Swedish study by Westerdahl et al. showed that one out of four patients received at least one shock during the last day of their life. It is noteworthy that this study also showed that ICD devices were active in half of patients with a do-not-resuscitate order [19].

Earlier studies have shown that patients and their family members - as well as healthcare professionals - are reluctant to speak about not replacing the battery or deactivation [17, 21, 39]. Our study underlines these findings and showed that remarkably few had discussed deactivation with their physician and/or family members. A study by van der Wal et al. found that many elderly and severly ill cardiac patients do not know what to expect for the future and some have unrealistic exectations on their long-term survival [40]. Older people obviously have a higher annual rate of death – with a 38% mortality rate 2 years after ICD replacement in octogenarians reported in a recent study [41], and this fact must be taken into consideration when discussing future expectations with the patient. Our study further showed that about one-forth of the participants had insufficient knowledge regarding the ethical aspects, function of the ICD, and practical consequences of withdrawing the ICD treatment in the end-of-life. We have previously shown that increased knowledge improve the compentences and skills of making a decision, in favour of deactivation or not [16]. Dodson et al., [42] found that providing information regarding the best current evidence on benefits and burdens of an ICD with focus on person-centered outcomes, triggered that ICD-recipients made a decision for deactivation in at least 1 out of 5 end-of-life scenarios [42]. However, the lack of knowledge is not just on the patient side. Many physicians, medically responsible for elderly patients with an ICD, have limited knowledge of ICD treatment and may therefore not be able to provide the best possible care from implantation to the end-of-life in the elderly ICD-recipients [19]. Thus, we see a need for more education on ICD care and communication about deactivation to physicians both in geriatrics, internal medicine and primary care as well as a more close collaboration with cardiologists and device nurses responsible for ICD follow-up.

Methodological issues

The study has several limitations with the design being cross sectional and data collected by self-report. Only one data collection point was used, therefore it is not known if the individual's psychological distress existed before the ICD-implantation. A longitudinal study of a large cohort of older ICD-recipients would be helpful in understanding the process of adjustment, changes in psychological distress and outlook on death over time. Even thought this is a national registry based study, we may have had a selection bias with those octo- and nonagenarian ICD-recipients responding to the survey being less burdened by psychosocial distress and having better QOL. However, a reasonable response rate and a large sample size contributed strength to the results. Lastly, more than 60% of participants had ICD implanted as secondary prevention. This is a relatively high rate for current practice which could be seen as a limitation, but could be explained by the rather long time since implantation ranging up to 23 years.

Conclusions

We found that most octo- and nonagenarian ICD-recipients report a good health with similar prevalence of psychological distress as younger ICD-recipients and other populations in the same age group. They view their ICD experience as positive and continue to desire ICD therapy in spite of age or serious illness. However, a significant majority of patients have not discussed possible future deactivation with their physician or family. Misunderstandings regarding withdrawing the ICD treatment in the end-of-life were evident, which may result in a potentially painful end-of-death with the ICD not being deactivated. Increasing numbers of elderly persons receive an ICD and geriatric care must remember involving assessments of life expectancy as well as the patients' knowledge and attitudes in relation to generator changes and deactivation. These conversations should continue over the course of the patient's lifespan, since patient preferences may change as illness progresses and deactivation needs to be a deliberate decision based on knowledge.

Abbreviations

CAS: The 4-item Control Attitudes Scale; CRT: Cardiac resynchronisation therapy; CRT-D: Cardiac resynchronisation therapy with defibrillator; EOL-ICDQ: The Experiences, Attitudes and Knowledge of End-of-Life Issues in Implantable Cardioverter Defibrillator Patients Questionnaire; EQ-5D: EuroQol-5 Dimensions; EQ-VAS: EQ-5D visual analogue scale; HADS: The Hospital Anxiety and Depression Scale; ICD: Implantable cardioverter defibrillator; ICDC: The 8-item Patient ICD Concerns questionnaire; MSPSS: The Multidimensional Scale of Perceived Social Support; QOL: Quality-of-life

Acknowledgments

We are grateful to the ICD-recipients who have made this work possible.

Funding

This study was funded with grants from the Medical Research Council of Southeast Sweden (FORSS) and the Swedish Heart and Lung Association. The funder had no role in study design, data collection and analysis, or preparation of the manuscript.

Authors' contributions

IT, DM and AS contributed to the conception and design of this study. IT conceptualized the research problem and did the statistical analyses. IT, DM and AS wrote the manuscript, provided literature review and participated in interpretation of results. IT, DM and AS critically revised and approved the final manuscript.

Competing interests

The authors declare that they have no competing interests.

Author details

[1]Department of Cardiology and Department of Medical and Health Sciences, Division of Nursing Sciences, Linköping University, S-581 83 Linköping, Sweden. [2]College of Nursing, University of Kentucky, Lexington, USA. [3]Sue and Bill Gross School of Nursing, University of California, Irvine, USA.

References

1. Tracy CM, et al. 2012 ACCF/AHA/HRS Focused Update Incorporated Into the ACCF/AHA/HRS 2008 Guidelines for Device-Based Therapy of Cardiac Rhythm Abnormalities: A Report of the American College of Cardiology Foundation/American Heart Association Task Force on Practice Guidelines and the Heart Rhythm Society. J Am Coll Cardiol. 2013;61(3):e6-e75.
2. Epstein AE, et al. Implantable cardioverter-defibrillator prescription in the elderly. Heart Rhythm. 2009;6(8):1136–43.
3. Russo AM, et al. ACCF/HRS/AHA/ASE/HFSA/SCAI/SCCT/SCMR 2013 appropriate use criteria for implantable cardioverter-defibrillators and cardiac resynchronization therapy: a report of the American College of Cardiology Foundation appropriate use criteria task force, Heart Rhythm Society, American Heart Association, American Society of Echocardiography, Heart Failure Society of America, Society for Cardiovascular Angiography and Interventions, Society of Cardiovascular Computed Tomography, and Society for Cardiovascular Magnetic Resonance. J Am Coll Cardiol. 2013; 61(12):1318–68.
4. Kurtz SM, et al. Implantation trends and patient profiles for pacemakers and implantable cardioverter defibrillators in the United States: 1993-2006. Pacing Clin Electrophysiol. 2010;33(6):705–11.
5. Kinch Westerdahl A, et al. Implantable cardioverter-defibrillator therapy before death: high risk for painful shocks at end of life. Circulation. 2014; 129(4):422–9.
6. Merchant FM, et al. Incidence of defibrillator shocks after elective generator exchange following uneventful first battery life. J Am Heart Assoc. 2014;3: e001289.
7. van der Heijden AC, et al. The clinical course of patients with implantable cardioverter-defibrillators: extended experience on clinical outcome, device replacements, and device-related complications. Heart Rhythm. 2015;12(6): 1169–76.
8. Erkapic D, et al. Long-term benefit of implantable cardioverter/defibrillator therapy after elective device replacement: results of the INcidence free SUrvival after ICD REplacement (INSURE) trial--a prospective multicentre study. Eur Heart J. 2013;34(2):130–7.
9. da Silva KR, et al. Quality of life in patients with implantable cardioverter-defibrillator: systematic review of randomized controlled trials. Eur J Cardiovasc Nurs. 2017. https://doi.org/10.1177/1474515117739619.
10. Magyar-Russell G, et al. The prevalence of anxiety and depression in adults with implantable cardioverter defibrillators: a systematic review. J Psychosom Res. 2011;71(4):223–31.
11. Padeletti L, et al. EHRA expert consensus statement on the management of cardiovascular implantable electronic devices in patients nearing end of life or requesting withdrawal of therapy. Europace. 2010;12(10):1480–9.
12. Goldstein NE, Back AL, Morrison RS. Titrating guidance: a model to guide physicians in assisting patients and family members who are facing complex decisions. Arch Intern Med. 2008;168(16):1733–9.
13. Lampert R, et al. HRS expert consensus statement on the Management of Cardiovascular Implantable Electronic Devices (CIEDs) in patients nearing end of life or requesting withdrawal of therapy. Heart Rhythm. 2010;7(7): 1008–26.
14. Thylén I, et al. Are ICD recipients able to foresee if they want to withdraw

therapy or deactivate defibrillator shocks? Int J Cardiol Heart Vessels. 2013. https://doi.org/10.1016/j.ijchv.2013.11.001.
15. Goldstein N, et al. Barriers to conversations about deactivation of implantable defibrillators in seriously ill patients: results of a nationwide survey comparing cardiology specialists to primary care physicians. J Am Coll Cardiol. 2009;54(4):371–3.
16. Stromberg A, et al. ICD recipients' understanding of ethical issues, ICD function, and practical consequences of withdrawing the ICD in the end-of-life. Pacing Clin Electrophysiol. 2014;37(7):834–42.
17. Sherazi S, et al. Physicians' preferences and attitudes about end-of-life care in patients with an implantable cardioverter-defibrillator. Mayo Clin Proc. 2008;83(10):1139–41.
18. Kelley, A.S., et al., Implantable cardioverter-defibrillator deactivation at the end of life: a physician survey. Am Heart J, 2009. 157(4): p. 702–8 e1.
19. Kinch Westerdahl A, Frykman V. Physicians' knowledge of implantable defibrillator treatment: are we good enough? Europace. 2017;19(7):1163–9.
20. Russo JE. Original research: deactivation of ICDs at the end of life: a systematic review of clinical practices and provider and patient attitudes. Am J Nurs. 2011;111(10):26–35.
21. Fluur C, et al. Patients' experiences of the implantable cardioverter defibrillator (ICD); with a focus on battery replacement and end-of-life issues. Heart Lung. 2013;42(3):202–7.
22. Herman D, et al. Deactivation of implantable cardioverter-defibrillators: results of patient surveys. Europace. 2013;15(7):963–9.
23. Miller J, Thylen I, Moser DK. Gender disparities in symptoms of anxiety, depression, and quality of life in defibrillator recipients. Pacing Clin Electrophysiol. 2015;00:1–11.
24. Thylen I, et al. Characteristics associated with anxiety, depressive symptoms, and quality-of-life in a large cohort of implantable cardioverter defibrillator recipients. J Psychosom Res. 2014;77(2):122–7.
25. Thylen I, et al. Concerns about implantable cardioverter defibrillator shocks mediate the relationship between actual shocks and psychological distress. Europace. 2015. https://doi.org/10.1093/europace/euv220.
26. EuroQol, G. EuroQol-a new facility for the measurement of health-related quality of life. Health Policy. 1990;16(3):199–208.
27. Zigmond AS, Snaith RP. The hospital anxiety and depression scale. Acta Psychiatr Scand. 1983;67(6):361–70.
28. Bjelland I, et al. The validity of the hospital anxiety and depression scale. An updated literature review. J Psychosom Res. 2002;52(2):69–77.
29. Pedersen SS, et al. Concerns about the implantable cardioverter defibrillator: a determinant of anxiety and depressive symptoms independent of experienced shocks. Am Heart J. 2005;149(4):664–9.
30. Pedersen SS, et al. Course of anxiety and device-related concerns in implantable cardioverter defibrillator patients the first year post implantation. Europace. 2010;12:1119–26.
31. Zimet GD, et al. Psychometric characteristics of the multidimensional scale of perceived social support. J Pers Assess. 1990;55(3–4):610–7.
32. Arestedt K, et al. A psychometric evaluation of the four-item version of the control attitudes scale for patients with cardiac disease and their partners. Eur J Cardiovasc Nurs. 2015;14(4):317–25.
33. Moser DK, et al. Impact of anxiety and perceived control on in-hospital complications after acute myocardial infarction. Psychosom Med. 2007; 69(1):10–6.
34. Thylen I, et al. Development and evaluation of the EOL-ICDQ as a measure of experiences, attitudes and knowledge in end-of-life in patients living with an implantable cardioverter defibrillator. Eur J Cardiovasc Nurs. 2014; 13(2):142–51.
35. Börjesson-Hansson A, et al. One-month prevalence of mental disorders in a population sample of 95-year-olds. Am J Geriatr Psychiatry. 2011; 19(3):284–91.
36. Cutitta KE, et al. Shocktivity: ability and avoidance of daily activity behaviors in ICD patients. J Cardiopulm Rehabil Prev. 2014;34:241–7.
37. Sears SF, et al. Examination of the differential impacts of antitachycardia pacing vs. shock on patient activity in the EMPIRIC study. Europace. 2015;17:417–23.
38. Kramer DB, et al. Patient activity and survival following implantable cardioverter-defibrillator implantation: the ALTITUDE activity study. J Am Heart Assoc. 2015;4:e001775.
39. Fluur C, et al. Spouses' reflections on implantable cardioverter defibrillator treatment with focus on the future and the end-of-life: a qualitative content analysis. J Adv Nurs. 2014;70(8):1758–69.
40. van der Wal MH, et al. Heart failure patients' future expectations and their association with disease severity, quality of life, depressive symptoms and clinical outcomes. Int J Clin Pract. 2016;70(6):469–76.
41. Goonewardene M, et al. Cardioverter defibrillator implantation and generator replacement in the octogenarian. Europace. 2015;17:409–16.
42. Dodson JA, et al. Patient preferences for deactivation of implantable cardioverter defibrillators. JAMA Intern Med. 2013;173(3):377–8.

21

Clinical outcomes and prognostic factors in patients directly transferred to the intensive care unit from long-term care beds in institutions and hospitals: a retrospective clinical study

Su Hwan Lee[1], Soo Jung Kim[1], Yoon Hee Choi[2], Jin Hwa Lee[1], Jung Hyun Chang[1] and Yon Ju Ryu[1*]

Abstract

Background: There has been a steady increase in the aging population and an increase in the need for long-term care beds in institutions and hospitals (LTCHs) in Korea. The aim of this study was to investigate prognosis and to identify factors contributing to mortality of critically ill patients with respiratory problems who were directly transferred to intensive care units (ICU) from LTCHs.

Methods: Following a retrospective review of clinical data and radiographic findings between July 2009 and September 2016, we included 111 patients with respiratory problems who had visited the emergency room (ER) transferred from LTCHs due to respiratory symptoms and who were then admitted to the ICU.

Results: The mean age of the 111 patients was 79 years, and 71 patients (64%) were male. Pneumonia developed in 98 patients (88.3%), pulmonary thromboembolism in 4 (3.6%) and pulmonary tuberculosis in 3 (2.7%). Overall mortality was 19.8% (22/111). Multiple-drug-resistant (MDR) pathogens (odds ratio [OR], 17.43; 95% confidence interval [CI], 1.96–155.40) and serum albumin levels < 2.15 g/dL, which were derived through ROC (sensitivity, 72.7%; specificity, 85.4%) (OR, 28.05; 95% CI, 5.47–143.75), were independent predictors for mortality. The need for invasive ventilation (OR, 2.74; 95% CI, 1.02–7.32) and history of antibiotic use within the 3 months (OR, 3.23; 95% CI, 1.32–7.90) were risk factors for harboring MDR pathogens.

Conclusions: The presence of MDR pathogens and having low serum albumin levels may be poor prognostic factors in patients with respiratory problems who are admitted to the ICU from LTCHs. A history of antibiotic use within the 3 months and the need for invasive ventilation can be helpful in choosing the appropriate antibiotics to combat MDR pathogens at the time of admission.

Keywords: Long-term care, Nursing homes, Intensive care units, Pneumonia

* Correspondence: medyon@ewha.ac.kr
[1]Division of Pulmonary and Critical Care Medicine, Department of Internal Medicine, College of Medicine, Ewha Womans University, Mokdong Hospital, 1071 Anyangcheon-ro, Yangcheon-gu, Seoul 07985, South Korea
Full list of author information is available at the end of the article

Background

According to a recent statistical report, the number of people aged ≥65 is predicted to increase more from approximately 500 million in 2010 to approximately 1.5 billion in 2050, and the number of people aged ≥65 is expected to surpass that of those under 5 years old by 2050 [1]. As the proportion of the elderly population increases, the prevalence of various chronic diseases increases concomitantly, and the percentage of individuals considered frail also increases [2].

In Korea, the average life span is increasing and the proportion of elderly people aged ≥65 thus continues to rise. Combined with decreasing in fertility rates, Korea is becoming an aging society similar to the rest of the world [3]. The prevalence of chronic diseases and various age-related conditions including Alzheimer disease and stroke have increased. Accordingly, the need for long-term care beds in institutions and hospitals (LTCHs), defined as nursing and residential care facilities providing accommodations and long-term care as a package, is growing for this frail population [4–8].

Elderly patients living in LTCHs have a high incidence of chronic degenerative diseases [9–11] and frequently develop urinary tract infections and pneumonia [12–15]. Furthermore, elderly patients frequently experience unplanned transfers to general hospitals for various reasons [16]. These transfers generally result in patients being evaluated or managed by an emergency department that is likely to hospitalize patients [16], and some patients may be admitted to the intensive care unit (ICU) for treatment.

In Korea, a study of patients who visited the emergency department from LTCHs was reported previously [17]. However, studies on patients who were admitted to ICUs via emergency departments from LTCHs have not been conducted. Hence, we performed this study to investigate the factors associated with mortality in patients with respiratory problems who were directly transferred to the ICU from LTCHs.

Methods

Study design and subjects

This single-center study was a retrospective clinical study of all patients with respiratory problems who had been transferred from LTCHs to the ICU via the Emergency Department of Ewha Womans University Mokdong Hospital, which is a referral hospital with a 759-bed capacity containing 55 ICU beds (cardiovascular ICU, 7 beds; medical ICU, 15 beds; neuro ICU 18 beds; surgical ICU 15 beds) in Korea between July 2009 and September 2016. During this period, a total of 211 patients who had been transferred to our emergency department from LTCHs were hospitalized in the Pulmonary Department due to respiratory problems. Among these patients, 52.6% (111 of 211) required ICU admission.

Data collection

Data from all patients admitted to the ICU were obtained through review the hospital's electronic medical records. Variables for analysis were determined based on previous ICU mortality and LTCH studies [17–19]. Clinical data such as demographic characteristics, development of acute respiratory distress syndrome (ARDS), blood culture positivity, and mortality were evaluated. Various laboratory data such as albumin, C-reactive protein, and triglyceride levels were collected based on the first available data within 24 h after ICU admission. Sputum and bronchoalveolar lavage cultures were only collected within 48 h after admission to exclude infections after hospitalization. The severity of each patient's condition was calculated according to the acute physiology and chronic health evaluation (APACHE) II score, and comorbidity was calculated using the Charlson comorbidity index [20, 21].

Definition

A LTCH was defined as a medical institution with more than 30 beds for patients who need long-term hospitalization [7]. We excluded patients with LTCH stays of less than 3 days to exclude problems that occurred prior to LTCH admission.

The definition of a multi-resistant pathogen is based on non-susceptibility to at least one agent in three or more antimicrobial categories [22]. We considered several multiple-drug-resistant (MDR) pathogens including drug-resistant strains of *Pseudomonas aeruginosa*, carbapenem-resistant *Acinetobacter baumanii* (CRAB), *Stenotrophomonas maltophilia*, extended-spectrum β-lactamase (ESBL)-producing *Enterobacteriaceae* and methicillin-resistant *Staphylococcus aureus* (MRSA), all of which can be acquired during ICU hospitalization [23].

Acute kidney injury was defined as an increase in serum creatinine of ≥0.3 mg/dL within 48 h or an increase in serum creatinine to 30% more than the baseline level. Brain problems were defined as including neurodegenerative disorders, stroke, and brain hemorrhage.

Statistical analysis

Demographic data are described as averages with standard deviation or numbers with percentage. For analysis between groups, data are described as medians with interquartile range or numbers with percentage. The Mann–Whitney U test or the chi-squared and Fisher's exact tests were used to assess differences between groups. Logistic regression was used to investigate multivariate analysis for study of risk factors. Cut-off values for albumin were measured using receiver operating characteristic (ROC). The Kaplan–Meier method was used to report ICU length of stay and the survival curve, which were analyzed using the log-rank test. In all cases, a *p*-value of < 0.05 was considered statistically significant. SPSS version 23 (IBM, Armonk, NY, USA) was used for statistical analysis.

Results

Demographic characteristics of the overall study population

The number of patients admitted to the ICU via the emergency department from LTCHs gradually increased during the study period (Fig. 1). The patient population comprised a higher proportion of males than females (64% vs. 36%) who were of advanced age (mean age, 79 years). Pneumonia ($n = 98$) was the leading cause requiring a visit to the hospital, followed by pulmonary thromboembolism ($n = 4$), active pulmonary tuberculosis ($n = 3$), idiopathic pulmonary fibrosis ($n = 1$), exacerbation of chronic obstructive pulmonary disease ($n = 1$), hemoptysis ($n = 1$), lung cancer ($n = 1$), and asphyxia ($n = 1$). Seventy-seven patients (69.4%) developed acute respiratory failure requiring invasive ventilation. The mean APACHE II score was 24.9, and the mean Charlson comorbidity index was 2.45. The incidence rates of ARDS and positive blood culture were 26.1% and 22.5%, respectively. Among the sputum cultures that were performed for patients within 48 h of admission, 66 patients had positive sputum cultures, and more than 2 pathogens were identified in 8 patients. The mean ICU length of stay was 11.8 days, and the mean hospital length of stay was 24.5 days. The 28-day mortality rate was 15.3% (17/111), and the all-cause mortality rate during hospitalization was 19.8% (22/111). Two of the surviving patients were discharged to their homes, while all other survivors were transferred to other LTCHs. Baseline characteristics were not significantly different from 2009 to 2016 except sputum MDR pathogen species. CRAB was not identified before 2012, but has been consistently identified since 2012. Other MDR pathogens were similarly identified during the study period. Table 1 shows the baseline characteristics of the study population.

Comparison of characteristics between survivors and non-survivors

Study populations were divided into survivor and non-survivor groups according to all-cause mortality. The results of this inter-group comparison are shown in Table 2. The variables of sex, median age, median severity score, tracheostomy or nasogastric tube insertion, use of antibiotics within 3 months, development of ARDS, and acute kidney injury did not significantly differ between the survivor and non-survivor groups. However, the non-survivor group had lower median body mass index (BMI) compared with the survivor group (18.3 vs. 20.8, $P = 0.016$). Identification of MDR pathogens was also significantly higher in the non-survivor group relative to the survivor group (86.4% vs. 38.2%, $P < 0.001$). Regarding the laboratory parameters that were routinely analyzed in ICU patients, serum albumin and fasting triglyceride levels both measured significantly low in the non-survivor group. In particular, the proportion of patients whose serum albumin levels were < 2.15 g/dL, which was derived through ROC (sensitivity, 72.7%;

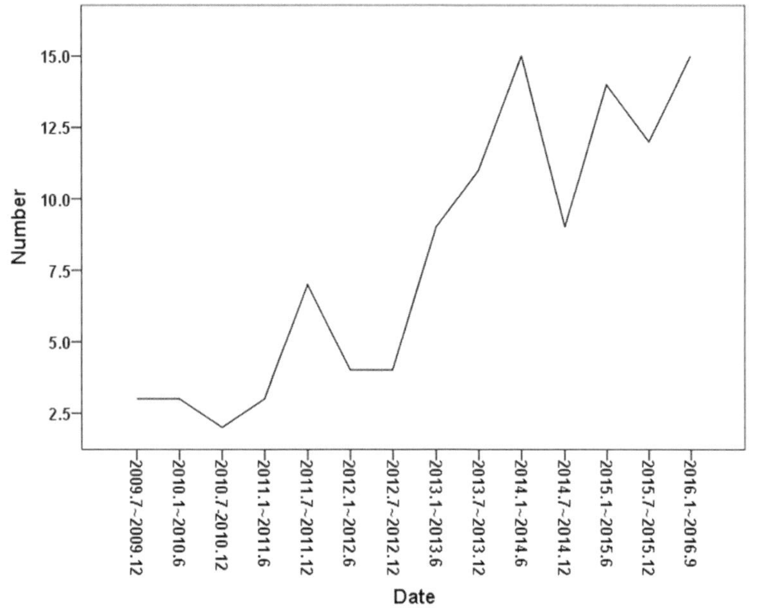

Fig. 1 Trends in the number of patients with respiratory problems admitted to the ICU from long-term care beds in institutions and hospitals

Table 1 Demographic and clinical characteristics of the study population

Characteristics	$N = 111$
Male sex	71 (64)
Age, years	79 ± 10
BMI, kg/m^2	20.7 ± 4.0
APACHE II score	24.9 ± 6.7
Charlson Comorbidity Index	2.45 ± 1.67
ICU length of stay, days	11.8 ± 1.3
Hospital length of stay, days	24.5 ± 3.0
Permanent tracheostomy status	28 (25.2)
Nasogastric tube insertion status	38 (34.2)
Bedridden status	50 (45)
ARDS	29 (26.1)
Use of antibiotics within 3 months	49 (44.1)
Blood culture positive	25 (22.5)
Sputum culture positive	66 (59.5)
MDR pathogen (sputum culture or blood culture)	53 (47.7)
Major cause of admission	
Pneumonia	98 (88.3)
Pulmonary thromboembolism	4 (3.6)
Pulmonary tuberculosis	3 (2.7)
Lung abscess	1 (0.9)
Idiopathic pulmonary fibrosis	1 (0.9)
Lung cancer	1 (0.9)
COPD exacerbation	1 (0.9)
Asphyxia	1 (0.9)
Hemoptysis	1 (0.9)

Values are presented as numbers (percentages) and as mean ± standard deviation, unless otherwise indicated. BMI, body mass index; APACHE, acute physiology and chronic health evaluation; ICU, intensive care unit; ARDS, acute respiratory distress syndrome; MDR, multiple-drug-resistant; COPD, Chronic Obstructive Pulmonary Disease

specificity, 85.4%), as compared with the proportion of patients with serum albumin levels ≥2.15 g/dL was higher in the non-survivor group than in the survivor group ($P < 0.001$).

Multivariate analysis showed that the MDR pathogen identification (odds ratio [OR], 17.43; 95% confidence interval [CI], 1.96–155.40) and serum albumin levels < 2.15 g/dL (OR, 28.05; 95% CI, 5.47–143.75) were associated with increased mortality. Statistical analysis of groups divided according to MDR pathogen or albumin level showed significant differences in survival rate and ICU length of stay (Fig. 2).

Risk factors for identification of MDR pathogens

Further analysis of MDR pathogens was performed, because the previous analysis demonstrated a difference between identification of MDR pathogens in the survivor and non-survivor groups. We identified 74 bacterial pathogens from the sputum cultures of 66 patients, and more than 2 bacterial pathogens were identified in 8 of the patients (Table 3). Among the 74 bacterial pathogens, 49 (66.2%) were MDR. The most common pathogens were CRAB (31.1%) followed by MRSA (23%).

In 25 patients with positive blood cultures, 12 MDR bacterial pathogens were identified including 3 MRSA, 3 methicillin-resistant coagulase-negative *Staphylococci* spp., 1 MDR *Streptococcus*, 2 CRAB and 3 ESBL-producing *Enterobacteriaceae* spp. There were 53 patients with MDR pathogens in sputum or blood cultures compared with 58 patients who did not have MDR pathogens.

A comparison of the MDR-negative and MDR-positive groups is shown in Table 4. The MDR-positive group had a higher proportion of males (77.4% vs. 51.7%, $P = 0.005$) and lower BMI (19.2 vs. 20.8, $P = 0.005$) than the MDR-negative group. At the time of admission, the presence of tracheostomy or nasogastric tube insertion did not differ between the two groups. The need for invasive ventilation, history of antibiotics use within the 3 months, and proportion of serum albumin level < 2.15 g/dL were higher in the MDR positive group. After multivariate analysis, the need for invasive ventilation (OR, 2.74; 95% CI, 1.02–7.32) and history of antibiotics use within the 3 months (OR, 3.23; 95% CI, 1.32–7.90) were shown to be risk factors for MDR pathogens.

Discussion

In this study, we found that the number of patients with respiratory problems admitted to the ICU from LTCHs increased gradually over the study period, and those who harbored MDR pathogens or had low serum albumin levels at the time of admission showed lower survival rates. A history of antibiotic use within 3 months and the need for invasive ventilation were risk factors for MDR pathogen infection.

The major cause of hospitalization for respiratory problems was pneumonia. Infection with MDR pathogens is associated with a worse prognosis than infection with susceptible pathogens, and the rapid administration of appropriate antibiotics is critical for a good prognosis [24–26]. In our study, the presence of MDR pathogens, which plays an important role in the selection of appropriate antibiotics, was also associated with mortality in patients from LTCHs. Previous studies about community-acquired pneumonia or healthcare-associated pneumonia reported that home infusion therapy, immunosuppression, chronic kidney disease, tube feeding, aspiration, LTCHs, a history of prior hospitalization, and a history of antibiotic use within the 3 months were risk factor for MDR pathogen infection [27–30]. Because our study subjects mostly had chronic diseases and brain problems or were frail, we supposed that only a history of antibiotics and the need for

Table 2 Predictors of mortality between survivors and non-survivors

Variable	Univariate			Multivariate	
	Survivor (*n* = 89)	Non-survivor (*n* = 22)	*P*	*OR (95% CI)*	*P*
Male sex	55 (61.8)	16 (72.7)	0.339	0.31 (0.06–1.75)	0.186
Age, years	78 (69.5–83.0)	81.5 (74.3–86.3)	0.064	1.07 (0.96–1.08)	0.143
BMI, kg/m^2	20.8 (18.7–23.7)	18.3 (15.9–22.3)	0.016	1.05 (0.85–1.31)	0.643
APACHE II score	25.0 (21.0–29.5)	25.5 (22.0–30.3)	0.459		
Charlson Comorbidity Index	2 (1–3)	2 (1–3)	1.000		
Blood culture positive	21 (23.6)	4 (18.2)	0.777		
Permanent tracheostomy status	26 (29.2)	2 (9.1)	0.052	0.35 (0.04–3.02)	0.340
Nasogastric tube insertion status	30 (33.7)	8 (36.4)	0.814		
Invasive ventilation	58 (65.2)	19 (86.4)	0.053	4.02 (0.68–23.76)	0.124
ARDS	21 (23.6)	8 (36.4)	0.222		
Use of antibiotics within 3 months	37 (41.6)	12 (54.5)	0.273		
MDR pathogen	34 (38.2)	19 (86.4)	< 0.001	17.43 (1.96–155.40)	0.010
MRSA	8 (9)	10 (45.5)	< 0.001		
CRAB	16 (18)	7 (31.8)	0.238		
Bedridden status	44 (49.4)	6 (27.3)	0.061	0.24 (0.05–1.13)	0.071
Brain problem[a]	69 (77.5)	15 (68.2)	0.36		
Diabetes mellitus	20 (22.5)	7 (31.8)	0.36		
Hypertension	37 (41.6)	7 (31.8)	0.402		
Acute kidney injury	27 (30.3)	4 (18.2)	0.255		
Albumin, g/dL	2.6 (2.3–2.9)	2.0 (1.7–2.2)	< 0.001		
Albumin < 2.15 g/dL	13 (14.6)	16 (72.7)	< 0.001	28.05 (5.47–143.75)	< 0.001
Total bilirubin, mg/dL[b]	0.5 (0.3–0.8)	0.6 (0.4–0.7)	0.627		
LDH, IU/L	239 (185.5–307.5)	258 (200.5–367.0)	0.184		
CRP, mg/dL	13.0 (7.3–23.6)	16.3 (12.8–21.3)	0.151		
NT-ProBNP pg/mL	1337 (410–4462)	2909.5 (1302.5–10,555.3)	0.124		
Triglyceride, mg/dL[c]	76.0 (55.0–106.3)	54.0 (43.0–83.0)	0.034		
ICU length of stay	7 (3–14.5)	5.5 (3.5–19)	0.801		

Values are presented as numbers (percentages), and as median (interquartile range), unless otherwise indicated. OR, odds ratio; CI, confidence interval; BMI, body mass index; APACHE, acute physiology and chronic health evaluation; ARDS, acute respiratory distress syndrome; MDR, multiple-drug resistant; MRSA, methicillin-resistant *Staphylococcus aureus*; CRAB, carbapenem-resistant *Acinetobacter baumannii*; LDH, lactate dehydrogenase; CRP, C-reactive protein; NT-ProBNP, N-terminal prohormone of brain natriuretic peptide; ICU, intensive care unit; [a]neurodegenerative disorders and stroke; [b]Five missing values; [c]Fourteen missing values

invasive ventilation were shown as risk factors. Many subjects in our study already had nasogastric tubes, tracheostomies, or were bedridden, all of which have been shown to be risk factors for developing MDR infections [28, 30]. The need for invasive ventilation indicates poor lung condition. Some patients transferred from our emergency department to LTCHs were already using antibiotics. Thus, the need for invasive ventilation may be a result of non-response to current antibiotic treatment, which may suggest the possibility of MDR pathogen infection.

Lastly, our study showed that male sex was associated with infection with MDR pathogens. In our study, males were not older than females, and there were no significant differences in ARDS, nasogastric tube, BMI, or other variables. Males showed higher a proportion of antibiotic use within 3 months than females; however, this difference was not statistically significant. It is possible that cigarette smoking have affected the results [31], because Korean males have a higher prevalence of smoking than Korean females [32]. A study reported male sex to be a risk factor for MDR pathogen infection similar to our results [28]. Unfortunately, we could not clarify the relevance because it was difficult to definitively document smoking history due to cognitive issues in many patients.

Serum albumin levels are a strong predictor of all-cause mortality in acutely admitted medical patients [19, 33, 34]. Our study also showed that hypoalbuminemia was correlated with mortality. As previous studies demonstrated that hypoalbuminemia is often associated with malnutrition and malnutrition is associated with mortality

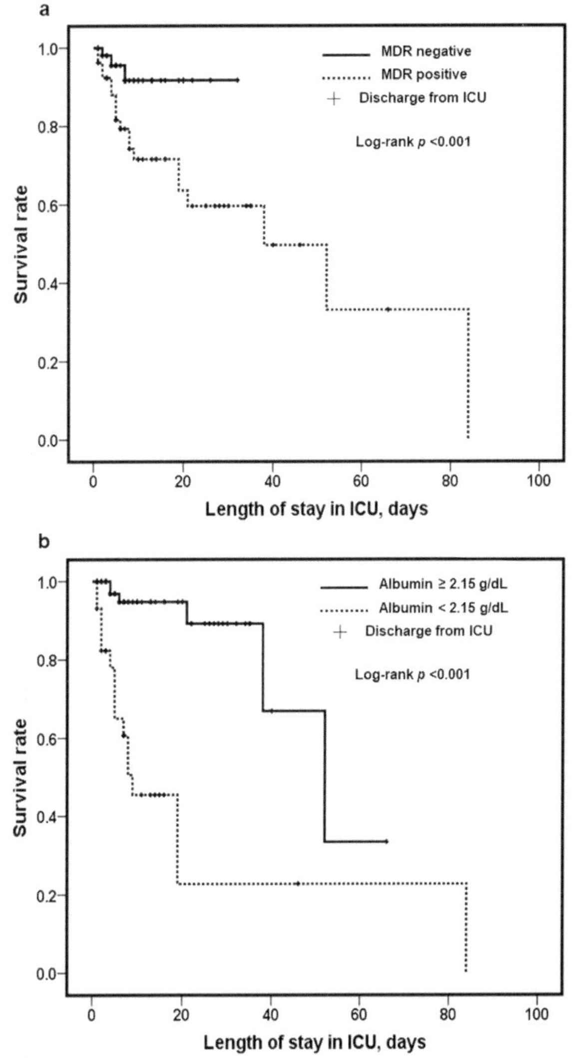

Fig. 2 **a**, **b** Kaplan-Meier survival analysis of mortality and ICU length of stay according to identification of MDR pathogen and albumin levels

[19, 35], we initially thought that the cause of the association of hypoalbuminemia and mortality was the nutritional status of the patients. Furthermore, univariate analysis demonstrated that the non-survivor group had a lower median BMI compared to the survivor group. However, other studies have reported that albumin is not a good marker of malnutrition for elderly patients [36, 37]; rather, they suggest that the decrease in albumin, which acts as a binding protein, increases the circulation of unbound drugs, which may lead to adverse events [33]. In addition, serum albumin can decrease dramatically in critical illness, which may cause problems such as transport of substances, anti-thrombotic effects, and maintenance of normal plasma oncotic pressure. In elderly patients, increases in the bioavailability of medications due to impaired protein homeostasis and taking various medications might explain adverse events [38]. In our study,

Table 3 Distribution of isolated sputum culture pathogens within 48 h after admission

Pathogen identified	$N = 74$
Gram-positive pathogen	
Staphylococcus aureus	20 (27.0)
MSSA	2 (2.7)
MRSA	18 (24.3)
Streptococcus pneumonia	5 (6.8)
Gram-negative pathogen	
Acinetobacter baumannii	24 (32.4)
Escherichia coli	2 (2.7)
Klebsiella pneumonia	7 (9.5)
Enterobacter cloacae	1 (1.4)
Stenotrophomonas maltophilia	2 (2.7)
Pseudomonas aeruginosa	5 (6.8)
Serratia marcescens	1 (1.4)
Proteus mirabilis	4 (5.4)
Mycobacterium tuberculosis	3 (4.1)
MDR pathogen	49 (66.2)
MRSA	18 (24.3)
ESBL producing *Enterobacteriae*	7 (9.5)
MDR-*Pseudomonas* spp.	1 (1.4)
CRAB	23 (31.1)

Values are presented as numbers (percentages) unless otherwise indicated; MSSA, methicillin-susceptible *Staphylococcus aureus*; MRSA, methicillin-resistant *Staphylococcus aureus*; MDR, multiple-drug-resistant; ESBL, extended-spectrum beta-lactamases; CRAB, carbapenem-resistant *Acinetobacter baumannii*

most patients from LTCHs were elderly; only 16 patients were under 65 years of age. We supposed that these several reasons induced serum albumin level was associated with mortality in patients who transferred from LTCHs. Furthermore, APACHE II score and Charlson comorbidity index did not vary between groups in this study. Albumin levels might be a better marker for severity or prediction of length of stay in ICU in elderly patients from LTCHs.

This study had some limitations. First, since this study was performed at a single center, it is difficult to generalize the trend to LTCHs throughout Korea. However, to the best of our knowledge, there are no other studies investigating patients with respiratory problems who were transferred to ICU from LTCHs in Korea. Therefore, this study may have important implications for aging societies such as Korea and other similar countries. Second, this was a retrospective study, thus we could only use data included in electronic medical records. The subjects' status and medication history at the time of admission were documented in records from LTCH doctors; however, some data were difficult to confirm due to patient cognitive difficulties, including the infectious history of subjects, the drug sensitivity of pathogens during LTCH hospitalization,

Table 4 Risk factors for MDR pathogens in patients who transferred from long-term care beds in institutions and hospitals

Variable	Univariate			Multivariate	
	MDR negative (*n* = 58)	MDR positive (*n* = 53)	*P*	*OR (95% CI)*	*P*
Male sex	30 (51.7)	41 (77.4)	0.005	2.65 (1.02–6.93)	0.046
Age, years	78 (70.8–82)	79 (71–84)	0.372	1.02 (0.97–1.07)	0.373
BMI, kg/m^2	20.8 (19.4–25.3)	19.2 (17.5–22.7)	0.005	0.9 (0.80–1.02)	0.102
Permanent tracheostomy status	17 (29.3)	11 (20.8)	0.300		
Nasogastric tube insertion status	16 (27.6)	22 (41.5)	0.123		
Invasive ventilation	34 (58.6)	43 (81.1)	0.010	2.74 (1.02–7.32)	0.045
Bedridden status	25 (43.1)	25 (47.2)	0.667		
Brain problem[a]	46 (79.3)	38 (71.7)	0.350		
Use of antibiotics within 3 months	16 (27.6)	33 (62.3)	< 0.001	3.23 (1.32–7.90)	0.010
Diabetes mellitus	16 (27.6)	11 (20.8)	0.402		
Hypertension	25 (43.1)	19 (35.8)	0.435		
Chronic pulmonary disease	7 (12.1)	13 (24.5)	0.088		
Acute kidney injury	19 (32.8)	12 (22.6)	0.235		
Albumin < 2.15 g/dL	8 (13.8)	21 (39.6)	0.002	2.85 (0.98–8.24)	0.054

Values are presented as numbers (percentages), and as median (interquartile rage), unless otherwise indicated; MDR, multiple-drug-resistant; OR, odds ratio; CI, confidence interval; BMI, body mass index; [a]neurodegenerative disorders and stroke

and survey data including smoking history and degree of symptoms. Third, we could not exclude colonization or contamination by the identified pathogens; thus, such pathogens may be included in our analysis. To overcome these challenges, more prospective studies are needed.

Conclusion

Identification of MDR pathogens and low serum albumin levels were associated with poor prognosis in patients with respiratory problems who were admitted to the ICU from LTCHs. A history of antibiotic use within the 3 months and the need for invasive ventilation were associated with infection with MDR pathogens; thus, these factors should be considered when selecting appropriate antibiotics at admission. Additionally, serum albumin levels at admission may be helpful for predicting prognosis.

Abbreviations

APACHE: Acute physiology and chronic health evaluation; ARDS: Acute respiratory distress syndrome; BMI: Body mass index; CI: Confidence interval; ESBL: Extended-spectrum β-lactamase; HCAP: Healthcare-associated pneumonia; ICH: Intensive care unit; LTCHs: Long-term care beds in institutions and hospitals; MDR: Multiple-drug-resistant; MRSA: Methicillin-resistant Staphylococcus aureus; OR: Odds ratio; ROC: Receiver operating characteristic

Funding

The authors received no specific funding for this work.

Authors' contributions

SHL and YJR contributed to the study design, analysis, and interpretation of data, and writing of the manuscript. SJK, JHL, JHC contributed to drafting the manuscript and to literature review. YHC contributed to analysis and interpretation of data. All authors contributed to the preparation and revision of the manuscript. All authors read and approved the final manuscript.

Competing interests

The authors have no financial or non-financial conflicts of interest with any company referred to in this article.

Author details

[1]Division of Pulmonary and Critical Care Medicine, Department of Internal Medicine, College of Medicine, Ewha Womans University, Mokdong Hospital, 1071 Anyangcheon-ro, Yangcheon-gu, Seoul 07985, South Korea.
[2]Department of Emergency Medicine, College of Medicine, Ewha Womans University, Mokdong Hospital, 1071 Anyangcheon-ro, Yangcheon-gu, Seoul 07985, South Korea.

References

1. Suzman R BJ: Glob Health and aging: National Institute on Aging website. http://www.who.int/ageing/publications/global_health/en. Accessed 2 October 2017.
2. Divo MJ, Martinez CH, Mannino DM. Ageing and the epidemiology of multimorbidity. Eur Respir J. 2014;44(4):1055–68.
3. Choi IA, Song YW. Perspectives and challenges for geriatric medicine. Korean J Med. 2017;92(3):225–34.
4. Choi H. Present and future of Korean geriatrics. J Korean Geriatr Soc. 2011; 15(2):71–9.
5. Song H. Long-term Care Hospital Systems in Developed Countries and the implications for Korea. J Korean Geriatr Soc. 2012;16(3):114–20.
6. OECD: Long-term care beds in institutions and hospitals: OECD Publishing. http://www.oecd-ilibrary.org/social-issues-migration-health/health-at-a-glance-2015/long-term-care-beds-in-institutions-and-hospitals_health_glance-2015-78-en. Accessed 1 Agust 2017.
7. Ga H, Won CW. Perspective on long term care hospitals in Korea. J Am Med Dir Assoc. 2013;14(10):770–2.
8. Hashimoto H, Horiguchi H, Matsuda S. Micro data analysis of medical and long-term care utilization among the elderly in Japan. Int J Environ Res Public Health. 2010;7(8):3022–37.
9. Sager MA, Rudberg MA, Jalaluddin M, Franke T, Inouye SK, Landefeld CS,

Siebens H, Winograd CH. Hospital admission risk profile (HARP): identifying older patients at risk for functional decline following acute medical illness and hospitalization. J Am Geriatr Soc. 1996;44(3):251–7.
10. Gill TM, Allore HG, Holford TR, Guo Z. Hospitalization, restricted activity, and the development of disability among older persons. JAMA. 2004; 292(17):2115–24.
11. Avelino-Silva TJ, Farfel JM, Curiati JA, Amaral JR, Campora F, Jacob-Filho W. Comprehensive geriatric assessment predicts mortality and adverse outcomes in hospitalized older adults. BMC Geriatr. 2014;14(1):129.
12. Fink R, Gilmartin H, Richard A, Capezuti E, Boltz M, Wald H. Indwelling urinary catheter management and catheter-associated urinary tract infection prevention practices in nurses improving Care for Healthsystem Elders hospitals. Am J Infect Control. 2012;40(8):715–20.
13. Montoya A, Cassone M, Mody L. Infections in nursing homes. Clin Geriatr Med. 2016;32(3):585–607.
14. Rossio R, Franchi C, Ardoino I, Djade CD, Tettamanti M, Pasina L, Salerno F, Marengoni A, Corrao S, Marcucci M, et al. Adherence to antibiotic treatment guidelines and outcomes in the hospitalized elderly with different types of pneumonia. Eur J Intern Med. 2015;26(5):330–7.
15. Nico T Mutters FG, Heininger A, Frank U. Device-related infections in long-term healthcare facilities: the challenge of prevention. Future Microbiol. 2014;9(4):487–95.
16. Dwyer R, Stoelwinder J, Gabbe B, Lowthian J. Unplanned transfer to emergency departments for frail elderly residents of aged care facilities: a review of patient and organizational factors. J Am Med Dir Assoc. 2015; 16(7):551–62.
17. Kim KW, Jang S. Characteristics and mortality risk factors in geriatric hospital patients visiting one region-wide emergency department. J Korean Acad Community Health Nurs. 2016;27(4):327–36.
18. Mattison ML, Rudolph JL, Kiely DK, Marcantonio ER. Nursing home patients in the intensive care unit: risk factors for mortality. Crit Care Med. 2006; 34(10):2583–7.
19. Tal S, Guller V, Shavit Y, Stern F, Malnick S. Mortality predictors in hospitalized elderly patients. Qjm. 2011;104(11):933–8.
20. Knaus WA, Draper EA, Wagner DP, Zimmerman JE. APACHE II: a severity of disease classification system. Crit Care Med. 1985;13(10):818–29.
21. Charlson ME, Pompei P, Ales KL, MacKenzie CR. A new method of classifying prognostic comorbidity in longitudinal studies: development and validation. J Chronic Dis. 1987;40(5):373–83.
22. Magiorakos AP, Srinivasan A, Carey RB, Carmeli Y, Falagas ME, Giske CG, Harbarth S, Hindler JF, Kahlmeter G, Olsson-Liljequist B, et al. Multidrug-resistant, extensively drug-resistant and pandrug-resistant bacteria: an international expert proposal for interim standard definitions for acquired resistance. Clin Microbiol Infect. 2012;18(3):268–81.
23. Nseir S, Blazejewski C, Lubret R, Wallet F, Courcol R, Durocher A. Risk of acquiring multidrug-resistant gram-negative bacilli from prior room occupants in the intensive care unit. Clin Microbiol Infect. 2011;17(8):1201–8.
24. Rhodes A, Evans LE, Alhazzani W, Levy MM, Antonelli M, Ferrer R, Kumar A, Sevransky JE, Sprung CL, Nunnally ME, et al. Surviving sepsis campaign: international guidelines for Management of Sepsis and Septic Shock: 2016. Crit Care Med. 2017;45(3):486–552.
25. Vardakas KZ, Rafailidis PI, Konstantelias AA, Falagas ME. Predictors of mortality in patients with infections due to multi-drug resistant gram negative bacteria: the study, the patient, the bug or the drug? The Journal of infection. 2013;66(5):401–14.
26. Bodi M, Ardanuy C, Rello J. Impact of gram-positive resistance on outcome of nosocomial pneumonia. Crit Care Med. 2001;29(4 Suppl):N82–6.
27. Poch DS, Ost DE. What are the important risk factors for healthcare-associated pneumonia? Semin Respir Crit Care Med. 2009;30(1):26–35.
28. Prina E, Ranzani OT, Polverino E, Cilloniz C, Ferrer M, Fernandez L, Puig de la Bellacasa J, Menendez R, Mensa J, Torres A. Risk factors associated with potentially antibiotic-resistant pathogens in community-acquired pneumonia. Ann Am Thorac Soc. 2015;12(2):153–60.
29. Aliberti S, Di Pasquale M, Zanaboni AM, Cosentini R, Brambilla AM, Seghezzi S, Tarsia P, Mantero M, Blasi F. Stratifying risk factors for multidrug-resistant pathogens in hospitalized patients coming from the community with pneumonia. Clin Infect Dis. 2012;54(4):470–8.
30. Sibila O, Rodrigo-Troyano A, Shindo Y, Aliberti S, Restrepo MI. Multidrug-resistant pathogens in patients with pneumonia coming from the community. Curr Opin Pulm Med. 2016;22(3):219–26.
31. Alberg AJ, Shopland DR, Cummings KM. The 2014 surgeon General's report: commemorating the 50th anniversary of the 1964 report of the advisory committee to the US surgeon general and updating the evidence on the health consequences of cigarette smoking. Am J Epidemiol. 2014;179(4):403–12.
32. Choi S, Kim Y, Park S, Lee J, Oh K. Trends in cigarette smoking among adolescents and adults in South Korea. Epidemiol Health. 2014;36:e2014023.
33. Jellinge ME, Henriksen DP, Hallas P, Brabrand M. Hypoalbuminemia is a strong predictor of 30-day all-cause mortality in acutely admitted medical patients: a prospective, observational, cohort study. PLoS One. 2014;9, e105983(8).
34. Lyons O, Whelan B, Bennett K, O'Riordan D, Silke B. Serum albumin as an outcome predictor in hospital emergency medical admissions. Eur J Intern Med. 2010;21(1):17–20.
35. Mogensen KM, Robinson MK, Casey JD, Gunasekera NS, Moromizato T, Rawn JD, Christopher KB. Nutritional status and mortality in the critically ill. Crit Care Med. 2015;43(12):2605–15.
36. Kuzuya M, Izawa S, Enoki H, Okada K, Iguchi A. Is serum albumin a good marker for malnutrition in the physically impaired elderly? Clin Nutr. 2007; 26(1):84–90.
37. Bouillanne O, Hay P, Liabaud B, Duche C, Cynober L, Aussel C. Evidence that albumin is not a suitable marker of body composition-related nutritional status in elderly patients. Nutrition. 2011;27(2):165–9.
38. López-Otín C. The hallmarks of aging. Cell. 2013;153(6):1194–217.

Pre-kidney transplant lower extremity impairment and transplant length of stay: a time-to-discharge analysis of a prospective cohort study

Anthony J. Nastasi[1,2†], Tyler S. Bryant[1†], Jimmy T. Le[1†], Jennifer Schrack[1], Hao Ying[2], Christine E. Haugen[2], Marlís González Fernández[3], Dorry L. Segev[1,2] and Mara A. McAdams-DeMarco[1,2*]

Abstract

Background: Few objective tests can be performed at admission for kidney transplantation [KT] to discern risk of increased length of stay [LOS], which is important for patient counseling and is associated with increased costs and mortality. The short physical performance battery [SPPB] is an easily administered, potentially modifiable, 3-part test of lower extremity function. SPPB score is associated with longer hospital LOS in older adults, and may provide similar utility in KT recipients given that ESRD is a disease of accelerated aging. The aim of this study was to characterize the association between SPPB-derived lower extremity function and LOS.

Methods: The SPPB was administered at KT admission in a prospective cohort of 595 recipients (8/2009–6/2016). The independent association between SPPB impairment (score ≤ 10) and LOS was tested with an adjusted conventional generalized gamma parametric survival model.

Results: Impaired recipients experienced longer LOS (median: 10 vs. 8 days; $P < 0.001$) with the greatest difference in percent discharged on day 10 (impaired: 54.5%, unimpaired: 73.3%). Discharge typically took 13% longer in the impaired group (relative time = 1.13; 95%CI: 1.05, 1.21, $P = 0.001$). Discharge for impaired recipients compared to unimpaired was least likely at day 5 (hazard ratio = 0.71; 95% CI:0.68, 0.74, $P < 0.001$). No differences in the SPPB impairment-LOS relationship were found by age (interaction $P = 0.74$).

Conclusions: Pre-KT SPPB impairment was independently associated with longer LOS regardless of age, indicating that it is a useful, objective tool for pre KT risk assessment in younger and older recipients that may help inform discharge planning.

Keywords: Kidney transplantation, Length of stay, Survival analysis

Background

Length of stay [LOS] is an important outcome associated with increased complications, death, and costs in transplant recipients [1–3]. A clear understanding of hospital LOS following kidney transplantation [KT] allows for appropriate informed consent, improved patient and caregiver counseling, as well as better discharge planning. We have recently identified transplant, recipient, and donor factors that are associated with LOS in KT recipients including pre-KT frailty [4]. Other than a frailty assessment [4–9], there is a dearth of inexpensive tests that can be performed successfully at admission for KT to identify recipients at risk of longer LOS [10].

The Short Physical Performance Battery [SPPB] is a well-validated, inexpensive, objective assessment tool of lower extremity function that was developed in community-dwelling older adults. Functional limitations,

* Correspondence: mara@jhu.edu
†Anthony J. Nastasi, Tyler S. Bryant and Jimmy T. Le contributed equally to this work.
[1]Department of Epidemiology, Johns Hopkins Bloomberg School of Public Health, 615 N. Wolfe St, Baltimore, MD 21205, USA
[2]Department of Surgery, Johns Hopkins School of Medicine, Baltimore, MD, USA
Full list of author information is available at the end of the article

including SPPB impairment, have been shown to be associated with many important health outcomes including mortality, quality of life, functional decline, and LOS in older adults [11–14]. Our group recently found that SPPB impairment is associated with a 2-fold increased risk of post-KT mortality [15]. Given this strong association, it is likely that SPPB impairment is also associated with other KT outcomes, such as longer LOS. The SPPB measures the modifiable risk factor of functional limitations and may provide a target for interventions to prevent longer LOS.

However, there is currently no consensus regarding the most appropriate way to model the relationship between LOS and predictors of functional limitations such as the SPPB [16–18]. Conventional regression modeling treats LOS as a count of the number of days in the hospital, but does not appropriately account for patients who die during the hospitalization (non-informative censoring) and the skewed distributions of extended LOS, both of which are more common in older populations. Treating LOS as a time-to-discharge (i.e. time-to-event) analysis is seldom carried out when examining LOS, yet it allows for the calculation of informative, novel metrics of high utility for patient counseling and discharge planning [17]. This method allows for more clinically meaningful metrics to be calculated; for example, it provides the probability of being discharged each day for patients with and without SPPB impairment.

The goals of this study were to: (1) quantify the association between SPPB-derived lower extremity function and KT LOS, (2) stratify KT recipients by LOS, and (3) estimate novel and more clinically meaningful metrics of LOS by SPPB impairment using time-to-discharge analyses. We hypothesized that recipients with SPPB impairment at admission for KT would be at increased risk of longer LOS.

Methods

Study design

We studied 652 KT recipients who were enrolled in a longitudinal cohort study at the Johns Hopkins Hospital, Baltimore, Maryland between August 2009 and June 2016. We excluded patients whose LOS was longer than 30 days post-KT as has been done previously due to methodological and generalizability concerns (n = 57), leaving 595 recipients in the analysis [19, 20]. We abstracted LOS from medical records along with the recipient, transplant, and donor factors that were previously identified as potential risk factors for longer LOS [4]. Recipient factors include age, sex, race, education, body mass index, hepatitis C status, preemptive KT (i.e., KT before patient initiates dialysis), years on dialysis, previous KT, and cause of end-stage renal disease (ESRD) including hypertension, diabetes, glomerulonephritis, or other cause. Additionally, we included recipient comorbidity (as measured by the Charlson Comorbidity Index [CCI] adapted for ESRD), which was both abstracted from the medical record and self-reported [21]. Transplant factors include panel reactive antibody, ABO incompatibility, human leukocyte antigen mismatches, cold ischemic time, and donor type (live vs. deceased). Donor factors include age, sex, race, donation after cardiac death, deceased expanded criteria, hypertension, diabetes, hepatitis C status, and creatinine. The Johns Hopkins Institutional Review Board approved this study (NA_00015758) and all participants provided written informed consent.

Short physical performance battery (SPPB)

The SPPB consists of 3 objective physical assessments (standing balance, walking speed, and repeated chair stands) of lower extremity function each with a score ranging from 0 to 4 with a summed composite score ranging from 0 to 12, as has been previously described [11]. For the balance portion, recipients were asked to stand and remain in several progressively more difficult positions (side-by-side, semi-, and full-tandem stances) for 10 s each. If a position could not be held, no further positions were attempted. For the walking speed test, recipients' usual walking speed was timed from the first foot fall over the starting line to the first foot fall over the finish line of an 8-ft course. Finally, for the chair stand portion, recipients were asked to fold their arms across their chest and rise from a chair 5 times as quickly as possible. The SPPB was measured at the time of hospital admission for KT, prior to the start of maintenance immunosuppressive medications and inpatient dialysis; a score of ≤10 was decided a priori to signify impaired lower extremity function based on previous work looking at post-KT mortality [15].

SPPB & LOS

We treated the LOS analysis as a time-to-event analysis and calculated the cumulative incidence of discharge using a Kaplan-Meier approach. This approach allows for a more detailed examination of discharge by impairment group with respect to time after KT and accounts for any non-informative censoring. Furthermore, using this approach we were able to calculate more clinically useful measures by estimating the changes in the relative hazard of discharge over time by SPPB impairment status as well as how many more days were needed for a given percent of impaired patients to be discharged compared to unimpaired.

We tested proportional hazards visually by graphing the log-log plot of survival and statistically using Schoenfeld residuals (P = 0.04), indicating the likelihood of non-proportional hazards. Therefore, we explored several parametric survival models and selected the generalized gamma [GG] model [22] based on a comparison of log likelihoods and Akaike Information Criteria. This model had the highest model quality, balancing fit and parsimony as has been previously demonstrated in LOS modeling [17]. For the GG model, we estimated 3 parameters, β (a location parameter that is related to median time to discharge), σ (a dispersion or scale parameter related to the interquartile ratio: third quartile divided by the first quartile of lengths of stay), and κ (shape). We modeled the relative hazard with time and the relative time to discharge, the factor by which times were expanded or contracted. For example, a relative time of 2 would mean that it generally took twice as long for SPPB impaired recipients to be discharged compared to the unimpaired recipients and would correspond with a relative hazard < 1.

We quantified the association between SPPB impairment and LOS after adjusting for age, sex, race, body mass index, years on dialysis, cause of ESRD, and donor type. These covariates were selected based on their relevance to LOS as well as their use in previous literature [4]. To assess the fit of this model, we graphically overlaid the GG cumulative discharge functions with the non-parametric Kaplan-Meier cumulative discharge functions for comparison. Death was not treated as a competing risk as only 2 patients died during hospitalization.

SPPB & LOS ≥14 days

In addition, we used logistic regression models to assess both the relationship between SPPB impairment and LOS ≥14 days adjusting for the same factors as in the GG model. LOS ≥14 days was selected as an a priori outcome because it is seen as clinically relevant and has been previously used as a threshold for longer LOS after KT [4]. Using a similar approach, we assessed the independent association between a 1-point decrease in SPPB score (worse function) as well as each individual component of the SPPB (balance, walking speed, and chair stands) and LOS ≥14 days.

Effect heterogeneity

Effect modification of the associations between SPPB impairment and LOS ≥14 days by recipient age, sex, race, diabetes status, and frailty status were tested using a Wald test. We used a similar approach to test for effect modification between as well as SPPB composite score and LOS ≥14 days.

Sensitivity analysis of SPPB and LOS

We assessed the robustness of the adjusted associations between SPPB performance (composite score, impairment) and LOS (logistic model with LOS ≥14 days, GG model with continuous LOS) by including KT recipients omitted previously from the primary analysis for having a LOS > 30 days due to generalizability concerns (i.e., these patients not representing the typical KT recipient) as well as additionally adjusting for comorbidities including cardiovascular disease (including any ischemic heart disease, cerebrovascular disease, or peripheral vascular disease), lung disease, diabetes status, and CCI adapted for ESRD.

Statistical analysis

A *P* value < 0.05 was considered statistically significant. All analyses were performed using Stata (version 14; StataCorp, College Station, TX) and R Statistical software version 3.3 (http://www.r-project.org).

Results

Study population

The mean age of the 595 KT recipients was 51.8 years (SD = 14.1, range: 18.7–86.0); 225 (37.8%) were female, 255 (42.9%) were African American, and 212 (35.6%) were live donor recipients. At time of KT, 47.1% of KT recipients were SPPB impaired. The median LOS was 8 days (IQR: 7–13, range: 2–30). Tacrolimus was associated with a shorter LOS (*P* = 0.02); no other association between immunosuppressive medication (thymoglobulin, mycophenolate mofetil, or prednisone) and LOS was found.

SPPB at the time of admission for KT

The median SPPB score for the 595 KT recipients was 11 (IQR: 9–12, range 0–12). On average, impaired recipients were significantly older (56.3 vs. 47.8 years; *P* < 0.001), had higher body mass indices (28.1 vs. 26.7; *P* = 0.004), were on dialysis for a longer duration (3.3 vs. 2.7 years; *P* = 0.01), were more likely to be black (*P* = 0.01) and have diabetes as their cause of ESRD (*P* < 0.001) compared to those who were unimpaired (Table 1). SPPB impaired individuals were more likely to have an expanded criteria donor (11.1% vs. 4.0%; *P* = 0.01), a donor with hypertension (21.8% vs. 13.0%; *P* = 0.02), and a donor with a creatinine > 1.5 mg/dL (27.5% vs. 20.0%; *P* = 0.03). No association was found between SPPB impairment and immunosuppressive medication (tacrolimus, thymoglobulin, mycophenolate mofetil, or prednisone; all *P* > 0.35).

SPPB & LOS

SPPB impaired recipients experienced a longer LOS compared to unimpaired recipients (*P* < 0.001) (Fig. 1) such that impaired recipients had a median LOS of 10 days (IQR; 7–14) while unimpaired recipients had a median LOS of 8 days (IQR; 6–11). From the Kaplan-Meier calculations of cumulative discharge, by 7 days post-KT, 43.2% of unimpaired and 34.1% of impaired recipients were discharged (Fig. 1, Table 2). By 14 days post-KT, 87.9% of unimpaired and 75.3% of impaired recipients were discharged. By 21 days, 97.1% of unimpaired and 92.8% of impaired recipients were discharged. The greatest difference in percent discharged between impaired and unimpaired recipients occurred 10 days post-KT at which time 18.8% more unimpaired recipients were discharged (Table 2). The conventional GG

Table 1 Baseline Characteristics of Kidney Transplant Recipients by Short Physical Performance Battery (SPPB) Impairment Status, Baltimore, Maryland, 2009–2016

Factors	Unimpaired (SPPB Score > 10) N = 315	Impaired (SPPB Score ≤ 10) N = 280	P Value
Recipient factors			
Age (years)	47.8 (14.1)	56.3 (12.6)	< 0.001
Female	39.4	36.1	0.41
Race			0.01
White	55.2	41.1	
Black	36.2	50.4	
Other	8.5	8.8	
Education			0.06
High school (9–12) or less	40.6	47.0	
2-year technical school	5.5	9.7	
College/technical school	31.5	23.9	
Post-college graduate degree	22.4	19.4	
Body mass index (kg/m^2)	26.7 (5.1)	28.1 (6.2)	< 0.01
Hepatitis C virus positive	7.0	7.6	0.8
Preemptive transplant	20.3	18.2	0.52
Years on dialysis[a]	1.7 (0.1–3.9)	2.4 (0.4–4.8)	0.01
Previous KT	20.3	15.4	0.12
Cause of end-stage renal disease			< 0.001
Hypertension	30.8	34.3	
Diabetes	10.5	21.1	
Glomerulonephritis	2.9	5.4	
Other	55.9	39.3	
Transplant factors			
0 Human leukoctye antigen mismatches	15.1 (14.0)	22.0 (15.5)	< 0.01
Cold ischemic time > 24 h	32.7	51.43	< 0.001
Live donor	44.1	26.1	< 0.001
Donor factors			
Age (years)	37.7 (13.9)	38.5 (15.4)	0.36
Female sex	49.5	43.9	0.17
Race			0.42
White	73.7	68.6	
Black	17.5	23.2	
Other	8.8	8.2	
Donation after cardiac death	19.4	22.2	0.5
Expanded criteria donor	4	11.1	0.01
Charlson Comorbidity Index[a]	0 (0–2)	1 (0–3)	< 0.001

Percentages and mean (SD) are presented unless otherwise noted
[a]Median and IQR are presented

models for impaired ($\beta = 1.87$, $\sigma = 0.41$, $\kappa = -0.56$) and unimpaired ($\beta = 1.75$, $\sigma = 0.41$, $\kappa = -0.56$) recipients closely mirrored the Kaplan-Meier cumulative discharge curves (Table 3, Fig. 1), confirming a good fit to describe the SPPB impairment-LOS relationship.

The adjusted hazard of discharge was lower for impaired recipients compared to unimpaired recipients until approximately 21 days post-KT as shown by an adjusted relative hazard < 1 during this time (Fig. 2a). By day 6, the adjusted relative hazard of discharge comparing impaired

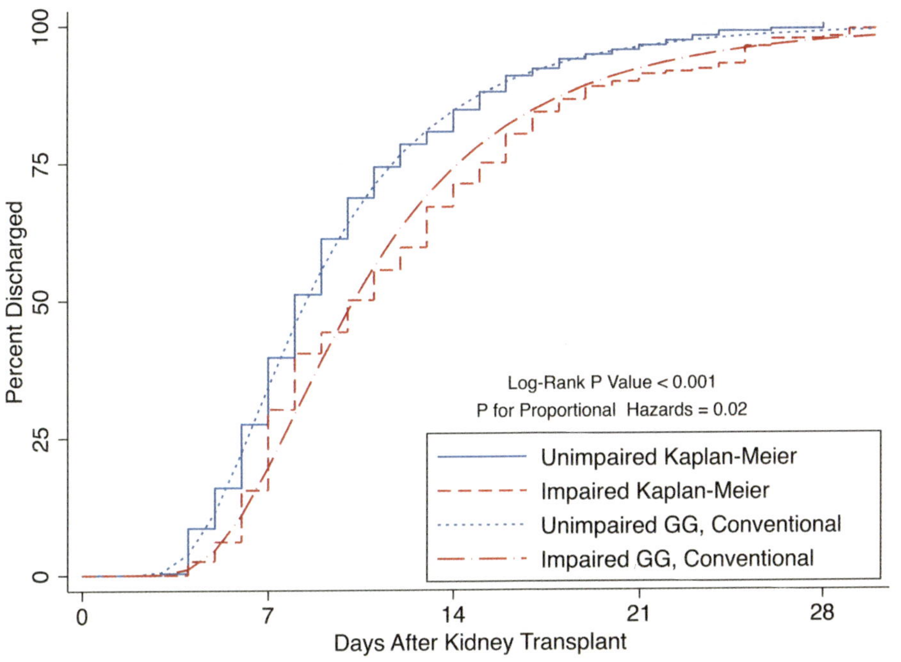

Fig. 1 Cumulative Percent Discharged by Short Physical Performance Battery (SPPB) Impairment Status Among Kidney Transplant Recipients (n = 595). SPPB impairment was defined as an SPPB score ≤ 10. The Kaplan-Meier and conventional Generalized Gamma (GG) cumulative incidences of discharge are shown

to unimpaired recipients was at its lowest at 0.71 (95% confidence interval (CI): 0.68, 0.74; $P < 0.001$), indicating that impaired recipients had a 29% lower chance of being discharged on this day. The adjusted relative time comparing impaired to unimpaired recipients was 1.13 (95% CI: 1.05, 1.21; $P = 0.001$), indicating that for the same percentage of recipients to be discharged, it typically took 13% longer in the impaired group compared to the unimpaired group (Table 3). Similarly, it took approximately 1 day, 2 days, and 3 days longer for impaired recipients to achieve 25, 50, and 75% discharged compared to unimpaired recipients, respectively (Fig. 2b).

SPPB & LOS ≥14 Days

SPPB impaired recipients experienced an adjusted 1.90-fold (95% CI: 1.23, 2.94; $P = 0.004$) higher odds of a LOS ≥14 days (Table 3). A 1-point decrease (worse function) in SPPB composite score was associated with an adjusted 1.16-fold (95% CI: 1.08, 1.27; $P < 0.001$) higher odds of a LOS ≥14 days (Table 3). Each 1-point decrease (worse function) in the balance, walking speed, and chair stand component scores were associated with 1.54-fold (95% CI: 1.27, 1.89; $P < 0.001$), 1.33-fold (95% CI: 1.08, 1.67; $P = 0.01$), and 1.23-fold (95% CI: 1.05, 1.45; $P = 0.01$) higher odds of a LOS ≥14 days, respectively.

Effect heterogeneity

No differences in the association between SPPB impairment status and LOS ≥14 days were found by age (interaction $P = 0.74$), race (interaction $P = 0.34$), sex (interaction $P = 0.20$), diabetes status (interaction $P = 0.71$), or frailty status (interaction $P = 0.20$). Similarly, no differences in the association between SPPB composite score and LOS ≥14 days were found by age (interaction $P = 0.67$), race (interaction $P = 0.23$), sex (interaction $P = 0.99$), diabetes status (interaction $P = 0.63$), or frailty status (interaction $P = 0.24$).

Sensitivity analysis of SPPB and LOS

SPPB impairment and composite score remained significantly associated with LOS ≥14 days in the fully adjusted logistic models that additionally adjusted for comorbidities including cardiovascular disease (including any ischemic heart disease, cerebrovascular disease, or peripheral vascular disease), lung disease, diabetes status, and CCI adapted for ESRD and included KT recipients with LOS > 30 days. Specifically, impairment was associated with a 1.74-fold (95% CI: 1.31, 2.65; $P = 0.01$) increase in risk of LOS ≥14 days; a one-point decrease in SPPB score was associated with a 1.19-fold (95% CI: 1.08, 1.30; $P < 0.001$) increase in risk. SPPB impairment also remained significantly associated with LOS in the conventional GG model such that the adjusted relative time comparing impaired to unimpaired recipients was 1.11 (95% CI: 1.03, 1.19; $P = 0.005$).

Table 2 Cumulative Percent of Kidney Transplant Recipients Discharged by Short Physical Performance Battery (SPPB) Impairment Status, Baltimore, Maryland, 2009–2016

Days Post-KT	SPPB Unimpaired[a] (%)	SPPB Impaired (%)
1	0	0
2	0	0
3	0.3	0
4	9.2	2.5
5	16.8	6.8
6	29.8	17.2
7	43.2	34.1
8	55.6	44.4
9	65.1	48.4
10	73.3	54.5
11	78.1	60.6
12	82.2	64.5
13	84.4	71.7
14	87.9	75.3
15	90.5	79.6
16	93.0	83.9
17	94.0	87.5
18	95.2	89.3
19	95.9	91.0
20	96.5	91.8
21	97.1	92.8
22	97.8	93.2
23	98.4	93.6
24	99.1	94.3
25	99.1	96.8
26	99.4	97.9
27	99.4	97.9
28	100	98.2
29	100	99.3
30	100	100

Abbreviations: *KT* Kidney Transplant, *SPPB* Short Physical Performance Battery
[a]SPPB impairment was defined as an SPPB score ≤ 10

Table 3 Independent Associations of Short Physical Performance Battery Impairment with Kidney Transplant Length of Stay, Baltimore, Maryland, 2009–2016

Model[a]	Association between SPPB and LOS	
Conventional Generalized Gamma (Time-to-Discharge)	Relative Time (95% CI)	
	Impaired Vs. Unimpaired[b]	1.13 (1.05, 1.21)
Logistic Regression	Odds Ratio (95% CI)	
(LOS ≥14 Days)	Impaired Vs. Unimpaired	1.90 (1.23, 2.94)
	One-point decrease in SPPB composite score	1.16 (1.08, 1.27)

Abbreviations: *CI* Confidence Interval, *LOS* Length of Stay, *SE* Standard Error, *SPPB* Short Physical Performance Battery
[a]Adjusted for age, sex, race, body mass index, years on dialysis, cause of end-stage renal disease, and donor type. GG model parameters were $\beta = 1.87$, $\sigma = 0.41$, $\kappa = -0.56$ and $\beta = 1.75$, $\sigma = 0.41$, $\kappa = -0.56$ for the impaired and unimpaired recipients, respectively. Parameters for the GG model define the shape of the curve; β (a location parameter that is related to median time to discharge), σ (a dispersion or scale parameter related to the interquartile ratio: third quartile divided by the first quartile of lengths of stay), and κ (shape)
[b]SPPB impairment was defined as an SPPB score ≤ 10

Discussion

In a prospective, longitudinal cohort study of 595 KT recipients, we found that pre-KT SPPB composite score and lower extremity functional impairment were independently associated with increased LOS. Physical functioning in ESRD patients is important, given that ESRD is a disease of accelerated aging [10]. By modeling the relationship between SPPB impairment and LOS with a conventional GG model, we estimated that it took 13% longer for SPPB impaired recipients to be discharged compared to unimpaired recipients, and that impaired recipients experienced a consistently and significantly lower chance of being discharged until approximately 21 days post-KT. The component of the SPPB with the strongest association with LOS was the balance test in which a one-point decrease in balance score was associated with a 1.54-fold increase in odds of LOS ≥14 days. These strong, independent, and consistent findings remained in both older and younger adults, highlighting the fact that ESRD is a disease of accelerated aging with outcomes strongly tied to function abilities. Our work also demonstrates the SPPB's great potential utility as a risk stratification tool in KT, making it one of a limited selection of tools with such potential particularly among older surgical patients.

Frailty, an aging-related syndrome marked by diminished physiologic reserve, has been studied in ESRD patients and is the main assessment tool for risk stratification in transplantation [4–9, 23–30]. Frailty is also a strong predictor of important transplant outcomes including quality of life, LOS, early hospital readmission, and mortality [4–7, 9, 23, 29–32]. The SPPB, a measure of functional limitation, consists of completely objective components and is less burdensome to measure than frailty given that it consists of fewer components and requires no additional tools. These qualities facilitate its use in non-research, clinical settings, permitting improved patient counseling and other clinical goals for which frailty may not be as easily administered. Furthermore, transplant centers tend to have their own procedures for evaluation, waitlisting, and pre-operative counseling, often relying on comorbidities and age. The SPPB, therefore, offers a standard, reliable tool across centers.

Functional limitation as measured by SPPB has been found to be predictive of important health outcomes in a variety of populations [11, 33]. To our knowledge, three other works have looked at the SPPB in transplant

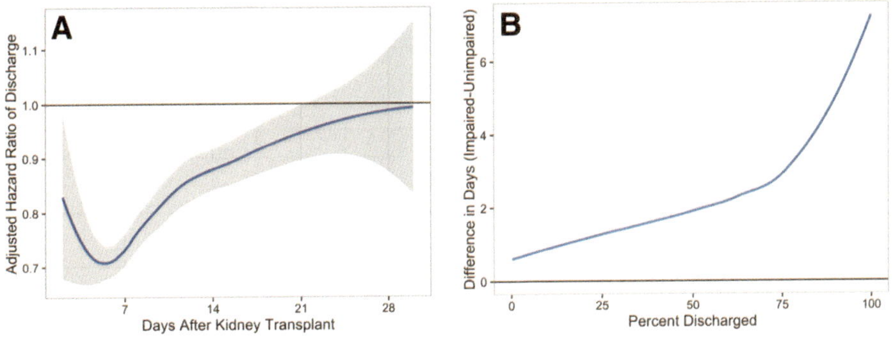

Fig. 2 a Relative Hazard (HR) of length of stay (LOS) over time, comparing kidney transplant (KT) recipients who are Short Physical Performance Battery (SPPB) impaired versus those who are not. The SPPB-impaired group has a significantly lower hazard of discharge compared to the unimpaired group until around day 21, when there is no longer a significant difference between the hazards of the two groups. **b** The number of days longer that SPPB impaired kidney transplant recipients needed to reach the same percentage discharged as the SPPB unimpaired recipients. Patients who are SPPB-impaired stay in the hospital longer regardless of the percentage of patients discharged in each group. The time to reach 50% discharge was 2 days longer in the impaired group. Lower extremity impairment was defined as an SPPB score ≤ 10

populations. Nastasi et al. and Wang et al. found an association between pre-KT or pre-liver transplant SPPB score, respectively, and waitlist death/delisting [34]. Lorenz et al. also found an association between pre-KT SPPB and LOS; however, this association was not explored in depth and was limited to a logistic regression of LOS >4 days [35]. Our findings extended this work to KT recipients in demonstrating a robust association between SPPB-measured lower extremity impairment and post-KT LOS.

Functional limitations is associated with worse outcomes in patients across the kidney disease spectrum. Longitudinal studies in aging have shown that functional limitation is a critical step in the pathway describing progression from disease to disability [36, 37]. This has been observe in patients with ESRD, where the trajectory of recovery is rapidly downward without efforts to improve or preserve physical functioning. For example, of the 366 patients who received a transplant within 24 months of initiating dialysis in the Dialysis Morbidity and Mortality Study, those with a lower self-reported physical functioning before KT were more likely to be rehospitalized after transplantation [38].

Functional limitation, however, can be modified through prehabilitiation. There is evidence that patients with higher physical functional capabilities before a surgical intervention will better tolerate a procedure such as KT. For example, a recent review of the literature by Cheng et al. identified a growing body of evidence documenting improved outcomes in cardiopulmonary fitness with exercise training in patients after cardiothoracic and orthopedic surgeries, including post-cardiac transplantation [39]. There is also evidence that most nephrologists, geriatricians, transplant surgeons, and ESRD patients agree that prehabilitation could make ESRD patients less frail [40]. Because functional limitations can be improved through intervention, pre-KT risk assessment with the SPPB may provide an opportunity to intervene by encouraging patient participation in a prehabilitation program.

To our knowledge, this was the first use of a parametric GG survival model to analyze LOS in a surgical population and to calculate novel LOS metrics, which provide a detailed and informative characterization of the differing trajectories of recipients with functional limitations over the course of hospital stay. These methods, in addition to being informative regarding clinical utility, appear to be the most appropriate methodologically when considering predictive ability and model quality [16, 17]. These are likely even more important methodologic weaknesses to consider when looking at older surgical populations because they take into account noninformative censoring (e.g., death) and better handle skewed distributions of extended LOS, issues likely more common in older adults. Using our methodologically appropriate approach, a recipient can know their absolute and relative chance of discharge on any given day post-KT, which provides the chance to better inform care of older adult surgical patients.

A limitation of our work is that we only had data from a single transplant center, which may limit generalizability of our findings. However, we believe the participants in this study are at least representative of the entire KT population at our institution as our cohort of participating KT recipients were not significantly different from those that did not agree to participate and likely represent the KT population in general. Additionally, we found no effect heterogeneity by major recipient characteristics, further suggesting that our findings are generalizable to other populations that might not share the same characteristics as ours.

This study has several important strengths including its prospective design, the representativeness of the cohort, and the measurement of the SPPB, a novel measure of functional limitation. Ascertainment and assessment of recipient factors in this cohort are strengths given that the national registry data of KT recipients lack granular measurements of specific gerontology concepts like the SPPB.

Conclusions

Pre-KT SPPB impairment and composite score were both independently associated with increased LOS, suggesting that the SPPB is a high-utility objective physical assessment capable of successful post-KT risk stratification for LOS and potentially other important KT outcomes. Furthermore, the use of a parametric survival model like the GG model allowed for a more informative and methodologically appropriate analysis of LOS and should thus be considered in place of conventional regression approaches especially in older adult surgical populations given their unique methodologic considerations. Based on these findings, SPPB impaired individuals should be identified at time of KT to facilitate successful patient discharge counseling and to potentially receive more careful follow-up to avoid adverse events associated with an increased LOS.

Abbreviations

CI: Confidence interval; ESRD: End-stage renal disease; GG: Generalized gamma; KT: Kidney transplantation; LOS: Length of stay; SPPB: Short Physical Performance Battery

Acknowledgements

A big "thank you" to Dr. Alvaro Muñoz, Dr. Christopher Cox, and the rest of the AMDACS team for their enlightening instruction and penetrating insight during the course of this work.

Funding

This work was supported by the National Institutes of Health [grant numbers R01 AG042504, K24 DK101828 to D.L.S.]; the National Institute on Aging and Johns Hopkins University Claude D. Pepper Older Americans Independence Center [grant number P30 AG021334 to M.M.D.]; and the National Institute on Aging [grant number R01 AG055781 to M.M.D.; K01 AG043501 to M.M.D., grant number K01 AG048765 to J.S., grant number T32 AG000247 to J.T.L., grant number F32 AG053025 to C.E.H.]. The funding bodies had no role in: 1) the design of the study, 2) the collection, analysis, and interpretation of the data or 3) the writing of the manuscript.

Authors' contributions

All authors have made substantial contributions to conception and design, or acquisition of data, or analysis and interpretation of data; been involved in drafting the manuscript or revising it critically for important intellectual content; read and given final approval of the version to be published. Each author participated sufficiently in the work to take public responsibility for appropriate portions of the content and agreed to be accountable for all aspects of the work in ensuring that questions related to the accuracy or integrity of any part of the work are appropriately investigated and resolved. Specifically, the authors contributed to: Data Acquisition (AJN, TSB, JTL, DLS, MMD). Study Design (AJN, TSB, JTL, JS, HY, CEH, MGF, DLS, MMD). Statistical Analysis (AJN, TSB, JTL, HY, MMD).

Competing interests

DLS reports receiving speaking honoraria from Sanofi, Genzyme, and CSL Behring. The other authors declare that they have no sources of funding or conflicts of interest relevant to the analysis to report.

Author details

[1]Department of Epidemiology, Johns Hopkins Bloomberg School of Public Health, 615 N. Wolfe St, Baltimore, MD 21205, USA. [2]Department of Surgery, Johns Hopkins School of Medicine, Baltimore, MD, USA. [3]Department of Physical Medicine and Rehabilitation, Johns Hopkins University School of Medicine, Baltimore, MD, USA.

References

1. Banga A, Mohanka M, Mullins J, Bollineni S, Kaza V, Ring S, Bajona P, Peltz M, Wait M, Torres F. Hospital length of stay after lung transplantation: independent predictors and association with early and late survival. J Heart Lung Transplant.
2. Smith JO, Shiffman ML, Behnke M, Stravitz RT, Luketic VA, Sanyal AJ, Heuman DM, Fisher RA, Cotterell AH, Maluf DG, et al. Incidence of prolonged length of stay after orthotopic liver transplantation and its influence on outcomes. Liver Transpl. 2009;15(3):273–9.
3. Villa M, Siskind E, Sameyah E, Alex A, Blum M, Tyrell R, Fana M, Mishler M, Godwin A, Kuncewitch M, et al. Shortened length of stay improves financial outcomes in living donor kidney transplantation. Int J Angiol. 2013;22(2):101–4.
4. McAdams-DeMarco MA, King EA, Luo X, Haugen C, DiBrito S, Shaffer A, Kucirka LM, Desai NM, Dagher NN, Lonze BE, et al. Frailty, length of stay, and mortality in kidney transplant recipients: a National Registry and prospective cohort study. Ann Surg. 2016.
5. McAdams-DeMarco MA, Law A, King E, Orandi B, Salter M, Gupta N, Chow E, Alachkar N, Desai N, Varadhan R, et al. Frailty and mortality in kidney transplant recipients. Am J Transplant. 2015;15(1):149–54.
6. McAdams-DeMarco MA, Law A, Salter ML, Chow E, Grams M, Walston J, Segev DL. Frailty and early hospital readmission after kidney transplantation. Am J Transplant. 2013;13(8):2091–5.
7. McAdams-DeMarco MA, Law A, Tan J, Delp C, King EA, Orandi B, Salter M, Alachkar N, Desai N, Grams M, et al. Frailty, mycophenolate reduction, and graft loss in kidney transplant recipients. Transplantation. 2015;99(4):805–10.
8. McAdams-DeMarco MA, Law A, Salter ML, Boyarsky B, Gimenez L, Jaar BG, Walston JD, Segev DL. Frailty as a novel predictor of mortality and hospitalization in individuals of all ages undergoing hemodialysis. J Am Geriatr Soc. 2013;61(6):896–901.
9. Garonzik-Wang JM, Govindan P, Grinnan JW, et al. Frailty and delayed graft function in kidney transplant recipients. Arch Surg. 2012;147(2):190–3.
10. Johansen KL, Chertow GM, Jin C, Kutner NG. Significance of frailty among Dialysis patients. J Am Soc Nephrol. 2007;18(11):2960–7.
11. Guralnik JM, Simonsick EM, Ferrucci L, Glynn RJ, Berkman LF, Blazer DG, Scherr PA, Wallace RB. A short physical performance battery assessing lower extremity function: association with self-reported disability and prediction of mortality and nursing home admission. J Gerontol. 1994;49(2):M85–94.
12. Oh B, Cho B, Choi H-C, Son K-Y, Park SM, Chun S, Cho S-I. The influence of lower-extremity function in elderly individuals' quality of life (QOL): an analysis of the correlation between SPPB and EQ-5D. Arch Gerontol Geriatr. 2014;58(2):278–82.
13. Vasunilashorn S, Coppin AK, Patel KV, Lauretani F, Ferrucci L, Bandinelli S, Guralnik JM. Use of the short physical performance battery score to predict loss of ability to walk 400 meters: analysis from the InCHIANTI study. J Gerontol Ser A. 2009;64A(2):223–9.
14. Fisher S, Ottenbacher KJ, Goodwin JS, Graham J, Ostir GV. Short physical performance battery in hospitalized older adults. Aging Clin Exp Res. 2009; 21(6):445.
15. Nastasi AJ, McAdams-DeMarco MA, Schrack J, Ying H, Olorundare I, Warsame F, Mountford A, Haugen CE, Gonzalez Fernandez M, Norman SP, et al. Pre-kidney transplant lower extremity impairment and post-kidney transplant mortality. Am J Transplant Off J Am Soc Transplant Am Soc Transplant Surg. 2017.
16. Austin PC, Rothwell DM, Tu JV. A comparison of statistical modeling strategies for analyzing length of stay after CABG surgery. Health Serv Outcomes Res Methodol. 2002;3(2):107–33.
17. Ravangard R, Arab M, Rashidian A, Akbarisari A, Zare A, Zeraati H. Comparison of the results of cox proportional hazards model and parametric models in the study of length of stay in a tertiary teaching Hospital in Tehran, Iran. Acta Med Iran. 2011;49(10):650–8.
18. Verburg IWM, de Keizer NF, de Jonge E, Peek N. Comparison of regression methods for modeling intensive care length of stay. PLoS One. 2014;9(10):e109684.
19. Kramer AA, Zimmerman JE. A predictive model for the early identification of patients at risk for a prolonged intensive care unit length of stay. BMC Med Inform Decis Making. 2010;10:27.

20. Weissman C. Analyzing the impact of long-term patients on ICU bed utilization. Intensive Care Med. 2000;26(9):1319–25.
21. Hemmelgarn BR, Manns BJ, Quan H, Ghali WA. Adapting the Charlson comorbidity index for use in patients with ESRD. Am J Kidney Dis. 2003;42(1):125–32.
22. Cox C, Chu H, Schneider MF, Muñoz A. Parametric survival analysis and taxonomy of hazard functions for the generalized gamma distribution. Stat Med. 2007;26(23):4352–74.
23. McAdams-DeMarco MA, Grams ME, Hall EC, Coresh J, Segev DL. Early hospital readmission after kidney transplantation: patient and center-level associations. Am J Transplant. 2012;12(12):3283–8.
24. McAdams-DeMarco MA, Isaacs K, Darko L, Salter ML, Gupta N, King EA, Walston J, Segev DL. Changes in frailty after kidney transplantation. J Am Geriatr Soc. 2015;63(10):2152–7.
25. McAdams-DeMarco MA, James N, Salter ML, Walston J, Segev DL. Trends in kidney transplant outcomes in older adults. J Am Geriatr Soc. 2014;62(12):2235–42.
26. McAdams-DeMarco MA, Suresh S, Law A, Salter ML, Gimenez LF, Jaar BG, Walston JD, Segev DL. Frailty and falls among adult patients undergoing chronic hemodialysis: a prospective cohort study. BMC Nephrol. 2013;14(1):224.
27. McAdams-DeMarco MA, Tan J, Salter ML, Gross A, Meoni LA, Jaar BG, Kao WH, Parekh RS, Segev DL, Sozio SM. Frailty and cognitive function in incident hemodialysis patients. Clin J Amer Soc Nephrol. 2015;10(12):2181–9.
28. McAdams-DeMarco MA, Ying H, Olorundare I, King EA, Haugen C, Buta B, Gross AL, Kalyani R, Desai NM, Dagher NN, et al. Individual frailty components and mortality in kidney transplant recipients. Transplantation. 2016.
29. Exterkate L, Slegtenhorst B, Kelm M, Seyda M, Schuitenmaker J, Quante M, Uehara H, El Khal A, Tullius S, Md P. Frailty and transplantation. Transplantation. 2016;100(4):727–33.
30. Lai JC, Feng S, Terrault NA, Lizaola B, Hayssen H, Covinsky K. Frailty predicts waitlist mortality in liver transplant candidates. Am J Transplant. 2014;14(8):1870–9.
31. Derck J, Thelen A, Cron D, Friedman J, Gerebics A, Englesbe M, Sonnenday C. Quality of life in liver transplant candidates: frailty is a better Indicator than severity of liver disease. Transplantation. 2015;99(2):340–4.
32. Fried LP, Tangen CM, Walston J, Newman AB, Hirsch C, Gottdiener J, Seeman T, Tracy R, Kop WJ, Burke G, et al. Frailty in older adults: evidence for a phenotype. J Gerontol A Biol Sci Med Sci. 2001;56(3):M146–56.
33. Ostir GV, Volpato S, Fried LP, Chaves P, Guralnik JM. Reliability and sensitivity to change assessed for a summary measure of lower body function: results from the Women's health and aging study. J Clin Epidemiol. 2002;55(9):916–21.
34. Wang CW, Covinsky KE, Feng S, Hayssen H, Segev DL, Lai JC. Functional impairment in older liver transplantation candidates: from the functional assessment in liver transplantation study. Liver Transpl. 2015;21(12):1465–70.
35. Lorenz EC, Cheville AL, Amer H, Kotajarvi BR, Stegall MD, Petterson TM, Kremers WK, Cosio FG, LeBrasseur NK. Relationship between pre-transplant physical function and outcomes after kidney transplant. Clin Transpl. 2017: e12952-n/a.
36. Guralnik JM, Ferrucci L. Assessing the building blocks of function: utilizing measures of functional limitation. Am J Prev Med. 2003;25(3 Suppl 2):112–21.
37. Verbrugge LM, Jette AM. The disablement process. Soc Sci Med. 1994;38(1):1–14.
38. Kutner NG, Zhang R, Bowles T, Painter P. Pretransplant physical functioning and kidney patients' risk for posttransplantation hospitalization/death: evidence from a national cohort. Clin J Amer Soc Nephrol. 2006;1(4):837–43.
39. Cheng XS, Myers JN, Chertow GM, Rabkin R, Chan KN, Chen Y, Tan JC. Prehabilitation for kidney transplant candidates: is it time? Clin Transpl. 2017;31(8).
40. Van Pilsum Rasmussen S, Konel J, Warsame F, Ying H, Buta B, Haugen C, King E, DiBrito S, Varadhan R, Rodriguez-Manas L, et al. Engaging clinicians and patients to assess and improve frailty measurement in adults with end stage renal disease. BMC Nephrol. 2018;19(1):8.

23

The effectiveness of an integrated care pathway in geriatric rehabilitation among older patients with complex health problems and their informal caregivers: a prospective cohort study

Irma H. J. Everink[1*], Jolanda C. M. van Haastregt[1], Frans E. S. Tan[2], Jos M. G. A. Schols[1,3] and Gertrudis I. J. M. Kempen[1]

Abstract

Background: To improve continuity and coordination of care in geriatric rehabilitation, an integrated care pathway was developed and implemented in The Netherlands. The purpose of this study was to assess the effects of this pathway on patients and informal caregivers.

Methods: Two cohorts of patients and their informal caregivers were prospectively recruited before implementation of the pathway (2011–2012) and after implementation of the pathway (2013–2014). Primary outcome measures were dependence in activities of daily living in patients (KATZ-15) and self-rated burden among informal caregivers (SRB-VAS). Secondary outcome measures were the frequency of performing extended daily activities, social participation, psychological well-being, quality of life and discharge location (patients) and quality of life and objective care burden (informal caregivers). Outcomes were measured at baseline, after three and after nine months.

Results: No effect was shown on the KATZ-15 after three and nine months. However, a larger percentage of patients were discharged home in the care pathway cohort (83% vs 58.1% after three months and 88.6% vs 67.4% after nine months; $p = 0.004$). Furthermore, after three months, patients from the care pathway cohort performed more extended daily activities ($p = 0.014$) and informal caregivers experienced a lower self-rated burden ($p = 0.05$). After nine months, these effects disappeared. No differences were found for the other outcome measures.

Conclusions: Due to the positive effects of the integrated care pathway, we are inclined to recommend implementing the care pathway in regular care. To have longer lasting effects among patients and informal caregivers, we suggest actively disseminating information about the pathway to primary care providers who are currently still unaware of its content.

Keywords: Aged, Geriatric rehabilitation, Subacute care, Integrated care, Pathway, Dependence in activities of daily living, Informal care

* Correspondence: i.everink@maastrichtuniversity.nl
[1]Department of Health Services Research and Care and Public Health Research Institute (CAPHRI), Maastricht University, P.O. Box 616, 6200, MD, Maastricht, The Netherlands
Full list of author information is available at the end of the article

Background

Functional decline and deterioration in self-care abilities are common consequences of hospitalization among older adults, and can be exacerbated by inactivity and immobility during hospital stay [1, 2]. As a result, after hospital admission a considerable number of community-living older patients are discharged to an inpatient geriatric rehabilitation facility where they receive short-term multidisciplinary care to restore functional independence, such as activities of daily living (ADL), to improve quality of life and to prepare them to return to their former living situation [3].

A meta-analysis revealed that geriatric rehabilitation has beneficial effects on functional status and prevents permanent admission to nursing homes [4]. However, the fact that patients transfer between care settings (hospital, geriatric rehabilitation facility and primary care) and are confronted with multiple caregivers, forms a challenge for the coordination and continuity of care [5]. Frequently mentioned problems in these transitional phases are care plans not being communicated from one organization to the other, the transfer of medication lists which are not up-to-date or incomplete, and lack of communication between professionals from different organizations [6–10]. Furthermore, patients and their informal caregivers are often not sufficiently prepared for the transition to the home situation [5]. These problems in continuity of care could result in adverse events among patients, such as insufficient functional improvement, unnecessary hospital readmissions and permanent admission to a nursing home [6, 8, 10]. Moreover, care transitions affect the emotional, social, financial and physical functioning of informal caregivers. Therefore, inadequate care transitions are a substantial risk factor for high informal caregiver burden [11].

Various transitional care interventions have been developed to deal with these problems; these interventions focus mainly on discharge planning and discharge support for older adults. A systematic literature review by Laugaland and colleagues showed that the majority of these programs have beneficial effects, but that most interventions focus on single groups of caregivers, such as nurses or occupational therapists. Furthermore, all studies in this review focused on discharge interventions from hospital to home and did not include transfer to post-acute care settings, such as geriatric rehabilitation facilities [12].

To deal with challenges in continuity and coordination of care for patients who go through the trajectory of hospitalization, admission to a geriatric rehabilitation facility and discharge back to the home situation, an integrated care pathway in geriatric rehabilitation was developed and implemented in an urban region in the southern part of the Netherlands [13]. Integrated care pathways describe a sequence and timing of activities or interventions performed by care providers to obtain clinical goals. They comprise detailed information about which professional is responsible for these interventions and activities [14]. The integrated care pathway in geriatric rehabilitation focused on improving communication, triage and transfers of patients between hospital, geriatric rehabilitation facility and primary care organizations. To evaluate the effectiveness of this pathway, a prospective cohort study was conducted with a usual care cohort and a care pathway cohort of patients and informal caregivers. This study assessed the effectiveness of this pathway in comparison with usual care with respect to the level of dependence in activities of daily living among patients and the self-rated burden among informal caregivers as primary outcomes. Furthermore, recent performance of extended daily activities, social participation, psychological well-being, quality of life and discharge location were assessed as secondary outcomes among patients, and, among informal caregivers, quality of life and objective care burden.

Methods

Study design

A prospective cohort study was used to assess the effects of the integrated care pathway. Two cohorts of patients and informal caregivers were prospectively recruited in the geriatric rehabilitation facility where the pathway was implemented. This geriatric rehabilitation facility was situated in the Maastricht area (in the southern part of the Netherlands). The first cohort of patients and informal caregivers (the care as usual cohort) was included in the period April 2011 – March 2012, prior to implementation of the care pathway. The second cohort (the care pathway cohort) was included in the period April 2013–August 2014, after implementation of the pathway. This study design and methods were approved by the Medical Ethics Committee of University Hospital Maastricht (#11–4-020).

Participants

The participants of this study were patients admitted to a geriatric rehabilitation facility in Maastricht, the Netherlands, and their informal caregivers. In the Netherlands, patients admitted to a geriatric rehabilitation facility are categorized into four groups: patients with stroke, trauma orthopedics, elective orthopedics and the residual, referred to as patients with complex health problems. The pathway described in the present study was developed for this heterogeneous group of patients with complex health problems. These patients often suffer from multi-morbidity, mostly involving cardiac problems, problems with the respiratory system, neurological problems, oncological problems and other internal medicine problems such as gastrointestinal problems. Disease exacerbations are common in this group, leading to hospital readmissions and the necessity for geriatric rehabilitation. All patients from this group were eligible for participation if they were admitted to the geriatric rehabilitation facility in the period April 2011–March 2012 or in the period April 2013–August 2014, aged ≥65 years, admitted to the hospital prior to admission to the geriatric rehabilitation facility and were community-dwelling prior to hospital admission. Patients in the two cohorts were not eligible to participate if the elderly care physician assessed their cognitive status as insufficient for participation, based on their expert opinion.

Informal caregivers were recruited by asking the included patients who their main informal caregiver was, and whether they permitted the researchers to invite them for participation in the study. Informal caregiving was defined as voluntary and unpaid care, delivered on a structural basis to people with physical, cognitive of mental deficiencies. This could be either a family member or not. If the patient approved contacting their informal caregiver, the latter was invited for participation by telephone. All patients and informal caregivers provided written informed consent.

Intervention

The integrated care pathway was developed by reviewing relevant literature and consulting experts. Furthermore, iterative meetings with two multidisciplinary workgroups of professionals and one workgroup of patients and informal caregivers were organized. During these meetings, current practice, barriers to and incentives for change were analyzed and proposals for improving the care process were generated. These proposals for improvement were critically discussed in the multidisciplinary workgroups, finally resulting in the integrated care pathway. The development and implementation process of the integrated care pathway is described in more detail elsewhere [13]. Due to the heterogeneity of this group of patients with complex health problems, the pathway is focused on the process of care instead of the contents of the rehabilitation treatment and involves the full trajectory of hospital admission, discharge to the geriatric rehabilitation facility and discharge back to the community. The key components of the pathway are the following:

1. A care pathway coordinator is appointed. The role of the care pathway coordinator is to act as a contact person for professionals involved in the pathway, to further streamline the care processes in the pathway and improve continuity and coordination of care.
2. A triage instrument is used by discharge nurses in the hospital. The instrument instructs discharge nurses to gather information for potential patients for geriatric rehabilitation about functional prognosis, endurability of the patient, teachability/trainability and patients' and informal caregiver's needs and abilities. This information should enable the nurses to decide if geriatric rehabilitation is indeed appropriate for a patient or not. If the discharge nurse has doubts about the appropriateness of geriatric rehabilitation for a patient, the elderly care physician from the geriatric rehabilitation facility is consulted, and makes the final decision.
3. Patients and their informal caregivers are always actively involved in the triage decision in the hospital, and in the establishment of their care and treatment plan in the geriatric rehabilitation facility and in primary care;
4. All patient discharge summaries (medical, nursing and from allied care professionals) from the hospital to the geriatric rehabilitation facility and from the geriatric rehabilitation facility to primary care are sent on the day of discharge and are of high quality (clear andcomprehensive);
5. Meetings between care professionals from the hospital and the geriatric rehabilitation facility are organized at least twice per year, and between the geriatric rehabilitation facility and primary care organizations at least once per year. These meetings focus on improving the triage process, the timing and quality of discharge summaries and the transfer of patients between the hospital, geriatric rehabilitation facility and primary care organizations.

The agreements in the care pathway can be retrieved in the Appendix.

As the integrated care pathway was regular care from April 2013 onwards in the participating geriatric rehabilitation facility, all patients in the group of complex health problems admitted after April 2013 received care according to the pathway. In the care as usual cohort, there was no care pathway coordinator appointed, the decision to refer someone to the geriatric rehabilitation facility was made without the use of an official triage instrument and there were no structural meetings between professionals of the hospital, the geriatric rehabilitation facility and the primary care organizations. Furthermore, the active involvement of patients and informal caregivers in their rehabilitation trajectory and the timeliness and high quality of discharge summaries were not established in agreements or protocols in the care as usual cohort.

Outcome measures

The primary outcome measure used to evaluate the effects of the pathway on patients was dependence in activities of daily living, measured with the Katz Index KATZ-15 [15]. This scale assesses one's ability to perform activities of daily living by asking 15 questions related to the (instrumental) activities of daily living, self-care and mobility. Each question could be answered with "no help needed" (0) or "help needed" (1) and a total score of 15 could be achieved. A higher score represents more dependence in activities of daily living.

Five secondary outcome measures were used to assess the effects of the pathway on the patients. The first secondary outcome measure was recent performance of extended daily activities, measured with the Frenchay Activities Index (FAI) [16]. This index consists of 15 items assessing the frequency with which activities are performed that reflect the extended activities of daily life. These activities range from domestic chores, to leisure and outdoor activities. The frequency of performing these activities can be scored on a scale ranging from "never" (1) to "often" (4). The second secondary outcome measure was social participation, assessed using two subscales of the Impact on Participation and Autonomy (IPA) questionnaire [17]. These subscales are "autonomy outdoors" and "social life and relationships" and consist, respectively, of 5 and 7 items. The questions examine the extent to which people are able to perform activities such as visiting friends and going on a trip or holiday whenever they want to (autonomy outdoors) and the degree to which they are able to interact with people on an equivalent level (social life and relationships). Answer options range from "very good" (1) to "poor" (5). Whereas the KATZ-15 thus mainly focuses on self-care and mobility, the FAI adds somewhat more complex leisure and outdoor activities. Finally, the IPA also focuses on interaction with other people. The third secondary outcome measure was psychological well-being, measured using a subscale from the RAND-36 item Health Survey (RAND-36) [18]. This subscale consists of five items focusing on feelings (such as happiness, sadness and nervousness) people experienced in the last month. These items have six answer categories each, ranging from "always" (1) to "never" (6). The fourth secondary outcome measure was quality of life, measured with a modified version of Cantril's Self Anchoring Ladder (CSAL) [15]. This measure asks patients to value their quality of life on a scale ranging from 0 to 100, with higher scores indicating a better quality of life. The fifth and last secondary patient outcome measure assessed was discharge location after inpatient geriatric rehabilitation. This was scored as back home (0) or not back home (1), the latter including institutionalization (admission to an elderly care home, a nursing home or palliative care in a hospice), hospital readmission or death.

The primary outcome measure used to assess the effects of the pathway on informal caregivers was self-rated burden of informal caregiving, measured with the Self-Rated Burden Visual Analogue Scale (SRB-VAS). The self-rated burden VAS assesses on a scale from 0 to 10 how burdensome informal caregiving is for the informal caregiver, with a higher score indicating a higher burden [19].

Secondary outcomes used to assess the effects of the pathway on informal caregivers were quality of life, assessed with a modified version of Cantril's Self Anchoring Ladder [15], and objective burden of caregiving, measured using the Erasmus iBMG instrument [15]. This instrument asks informal caregivers how many hours per week they spend on various caregiving tasks.

Data collection

Primary and secondary outcome measures for this effect evaluation were collected through structured face-to-face interviews by a trained research assistant with patients, and, for informal caregivers, through written questionnaires. The interviews with patients were conducted at admission in the geriatric rehabilitation facility (baseline), after 3 months and after 9 months. The written questionnaires were sent to the informal caregivers using the same timeframes. Discharge location was assessed by reviewing patient files in the geriatric rehabilitation facility.

Statistical analysis

Statistical analyses were performed using the statistical software package SPSS for Windows, version 22. Descriptive statistics, independent t-tests and chi square tests were used to describe and compare the baseline characteristics of patients and informal caregivers in the two cohorts. Because data was collected longitudinally, a two-level mixed model was used to compare the two cohorts of patients and informal caregivers with respect to the continuous primary and secondary outcome measures. Repeated measurements were the first level observations and respondents were the second level observations. A longitudinal model was specified with the outcome variable as a function of all three time points treated as dependent. Adjusted mean differences were calculated to express the differences between groups and were fully corrected for baseline differences (by specifying group and time as main effects as well as the interaction between time and group). The group differences were also corrected for age, sex, living situation (not living alone vs. living alone), educational level (lower than vocational school vs. vocational school or higher), multi-morbidity (one condition vs. the presence of two or more conditions). As the secondary outcome measure "discharge location" is dichotomous (home vs. not home), this outcome measure was analyzed with a standard logistic regression model. The previously mentioned covariates for patients (i.e. age, sex, living situation, educational level, and multi-morbidity) were also included in this model.

For the informal caregivers, covariates included in each multilevel model were age, sex and living situation (not living with care receiver vs. living with care receiver). Adjusted mean differences were calculated to express the differences between groups, fully corrected for baseline differences. Missing data among patients and among informal caregivers were assumed to be missing at random.

Results

Patients

In total, 260 patients in the two cohorts were eligible for participation in the study: 71 in the care as usual cohort and 189 in the care pathway cohort. In the care as usual cohort, 49 patients agreed to participate (69%) and in the care pathway cohort this number was 113 (60%). The reasons for not participating were rather similar in both cohorts. Figure 1 shows the flowchart of the patient study population.

All interviews with patients were performed face-to-face. Because six patients in the care as usual cohort and seven patients in the care pathway cohort did not participate in the baseline measurement (because they dropped out of the study prior to their first interview or had only follow-up measurements), these patients were not included in the analyses. Thus the total number of patients in the analyses was 43 and 106, respectively. Total dropout during the course of the study in the care as usual cohort was 24 (56%) and 38 (36%) in the care pathway cohort. The reasons for dropout are provided in Fig. 1 as well.

Table 1 shows the baseline characteristics of the patients. More patients in the care pathway cohort suffered from diseases of the locomotor system in comparison with the care as usual cohort (18.1% versus 4.7%). Furthermore, the difference between the two groups in the number of patients suffering from cardiovascular diseases is borderline significant (37.2% in the care as usual cohort versus 22.9% in the care pathway cohort; $p = 0.074$).There are no other statistically significant differences between the two cohorts.

Informal caregivers

In total, 26 informal caregivers were included in the care as usual cohort and 28 informal caregivers in the care pathway cohort. In the care as usual cohort, 9 patients (20.9%) indicated not having an informal caregiver. Furthermore, 9 informal caregivers did not participate because the person they cared for died ($n = 4$) or they were not interested in participating ($n = 4$). In the care pathway cohort, the main reasons for not participating were that (a) the patient indicated not having a caregiver ($n = 32$), (b) the caregiver was not interested in participating ($n = 24$), or (c) the patient did not want to burden the informal caregiver ($n = 10$).

In Table 2, the background characteristics of the informal caregivers are displayed. In the care as usual cohort, two informal caregivers participated only in follow-up measurements, and in the care pathway cohort, six informal caregivers participated only in follow-up measurements. Therefore, these informal caregivers did not have scores on the primary and secondary outcome measures at baseline. As shown in Table 2, the differences in baseline characteristics between the two groups at baseline are not statistically different.

In the care as usual cohort, 10 informal caregivers dropped out during the study due to variable reasons: the patient died ($n = 6$), the informal caregiver did not return the questionnaire ($n = 3$) or lost interest ($n = 1$). In the care pathway cohort, 14 informal caregivers dropped out for the following reasons: the patient died ($n = 7$), the caregivers indicated they no longer had informal care tasks ($n = 3$), they simply did not return the questionnaire ($n = 2$), they lost interest ($n = 1$), or were too ill ($n = 1$).

Effects of the integrated care pathway on patients

The mixed model analysis showed no difference after 3 and 9 months in the primary outcome measure, dependence in activities of daily living as measured with the KATZ-15. The adjusted mean difference was − 0.51 ($p = 0.360$) after 3 months and − 0.14 ($p = 0.862$) after 9 months (Table 3). Furthermore, a significant adjusted mean difference of 4.14 ($p = 0.014$) was found for the secondary outcome measure as measured with the FAI – the frequency of performing extended daily activities - after 3 months. This significant difference disappeared after 9 months (adjusted mean difference = 1.84, $p = 0.288$). No significant differences were found for

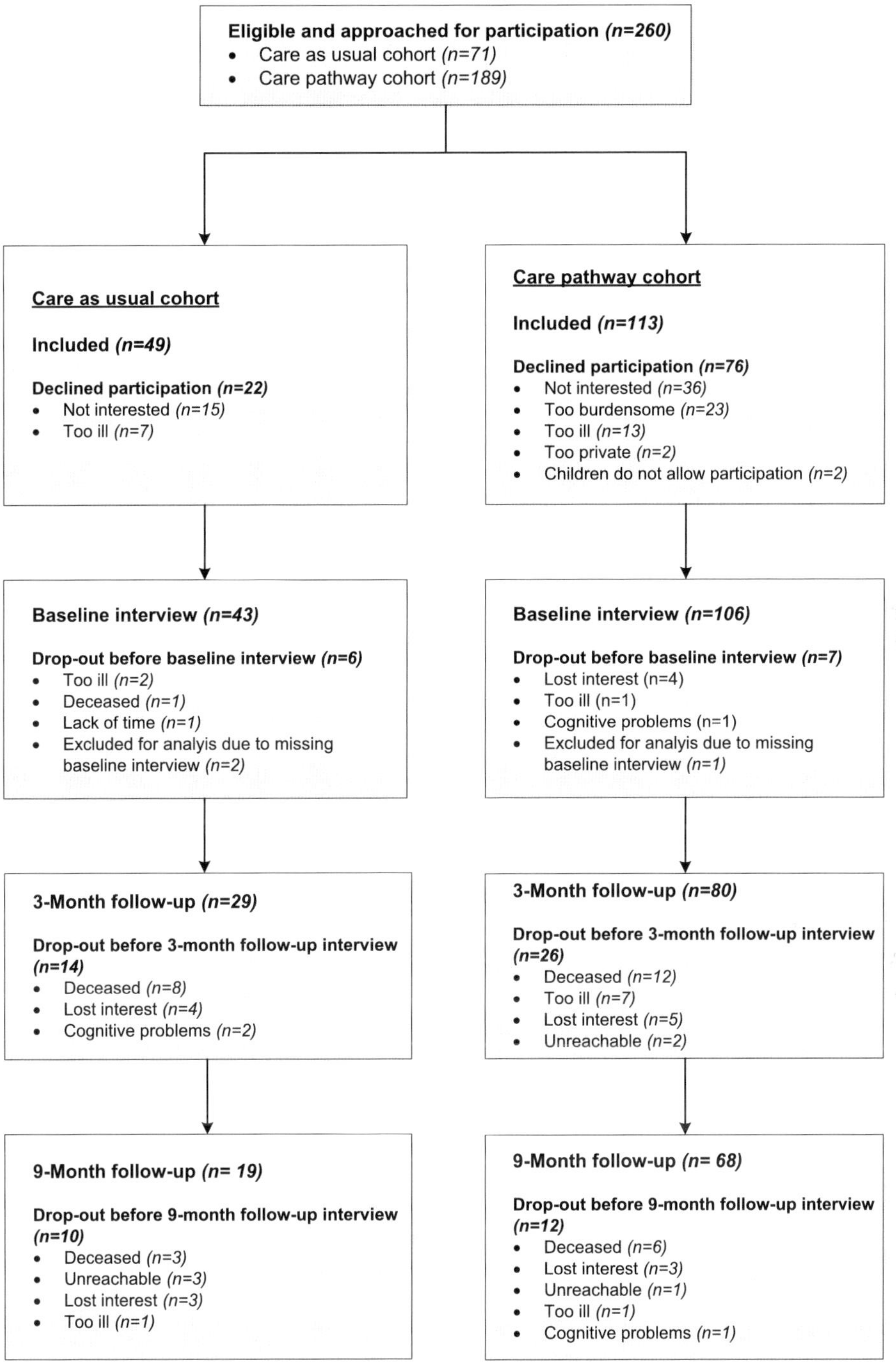

Fig. 1 Flowchart of Patients through the Study

social participation, psychological well-being and quality of life after 3 and 9 months.

As shown in Table 4, a significantly higher proportion of patients in the care pathway cohort were discharged to their home situation compared to patients in the care as usual cohort. This difference between the two cohorts is visible after 3 months (83.0% vs 58.1%; $p = 0.004$) as well as after 9 months (88.6% vs 67.4%; $p = 0.004$).

Effects of the integrated care pathway on informal caregivers

As shown in Table 5, after 3 months there was a significant adjusted mean difference for the primary outcome measure self-rated burden (SRB-VAS) among informal

Table 1 Baseline Characteristics of Patients in Both Cohorts

Characteristics	Care as usual cohort $n = 43$	Care pathway cohort $n = 106$	p-value
Mean age (sd)	79.6 (7.1)	80.7 (6.9)	0.370
Sex (% female)	65.0%	67.9%	0.471
Living situation (% living alone)	67.4%	68.9%	0.865
Education (% ≥ vocational school)	60.5%	67.9%	0.385
Multi-morbidity (% having at least 2 conditions)	87.8%	88.7%	0.882
Medical diagnosis			
• Cardiovascular diseases (n, %)	16 (37.2%)	24 (22.9%)	0.074
• Internal medicine diseases (n, %)	15 (34.9%)	30 (28.6%)	0.449
• Oncological diseases (n, %)	5 (11.6%)	7 (6.7%)	0.331
• Respiratory diseases (n, %)	4 (9.3%)	11 (10.5%)	0.547
• Diseases of locomotor system (n, %)	2 (4.7%)	19 (18.1%)	0.033[†]
• Neurological diseases (n, %)	1 (2.3%)	8 (7.6%)	0.448
• Other (n, %)	0 (0%)	6 (5.7%)	0.181
Primary outcome measure			
Dependence in activities of daily living (mean score KATZ-15; range 0–15*) (sd)	6.6 (3.7)	5.7 (3.3)	0.179
Secondary outcome measures			
Extended daily activities (mean score FAI; range 15–60) (sd)	33.5 (9.6)	32.2 (8.7)	0.411
Social participation (mean score IPA; range 12–60) (sd)	30.5 (6.5)	29.2 (6.2)	0.310
Psychological well-being (mean score subscale RAND-36; range 5–30) (sd)	21.1 (6.2)	21.8 (5.6)	0.481
Quality of life (mean score CSAL; range 1–100) (sd)	66.4 (12.9)	65.6 (14.8)	0.768

Internal medicine diseases are diseases of the internal organs such as renal diseases, gastrointestinal diseases and infections
KATZ-15 modified version of the Katz Index of Independence in Activities of Daily Living, *FAI* Frenchay Activities Index, *IPA* Impact on Participation and Autonomy, *CSAL* Cantril's Self Anchoring Ladder
[a]The underlined score represents the most favorable score
[†]Statistically significant (p-value < 0.05)

Table 2 Baseline Characteristics of Informal Caregivers in Both Cohorts

Characteristics	Care as usual cohort $n = 26$	Care pathway cohort $n = 28$	p-value
Mean age (sd)	58.9 (14.4)	61.3 (13.9)	0.537
Sex (% female)	20 (76.9%)	20 (71.4%)	0.645
Living together with patient (%)	8 (30.8%)	5 (17.9%)	0.267
Primary outcome measure	n = 24	$n = 22$	
Self-rated burden of informal caregiving (mean score SRB-VAS; 0-10[a]) (sd)	4.7 (2.8)	5.5 (2.5)	0.289
Secondary outcome measures			
Quality of life (Mean score CSAL; range 0-100[a]) (sd)	70.9 (13.8)	71.0 (12.1)	0.991
Mean (sd) objective burden of caregiving (Erasmus iBMG)			
• Domestic duties (hours/week)	6.1 (9.3)	7.7 (13.6)	0.654
• Personal care (hours/week)	1.7 (4.3)	0.17 (0.76)	0.121
• Moving outside the house (hours/week)	4.2 (3.8)	5.3 (4.0)	0.401
• Number of hours help of other informal caregivers / volunteers (hours/week)	1.6 (2.8)	1.1 (2.3)	0.610

SRB Self-Rated Burden visual analogue scale, *CSAL* Cantril's Self Anchoring Ladder
[a]The underlined score represents the most favorable score

Table 3 Multilevel Analysis for Differences between Patients in the Two Cohorts at 3 and 9-Month Follow-up ($n = 149$)

	3-month follow-up Mean (SD) [a]		Adj. mean difference[b] (95% CI)	p-value	9-month follow-up Mean (SD) [a]		Adj. mean difference[b] (95% CI)	p-value
Primary outcome measure	CUC; $n = 26$	CPC; $n = 75$	$n = 147$		CUC; $n = 19$	CPC; $n = 68$	$n = 147$	
Dependence in activities of daily living (KATZ-15; range 0-15[c])	5.7 (2.8)	4.6 (2.4)	−0.51 (−1.60, 0.59)	0.360	5.0 (3.0)	4.4 (2.9)	−0.14 (− 1.41, 1.12)	0.862
Secondary outcome measures								
Extended daily activities (FAI; range 15–60)	27.4 (9.7)	31.1 (9.4)	4.14 (0.86, 7.42)	0.014†	29.4 (11.2)	31.0 (9.4)	1.84 (−1.58, 5.26)	0.288
Social participation (IPA; range 12–60)	31.0 (6.2)	28.9 (6.8)	−1.20 (−4.28, 1.88)	0.441	30.8 (8.0)	30.8 (8.3)	−0.27 (−4.70, 4.16)	0.903
Psychological well-being (Subscale RAND-36; range 5–30)	22.8 (5.0)	23.7 (4.7)	−0.53 (−2.61, 1.54)	0.610	22.8 (6.3)	22.9 (5.6)	−0.91 (−3.67, 1.94)	0.529
Quality of life (CSAL; range 0–100)	67.9 (14.1)	70.7 (9.4)	4.95 (−2.17, 12.08)	0.171	71.4 (9.2)	68.9(16.4)	1.54 (−7.29, 10.37)	0.730

CUC Care as Usual Cohort, *CPC* Care Pathway Cohort, *KATZ-15* modified version of the Katz Index of Independence in Activities of Daily Living, *FAI* Frenchay Activities Index, *IPA* Impact on Participation and Autonomy, *CSAL* Cantril's Self Anchoring Ladder
†Statistically significant (p-value < 0.05)
[a]Unadjusted means
[b]Adjusted for age, sex, living situation, educational level, multi-morbidity and the interaction term "group*time"
[c]The underlined score represents the most favorable score

caregivers (− 1.54; $p = 0.05$). The significance of this difference disappeared after 9 months ($p = 0.077$). Table 5 shows that implementation of the integrated care pathway did not result in significant differences between the two cohorts of informal caregivers on the secondary outcome measures after 3 and 9 months (Table 5).

Discussion

This study examined if implementation of an integrated care pathway in geriatric rehabilitation resulted in lower dependence in activities of daily living among patients and decreased self-rated burden among informal caregivers. The results of this study show that implementation of the pathway had no significant effect on level of dependence in activities of daily living among patients over a period of 3 and 9 months. A statistically significant effect was found for self-rated burden among informal caregivers after 3 months. However, this effect disappeared after 9 months. With respect to secondary outcome measures, our study showed that the pathway had a significant effect on the frequency of performing extended daily activities among patients after 3 months. This effect also disappeared after 9 months. No significant effect was found for the secondary outcome measures social participation, psychological well-being and quality of life among patients, or on quality of life and objective care burden among informal caregivers after 3 and 9 months. Therefore, it can be stated that overall, only small effects were found on the functional outcome measures. However, a significantly higher proportion of patients in the care pathway cohort were discharged back home in comparison with patients in the care as usual cohort. Overall, if patients are discharged home, their functional status is higher compared to patients who are still in the geriatric rehabilitation facility or patients who are admitted to nursing homes. This is also shown by the difference in score on the FAI after 3 months. Furthermore, in addition to the effects on these functional outcome measures, the economic evaluation executed alongside this study showed that implementation of the pathway resulted in a shorter length of stay in the hospital and the geriatric rehabilitation facility [20]. As a consequence, large cost savings were achieved.

It is noteworthy to mention that an effect was found on the secondary outcome measure performance of extended activities of daily living, while no effect was found on the primary outcome measure independence in activities of daily living. A reason could be that the integrated care pathway is focused on the active involvement of patients in the establishment of their

Table 4 Discharge Location after Geriatric Rehabilitation at 3 and 9 Month Follow-up (n=149)

	3 months follow-up			9 months follow-up		
	CUC $n = 43$	CPC $n = 106$	P-value*	CUC $n = 43$	CPC $n = 106$	P-value*
Home	25 (58.1%)	88 (83.0%)	0.004†	29 (67.4%)	94 (88.6%)	0.004†
Not home	18 (41.9%)	18 (17.0%)		14 (32.6%)	12 (11.4%)	

CUC Care as Usual Cohort, *CPC* Care Pathway Cohort
*Adjusted for age, sex, living situation, educational level and multi-morbidity
†Statistically significant (p-value < 0.05)

Table 5 Multilevel Analysis for Differences between Informal Caregivers in the Two Cohorts at 3 and 9-Month Follow-up ($n = 54$)

	3-month follow-up Mean (SD)[a]		Adj. mean difference[b] (95% CI)	*p*-value	9-month follow-up Mean (SD)[a]		Adj. mean difference[b] (95% CI)	*p*-value
Primary outcome measure	CUC; $n = 18$	CPC; $n = 19$	$n = 54$		CUC; $n = 16$	CPC; $n = 14$	$n = 54$	
Self-rated burden of informal caregiving (SRB-VAS; 0-10[c])	5.4 (2.2)	4.1 (2.4)	−1.54 (−3.08, −0.00)	0.050[†]	4.4 (2.2)	3.5 (2.6)	−1.54 (−3.25, 0.17)	0.077
Secondary outcome measures								
Quality of life (CSAL; range 0–100)	68.2 (14.3)	73.2 (15.2)	3.11 (−3.86, 10.01)	0.371	68.7 (11.3)	73.2 (8.2)	5.26 (−2.24, 12.77)	0.158
Mean objective burden of caregiving (Erasmus iBMG)								
• Domestic duties (hours/week)	11.7 (20.9)	9.7 (14.0)	−3.15 (−13.14, 6.84)	0.525	10.4 (12.8)	9.1 (12.5)	−4.54 (−14.54, 5.46)	0.361
• Personal care (hours/week)	2.0 (3.9)	0.9 (2.4)	0.54 (−1.80, 2.87)	0.646	4.1 (10.5)	5.6 (12.4)	2.99 (−5.36, 11.33)	0.470
• Moving outside the house (hours/week)	3.2 (2.7)	3.8 (2.6)	−0.72 (−3.33, 1.90)	0.583	3.9 (4.2)	5.6 (8.1)	1.65 (−3.40, 6.71)	0.510
• Number of hours help from other informal caregivers / volunteers (hours/week)	1.9 (3.0)	1.0 (1.7)	−0.67 (−2.67, 1.32)	0.500	6.4 (20.8)	2.9 (4.8)	−1.92 (−11.73, 7.89)	0.684

CUC Care as Usual Cohort, *CPC* Care Pathway Cohort
[†]Statistically significant (*p*-value < 0.05)
[a]Unadjusted means
[b]Adjusted for age, sex, living situation and the interaction term "group*time"
[c]The underlined score represents the most favorable score

rehabilitation goals. When rehabilitation goals are tailored and more personalized towards the patient's wishes and preferences, patients will probably be better prepared to restart leisure and outdoor activities once discharged to the home situation. This might indicate that patients are taught how to resume these extended daily activities, irrespective of their limitations or level of dependence in activities of daily living. Another remarkable finding is that although more patients were discharged home in the care pathway cohort, the self-rated burden among informal caregivers after 3 months was significantly lower. This might indicate that patients are either less dependent on the informal caregivers, or the informal caregivers are better prepared at the moment the patients are discharged home.

The statistically significant favorable outcomes on 'frequency of performing extended daily activities' among patients and 'self-rated burden' among informal caregivers after 3 months, disappeared after 9 months. An explanation for the disappearance of these effects could be that the pathway is focused on patients who transfer between hospital, geriatric rehabilitation facility and home. After patients returned home, the integrated care pathway turns into regular primary care. This means that the reach of the pathway (i.e. the active involvement of the care pathway coordinator) extends to approximately 1 month after discharge of a patient from the geriatric rehabilitation facility. Thus, after 9 months, the pathway activities are no longer active. Still, it was expected that due to the improved transfer phases and improved coordination of follow-up care, the effects of the integrated care pathway would carry on for a longer period of time. Another explanation could be that the number and variety of professionals providing primary care in the Maastricht region is large (i.e. home care providers, general practitioners, physiotherapists, occupational therapists, etc.) and rather dispersed. This might have affected the extent to which multidisciplinary and coordinated care was provided in the home situation. Although we tried to reach all primary care providers via their professionals associations, it is possible that not all providers were aware of the content of the integrated care pathway. In addition it is possible that the care providers who were aware of the agreements of the pathway did not always act upon these agreements, due to lack of time, motivation or other hindering factors. Therefore, in the future it should be more closely monitored to which extent primary care professionals are actually aware of the pathway and have implemented its different components in daily practice. Targeted implementation strategies should then be deployed to improve the implementation of the care pathway in primary care.

Finally, a process evaluation executed alongside this study (described elsewhere) showed that this care pathway is a promising start, but there seems to be room for optimization as well [20].

Due to a lack of studies in the area of geriatric rehabilitation, it is not possible to compare our results to related studies within the domain. However, several studies concerning inter-organizational care pathways involving hospital and primary care showed positive results regarding care coordination, morbidity, drug-related adverse events, hospital readmission rates, emergency department visits and healthcare costs [21–25]. Patient-related outcomes such as dependence in activities of daily living and perceived burden of care for informal caregivers were not assessed in these studies.

Although this pathway was developed in the Netherlands, the majority of its content is relevant internationally as well. As an increasing number of older people suffer from multi-morbidity, they mostly receive care from a range of professionals in various organizations [22]. The principles of this pathway regarding inter-organizational collaboration and improved communication between providers can be used to facilitate continuity and coordination of care between these organizations.

Some limitations of our study should be mentioned. First, because the effects of the pathway were studied in a prospective cohort study where the care as usual cohort was included in 2011–2012 and the care pathway cohort was included in 2013–2014, the possible influence of external factors on the results has to be considered. Although the use of the triage instrument by discharge nurses in the hospital was a fundamental part of the integrated care pathway, the stricter admission criteria for geriatric rehabilitation enforced by this triage instrument were accompanied by the nationwide introduction of stricter admission criteria in 2013. These criteria were used to facilitate the development and implementation of the triage instrument. This has probably influenced the type of patients who were eligible for geriatric rehabilitation. Although the two cohorts were comparable on their baseline characteristics, there is a reasonable chance that selection bias occurred. This might explain (part of) the effect on discharge destination. Second, because our patient population was highly frail (as indicated by the fact that almost 20% of the patients died during the course of the study; Fig. 1), the number of patients included was relatively low and the number of dropouts was large. This is also true for the group of informal caregivers: many patients in the care pathway cohort stated that they were independent prior to hospital admission and therefore did not have an informal caregiver. This resulted in smaller numbers for inclusion which also could have resulted in the failure to detect an effect. Third, we do not have data of patients and informal caregivers who declined participation. Therefore, we cannot compare this group to our participants. Furthermore, selective dropout might have resulted in underestimation or overestimation of our results. However, because the reasons for non-participation and dropout are rather similar across cohorts we have no reason to assume that they are disproportionately related to the primary or secondary outcome measures. Furthermore, because multilevel analyses were performed, the risk of bias due to missing values decreased.

Our study has two important strengths as well. First, as an observational design was used to assess the effects of the pathway, there was room for optimization and adjustment of the pathway during the implementation phase based on the needs and circumstances of the organizations involved. Therefore, results of this evaluation can be interpreted as 'real world' results, which makes it more likely that results are generalizable towards other geriatric rehabilitation settings. Furthermore, because thorough research into the effects of integrated care pathways across organizational and disciplinary borders is scarce [26], this study forms a unique and valuable contribution to existing knowledge in the complex domain of integrated care pathways and geriatric rehabilitation care.

Conclusions

We conclude that implementation of the integrated care pathway resulted in a significantly higher proportion of patients being discharged to the home situation after geriatric rehabilitation. Furthermore, the frequency of performing extended daily activities among patients in the care pathway cohort was significantly higher after 3 months compared to patients in the care as usual cohort, and the self-rated burden of informal caregivers was significantly lower after 3 months. Based on the positive results on these outcome measures, together with a shorter length of stay in hospital and geriatric rehabilitation facility [20], we are recommend implementing the integrated care pathway in regular care. When implementing the pathway in regular care, it is important to keep monitoring the effects on patients and informal caregivers, but also on process related factors such as length of stay in hospital and in geriatric rehabilitation facility. It is also recommended to optimize the pathway elements which were not fully implemented according to plan, and to explore if all primary care providers in the Maastricht region are aware of the content of the integrated care pathway. Based on this exploration, targeted implementation strategies should be used for those primary care professionals who are unaware of its content or have not implemented it in daily practice. It is expected that this may prolong effects on patients and informal caregivers. Finally, more studies in the field of integrated care pathways in geriatric rehabilitation are needed to assess its impact on functional gains, discharge destination and length of stay in hospital and geriatric rehabilitation facility.

Appendix

Table 6 Integrated care pathway for geriatric rehabilitation

Setting	No.	Care pathway element
Hospital	1	If the main treatment provider believes that the patient is eligible for geriatric rehabilitation, the discharge nurses of the hospital will be consulted. Preferably, this consultation takes place well in advance of discharge.
	2	Dismissal from the hospital is preceded by a triage by a discharge nurse. Information about the patient's functional prognosis, endurability, teachability and trainability and the patient's and informal caregiver's needs and abilities needs to be gathered to make this triage decision.
	3	The triage is always performed under the responsibility of an elderly care physician from the geriatric rehabilitation facility. If the discharge nurse has doubts about the patient's eligibility for geriatric rehabilitation, the elderly care physician should be consulted.
	4	Information about functional prognosis, endurability, teachability and trainability and needs and abilities of the patient should be gathered by consulting professionals in the hospital who have been involved in the patient's care.
	5	The patient should always be asked about their needs and abilities and this should explicitly be taken into account when making the triage decision.
	6	The informal caregiver should (if applicable) be asked about their ability to provide informal care and this should explicitly be taken into account when making the triage decision.
	7	The discharge nurse should always provide oral and written information about geriatric rehabilitation to the patient and the informal caregiver.
	8	On the day the patient is discharged from the hospital, an up-to-date list of medications, a medical and nursing discharge summary and, if necessary, a discharge summary from allied health professionals should be available for the professionals in the geriatric rehabilitation facility.
Geriatric rehabilitation facility	9	In the cases where the patient discharge summaries are not available on the day the patient is admitted to the geriatric rehabilitation facility, professionals from the geriatric rehabilitation facility should contact the hospital directly.
	10	All patients with complex care needs admitted to the geriatric rehabilitation facility receive a systematic and multidisciplinary examination to determine which rehabilitation program is suitable for the patient.
	11	The patient's rehabilitation program will be established in close consultation with patient and (if applicable) informal caregiver. The patient's wishes and abilities and their informal caregiving situation will be taken into account when determining this program.
	12	Multidisciplinary meetings are organized at least twice during the patient's stay.
	13	Patients and (if applicable) informal caregivers should always receive feedback on the issues discussed during the multidisciplinary meetings. In those cases where a modification to the patient's rehabilitation program is desirable, this will be discussed with the patient and informal caregiver.
	14	Within two weeks after admission to the geriatric rehabilitation facility, the patient and (if applicable) informal caregiver will be informed about the patient's provisional discharge date.
	15	The treatment intensity should be adjusted (decreased or increased) if this is required by the progress the patient is making.
	16	The provisional discharge date should be adjusted (decreased or increased) if this is required by the progress the patient is making.
	17	Well before discharge, the patient's home situation should be mapped out by a physiotherapist or occupational therapist.
	18	After the home visit, advice should be given to the patient about required adjustments and aids in the home.
	19	The nurses in the geriatric rehabilitation facility should arrange home care prior to discharge of the patient.
	20	If the situation of the patient is complex, a professional of the home care organization will visit the geriatric rehabilitation facility for an intake.
	21	A professional of the home care organization will visit the geriatric rehabilitation facility for an intake if this is preferred by the patient.
	22	An up-to-date nursing discharge summary will be sent to the home care organization on the day of discharge.
	23	An up-to-date prescription for medication will be sent to the patient's pharmacy on the day of discharge.
	24	An up-to-date discharge summary by allied health professionals will be given to the patient on the day of discharge.
	25	An up-to-date medical discharge summary and medication list will be sent to the patient's general practitioner on the day of discharge.
	26	The discharge summary to the general practitioner includes information on the follow-up care advised.

Table 6 Integrated care pathway for geriatric rehabilitation *(Continued)*

Setting	No.	Care pathway element
Primary care	27	In those cases where the patient discharge summaries are not available to the primary care providers on the day the patient is discharged from the geriatric rehabilitation facility, professionals from the primary care organizations should directly contact the geriatric rehabilitation facility.
	28	Once the patient is discharged from the geriatric rehabilitation facility, the nurse practitioner or district nurse in primary care should act as the patient's case manager.
All settings	29	A care pathway coordinator is appointed. The role of the care pathway coordinator is to act as a port of call for professionals involved in the pathway, to improve communication between professionals from different settings, improve continuity and coordinate care and to further streamline the pathway.
	30	At least twice per year, a meeting is organized between professionals from the hospital and from the geriatric rehabilitation facility who are involved in the triage process. The aim of this meeting is to evaluate whether or not the triage process, the medical discharge summaries and the transfer of patients between the hospital and the geriatric rehabilitation facility are satisfactory.
	31	At least once a year a meeting is organized between professionals from the geriatric rehabilitation facility and from primary care to evaluate the timing and quality of the medical discharge summaries and patient transfers.

Abbreviations
ADL: Activities of daily living; CSAL: Cantril's Self Anchoring Ladder; Erasmus iBMG: Erasmus Instituut Beleid & Management Gezondheidszorg; FAI: Frenchay Activities Index; IPA: Impact on Participation and Autonomy; KATZ-15: KATZ Index of independence in activities of daily living; RAND-36: RAND-36 item Health Survey; SRB-VAS: Self rated burden – visual analogue scale

Acknowledgements
This study is part of a PhD thesis, written by the first author IHJE (ISBN 978 94 6159 719 9), funded by the Dutch National Care for the Elderly Programme and sponsored by the Dutch Organization for Health Research and Development (ZonMw #314070401).

Funding
This study was funded by the Dutch National Care for the Elderly Programme and sponsored by the Dutch Organization for Health Research and Development (ZonMw #314070401).

Authors' contributions
IHJE is the guarantor of the article. All authors take responsibility for the truthfulness of the data and the precision of the data analysis, the outline and critical revision of the manuscript. IHJE contributed to the design, data collection, data analysis, data interpretation and drafting of the manuscript. JCMvH contributed to the design, data interpretation, drafting and critical revision of the manuscript. FEST contributed to the data analysis, data interpretation and critical revision of the manuscript. JMGAS contributed to the design and critical revision of the manuscript. GIJMK contributed to the design and critical revision of the manuscript. All authors read and approved the final manuscript and agree to be accountable for all aspects of the work.

Competing interests
The authors declare that they have no competing interests.

Author details
[1]Department of Health Services Research and Care and Public Health Research Institute (CAPHRI), Maastricht University, P.O. Box 616, 6200, MD, Maastricht, The Netherlands. [2]Department of Methodology and Statistics and Care and Public Health Research Institute (CAPHRI), Maastricht University, P.O. Box 616, 6200, MD, Maastricht, The Netherlands. [3]Department of Family Medicine and Care and Public Health Research Institute (CAPHRI), Maastricht University, P.O. Box 616, 6200, MD, Maastricht, The Netherlands.

References
1. McCloskey R. Functional and self-efficacy changes of patients admitted to a geriatric rehabilitation unit. J Adv Nurs. 2004;46(2):186–93.
2. Stucki G, Stier-Jarmer M, Grill E, Melvin J. Rationale and principles of early rehabilitation care after an acute injury or illness. Disabil Rehabil. 2005;27(7–8):353–9.
3. Patrick L, Knoefel F, Gaskowski P, Rexroth D. Medical comorbidity and rehabilitation efficiency in geriatric inpatients. J Am Geriatr Soc. 2001;49(11): 1471–7.
4. Bachmann S, Finger C, Huss A, Egger M, Stuck AE, Clough-Gorr KM. Inpatient rehabilitation specifically designed for geriatric patients: systematic review and meta-analysis of randomised controlled trials. BMJ. 2010;340:c1718.
5. Storm M, Siemsen IM, Laugaland K, Dyrstad DN, Aase K. Quality in transitional care of the elderly: key challenges and relevant improvement measures. Int J Integr Care. 2014;14:e013.
6. Hesselink G, Schoonhoven L, Barach P, Spijker A, Gademan P, Kalkman C, Liefers J, Vernooij-Dassen M, Wollersheim H. Improving patient handovers from hospital to primary care: a systematic review. Ann Intern Med. 2012; 157(6):417–28.
7. Mesteig M, Helbostad JL, Sletvold O, Rosstad T, Saltvedt I. Unwanted incidents during transition of geriatric patients from hospital to home: a prospective observational study. BMC Health Serv Res. 2010;10:1.
8. Naylor MD, Kurtzman ET, Pauly MV. Transitions of elders between long-term care and hospitals. Policy Polit Nurs Pract. 2009;10(3):187–94.
9. Forster AJ, Clark HD, Menard A, Dupuis N, Chernish R, Chandok N, Khan A, van Walraven C. Adverse events among medical patients after discharge from hospital. CMAJ. 2004;170(3):345–9.
10. Coleman EA. Falling through the cracks: challenges and opportunities for improving transitional care for persons with continuous complex care needs. J Am Geriatr Soc. 2003;51(4):549–55.
11. Adelman RD, Tmanova LL, Delgado D, Dion S, Lachs MS. Caregiver burden: a clinical review. JAMA. 2014;311(10):1052–60.
12. Laugaland K, Aase K, Barach P. Interventions to improve patient safety in transitional care--a review of the evidence. Work (Reading, Mass). 2012; 41(Suppl 1):2915–24.
13. Everink I, van Haastregt J, Kempen G, Dielis L, Maessen J, Schols J. Challenges in geriatric rehabilitation: the development of an integrated care pathway. Tijdschr Gerontol Geriatr. 2015;46(2):104–12.
14. Huttin C. The use of clinical guidelines to improve medical practice: main issues in the United States. International journal for quality in health care. Journal of the international society for. Qual Health Care. 1997;9(3):207–14.
15. Lutomski JE, Baars MA, Schalk BW, Boter H, Buurman BM, den Elzen WP, Jansen AP, Kempen GI, Steunenberg B, Steyerberg EW, et al. The development of the older persons and informal caregivers survey minimum DataSet (TOPICS-MDS): a large-scale data sharing initiative. PLoS One. 2013; 8(12):e81673.
16. Schuling J, de Haan R, Limburg M, Groenier KH. The Frenchay activities

index. Assessment of functional status in stroke patients. Stroke. 1993;24(8): 1173–7.
17. Cardol M, de Haan RJ, van den Bos GA, de Jong BA, de Groot IJ. The development of a handicap assessment questionnaire: the impact on participation and autonomy (IPA). Clin Rehabil. 1999;13(5):411–9.
18. Hays RD, Sherbourne CD, Mazel RM. The RAND 36-item health survey 1.0. Health Econ. 1993;2(3):217–27.
19. van Exel NJ, Scholte op Reimer WJ, Brouwer WB, van den Berg B, Koopmanschap MA, van den Bos GA. Instruments for assessing the burden of informal caregiving for stroke patients in clinical practice: a comparison of CSI, CRA, SCQ and self-rated burden. Clin Rehabil. 2004;18(2):203–14.
20. Everink I, van Haastregt JC, Maessen JM, Schols JM, Kempen GI. Process evaluation of an integrated care pathway in geriatric rehabilitation for people with complex health problems. BMC Health Serv Res. 2017;17(1):34.
21. Van Houdt S, Heyrman J, Vanhaecht K, Sermeus W, De Lepeleire J. Care pathways across the primary-hospital care continuum: using the multi-level framework in explaining care coordination. BMC Health Serv Res. 2013;13:296.
22. Coleman EA, Parry C, Chalmers S, Min SJ. The care transitions intervention: results of a randomized controlled trial. Arch Intern Med. 2006;166(17):1822–8.
23. Courtney M, Edwards H, Chang A, Parker A, Finlayson K, Hamilton K. Fewer emergency readmissions and better quality of life for older adults at risk of hospital readmission: a randomized controlled trial to determine the effectiveness of a 24-week exercise and telephone follow-up program. J Am Geriatr Soc. 2009;57(3):395–402.
24. Jack BW, Chetty VK, Anthony D, Greenwald JL, Sanchez GM, Johnson AE, Forsythe SR, O'Donnell JK, Paasche-Orlow MK, Manasseh C, et al. A reengineered hospital discharge program to decrease rehospitalization: a randomized trial. Ann Intern Med. 2009;150(3):178–87.
25. Voss R, Gardner R, Baier R, Butterfield K, Lehrman S, Gravenstein S. The care transitions intervention: translating from efficacy to effectiveness. Arch Intern Med. 2011;171(14):1232–7.
26. Everink I, van Haastregt JC, Evers SM, Kempen GI, Schols JM. An economic evaluation of an integrated care pathway in geriatric rehabilitation for older patients with complex health problems. PLoS One. 2017;13(2):e0191851.

Trajectories of allostatic load among older Americans and Britons: longitudinal cohort studies

Gindo Tampubolon[1*] and Asri Maharani[2]

Abstract

Background: Difference in life expectancy between males and females has been suggested to rest on sex difference in physiological dysregulation. But allostatic load, a physiological index, has not been carefully examined for an extended period beyond middle age. We aim to draw longitudinal trajectories of allostatic load in a national sample of older Americans and Britons; also to examine sex-based trajectories and factors behind their differences.

Methods: We studied men and women aged ≥50 years participating in the Health and Retirement Study Waves 8–11, 2006–2012 (*N* = 15,583 person-years) and the English Longitudinal Study of Ageing Waves 2, 4 and 6, 2004–2012 (*N* = 14,765 person-years). Because of the difference in provenance, we included different number of biomarkers to calculate allostatic load in HRS and ELSA. In HRS we used 8 biomarkers (systolic and diastolic blood pressure, haemoglobin A1c, high-density lipoprotein, total cholesterol, waist circumference, cystatin C, and C-reactive protein) , while ELSA allostatic load was constructed from 10 biomarkers (systolic and diastolic blood pressure, haemoglobin A1c, high-density lipoprotein, total cholesterol, waist circumference, BMI, triglyceride, fibrinogen and C-reactive protein). A growth curve model was fitted to repeated observations of allostatic load, demographic characteristics, socioeconomic position, comorbidities and health behaviours (smoking, drinking, and physical exercise). To account for attrition, a joint model was applied.

Results: The analysis showed that allostatic load increases linearly with age in the U.S. However, there are different levels for males and females. In England allostatic load follows such different paths that their trajectories cross in later life.

Conclusions: Sex-based trajectories of allostatic load showed distinct female advantage and are mostly consistent with female advantage in life expectancy.

Keywords: Allostatic load, Ageing, Longitudinal analysis, Attrition

Background

The increasing proportion of older people in the population and their increasing life expectancy give larger number of older people longer lives [1]. This prospect raises the challenge of ensuring that the bulk of their lives is lived in a state of good health, free of morbidity and frailty, that will facilitate their continuing contributions to society, polity and the economy. Between the sexes, however, life expectancy differs with an advantage to females. Both in the US and the UK, government actuaries listed different life expectancies at various ages for males and females, with higher values for females. This advantage narrows down with age; thus sex difference in life expectancy converges with age [2, 3].

Despite the female advantage in life expectancy, they have higher morbidity rates and a declined quality of life than males in later life [4]. Literature has reported lower performance of older women on balance and gait tasks than men [5–7]. Older women also had higher prevalence of falling [8, 9] and the incidence of physical ability [10, 11] than their male counterparts. Sex differences in body composition, physical activity, and aerobic fitness are among the

* Correspondence: tampubolon@manchester.ac.uk
[1]Sociology and Cathie Marsh Institute for Social Research, University of Manchester, Humanities Bridgeford Street Building, Oxford Road, Manchester M13 9PL, UK
Full list of author information is available at the end of the article

plausible explanations of these differences. Prior studies found that female respondents reported less habitual physical activity and had lower cardiorespiratory fitness than male respondents [12, 13], which may result in have greater adiposity and less lean mass among older women [14]. The paradoxical differences physical health among males and females may also related to underlying physiological dysregulation, particularly allostatic load [15]. Yang and Kozloski reported that allostatic load is higher for females throughout adulthood (17+ years), showing a female disadvantage in allostatic load. The female advantage in life expectancy sits uneasily with female disadvantage in allostatic load.

Allostatic load captures the notion that the human physiological system is not a fixed and stable system but a dynamically stable one, especially in the face of insults, hazards and injuries to various organ systems [16–21]. Allostatic load is the physiological wear and tear that the body sustains throughout the life course. Allostatic load has been found to longitudinally predict self-rated health, physical function, frailty and ultimately mortality in the US and UK [22, 23]. It also shows gradients along markers of socioeconomic position [23]. Allostatic load is therefore useful not only as a risk factor for morbidity, frailty and mortality, but also in understanding the mechanism of ageing throughout the life course [22].

Few studies have been devoted to uncovering the longitudinal pattern of allostatic load based on repeated measurements. As to socioeconomic gradient in allostatic load, what role the gradient plays in longitudinal change remains relatively uncharted. When examining longitudinal patterns of allostatic load in later life, a study must also contend with the problem of attrition: i.e. when participants are lost to follow up for various reasons, some to do with health and death. This attrition problem is pervasive in ageing studies [24], and to deal with this various models have been applied [25–29], including joint model as applied to the English Longitudinal Study of Ageing [25, 26].

To focus our efforts four questions will be answered. First, is there a sex difference in longitudinal trajectories of allostatic load? Second, given the female advantage in life expectancy, do these trajectories show a female advantage, i.e. a lower allostatic load trajectory for females? Third, given that psychosocial factors get under the skin and affect physiological regulation [20, 30, 31], what social factors are linked with the trajectories? Lastly, are there any differences between the two countries?

This work makes three contributions. It is the first to draw longitudinal trajectories of allostatic load for males and females based on the major study of ageing in America and Britain. Second, in drawing these trajectories, it has uncovered unique patterns that are consistent with the female advantage in life expectancy. Lastly, it showed perceptibly advantageous trajectories of allostatic load in older Americans consistent with emerging comparative research [32–34].

Methods

We used two nationally longitudinal studies of aging: the U.S. Health and Retirement Study (HRS) [35] and The English Longitudinal Study of Ageing (ELSA) [36]. HRS is a multinational biannual household panel survey that collects information on the demographic characteristics, socioeconomic position, comorbidities and health behaviours of individuals aged 50+ in the U.S., while ELSA provided similar information among individuals in the same age range in England. HRS study was started in 1992, while the first wave of ELSA data was collected in 2002. So far there are twelve and seven waves of HRS and ELSA, respectively. This study used waves 8 to 11 of HRS (2006–2012) and every even-numbered wave (2004, 2008 and 2012/2013) of ELSA as the biomarker information was collected in those waves.

Dependent variable

Due to the availability of the data, we included different numbers of biomarkers in HRS and ELSA. Eight biomarkers (systolic and diastolic blood pressure, haemoglobin A1c, high-density lipoprotein/total cholesterol, waist circumference, cystatin C, and C-reactive protein) in the HRS and ten biomarkers (systolic and diastolic blood pressure, haemoglobin A1c, high-density lipoprotein/total cholesterol, waist circumference, BMI, triglyceride, fibrinogen and C-reactive protein) in the ELSA were included in the analysis. Following Stephan et al. (2016) [37], we calculated allostatic load scores in HRS and ELSA in two stages. Firstly, we standardised each of the marker scores to have a mean of zero and a standard deviation of one. Secondly, we took the average of those standardised scores, resulting in a summary allostatic load scores that can be interpreted in terms of standard deviation units. Higher values indicate higher multisystem physiological dysregulation.

Covariates

Demographic covariates include sex and age. Since age is capped at 90 in ELSA, information from respondents aged 50 to 89 in both surveys was used. Like other health functions, allostatic load is also shaped by social determinants of health. These include wealth tertiles (top, middle and bottom as reference), education (some college and high school or less as reference), and marital status (married/cohabiting and other as reference) [25, 38, 39].

Based on positive medical history (self-report of 'has been diagnosed by professionals'), a sum of indicators about comorbidities were included, covering diabetes, cancer, hypertension, lung disease, heart condition, and stroke. Behavioural risk factors known to be important in other studies include smoking (current smoker versus not current smoker as reference), drinking (days in a week having a drink) and physical activity (rigorous, moderate and mild or less as reference) [40].

We included only observation of respondents with complete information on the allostatic load components and the covariates in HRS ($N = 15{,}583$ observations) and ELSA ($N = 14{,}765$ observations) in the analysis. Differences between those included and left out were tested using t-test (continuous variables) or χ^2 test (categorical variables). At baseline, compared to those left out the analytic sample is younger (67 versus 73 year, $p < 0.001$ in the U.S and 65 versus 67 year, $p < 0.001$ in England), has fewer women (50% versus 57%; $p < 0.001$ in the U.S. and 53% versus 54%; $p = 0.338$ in England), and has lower levels of allostatic load (– 0.01 versus 0.008, $p = 0.039$ in the U.S. and 1.8 versus 2, $p < 0.001$ in England).

Statistical analysis

To model how allostatic load changes over time using repeated observations, a growth curve model with random intercepts is applied. This model gives consistent estimates of the effects of risk factors when some participants are lost in subsequent visits, assuming attrition at random. We fit two models to address the questions above. First the main *allostatic* model built one trajectory for both sexes. Second, to check whether there is a difference in the rate of change between the sexes, the *interaction* model has an additional sex-age interaction term. To deal with attrition bias, a joint model is used [24, 26, 27, 41]. This model has recovered robust estimates of cognitive ageing in Australia [27], quality of life and cognition among older adults in England [25, 26]. We used the joint model to deal with the attrition in the longitudinal study. The random effects (*h(.)* below) in the joint model influence both allostatic load, y, and attrition, t, given these, allostatic load and attrition are independent. A joint model has two parts: the growth curve model (*f(.)* below) and the survival model (*g(.)* below)with gender, age polynomial of degree three and the random intercepts from the first partt [25, 26].

$$L = \int f(y_i|b_i, x_i)g(t_i|b_i, x_i)h(b_i)db_i$$

We compare the results of growth curve models with those of joint or attrition-corrected models. The analyses were done in Stata 14 (StataCorp LP, College Station, Texas) and Latent Gold Syntax 5.1.

We carried out three supplementary analyses to check the robustness of our results. In the first supplementary analysis, we followed Read and Grundy (2014) by computing allostatic load score in ELSA using 13 indicators of whether biomarker values fell into their high risk quartiles [23]. The indicators cover five organ systems, including cardiovascular (diastolic blood pressure, systolic blood pressure), inflammation (CRP and fibrinogen), metabolic (haemoglobin A1c, high-density lipoprotein/total cholesterol ratio, triglycerides, and fasting glucose), body fat (BMI, waist circumference), and respiratory systems (forced expiratory volume, forced vital capacity and passive expired volume). Within each organ system each indicator receives the same proportion, for example the inflammation system has two biomarkers, each potentially contributing half a point when the biomarker value is found in the high risk quartile (zero otherwise) [22, 23]. The threshold of the high risk quartile is replaced with a clinical cut-off when there is one, for example the cut-off for male waist circumference is 102 cm. Finally, medication was considered, so that the value is automatically considered as high risk if the participant is using medication. The medication includes blood pressure lowering medication, anticoagulants, lipid lowering medication, diabetes medication and lung function medication. The scores range from 0 to 5.

In the second supplementary analyses, we analysed only the post-war cohort (those who were born on 1946 onwards) of ELSA to examine the effect of cohort on the allostatic load. Our previous work found that the trajectories of depressive symptoms between cohorts (pre-war, war, and post-war cohorts) in the US and England took different shapes [32]. The trajectories of pre-war cohorts in both countries and war cohort in England took a U-shape, while those of war cohort in England and post-war cohorts in both countries followed an inverted U-shape. We thus hypothesised that the allostatic load trajectory of the post-war cohort in ELSA follows that in HRS. In the final sensitivity analysis, we included the relevant medications taken by the respondents (medications for hypertension, hyperlipidaemia, and diabetes mellitus in ELSA and medication prescribed by the health professionals in HRS), and height (in cm).

Results

The sample for analysis consists of 56% and 54% females in HRS and ELSA data, respectively (Table 1). The table also contains distribution across age groups, only for description and not for modelling, which shows that for either males or females there is an increasing age gradient in allostatic load in both data. In particular it shows that before 70 years in ELSA

Table 1 Descriptive summaries of allostatic load scores (means) in different groups

	HRS				ELSA			
	N	All $N = 15,583$	Male $N = 6787$	Female $N = 8796$	N	All $N = 14,765$	Male $N = 6721$	Female $N = 8044$
All		0.006	0.027	− 0.009		1.926	1.92	1.932
Age group								
50-	3752	− 0.044	0.006	− 0.084	4109	1.554	1.592	1.523
60-	4532	−0.002	0.025	−0.023	5843	1.834	1.850	1.821
70-	4735	0.028	0.035	0.023	3648	2.255	2.210	2.291
80-	2564	0.056	0.047	0.064	1165	2.676	2.553	2.771
Married/cohabit								
Not married	4753	0.047	0.067	0.04	4555	2.116	2.07	2.139
Married	10,830	−0.011	0.017	−0.041	10,210	1.842	1.876	1.807
Wealth tertiles								
Poorest	4891	0.069	0.098	0.049	4135	2.251	2.198	2.289
Middle	5303	0.001	0.024	−0.016	5089	1.97	1.968	1.971
Wealthiest	5389	−0.045	−0.025	− 0.062	5541	1.645	1.696	1.598
Education								
< High school	2569	0.077	0.087	0.069	4561	2.252	2.249	2.254
High school	5080	0.029	0.059	0.011	5692	1.884	1.922	1.855
Some college	7934	−0.031	− 0.007	− 0.051	4512	1.651	1.692	1.6
Num. comorbidities								
0	4160	− 0.121	− 0.086	−0.143	6401	1.304	1.306	1.302
1	5270	−0.000	0.011	−0.009	5667	2.247	2.238	2.254
2	3671	0.065	0.074	0.057	2016	3.044	2.634	2.585
3+	2482	0.148	0.136	0.161	681	3.193	3.202	3.187
Current smoker								
No	13,611	0.006	0.024	−0.007	12,979	1.902	1.889	1.912
Yes	1972	0.009	0.049	−0.022	1786	2.107	2.147	2.074
Drinking								
Less	14,001	0.008	0.031	−0.008	9098	2.057	2.054	2.059
Daily	1582	−0.007	0.001	−0.021	5667	1.716	1.763	1.66
Vigorous physical activity								
No	9994	0.042	0.07	0.024	12,026	2.027	2.037	2.02
Yes	5589	−0.057	− 0.03	− 0.086	2739	1.483	1.51	1.451

and before 80 years in HRS, females have lower allostatic load than males, but beyond this age the order changes. So although both sexes appear to have comparable levels of allostatic load, its age distribution is quite different in the two sexes.

Married, better-educated and wealthy participants have lower allostatic load compared to reference categories in both data. Lastly (bottom block), to pick one behavioural factor, more physical activity inversely associates with allostatic load.

Table 2 collects the results of the growth curve and joint models using HRS and ELSA. The first model, labelled *Main*, showed that allostatic load increases with age in HRS ($\beta = 0.003$, $p < 0.001$), and ELSA (0.002, $p < 0.001$). To check for different trajectories for females and males, a sex-age interaction term was added in the *Interaction* model. This model gave the interaction terms positive and significant coefficients in both data, suggesting the trajectories are significantly different for females and for males.

To ease interpretation and comparison, the coefficients for the two joint models are plotted together in a figure of two panes corresponding to the two models (Fig. 1 for HRS and Fig. 2 for ELSA). Being female is associated with lower allostatic score in all

Table 2 Models of age trajectories of allostatic load, coefficients and standard errors: main and interaction models. Source HRS wave 8–11 (2006–2012) and ELSA Wave 2, 4 and 6 (2004–2012)

	HRS		*ELSA*	
	Main	*Interaction*	*Main*	*Interaction*
Age	0.003 ± 0.000***	0.001 ± 0.000***	0.002 ± 0.000***	−0.0001 ± 0.000
Sex, Female	−0.104 ± 0.007***	− 0.251 ± 0.047***	− 0.093 ± 0.009***	− 0.376 ± 0.062***
Age*gender		0.002 ± 0.000***		0.004 ± 0.000***
Married/cohabit	−0.023 ± 0.008***	−0.019 ± 0.008**	−0.007 ± 0.009	−0.002 ± 0.009
Middle wealth	− 0.042 ± 0.008***	− 0.042 ± 0.008***	− 0.043 ± 0.008***	− 0.043 ± 0.008***
Wealthiest	− 0.068 ± 0.009***	− 0.067 ± 0.009***	−0.091 ± 0.009***	− 0.090 ± 0.009***
High school	− 0.006 ± 0.011	− 0.007 ± 0.011	− 0.056 ± 0.011***	− 0.053 ± 0.011***
Some college	− 0.047 ± 0.01***	−0.048 ± 0.01***	− 0.102 ± 0.012***	− 0.101 ± 0.012***
Num. comorbidities	0.093 ± 0.003***	0.093 ± 0.003***	0.033 ± 0.003***	− 0.043 ± 0.008***
Current smoker	− 0.032 ± 0.011***	− 0.031 ± 0.011***	− 0.011 ± 0.013	−0.011 ± 0.013
Past smoker	0.006 ± 0.007	0.008 ± 0.007	0.089 ± 0.014***	0.088 ± 0.014***
Drink > 5 days/week	− 0.008 ± 0.011	−0.008 ± 0.011	− 0.021 ± 0.007***	−0.021 ± 0.007***
Vigorous exercise	−0.076 ± 0.007***	− 0.076 ± 0.007***	− 0.044 ± 0.008***	− 0.044 ± 0.008***
Constant	−0.159 ± 0.03**	−0.079 ± 0.039**	− 0.001 ± 0.038	0.147 ± 0.050***

Note: Sig.: * = 10% or less; ** = 5% or less; *** = 1% or less

models. The positive and significant coefficient for age and its interaction terms suggest different trajectories for females and for males. Other coefficients are not so different in the two survey data. Being wealthy and having high educational attainment have inverse relationships with allostatic score. The comorbidities and behavioural covariates (bottom block) also show similar patterns: comorbidities associate positively with allostatic load while rigorous physical exercise strongly associates with lower allostatic load.

Given that an extensive set of covariates is controlled, a summary of the trajectories based on the predicted allostatic load from the joint models can be drawn (Fig. 3). Comparing HRS (left) and ELSA (right) highlights striking similarities and differences. Older people on the west and east sides of the Atlantic accumulates allostatic load in a linear fashion as they age. In the US, females have lower allostatic load throughout later life, consistent with female advantage in life expectancy. A similar pattern characterises Britain although there is a

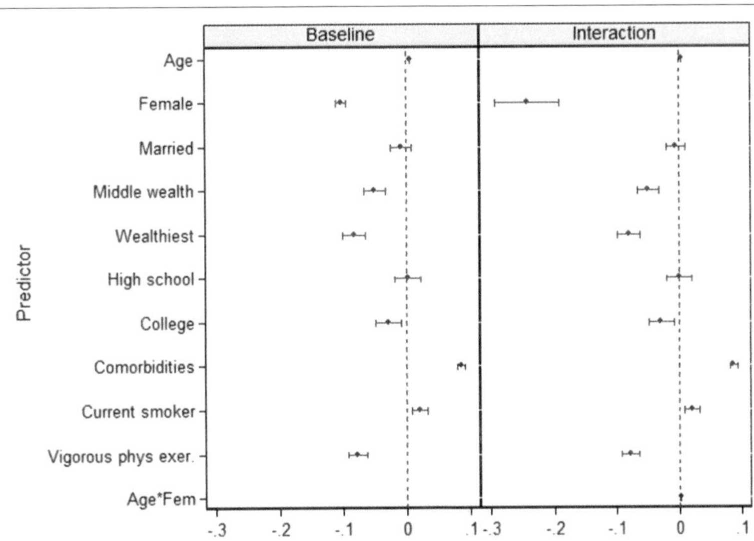

Fig. 1 Attrition corrected models of age trajectories of allostatic load, coefficients and 95% confidence intervals: Main Allostatic and Sex interaction models. Source HRS 2004–2013

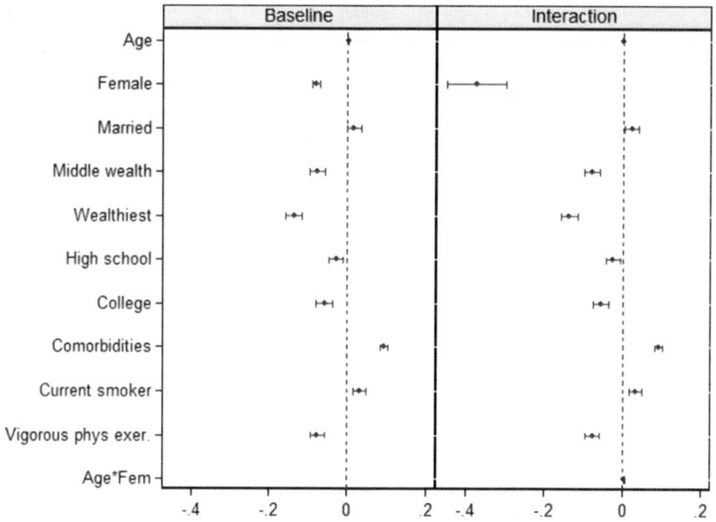

Fig. 2 Attrition corrected models of age trajectories of allostatic load, coefficients and 95% confidence intervals: Main Allostatic and Sex interaction models. Source ELSA 2004–2013

crossover in the latter half when female advantage disappeared. Nonetheless, the sex difference throughout later life is slight and unlikely to be a clinically significant dysregulation [42]. Particularly the sex difference in Britain is negligible compared to that in America. Similar trajectories are found in our supplementary analyses using ELSA data. Being female is associated with lower allostatic load ($\beta = -0.451$, $p < 0.001$) (see Appendix 1), we find a crossover of the allostatic load trajectories of males and females in the age of 57 ($\beta = 0.005$, $p < 0.001$) in which the allostatic load of the males is higher than that of females afterwards (see Appendix 2). The effect of cohort was shown in our analysis including only the post-war cohort of ELSA (see the Appendix 3). Supporting our previous work [32], the allostatic load trajectories of the post-war cohort of ELSA followed those of HRS: females have lower allostatic load throughout later life. The final sensitivity analysis demonstrated that the relationships between gender and allostatic load remained significant after controlling by height and the relevant medication (see Appendix 4). This sensitivity analysis shows that the results are robust.

Discussion

We set out to draw the sex-based trajectories of allostatic load in samples representing the American and British older populations. Upward trajectories of allostatic load for both males and females are found, but the rates of change differ for the two sexes. This led to allostatic load incline among older Americans and additionally a cross-over in older British allostatic load trajectories at the mid-60s. Allostatic load trajectory as a

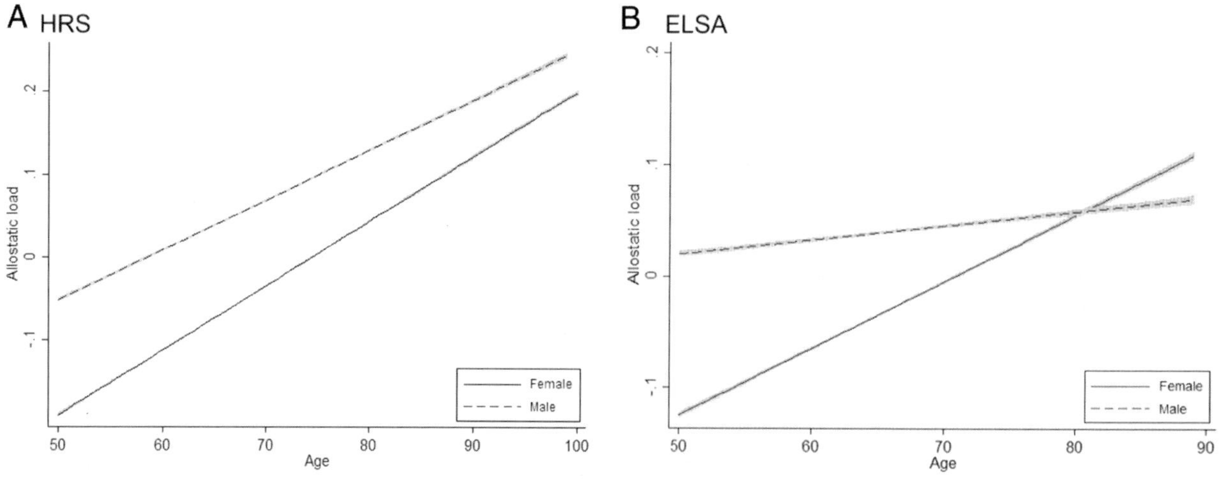

Fig. 3 Predicted trajectories of allostatic load for females and males. Source HRS 2004–2013 and ELSA 2004–2013

physiological signature of ageing unfolds differently for males and females. This is a novel finding that deserves replication and reflection, some of which are offered later.

The patterns in America, i.e. linear accumulation and female advantage, are consistent with the patterns of life expectancy worldwide. These patterns also showed a gentler incline of allostatic load overtime, compared to those in Britain. The somewhat advantageous patterns revealed in America is consistent with recent evidence uncovered using the HRS and ELSA. Tampubolon and Maharani [32] showed that today older Americans are composed of sociohistorical cohorts (pre-war, war and post-war) that have an advantageous mental health. The majority (war and post-war cohorts) have advantageous trajectory depression in later life. Not so in older Britons: only the post-war cohort attains this advantage (ibid, Fig. 1). A larger proportion of older Americans than older Britons has a better mental health trajectory. Consistent with this, the HRS patterns on the left pane of Fig. 3 and the post-war cohort patterns on the Appendix 3 suggest a lower allostatic load trajectory among female than male at any age.

This study has a number of limitations. Direct measures of the stress response system such as urinary norepinephrine, epinephrine and salivary cortisol are not available. Including these is wholly desirable [18] but would no doubt be challenging. These older adult participants have given many physical and blood measurements over the years; therefore this study and others on allostatic load [23, 37] have tried to make the most of what the participants have already contributed. Another limitation is the handling of attrition. The joint model is only one solution; two other alternatives are pattern mixture model and selection models [24, 28]. Accounting for attrition with these alternatives is worth considering. Finally, one limitation of large samples is that the beta weights are very low, but the p values are statistically significant. Although there is a statistically significant change, the change is not strong.

An advantage of this study is the nationally representative nature of both HRS and ELSA, ensuring that the accumulation of physiological wear and tear in these populations can be uncovered without being unduly influenced by specific patterns in some clinical or patient samples. Another strength arises from its longitudinal design, with repeated measures not only of allostatic load but also of an extensive set of covariates.

The similar increase of allostatic load found among older Americans and older Britons stands in contrast with the trajectories found in American adults [15]. There the pattern is of female disadvantage and of divergence: females carry heavier allostatic load throughout adulthood and the difference continues to widen with age. The pattern was derived from cross-sectional data, and this may explain the contrast, since cross-sectional design has been found to give overestimates of changes in health functioning [43].

The socio-economic gradient in trajectories of allostatic load found here is consistent with results from an earlier study using a shorter period of the ELSA sample [23]. Similarly, the associations with health behaviours such as levels of physical exercise and smoking are consistent in the two studies. These behaviours regulate trajectories in comparable ways in both sexes. Our findings extend their results by including comorbidities, enabling net associations with socio-economic factors to be recovered.

Conclusions

The trajectories of allostatic load in later life show distinct signatures for males and females. To uncover them not only is it necessary to use longitudinal data but also to account for attrition. With these done, both trajectories show clear social gradients in physiological wear and tear for an extended period in later life. Efforts to reduce these gradients earlier may yield fruit in later life by lightening the allostatic load, thus giving a healthier ageing experience to an increasingly large proportion of the population.

Appendix 1

Table 3 Models of age trajectories of allostatic load, coefficients and standard errors: main and interaction models. Source ELSA Wave 2, 4 and 6 (2004–2012). The Allostatic load score was calculated based on Read and Grundy (2014) [23]

	Main	Interaction
Age	0.036 ± 0.001***	0.032 ± 0.001***
Sex, Female	− 0.066 ± 0.018***	− 0.451 ± 0.126***
Age*gender		0.005 ± 0.001***
Married/cohabit	−0.027 ± 0.019	− 0.02 ± 0.019
Middle wealth	−0.16 ± 0.018***	− 0.159 ± 0.018***
Wealthiest	−0.304 ± 0.02***	− 0.303 ± 0.02***
High school	−0.086 ± 0.022***	− 0.083 ± 0.022***
Some college	−0.164 ± 0.025***	− 0.163 ± 0.025***
Num. comorbidities	0.389 ± 0.008***	0.39 ± 0.008***
Current smoker	0.125 ± 0.025***	0.126 ± 0.025***
Past smoker	0.004 ± 0.032	0.003 ± 0.032
Drink > 5 days/week	−0.102 ± 0.016***	−0.102 ± 0.016***
Vigorous exercise	−0.2 ± 0.017***	−0.201 ± 0.017***
Constant	−0.388 ± 0.077***	−0.185 ± 0.102

Note: Sig.: * = 10% or less; **: 5% or less; ***: 1% or less

Appendix 2

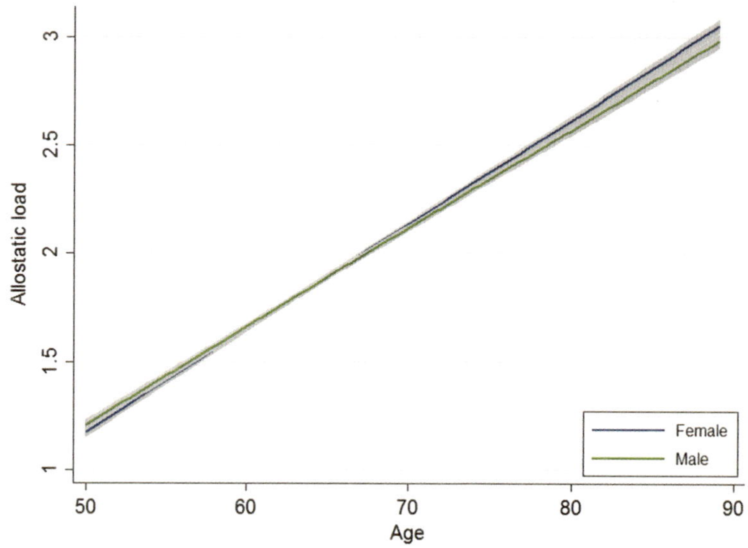

Fig. 4 Predicted trajectories of allostatic load for females and males. Source ELSA 2004–2013. The Allostatic load score was calculated based on Read and Grundy (2014)

Appendix 3

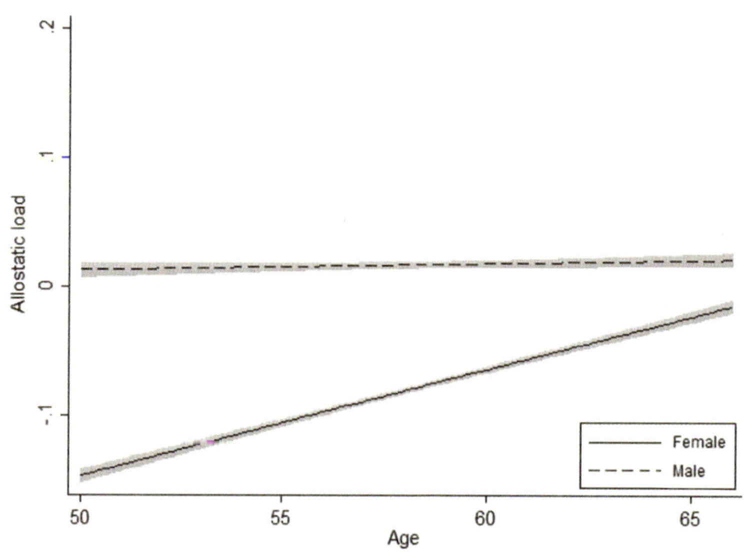

Fig. 5 Predicted trajectories of allostatic load among post-war cohort for females and males. Source ELSA 2004–2013

Appendix 4

Table 4 Models of age trajectories of allostatic load, coefficients and standard errors: main and interaction models. Source HRS wave 8–11 (2006–2012) and ELSA Wave 2, 4 and 6 (2004–2012)

	HRS		*ELSA*	
	Main	*Interaction*	*Main*	*Interaction*
Age	0.003 ± 0.000***	0.001 ± 0.000***	−0.000 ± 0.000	−0.002 ± 0.000***
Sex, Female	−0.071 ± 0.011***	−0.226 ± 0.048***	−0.110 ± 0.012***	− 0.408 ± 0.061***
Age*gender		0.002 ± 0.000***		0.004 ± 0.000***
Married/cohabit	−0.024 ± 0.008***	−0.020 ± 0.008**	−0.008 ± 0.009	−0.003 ± 0.009
Middle wealth	− 0.045 ± 0.008***	−0.044 ± 0.008***	−0.040 ± 0.008***	− 0.040 ± 0.008***
Wealthiest	−0.070 ± 0.009***	− 0.069 ± 0.009***	−0.083 ± 0.009***	− 0.082 ± 0.009***
High school	−0.006 ± 0.011	−0.008 ± 0.011	−0.054 ± 0.011***	−0.051 ± 0.011***
Some college	− 0.050 ± 0.010***	−0.050 ± 0.010***	−0.097 ± 0.012***	− 0.096 ± 0.012***
Num. comorbidities	0.093 ± 0.003***	0.094 ± 0.003***	0.033 ± 0.003***	− 0.033 ± 0.003***
Current smoker	−0.031 ± 0.011***	− 0.030 ± 0.011**	−0.006 ± 0.012	−0.006 ± 0.012
Past smoker	0.005 ± 0.007	0.007 ± 0.007	0.093 ± 0.014***	0.092 ± 0.014***
Drink > 5 days/week	−0.008 ± 0.011	−0.008 ± 0.011	− 0.015 ± 0.007**	−0.015 ± 0.007**
Vigorous exercise	−0.076 ± 0.007***	−0.076 ± 0.007***	−0.038 ± 0.008***	− 0.039 ± 0.008***
Height	0.216 ± 0.052***	0.218 ± 0.005***	−0.002 ± 0.000***	− 0.002 ± 0.000***
Taking prescribed medication	−0.007 ± 0.022	−0.008 ± 0.022		
Taking medication for hypertension			0.051 ± 0.008***	0.050 ± 0.008***
Taking medication for hyperlipidaemia			0.050 ± 0.009***	0.050 ± 0.009***
Taking medication for diabetes mellitus			0.207 ± 0.016***	0.209 ± 0.016***
Constant	−0.557 ± 0.102***	−0.476 ± 0.104***	0.464 ± 0.129***	0.616 ± 0.132***

Note: Sig.: * = 10% or less; ** = 5% or less; *** = 1% or less

Abbreviations
BMI: Body Mass Index; CRP: C-Reactive Protein; ELSA: English Longitudinal Study of Ageing; HRS: Health and Retirement Study; UK: United Kingdom; US: United States

Acknowledgments
No acknowledgment.

Funding
This work was supported by grants from the Medical Research Council and Economic & Social Research Council (grant no. G1001375/1), the National Institute of Health Research (grant no. ES/L001772/1) and the European Union's Horizon 2020 Research and Innovation Programme (grant no. 668648) to Gindo Tampubolon. Asri Maharani was supported by SENSE-Cog project, European Union's Horizon 2020 research and innovation programme under grant agreement No 668648.

Authors' contributions
GT designed the study. GT and AM analysed the data and wrote the manuscript. All authors read and approved the final manuscript.

Competing interests
The authors declare that they have no competing interests.

Author details
[1]Sociology and Cathie Marsh Institute for Social Research, University of Manchester, Humanities Bridgeford Street Building, Oxford Road, Manchester M13 9PL, UK. [2]Division of Neuroscience and Experimental Psychology, School of Biological Sciences, Faculty of Biology, Medicine and Health, University of Manchester, Manchester Academic Health Science Centre, Manchester M13 9PL, UK.

References
1. Mathers CD, Loncar D. Projections of global mortality and burden of disease from 2002 to 2030. PLoS Med. 2006;3(11):e442.
2. Office of National Statistics. Statistical bulletin: health state life expectancies by national deprivation deciles, England and Wales: 2014 to 2016. 2018.
3. National Center for Health Statistics. National Vital Statistics Reports: United States Life Tables 2014. 2017.
4. Rieker PP, Bird CE. Rethinking gender differences in health: why we need to integrate social and biological perspectives. J Gerontol Ser B Psychol Sci Soc Sci. 2005;60:S40–7.
5. Hageman PA, Leibowitz JM, Blanke D. Age and gender effects on postural control measures. Arch Phys Med Rehabil. 1995;76(10):961–5.
6. Wolfson L, Whipple R, Dreby CA, Amerman P, Nashner L. Gender differences in the balance of healthy elderly as demonstrated by dynamic posturography. J Gerontol. 1994;49(4):M160–7.
7. Musselman K, Brouwer B. Gender-related differences in physical performance among seniors. J Aging Phys Act. 2005;13(3):239–53.
8. Colledge NR, Cantley P, Peaston I, Brash H, Lewis S, Wilson JA. Ageing and balance: the measurement of spontaneous sway by posturography. Gerontology. 1994;40(5):273–8.
9. Prudham D, Evans JG. Factors associated with falls in the elderly: a community study. Age Ageing. 1981;10(3):141–6.

10. Leveille SG, Penninx BW, Melzer D, Izmirlian G, Guralnik JM. Sex differences in the prevalence of mobility disability in old age: the dynamics of incidence, recovery, and mortality J Gerontol Series B, 2000. 55(1): S41-S50.
11. Murtagh KN, Hubert HB. Gender differences in physical disability among an elderly cohort. Am J Public Health. 2004;94(8):1406–11.
12. Vogel JA, Patton JF, Mello RP, Daniels WL. An analysis of aerobic capacity in a large United States population. J Appl Physiol. 1986;60(2):494–500.
13. Caspersen CJ, Pereira MA, Curran KM. Changes in physical activity patterns in the United States, by sex and cross-sectional age. Med Sci Sports Exerc. 2000;32(9):1601–9.
14. Heyward VH, Wagner DR. Applied body composition assessment. Champaign: Human Kinetics; 2004.
15. Yang Y, Kozloski M. Sex differences in age trajectories of physiological dysregulation: inflammation, metabolic syndrome, and allostatic load. J Gerontol A Biol Sci Med Sci. 2011;66(5):493–500.
16. Seeman TE, McEwen BS, Rowe JW, Singer BH. Allostatic load as a marker of cumulative biological risk: MacArthur studies of successful aging. Proc Natl Acad Sci. 2001;98(8):4770–5.
17. Seeman TE, Epel E, Gruenewald T, Karlamangla A, BS ME. Socio-economic differentials in peripheral biology: cumulative allostatic load. Ann N Y Acad Sci. 2010;1186(1):223–39.
18. Seeman TE, Singer BH, Rowe JW, Horwitz RI, BS ME. Price of adaptation—allostatic load and its health consequences: MacArthur studies of successful aging. Arch Intern Med. 1997;157(19):2259–68.
19. McEwen BS. Protective and damaging effects of stress mediators. N Engl J Med. 1998;338(3):171–9.
20. Seeman T. How do others get under our skin? Social relationships and health. 2001.
21. McEwen BS, Stellar E. Stress and the individual: mechanisms leading to disease. Arch Intern Med. 1993;153(18):2093–101.
22. Gruenewald TL, Karlamangla AS, Hu P, Stein-Merkin S, Crandall C, Koretz B, Seeman TE. History of socioeconomic disadvantage and allostatic load in later life. Soc Sci Med. 2012;74(1):75–83.
23. Read S, Grundy E. Allostatic load and health in the older population of England: a crossed-lagged analysis. Psychosom Med. 2014;76(7):490.
24. Hardy SE, Allore H, Studenski SA. Missing data: a special challenge in aging research. J Am Geriatr Soc. 2009;57(4):722–9.
25. Tampubolon G. Delineating the third age: joint models of older people's quality of life and attrition in Britain 2002–2010. Aging Ment Health. 2015;19(7):576–83.
26. Tampubolon G. Cognitive ageing in Great Britain in the new century: cohort differences in episodic memory. PLoS One. 2015;10(12):e0144907.
27. Graham PL, Ryan LM, Luszcz MA. Joint modelling of survival and cognitive decline in the Australian longitudinal study of ageing. J R Stat Soc: Ser C: Appl Stat. 2011;60(2):221–38.
28. Tampubolon G. Trajectories of the healthy ageing phenotype among middle-aged and older Britons, 2004–2013. Maturitas. 2016;88:9–15.
29. Newman AB. An overview of the design, implementation, and analyses of longitudinal studies on aging. J Am Geriatr Soc. 2010;58:S287–91.
30. Ryff CD, Singer BH, Wing E, Love GD. Elective affinities and uninvited agonies. In: Emotion, social relationships, and health; 2001. p. 133–75.
31. Ryff CD, Singer BH. Emotion, Social Relationships, and Health. Oxford University Press; 2001.
32. Tampubolon G, Maharani A. When did old age stop being depressing? Depression trajectories of older Americans and Britons 2002-2012. Am J Geriatr Psychiatry. 2017;25(11):1187–95.
33. Tampubolon G, Maharani A. Depression trajectories of older Americans and Britons 2002-2013;2012: a rejoinder and a Hope. Am J Geriatr Psychiatry. 2017;25(11). https://doi.org/10.1016/j.jagp.2017.07.010.
34. Tampubolon G. Could cohort composition be driving this? Re: Temporal trend in dementia incidence since 2002 and projections for prevalence in England and Wales to 2040: modelling study. BMJ. 2017;358:j2856.
35. Sonnega A, Weir D. The health and retirement study: a public data resource for research on aging. Open Health Data. 2014;2(1).
36. Marmot M, Oldfield Z, Clemens S, Blake M, Phelps A, Nazroo J, Steptoe A, Rogers N, Bank J. English Longitudinal Study of Ageing: Waves 0–6, 1998–2013. Secondary English Longitudinal Study of Ageing: Waves 0–6, 1998. 2013: 2015.
37. Stephan Y, Sutin AR, Martina L, Antonio T. Allostatic load and personality: a 4-year longitudinal study. Psychosom Med. 2016;78(3):302–10.
38. Wilkinson RG, Marmot M. Social determinants of health: The solid facts: World Health Organization; 2003.
39. Marmot M. The health gap: The challenge of an unequal world. 2015: Bloomsbury Publishing.
40. Skelton D, Young A, Walker A, Hoinville E. Physical activity in later life: Further analysis of the Allied Dunbar national fitness survey and the Health Educ Authority national survey of activity and health. London: Health Educ Authority; 1999.
41. Rabbitt P, Diggle P, Smith D, Holland F, Mc Innes L. Identifying and separating the effects of practice and of cognitive ageing during a large longitudinal study of elderly community residents. Neuropsychologia. 2001; 39(5):532–43.
42. Karlamangla AS, Singer BH, BS ME, Rowe JW, Seeman TE. Allostatic load as a predictor of functional decline: MacArthur studies of successful aging. J Clin Epidemiol. 2002;55(7):696–710.
43. Singh-Manoux A, Kivimaki M, Glymour MM, Elbaz A, Berr C, Ebmeier KP, Ferrie JE, Dugravot A. Timing of onset of cognitive decline: results from Whitehall II prospective cohort study. BMJ. 2012;344:d7622.
44. Sonnega A, Faul JD, Ofstedal MB, Langa KM, Phillips JWR, Weir DR. Cohort profile: the health and retirement study (HRS). Int J Epidemiol. 2014;43(2):576–85.

Sedative-hypnotic initiation and renewal at discharge in hospitalized older patients: an observational study

Elsa Bourcier[1,2,3*], Amandine Baptiste[4], Adrien Borowik[2], Lucas Zerbib[2], Dominique Bonnet-Zamponi[5,6], Florence Tubach[7], Christine Fernandez[1,2,3] and Patrick Hindlet[1,2,3]

Abstract

Background: Sedative-hypnotics (SHs) are widely used in France but there are no available data addressing their prescription specifically in hospitalized older patients. The objective is thus to determine the cumulative incidence of sedative-hypnotic (SH) medications initialized during a hospital stay of older patients, the proportion of SH renewal at discharge among these patients and to study associated risk factors.

Methods: We conducted a retrospective observational study in six internal medicine units and six acute geriatric units in eight hospitals (France). We included 1194 inpatients aged 65 and older without SH medications prior to hospitalization. Data were obtained from patients' electronic pharmaceutical records. Primary outcome was the cumulative incidence of SH initiation in the study units. Secondary outcomes were the proportion of SH renewal at discharge and risk factors for SH initiation and renewal at discharge (patient characteristics, hospital organization). A Cox regression model was used to study risk factors for SH initiation. A mixed effects logistic regression was used to study risk factors for SH renewal at discharge.

Results: SH initiation occurred in 21.5% of participants 20 days after admission. SH renewal at discharge occurred in 38.7% of patients who had initiated it during their stay and were discharged home and in 56.0% of patients discharged to rehabilitation facilities. Neither patients' characteristics nor hospital organization patterns was associated with SH initiation. SH initiation after the first six days after admission was associated with a lower risk of SH renewal in patients discharged to rehabilitation facilities (OR = 0.19, 95% CI: [0.04–0.80]).

Conclusions: Hospitalization is a period at risk for SH initiation. The implementation of interventions promoting good use of SHs is thus of first importance in hospitals. Specific attention should be paid to patients discharged to rehabilitation facilities.

Keywords: Sedative-hypnotics, Initiation, Older adults, Hospitalization, Risk factors

Background

According to the International Narcotics Control Board, France ranked 6th for Sedative-Hypnotic (SH) consumption worldwide in 2015 [1]. According to the French National Agency for Medicines Safety, France ranked 3rd in Europe for SH consumption in 2015 with 3.5 million people exposed at least once to hypnotic benzodiazepines (BZDs) or z-drugs (zolpidem, zopiclone) [2]. Regarding the consumption of these drugs in older people, most recent data indicate that 18% of French women and 11% of French men aged 65 and older were prescribed a hypnotic BZD or a z-drug in 2012 [3]. There are no data specifically addressing the consumption of first-generation antihistamines as insomnia medications apart from the consumption of the other SHs. This situation is particularly worrying since hypnotic BZDs, z-drugs and first-generation antihistamines are associated with serious adverse drug events (ADE) in this population, such as falls and cognitive impairment, with an unfavorable benefit-risk balance

* Correspondence: elsa.bourcier@aphp.fr
[1]Sorbonne Université, INSERM, Institut Pierre Louis d'épidémiologie et de Santé Publique, IPLESP UMR-S1136, F-75012 Paris, France
[2]Assistance Publique – Hôpitaux de Paris, Hôpital Saint-Antoine, Service de Pharmacie, 184, rue du Faubourg Saint Antoine, F-75012 Paris, France
Full list of author information is available at the end of the article

[4–9]. Importantly, these drugs are cited in several tools as Potentially Inappropriate Medications (Beers, STOPP/START, EU (7)-PIM list) [10–12].

Very few studies addressed SH consumption in the hospital setting. During hospitalization, the prevalence of sleep disorders increases and is reported by 36.7 to 62.7% of hospitalized older patients [13, 14]. Hospitalization could thus be a period at risk for SH initiation. Studies published from 1996 to 2014 report an initiation of SHs for 8.3 to 44.6% of hospitalized patients, all ages combined [15–22]. Moreover, initiation of SHs during hospitalization has been shown to be a risk factor for long-term SH prescription after discharge (OR = 4.65, 95% confidence interval: [1.95–11.09]) [20]. There are no available data specifically about hospitalized older patients in France.

The primary objective of our study was thus to estimate the cumulative incidence of SH initiation among older hospitalized patients in a French hospital setting. Secondary objectives were (1) to estimate the proportion of SH prescription renewal at discharge among patients who initiated it during their stay (2) to study risk factors for SH initiation during hospitalization and (3) to study risk factors for SH prescription renewal at discharge among older patients who initiated it during their hospitalization.

Methods

Study design

We conducted a retrospective observational multicenter cohort study.

Setting

This study retrospectively addressed the period 2016/03/15 to 2016/06/15 in six internal medicine units and six acute geriatric units of eight hospitals located in Paris and its suburbs (France). All types of hospitals were represented: teaching hospitals ($n = 4$), general public hospitals ($n = 2$), non-profit private hospitals ($n = 1$), private clinics ($n = 1$).

Participants

All patients admitted into participating units during the study period were screened for eligibility. Eligible patients were patients aged 65 and older, with no mention of SH in the "medications taken before hospitalization" section of their hospitalization report and discharged to home or into rehabilitation facilities. Patients transferred to another acute care unit or enrolled in a clinical trial involving SHs were excluded. Patients for whom the prescriptions or the medical chart were unavailable were also excluded.

Data sources

All data were obtained retrospectively.

Data related to SH prescription during the stay were obtained from the Computerized Physician Order Entry.

Data related to patient characteristics (age, gender), medications taken before hospitalization, reason for admission, length of stay, SH prescription at discharge and type of discharge were obtained from the hospitalization report which is a mandatory document that contains all these data and is inserted in the medical chart at the end of the stay. These data were collected by a trained pharmacist in each center, using a standardized collection grid (Additional file 1).

Data related to hospital organization were collected by a trained pharmacist in each center and obtained from the head nurse of each unit, using a standardized collection grid (Additional file 2).

Bias related to data sources

This mainly concerns the "medications taken before admission" part of the hospitalization report which is the main data source used for this retrospective study. To guarantee the accuracy of this part of the hospitalization report, we ensured that physicians of the twelve study units used at least three sources of information (patient interview, call to the general practitioner, call to the community pharmacist for example) to complete it. We also conducted an independent pilot study on 50 patients hospitalized in study units: the list of medications taken before admission as written in their hospitalization report was compared to the list of medications taken before admission obtained from these 50 patients' community pharmacists. The agreement between these two data sources was assessed through the Cohen's kappa coefficient. With a coefficient of 0.66 the degree of agreement was considered as intermediate, with a tendency for physicians to underestimate medicationss taken before hospitalization in the hospitalization report [23].

Variables

Primary outcome

The primary outcome was SH initiation.

SH definition: prescription of any bedtime medications cited in the following list of SH medications established by the French Health Authority (FHA):

- Long half-life BZD (≥ 20 h as defined by the National French Health insurance system) (Anatomical Therapeutic Chemical classification): Diazepam (N05BA01), Clorazepate (N05BA05), Bromazepam (N05BA08), Clobazam (N05BA09), Prazepam (N05BA11), Nordazepam (N05BA16), Loflazepate (N05BA18), Nitrazepam (N05CD02), Triazolam (N05CD05).
- Short half-life BZD (< 20 h as defined by the National French Health insurance system) (Anatomical Therapeutic Chemical classification):

Oxazepam (N05BA04), Lorazepam (N05BA06), Alprazolam (N05BA12), Clotiazepam (N05BA21), Estazolam (N05CD04), Lormetazepam (N05CD06), Loprazolam (N05CD11).
- Z-drugs (ATC classification): Zopiclone (N05CF01), Zolpidem (N05CF02).
- Other (ATC classification): Hydroxyzine (N05BB01), Captodiame (N05BB02), Buspirone (N05BE01), Etifoxine (N05BX03), Alimemazine (R06AD01), Doxylamine (R06AA09), Promethazine (R06AD02).

SH initiation: prescription (systematic or "as needed") of at least one SH of the above-mentioned list in patients for whom there was no mention of SH in the list of "medications taken before hospitalization" section of their hospitalization report (this section being completed by the physician based on the latest available prescription from primary care before hospitalization).

Secondary outcomes

- SH prescription renewal at discharge among patients who had initiated this medication during their stay. SH prescription renewal was defined as the mention of prescription of any bedtime SH at discharge on the hospitalization report (either the same as the one prescribed during the stay or another, either systematic or as needed).
- Potential risk factors for SH initiation:
  Risk factors related to patient characteristics: age, gender, patients' type of admission (from home, emergency unit or transfer from another acute care unit), reason for admission as indicated by the physician in the hospitalization report, number of medications taken before hospitalization (total number of active ingredients, including oral, parenteral and topical route, over-the-counter medication, excluding homeopathy and phytotherapy), type of room (single or double) during the stay, medical specialty (internal medicine or geriatric unit).
  Risk factors related to hospital organization: type of hospital (general hospital, teaching hospital, non-profit private hospital, private clinic), number of patients per nurse at night, number of patients per nursing assistant at night.
- Potential risk factors for SH prescription renewal at discharge among patients who initiated this medication during their stay:
  Risk factors related to patients' characteristics: age, gender, length of stay, main reason for admission, time between admission and SH initiation, type of discharge (to home, nursing home, rehabilitation facilities).
  Risk factors related to hospital organization: pharmaceutical review of prescriptions during the stay (pharmaceutical review defined as technical review of the list of patient's medications (level 1) or review of medications with patient's full note (level 2) by the pharmacist [24]).

Statistical analysis

Descriptive analysis: results are presented as mean and standard deviation (sd) or median with interquartile range [IQR] for continuous variables and as absolute number and percentage (%) for categorical variables.

The graphical representation of SH initiation cumulative incidence was performed with the Kaplan Meier approach.

Risk factors for SH initiation: a time to event analysis was performed. Time to event was defined as the duration between hospital admission and the date of SH initiation or date of discharge if no SH initiation. The log-linearity of continuous variables was checked; covariates violating this assumption were transformed into categorical covariates. Proportional hazards assumption was checked plotting the scaled Schoenfeld residuals. Bivariable relationship between each potential risk factor and time to SH initiation was analyzed using a Cox model. Results are presented as Hazard Ratio (HR) and 95% Confidence Interval (CI). Covariates with a p value ≤ 0.20 (log rank test) were entered in the multivariate Cox regression model. A p value < 0.05 (likelihood ratio test) in the multivariate model was considered significant.

Risk factors for SH renewal at discharge: In all analyses, the population was stratified based on discharge disposition: home or rehabilitation facilities. Bivariate analyses were performed with the Wilcoxon-Mann Whitney test or the Student test for quantitative variables and the Chi-squared test or the Fisher's exact test for categorical variables, according to validity conditions of these tests. Variables with a p value ≤ 0.20 were included in the logistic regression model with a random center effect. To avoid convergence failure in the logistic regression model and to respect the assumption of having at least 5 to 10 events per variable, variables having a large number of categories and a very small number of cases within some categories (thus leading to complete or quasi complete separation) were re-scaled with a smaller number of categories. Important variables were forced into the model according to their clinical significance when the p value was ≥ 0.20. Results are presented as Odds Ratio (OR) and 95% Confidence Interval (CI). P values < 0.05 in the logistic regression model were considered statistically significant.

All analyses were performed using R software (version 3.1.2).

Results

Study population

Major baseline characteristics of patients are presented in Table 1. Among the 3202 patients admitted to the twelve units during the study period, 2315 were aged 65 and older and 1194 were included in the study. The flowchart with reasons for exclusion is presented in Fig. 1. The mean age of patients was 83.8 ± 8.3 years, 702 were women (58.8%). The mean length of stay was 11.4 ± 7.7 days. The mean number of medications taken before hospitalization was 6.0 ± 3.4. Regarding psychotropic medications taken before hospitalization other than SHs, 19.4% of patients had an antidepressant ($n = 232$), 3.8% had a medication indicated in Alzheimer's disease ($n = 45$), 2.6% had an antipsychotic ($n = 31$) and 1.9% ($n = 23$) had a major opioid analgesic (morphine, oxycodone, fentanyl).

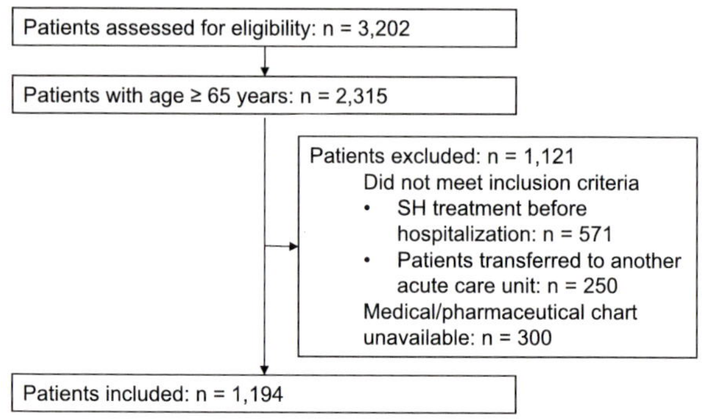

Fig. 1 Study flowchart. Legend: SH: Sedative-Hypnotic

Sedative-hypnotic initiation

The median hospitalization duration was 10 days [9-10]. The cumulative incidence of SH initiation is presented in Fig. 2 with a focus on day 0 to day 20 of hospitalization since no initiation occurred after 20 days (maximum duration of hospitalizatio$n = 77$ days). The cumulative incidence of SH initiation two days after admission was 9.4%. It raised to 11.5% 4 days after admission and 21.5% 20 days after admission. The most commonly prescribed SHs were z-drugs ($n = 116$, 62.7%), short half-life BZDs ($n = 38$, 20.5%), hydroxyzine ($n = 24$, 13.0%) and long half-life BZDs ($n = 7$, 3.8%). The SH was prescribed as needed in 42.2% of cases ($n = 78$).

Table 1 Patients' baseline characteristics ($n = 1194$)

Characteristics	Value
Demographic	
Age, mean ± standard deviation (years)	83.8 ± 8.3
80–89 years old, n (%)	522 (43.7)
≥ 90 years old, n (%)	351 (29.4)
Women, n (%)	702 (58.8)
Type of health facility, n (%)	
Teaching hospital	618 (51.8)
General hospital	262 (21.9)
Non-profit private hospital	228 (19.1)
Private clinic	86 (7.2)
Type of hospitalization unit, n (%)	
Geriatric unit	588 (49.2)
Internal medicine unit	606 (50.8)
Reason for admission, n (%)	
Cardiopulmonary disease	238 (19.9)
Fall	192 (16.1)
Infectious disease	161 (13.5)
Altered General state	139 (11.6)
Neurological disorder	133 (11.1)
Other	331 (27.7)

Risk factors for SH initiation during hospitalization

Bivariate relationship between each potential risk factor and time to initiation is presented in Additional file 3. Two variables were associated ($p \leq 0.20$) with the initiation of a SH during the stay: number of medications before admission (HR = 1.04, 95%CI [1.00–1.08], $p = 0.06$] and number of patients per nursing assistant at night ($HR_{21-40\ patients} = 1.23$, 95%CI [0.90–1.68], $p = 0.20$). However, in the multivariable Cox model regression, neither the number of medications before admission (HR = 1.04, 95%CI [1.00–1.09], $p = 0.05$) nor the number of patients per nursing assistant (HR = 1.25, 95%CI [0.91–1.70], $p = 0.17$) remained significantly associated with SH initiation.

Sedative-hypnotic renewal at discharge

Proportion of sedative-hypnotic prescription renewal at discharge

Considering the global population ($n = 1194$), 7.0% of patients aged 65 and older had an initial SH prescription

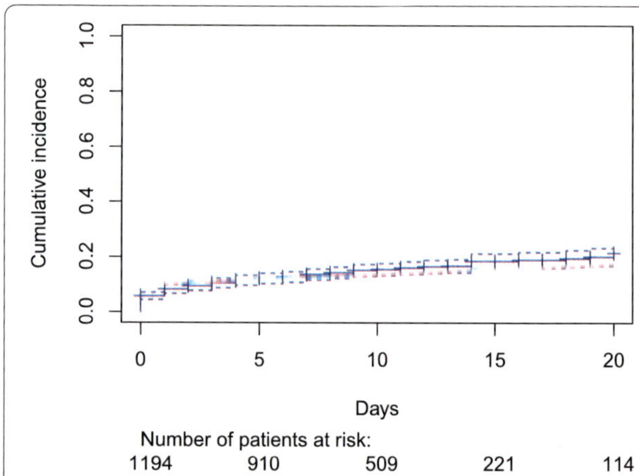

Fig. 2 Kaplan Meier graphical representation of SH initiation cumulative incidence. Legend: SH: Sedative-Hypnotic

in the hospital and were discharged home with it. Focusing on patients aged 65 and older who initiated a SH during their hospitalization ($n = 185$), the proportion of SH prescription renewal at discharge was 44.9% ($n = 83$). When stratifying the population based on discharge disposition, the proportion of SH renewal at discharge was 38.7% in patients discharged home ($n = 46/119$) and 56.0% in patients discharged to rehabilitation facilities ($n = 37/66$). Among patients discharged home, SH renewal reached 42.2% ($n = 35/83$) in patients aged 80 and older and 38.9% ($n = 14/36$) in patients aged 90 and older. Among patients discharged to rehabilitation facilities, SH renewal reached 53.8% ($n = 28/52$) in patients aged 80 and older and 50.0% ($n = 12/24$) in patients aged 90 and older.

Risk factors for SH prescription renewal at discharge

Patients discharged home The length of stay was the only variable associated with the renewal of SH prescription at discharge in the bivariate analysis ($p = 0.10$) (detailed results in Additional file 4). In the logistic regression with random center effect, this variable was not associated anymore with the renewal of SH prescription at discharge. Detailed results are presented in Table 2.

Patients discharged to rehabilitation facilities

In this population, the time between admission and SH initiation was the only variable associated with the renewal of SH prescription at discharge in the bivariate analysis (detailed results in Additional file 4). The main result of the logistic regression with random center effect is that when the SH was initiated after the first six days of hospitalization, patients were less likely to be prescribed a SH at discharge (OR = 0.19, 95%CI: [0.04–0.80], $p = 0.02$). Detailed results are presented in Table 3.

Discussion

Key results

This multicenter study assessed SH initiation and prescription renewal at discharge among older adults hospitalized in six geriatric units and six internal medicine units in France. Four days after admission, the cumulative incidence of SH initiation was 11.5%. It raised to 21.5% 20 days after admission. This is in the range of findings from other studies reporting an initiation of SH for 8.3 to 44.6% of hospitalized patients, all ages combined between 1996 and 2014 in Australia, Belgium, Canada, France, Israel and the USA [15–21]. In 83.2% of cases, the SH initiated was a z-drug or a short half-life benzodiazepine, thus in agreement with international guidelines [25, 26]. This is only partly reassuring since these drugs also have a high potential for ADE such as falls [27–29]. The persistence of hydroxyzine and long half-life benzodiazepine prescriptions for 16.8% of patients is also a matter of concern, reflecting a misreading of recommendations and potential ADE related to these drugs.

Table 2 Risk factors for SH prescription renewal among older patients who had an initiation and were discharged home

Variable	OR [95% CI]	*P* value
Length of stay		
≤ 7 days[a]	1	
8–14 days	1.30 [0.49–3.46]	0.59
> 14 days	2.33 [0.84–6.50]	0.10

OR: Odds Ratio (logistic regression with random effect at the center level); *CI*: Confidence Interval; [a]Reference category; *SH*: Sedative-hypnotics

Table 3 Risk factors for SH prescription renewal among older patients who had an initiation and were discharged to rehabilitation facilities

Variable	OR [95% CI]	*P* value
Time between admission and SH initiation		
≤ 2 days[a]	1	
3–6 days	0.28 [0.05–1.55]	0.14
> 6 days	0.19 [0.04–0.80]	0.02

OR: Odds Ratio (logistic regression with random effect at the center level); *CI*: Confidence Interval; [a]Reference category; *SH*: Sedative-hypnotics

Another important finding of this study is that the initiation occurred during the first 48 h of hospitalization for 50% of patients, with only 42.2% of prescriptions with the mention "as needed", suggesting systematic prescriptions at the acute phase of the hospitalization rather than rational prescriptions after non-pharmacological options attempts (e.g. noise and pain control).

This study also addressed the crucial point of SH prescription management at discharge for older patients who initiated this medication during hospitalization. The proportion of SH prescription renewal at discharge achieved 38.7% in patients discharged home and 56.0% in patients discharged to rehabilitation facilities. This is a particularly high proportion compared to two other French studies (population: adult inpatients all ages), one Australian study (population: adult inpatients all ages) and one Canadian study (population: adult aged 65 and over) who reported a proportion of renewal at discharge comprised between 10.1 and 35.7% [16, 18, 19, 22]. According to Zisberg et al., about one third of post-discharge new SH users had the first prescription of it during hospital stay, making hospitalization a turning point for new SH use in older people [20]. This makes our results even more alarming, considering the high cumulative incidence of SH initiation during hospital stay. Moreover, our results show that the final proportion of patients discharged with a new SH prescription comes to 7%, which is considerable compared to the proportion of SH initiation reported by the National French Health Insurance for the community in 2015 that was 1.2% [2].

Beyond these results, identifying specific risk factors for SH initiation and renewal prescription at discharge was of first importance to understand the situation and propose targeted actions to improve it. In our study, the number of medications taken before hospitalization was not significantly associated with an increased risk of SH initiation. However, the HR was 1.04 with a 95% CI comprised between 1.00 and 1.09 ($p = 0.05$). This tends to be in agreement with literature data that report polypharmacy as a risk factor for SH initiation during hospitalization [15, 18]. However, this is of particular concern since these patients are the most at risk for severe ADE. On the contrary, we found no effect of gender, patient type of hospitalization, whereas two studies found an increased risk for women and for patients not coming from home [15, 18].

Surprisingly, none of the following parameters: type of room, number of patients per nurse or per nursing assistant or type of unit (geriatric vs internal medicine) influenced the risk of SH initiation.

Regarding the risk of SH prescription renewal at discharge, a specific attention should be paid to patients discharged to rehabilitation facilities. In this population, the proportion of SH renewal at discharge reached 56.0% whereas it was 38.7% in patients discharged home. This could be explained by the fact that prescriptions may not be as carefully revised as for patients discharged to home. This could also be explained by the fact that unlike patients discharged home that are supposed to recover normal sleep conditions, factors responsible for sleep disorders are expected to persist in patients discharged to rehabilitation facilities [30]. If no specific risk factor could be highlighted for SH renewal at discharge in patients discharged home, an initiation of SH occurring after the first six days of hospitalization was protective (OR = 0.19, 95%CI [0.04–0.80], $p = 0.02$) in patients discharged to rehabilitation facilities. One hypothesis is that, compared to prescriptions occurring during the first two days, the benefit/risk ratio of a SH prescription occurring after the first six days has been well weighed and prescribers are more aware of proper use rules of these medications. Another hypothesis is that the initiation occurred so close to discharge that it was a very punctual prescription and that renewal at discharge was unnecessary. Further prospective studies are needed to underpin these hypotheses. Pharmaceutical review of prescriptions had no influence on renewal at discharge. This may be due to the fact that it only addressed prescriptions during the stay and was not followed up with discharge medication reconciliation by the pharmacist to alert on the risk of SH renewal at discharge.

Strengths, generalizability and limitations

This study has several strengths: in addition to the large sample size, it addressed different types of hospitals and was implemented in a large geographical area, reflecting an important socio-economic diversity. To our knowledge, this is the first multicenter study to specifically address the cumulative incidence of SH initiation and the proportion of prescription renewal at discharge in hospitalized older patients in France. At the international level, this is also one of the first studies to address risk factors related to hospital organization for SH initiation and renewal at discharge.

However, some limitations must be discussed. First, the retrospective design prevented us from collecting data such as more precise socio-economic characteristics of patients, comorbidities, degree of insomnia, number of SH intakes for patients with "as needed" prescriptions, grade of the prescriber (junior/senior), and precise reason for SH prescription. The lack of comorbidity reporting and precise reason for SH prescription could have led us to overestimate the cumulative incidence of SH initiation since bedtime SHs may have been prescribed to treat anxiety or agitation more than insomnia itself in some cases. However, 62.7% of SHs initiated were z-drugs which are exclusively prescribed in insomnia disorders. Regarding benzodiazepines and antihistamines that can have two indications, the fact that we only considered the one that were prescribed at bedtime exclusively should have limited the risk of classification bias. The fact that 300 potentially eligible patients could not be included due to missing hospitalization report is also a limitation but it is unlikely that the fact that the report was missing was associated with the initiation of SH. The use of the hospitalization report, which is known to slightly underestimate medications taken, to collect history of SH medication before hospitalization could also have led us to overestimate the proportion of patients considered as formerly free from SHs, depending on the quality of charts and patients' accuracy regarding self-medication reporting. However, as mentioned in the method, the pilot study allowed us to assess this point and showed that the quality of hospitalization reports was sufficient to consider these reports as data sources. Similarly, the fact that 42.2% of SHs initiated were prescribed "as needed" (thus maybe never administered) is potentially another source of overstatement of the actual SH initiation cumulative incidence. Further prospective studies monitoring all these factors are thus needed to confirm our results. Regarding SH renewal at discharge, our objective was to explore risk factors related to patients' characteristics and hospital organization that were associated with it. Therefore, we did not investigate the impact of these discharge prescriptions on long term consumption of SH: number of refills, adverse events, re-hospitalization for example. Further studies based on the French Health Insurance databases should help us to obtain these data that address the period post discharge and to provide more detailed results.

Conclusions

This study highlighted that hospitalization is a period at risk for SH initiation in older patients and that the renewal of SHs on discharge prescriptions affected more than half of the patients who initiated this medication during their stay and were discharged to rehabilitation facilities and more than one third of patients discharged home. As recommended by the FHA, the promotion of SH good use should thus be implemented in hospital setting and at the time of discharge. In addition to awareness campaigns directed towards general practitioners in the community, interventions should be implemented in hospitals to reduce both SH initiation and prescription renewal at discharge. If this study did not lead to the detection of specific risk factors regarding SH initiation during hospitalization, it did however highlight that a specific attention should be paid to patients discharged to rehabilitation facilities.

Additional files

Additional file 1: Data collection grid (patient characteristics). Collection grid for data related to patient characteristics and medications taken before, during and after hospitalization.

Additional file 2: Data collection grid (hospital organization). Collection grid for data related to hospital organization.

Additional file 3: Risk factors for sedative-hypnotic initiation among hospitalized patients aged 65 and older: bivariate analysis (Cox regression model). Risk factors for sedative-hypnotic initiation among hospitalized patients aged 65 and older: bivariate analysis (Cox regression model).

Additional file 4: Risk factors for sedative-hypnotic prescription renewal at discharge among hospitalized patients aged 65 and older who initiated a SH during their stay: bivariate analysis. Risk factors for sedative-hypnotic prescription renewal at discharge among hospitalized patients aged 65 and older who initiated a SH during their stay: bivariate analysis.

Abbreviations

ADE: Adverse Drug Event; ATC: Anatomical Therapeutic Chemical classification; BZD: Benzodiazepine; CI: Confidence Interval; FHA: French Health Authority; HR: Hazard Ratio; IQR: Interquartile Range; OR: Odds ratio; Sd: Standard deviation; SH: Sedative-Hypnotic

Acknowledgments

We gratefully acknowledge pharmacists, physicians and head nurses from the twelve centers for their participation to this study. The kind assistance of Stella Ghouti, qualified translator is gratefully acknowledged.

Funding

No funding was received for this study. This study had no sponsor.

Authors' contributions

EBR: study concept and design, analysis and interpretation of data, drafted the article. ABK and LZB: data analysis. PHT, CFZ, ABE, DBZ, FTH: study concept and design, interpretation of data, revision of the manuscript for important intellectual content. All authors read and approved the final manuscript.

Competing interests

The authors declare that they have no competing interests.

Author details

[1]Sorbonne Université, INSERM, Institut Pierre Louis d'épidémiologie et de Santé Publique, IPLESP UMR-S1136, F-75012 Paris, France. [2]Assistance Publique – Hôpitaux de Paris, Hôpital Saint-Antoine, Service de Pharmacie, 184, rue du Faubourg Saint Antoine, F-75012 Paris, France. [3]Université Paris-Sud, Faculté de Pharmacie, 5, rue Jean-Baptiste Clément, F-92296 Chatenay-Malabry, France. [4]AP-HP, Hôpital Pitié-Salpêtrière, Département Biostatistique Santé Publique et Information Médicale, Centre de pharmacoépidémiologie (Céphépi), INSERM, CIC-P 1421, 75013 Paris, France. [5]AP-HP, Hôpital Pitié-Salpêtrière, Centre de pharmacoépidémiologie (Céphépi), INSERM, UMR 1123, CIC-P 1421, 75013 Paris, France. [6]Observatoire du Médicament des Dispositifs Médicaux et de l'Innovation Thérapeutique Ile de France, Paris, France. [7]Sorbonne Université, Faculté de médecine Sorbonne Université, AP-HP, Hôpital Pitié-Salpêtrière, Département Biostatistique Santé Publique et Information Médicale, Centre de pharmacoépidémiologie (Céphépi), INSERM, UMR 1123, CIC-P 1421, 75013 Paris, France.

References

1. International Narcotics Control Board: Psychotropic Substances. Statistics for 2015. 2016.https://www.incb.org/documents/Psychotropics/technical-publications/2016/Technical_Publication_2016.pdf. Accessed 24 Nov 2017.
2. ANSM: État des lieux de la consommation des benzodiazépines en France. 2017.http://ansm.sante.fr/S-informer/Points-d-information-Points-d-information/Etat-des-lieux-de-la-consommation-des-benzodiazepines-Point-d-Information. Accessed 4 Jan 2018.
3. ANSM: Etat des lieux de la consommation des benzodiazépines en France (online). 2013.http://ansm.sante.fr/var/ansm_site/storage/original/application/3e06749ae5a50cb7ae80fb655dee103a.pdf. Accessed 4 jan 2018.
4. Glass J, Lanctot KL, Herrmann N, Sproule BA, Busto UE. Sedative hypnotics in older people with insomnia: meta-analysis of risks and benefits. BMJ. 2005;331(7526):1169.
5. Airagnes G, Pelissolo A, Lavallee M, Flament M, Limosin F. Benzodiazepine misuse in the elderly: risk factors, consequences, and Management. Curr Psychiatry Rep. 2016;18(10):89.
6. Billioti de Gage S, Pariente A, Begaud B. Is there really a link between benzodiazepine use and the risk of dementia? Expert Opin Drug Saf. 2015; 14(5):733–47.
7. Kaufmann CN, Spira AP, Alexander GC, Rutkow L, Mojtabai R. Emergency department visits involving benzodiazepines and non-benzodiazepine receptor agonists. Am J of Emerg Med. 2017;35(10):1414–9.
8. Shash D, Kurth T, Bertrand M, Dufouil C, Barberger-Gateau P, Berr C, et al. Benzodiazepine, psychotropic medication, and dementia: a population-based cohort study. Alzheimers Dement. 2015;12(5):604–13.
9. Billioti de Gage S, Moride Y, Ducruet T, Kurth T, Verdoux H, Tournier M, et al. Benzodiazepine use and risk of Alzheimer's disease: case-control study. BMJ. 2014;349:g5205.
10. American Geriatrics Society. American Geriatrics Society 2015 updated beers criteria for potentially inappropriate medication use in older adults. JAGS. 2015;63(11):2227–46.
11. O'Mahony D, O'Sullivan D, Byrne S, O'Connor MN, Ryan C, Gallagher P. STOPP/START criteria for potentially inappropriate prescribing in older people: version 2. Age Ageing. 2015;44(2):213–8.
12. Renom-Guiteras A, Meyer G, Thurmann PA. The EU (7)-PIM list: a list of potentially inappropriate medications for older people consented by experts from seven European countries. Eur J Clin Pharmacol. 2015;71(7):861–75.
13. Isaia G, Corsinovi L, Bo M, Santos-Pereira P, Michelis G, Aimonino N, et al. Insomnia among hospitalized elderly patients: prevalence, clinical characteristics and risk factors. Arch Gerontol Geriatr. 2011;52(2):133–7.
14. Enomoto M, Tsutsui T, Higashino S, Otaga M, Higuchi S, Aritake S, et al. Sleep-related problems and use of hypnotics in inpatients of acute hospital wards. Gen Hosp Psychiatry. 2010;32(3):276–83.
15. Somers A, Robays H, Audenaert K, Van Maele G, Bogaert M, Petrovic M. The use of hypnosedative drugs in a university hospital: has anything changed in 10 years? Eur J Clin Pharmacol. 2011;67(7):723–9.

16. Fagnoni P, Limat S, Haffen E, Henon T, Jacquet M, Sechter D, et al. Does hospitalisation affect hypnotic and anxiolytic drug prescribing? Pharm World Sci. 2007;29(6):611–8.
17. Frighetto L, Marra C, Bandali S, Wilbur K, Naumann T, Jewesson P. An assessment of quality of sleep and the use of drugs with sedating properties in hospitalized adult patients. Health Qual Life Outcomes. 2004;2:17.
18. Lagnaoui R, Moore N, Longy-Boursier M, Baumevieille M, Begaud B. Benzodiazepine use in patients hospitalized in a department of internal medicine: frequency and clinical correlates. Pharmacoepidemiol Drug Saf. 2001;10(6):531–5.
19. Howes JB, Ryan J, Fairbrother G, O'Neill K, Howes LG. Benzodiazepine prescribing in a Sydney teaching hospital. Med J Aust. 1996;165(6):305–8.
20. Zisberg A, Shadmi E, Sinoff G, Gur-Yaish N, Srulovici E, Shochat T. Hospitalization as a turning point for sleep medication use in older adults: prospective cohort study. Drugs Aging. 2012;29(7):565–76.
21. Gillis CM, Poyant JO, Degrado JR, Ye L, Anger KE, Owens RL. Inpatient pharmacological sleep aid utilization is common at a tertiary medical center. J Hosp Med. 2014;9(10):652–7.
22. Pek EA, Remfry A, Pendrith C, Fan-Lun C, Bhatia RS, Soong C. High prevalence of inappropriate benzodiazepine and sedative hypnotic prescriptions among hospitalized older adults. J Hosp Med. 2017;12(5):310–6.
23. Cohen J. A coefficient of agreement for nominal scales. Educ Psychol Meas. 1960;20(1):37–46.
24. Geurts MM, Talsma J, Brouwers JR, de Gier JJ. Medication review and reconciliation with cooperation between pharmacist and general practitioner and the benefit for the patient: a systematic review. Br J Clin Pharmacoll. 2012;74(1):16–33.
25. Riemann D, Baglioni C, Bassetti C, Bjorvatn B, Dolenc Groselj L, Ellis JG, et al. European guideline for the diagnosis and treatment of insomnia. J Sleep Res. 2017;26(6):675–700.
26. Sateia MJ, Buysse DJ, Krystal AD, Neubauer DN, Heald JL. Clinical practice guideline for the pharmacologic treatment of chronic insomnia in adults: an American Academy of sleep medicine clinical practice guideline. J Clin Sleep Med. 2017;13(2):307–49.
27. Wang PS, Bohn RL, Glynn RJ, Mogun H, Avorn J. Hazardous benzodiazepine regimens in the elderly: effects of half-life, dosage, and duration on risk of hip fracture. Am J Psychiatry. 2001;158(6):892–8.
28. Wang PS, Bohn RL, Glynn RJ, Mogun H, Avorn J. Zolpidem use and hip fractures in older people. JAGS. 2001;49(12):1685–90.
29. Landi F, Onder G, Cesari M, Barillaro C, Russo A, Bernabei R. Psychotropic medications and risk for falls among community-dwelling frail older people: an observational study. J Gerontol A Biol Sci Med Sci. 2005;60(5):622–6.
30. Martin JL, Jouldjian S, Mitchell MN, Josephson KR, Alessi CA. A longitudinal study of poor sleep after inpatient post-acute rehabilitation: the role of depression and pre-illness sleep quality. Am J Geriatr Psychiatry. 2012;20(6):477–84.

Permissions

All chapters in this book were first published in GERIATRICS, by BioMed Central; hereby published with permission under the Creative Commons Attribution License or equivalent. Every chapter published in this book has been scrutinized by our experts. Their significance has been extensively debated. The topics covered herein carry significant findings which will fuel the growth of the discipline. They may even be implemented as practical applications or may be referred to as a beginning point for another development.

The contributors of this book come from diverse backgrounds, making this book a truly international effort. This book will bring forth new frontiers with its revolutionizing research information and detailed analysis of the nascent developments around the world.

We would like to thank all the contributing authors for lending their expertise to make the book truly unique. They have played a crucial role in the development of this book. Without their invaluable contributions this book wouldn't have been possible. They have made vital efforts to compile up to date information on the varied aspects of this subject to make this book a valuable addition to the collection of many professionals and students.

This book was conceptualized with the vision of imparting up-to-date information and advanced data in this field. To ensure the same, a matchless editorial board was set up. Every individual on the board went through rigorous rounds of assessment to prove their worth. After which they invested a large part of their time researching and compiling the most relevant data for our readers.

The editorial board has been involved in producing this book since its inception. They have spent rigorous hours researching and exploring the diverse topics which have resulted in the successful publishing of this book. They have passed on their knowledge of decades through this book. To expedite this challenging task, the publisher supported the team at every step. A small team of assistant editors was also appointed to further simplify the editing procedure and attain best results for the readers.

Apart from the editorial board, the designing team has also invested a significant amount of their time in understanding the subject and creating the most relevant covers. They scrutinized every image to scout for the most suitable representation of the subject and create an appropriate cover for the book.

The publishing team has been an ardent support to the editorial, designing and production team. Their endless efforts to recruit the best for this project, has resulted in the accomplishment of this book. They are a veteran in the field of academics and their pool of knowledge is as vast as their experience in printing. Their expertise and guidance has proved useful at every step. Their uncompromising quality standards have made this book an exceptional effort. Their encouragement from time to time has been an inspiration for everyone.

The publisher and the editorial board hope that this book will prove to be a valuable piece of knowledge for researchers, students, practitioners and scholars across the globe.

List of Contributors

Dries Debeer
University of Zurich, Binzmuehlestr, 14, 8050 Zurich, Switzerland

Andreas Maercker
University of Zurich, Binzmuehlestr, 14, 8050 Zurich, Switzerland
University Research Priority Program "Dynamics of Healthy Aging", University of Zurich, Zurich, Switzerland

Simon Forstmeier
University of Zurich, Binzmuehlestr, 14, 8050 Zurich, Switzerland
University of Siegen, Faculty II, Developmental Psychology, Adolf-Reichwein-Str. 2, 57068 Siegen, Germany

Myriam V. Thoma
University of Zurich, Binzmuehlestr, 14, 8050 Zurich, Switzerland
University Research Priority Program "Dynamics of Healthy Aging", University of Zurich, Zurich, Switzerland
Psychopathology and Clinical Intervention, University of Zurich, Binzmuehlestr. 14/17, CH-8050 Zurich, Switzerland

Roger Schmid
Psychiatrische Klinik Zugersee, Zug, Switzerland

Oliver Kellner
Integrierte Psychiatrie Winterthur, Winterthur, Switzerland.
Present Address: Alterspsychiatrische Praxis, Buehlach, Switzerland

Franziskos Xepapadakos
Clienia Schloessli AG, Oetwil am See, Switzerland

Ursula Schreiter Gasser
Praxis für Psychiatrie Rehalp, Zurich, Switzerland

Andreas Blessing
Psychiatrische Dienste Thurgau, Muensterlingen, Switzerland

Axel Ropohl
Sanatorium Kilchberg AG, Kilchberg, Switzerland
Present Address: KMG – Kompetenz mentale Gesundheit GmbH, Baar, Switzerland

Gabriela Bieri-Brüning
Geriatric service of the city of Zurich, Zurich, Switzerland

Lourdes Moral-Fernández, Antonio Frías-Osuna, Sara Moreno-Cámara, Pedro A. Palomino-Moral and Rafael Del-Pino-Casado
Department of Nursing, School of Health Sciences, University of Jaén, Campus Las Lagunillas, s/n, 23071 Jaén, Spain

Hannah M. O'Rourke
Faculty of Nursing Level 3, Edmonton Clinic Health Academy, University of Alberta, 11405-87 Avenue, Edmonton, Alberta T6G 1C9, Canada

Laura Collins and Souraya Sidani
Daphne Cockwell School of Nursing, Ryerson University, 350 Victoria Street, Toronto, ON M5B 2K3, Canada

Jing Yang, Fei Wang, Jing Wang, Xu Han, Hua Hu, Caizheng Yu, Jing Yuan, Ping Yao, Youjie Wang, Weihong Chen, Yuan Liang, Huan Guo, Xiaomin Zhang, Dan Zheng, Yuhan Tang and Meian He
Department of Occupational and Environmental Health and State Key Laboratory of Environmental Health for Incubating, School of Public Health, Tongji Medical College, Huazhong University of Science and Technology, 13 Hangkong Rd, Wuhan 430030, Hubei, China

Xiaoping Miao and Sheng Wei
Department of Epidemiology and Biostatistics, School of Public Health, Tongji Medical College, Huazhong University of Science and Technology, Wuhan, China

Handong Yang
Dongfeng Central Hospital, Dongfeng Motor Corporation and Hubei University of Medicine, Shiyan, Hubei, China

Fiona Höbler
Toronto Rehabilitation Institute-University Health Network, 130 Dunn Ave, Toronto M6K 2R7, Canada

Rehabilitation Sciences Institute, University of Toronto, Toronto, ON, Canada

Katherine S. McGilton
Toronto Rehabilitation Institute-University Health Network, 130 Dunn Ave, Toronto M6K 2R7, Canada
Lawrence S. Bloomberg Faculty of Nursing, University of Toronto, 130 Dunn Ave, Toronto M6K 2R7, Canada

Astrid Escrig-Pinol
Toronto Rehabilitation Institute-University Health Network, 130 Dunn Ave, Toronto M6K 2R7, Canada
Dalla Lana School of Public Health, University of Toronto, Toronto, ON, Canada

Xochil Argueta-Warden
Lawrence S. Bloomberg Faculty of Nursing, University of Toronto, 130 Dunn Ave, Toronto M6K 2R7, Canada

Miriam Rodríguez-Monforte
FCS Blanquerna-Universitat Ramon Llull, Carrer de Padilla, 326-332, 08025 Barcelona, Spain

Walter Wittich
School of Optometry, Université de Montréal, 3744, rue Jean-Brillant, 260-7, Montréal, Québec H3T 1P1, Canada
CRIR/Centre de réadaptation MAB-Mackay du CIUSSS du Centre-Ouest-de-l'Île-de-Montréal, Montréal, Québec, Canada
CRIR/Institut Nazareth et Louis-Braille du CISSS de la Montérégie-Centre, Longueuil, Québec, Canada

Francesca Cecchi, Silvia Pancani, Desiderio Antonioli, Lucia Avila, Manuele Barilli, Massimo Gambini, Lucilla Landucci Pellegrini, Emanuela Romano, Chiara Sarti, Margherita Zingoni, Maria Assunta Gabrielli, Federica Vannetti and Guido Pasquini
Don Carlo Gnocchi Foundation, IRCSS, Via di Scandicci, 269, 50143 Florence, Italy

Claudio Macchi
Don Carlo Gnocchi Foundation, IRCSS, Via di Scandicci, 269, 50143 Florence, Italy
Department of Experimental and Clinical Medicine, University of Florence, Florence, Italy

Ana Rivera-Almaraz, Betty Manrique-Espinoza and Aarón Salinas-Rodríguez
National Institute of Public Health, Avenida Universidad #655, Colonia Santa María Ahuacatitlán, ZC, 62100 Cuernavaca, Morelos, Mexico

José Alberto Ávila-Funes
Department of Geriatrics, Salvador Zubirán National Institute of Medical Sciences and Nutrition, Mexico City, Mexico

Somnath Chatterji and Nirmala Naidoo
Department of Health Statistics and Information Systems, World Health Organization, Geneva, Switzerland

Paul Kowal
Department of Health Statistics and Information Systems, World Health Organization, Geneva, Switzerland
University of Newcastle Research Centre on Gender, Health and Ageing, Newcastle, Australia
Chiang Mai University Research Institute for Health Sciences, Chiang Mai, Thailand

Gabrielle Lindsay-Smith and Grant O'Sullivan
Institute for Health and Sport, Victoria University, Melbourne, Australia

Rochelle Eime and Jack Harvey
Institute for Health and Sport, Victoria University, Melbourne, Australia
School of Health and Life Sciences, Federation University, Ballarat, Australia

Jannique G. Z. van Uffelen
Institute for Health and Sport, Victoria University, Melbourne, Australia
Department of Movement Sciences, Physical Activity, Sports and Health Research Group, KU Leuven - University of Leuven, Leuven, Belgium

Esther Katharina Kiesel and Yvonne Marina Hopf
Department of Pharmacy, University Hospital, LMU Munich, Munich, Germany

Michael Drey
Department of Medicine IV, University Hospital, LMU Munich, Munich, Germany

François Béland
Groupe de recherche Solidage, CSSS de la Montagne, site Metro, 1801, boulevard de Maisonneuve Ouest, bureau 600, Montréal, Québec H3H 1J9, Canada

École de santé publique, Département d'administration de la santé, Université de Montréal, C.P. 6128, succ. Centre-Ville, Montréal, Québec H3C 3J7, Canada
Faculté de médecine, Division de médecine gériatrique, Université McGill, Hôpital général juif, 3755, chemin de la Côte-Ste-Catherine, Montréal, Québec H3T 1E2, Canada

Dominic Julien
Groupe de recherche Solidage, CSSS de la Montagne, site Metro, 1801, boulevard de Maisonneuve Ouest, bureau 600, Montréal, Québec H3H 1J9, Canada
Département de psychologie, Université de Montréal, Pavillon Marie-Victorin, C. P. 6128, succ. Centre-Ville, Montréal, Québec H3C 3J7, Canada
Centre de recherche, Institut universitaire en santé mentale de Montréal, 7331, rue Hochelaga, Montréal, Québec H1N 3V2, Canada

Nathalie Bier and Louise Demers
Centre de recherche, Institut Universitaire de Gériatrie de Montréal, 4545, Chemin Queen Mary, Montréal, Québec H3W 1W5, Canada
Faculté de médecine, École de réadaptation, Université de Montréal, C.P. 6128, succ. Centre-Ville, Montréal, Québec H3C 3J7, Canada

Marie-Jeanne Kergoat
Centre de recherche, Institut Universitaire de Gériatrie de Montréal, 4545, Chemin Queen Mary, Montréal, Québec H3W 1W5, Canada
Faculté de médecine, Département de médecine, Université de Montréal, C.P. 6128, succ. Centre-Ville, Montréal, Québec H3C 3J7, Canada

Johanne Desrosiers
École de réadaptation, Faculté de médecine et des sciences de la santé, Université de Sherbrooke, 3001, 12e Avenue Nord, Sherbrooke, Québec J1H 5N4, Canada
Centre de recherche sur le vieillissement, Centre intégré universitaire de santé et de services sociaux de l'Estrie, Centre hospitalier universitaire de Sherbrooke, 1036, rue Belvédère Sud, Sherbrooke, Québec J1H 4C4, Canada

Xiaoming Zhang, Wenwu Zhang, Conghua Wang, Wuyuan Tao, Qingli Dou and Yunzhi Yang
Department of Emergency Medicine, the Baoan Hospital affiliated with Southern Medical University, People's Hospital of Baoan District of Shenzhen, No. 118, Longjing, Baoan District, Shenzhen 518101, China

Christian G. G. Schwab and Martin Nikolaus Dichter
German Center for Neurodegenerative Diseases (DZNE), Stockumer Straße 12, 58453 Witten, Germany
School of Nursing Science, Witten/Herdecke University, Stockumer Straße 12, 58453 Witten, Germany

Martin Berwig
Clinic for Cognitive Neurology, Medical Faculty, Leipzig University, Liebigstraße 16, 04103 Leipzig, Germany
German Center for Neurodegenerative Diseases (DZNE), Stockumer Straße 12, 58453 Witten, Germany

Antonio Lopez-Villegas
Social Involvement of Critical and Emergency Medicine, CTS-609 Research Group, Hospital de Poniente, Almeria, Spain
Division of Medicine, Nordland Hospital, Bodø, Norway
Institute of Clinical Medicine, Faculty of Health Sciences, University of Tromsø, Tromsø, Norway

Terje Enebakk and Hilde Thunhaug
Division of Medicine, Nordland Hospital, Bodø, Norway

Knut Tore Lappegård
Division of Medicine, Nordland Hospital, Bodø, Norway
Institute of Clinical Medicine, Faculty of Health Sciences, University of Tromsø, Tromsø, Norway

Daniel Catalan-Matamoros
Department of Journalism and Communication, Universidad Carlos III de Madrid, Calle Madrid 133, 28903 Getafe, Madrid, Spain
Health Sciences CTS-451 Research Group, University of Almeria, Almería, Spain

Remedios Lopez-Liria
Nursing Science, Physiotherapy and Medicine, Faculty of Health Sciences, University of Almeria, Almería, Spain

Prasun Chatterjee, Prakash Kumar, Ruchika Madan, Meenakshi Tyagi, Gaurav Desai, Preeti Chaudhary and Aparajit Ballav Dey
Department of Geriatric Medicine, All India Institute of Medical Sciences, New Delhi, India

Ramesh Kandel
Division of Geriatric Medicine, Patan Academy of Health Sciences, Patan, Nepal

Deepa Anil Kumar
Healthy Aging India, New Delhi, India

Maroof Ahmad Khan
Department of Biostatistics, All India Institute of Medical Sciences, New Delhi, India

Shyama Gupta
Corner Office Advisors, New Delhi, India

Kanika Grover
University of Manitoba, Winnipeg, Canada

Su-min Jeong and Seulggie Choi
Department of Family Medicine, Seoul National University Hospital, 101 Daehak-ro, Jongno-gu, Seoul, South Korea

Sang Min Park
Department of Family Medicine, Seoul National University Hospital, 101 Daehak-ro, Jongno-gu, Seoul, South Korea
Department of Biomedical Sciences, Seoul National University Graduate School, 101 Daehak-ro, Jongno-gu, Seoul, South Korea

Kyuwoong Kim and Sung Min Kim
Department of Biomedical Sciences, Seoul National University Graduate School, 101 Daehak-ro, Jongno-gu, Seoul, South Korea

Sujin Kim
Korea Institute for Health and Social Affairs, Sejong, South Korea

K. L. Abdullah
Department of Nursing Sciences, Faculty of Medicine, University of Malaya, Kuala Lumpur, Malaysia

H. D. W. T. Damayanthi
Department of Nursing Sciences, Faculty of Medicine, University of Malaya, Kuala Lumpur, Malaysia
Department of Nursing, Faculty of Allied Health Sciences, University of Peradeniya, Peradeniya, Sri Lanka

F. M. Moy
Julius Centre University of Malaya, Department of Social and Preventive Medicine, Faculty of Medicine, University of Malaya, Kuala Lumpur, Malaysia

S. D. Dharmaratne
Department of Community Medicine, Faculty of Medicine, University of Peradeniya, Peradeniya, Sri Lanka
Department of Family and Community Medicine, College of Medicine, University of Kentucky, Kentucky, USA
Department of Health Metric Sciences, School of Medicine, University of Washington, Seattle, USA

Helen R Lam, Kate Taylor, Ronald Chow, Henry Lam, Katija Bonin and Leigha Rowbottom
Sunnybrook Health Sciences Centre, University of Toronto, 2075 Bayview Avenue, Toronto, ON M4N 3M5, Canada

Selina Chow and Nathan Herrmann
Sunnybrook Health Sciences Centre, University of Toronto, 2075 Bayview Avenue, Toronto, ON M4N 3M5, Canada
Division of Geriatric Psychiatry, Sunnybrook Health Sciences Centre, University of Toronto, 2075 Bayview Avenue, Room FG19, Toronto, ON M4N 3M5, Canada

Richard Walker and Catherine Dotchin
Institute of Health and Society, Faculty of Medical Sciences, Newcastle University, Newcastle upon Tyne, UK
Northumbria Healthcare NHS Foundation Trust, North Tyneside General Hospital, North Shields, UK

Emma Grace Lewis
Institute of Health and Society, Faculty of Medical Sciences, Newcastle University, Newcastle upon Tyne, UK
Northumbria Healthcare NHS Foundation Trust, North Tyneside General Hospital, North Shields, UK
Education centre, North Tyneside General Hospital, Rake Lane, North Shields NE29 8NH, UK

Kate Howorth and William Gray
Northumbria Healthcare NHS Foundation Trust, North Tyneside General Hospital, North Shields, UK

Selina Coles
The Medical school, Faculty of Medical Sciences, Newcastle University, Newcastle upon Tyne, UK

John Kissima
Hai District Hospital, Boma Ng'ombe, Hai, Kilimanjaro, Tanzania

Sarah Urasa
Kilimanjaro Christian Medical Centre, Moshi, Kilimanjaro, Tanzania

Jepchirchir Kiplagat
Moi University, College of Health Sciences, School of Medicine, Nandi Road, Eldoret, Kenya
Academic Model Providing Access to Healthcare (AMPATH) Program, Moi Teaching and Referral Hospital Campus, Nandi Road, Eldoret, Kenya
The University of Witwatersrand, School of Public Health, 27 St Andrews Road, Parktown, Johannesburg 2193, South Africa

Susann Huschke
Graduate Entry Medical School, University of Limerick, Castletroy, Limerick V94 T9PX, Ireland
School of History, Anthropology, Philosophy and Politics, Queen's University Belfast, 25 University Square, Belfast BT7 1NN, UK

Ingela Thylén
Department of Cardiology and Department of Medical and Health Sciences, Division of Nursing Sciences, Linköping University, S-581 83 Linköping, Sweden

Anna Strömberg
Department of Cardiology and Department of Medical and Health Sciences, Division of Nursing Sciences, Linköping University, S-581 83 Linköping, Sweden
Sue and Bill Gross School of Nursing, University of California, Irvine, USA

Debra K. Moser
College of Nursing, University of Kentucky, Lexington, USA

Su Hwan Lee, Soo Jung Kim, Jin Hwa Lee, Jung Hyun Chang and Yon Ju Ryu
Division of Pulmonary and Critical Care Medicine, Department of Internal Medicine, College of Medicine, Ewha Womans University, Mokdong Hospital, 1071 Anyangcheon-ro, Yangcheon-gu, Seoul 07985, South Korea

Yoon Hee Choi
Department of Emergency Medicine, College of Medicine, Ewha Womans University, Mokdong Hospital, 1071 Anyangcheon-ro, Yangcheon-gu, Seoul 07985, South Korea

Tyler S. Bryant, Jimmy T. Le and Jennifer Schrack
Department of Epidemiology, Johns Hopkins Bloomberg School of Public Health, 615 N. Wolfe St, Baltimore, MD 21205, USA

Anthony J. Nastasi, Dorry L. Segev and Mara A. McAdams-DeMarco
Department of Epidemiology, Johns Hopkins Bloomberg School of Public Health, 615 N. Wolfe St, Baltimore, MD 21205, USA
Department of Surgery, Johns Hopkins School of Medicine, Baltimore, MD, USA

Hao Ying and Christine E. Haugen
Department of Surgery, Johns Hopkins School of Medicine, Baltimore, MD, USA

Marlís González Fernández
Department of Physical Medicine and Rehabilitation, Johns Hopkins University School of Medicine, Baltimore, MD, USA

Irma H. J. Everink, Jolanda C. M. van Haastregt and Gertrudis I. J. M. Kempen
Department of Health Services Research and Care and Public Health Research Institute (CAPHRI), Maastricht University, 6200, MD, Maastricht, The Netherlands

Jos M. G. A. Schols
Department of Health Services Research and Care and Public Health Research Institute (CAPHRI), Maastricht University, 6200, MD, Maastricht, The Netherlands
Department of Family Medicine and Care and Public Health Research Institute (CAPHRI), Maastricht University, 6200, MD, Maastricht, The Netherlands

Frans E. S. Tan
Department of Methodology and Statistics and Care and Public Health Research Institute (CAPHRI), Maastricht University, 6200, MD, Maastricht, The Netherlands

Gindo Tampubolon
Sociology and Cathie Marsh Institute for Social Research, University of Manchester, Humanities Bridgeford Street Building, Oxford Road, Manchester M13 9PL, UK

Asri Maharani
Division of Neuroscience and Experimental Psychology, School of Biological Sciences, Faculty of Biology, Medicine and Health, University of Manchester, Manchester Academic Health Science Centre, Manchester M13 9PL, UK

Elsa Bourcier, Christine Fernandez and Patrick Hindlet
Sorbonne Université, INSERM, Institut Pierre Louis d'épidémiologie et de Santé Publique, IPLESP UMR-S1136, F-75012 Paris, France
Assistance Publique - Hôpitaux de Paris, Hôpital Saint-Antoine, Service de Pharmacie, 184, rue du Faubourg Saint Antoine, F-75012 Paris, France
Université Paris-Sud, Faculté de Pharmacie, 5, rue Jean-Baptiste Clément, F-92296 Chatenay-Malabry, France

Adrien Borowik and Lucas Zerbib
Assistance Publique - Hôpitaux de Paris, Hôpital Saint-Antoine, Service de Pharmacie, 184, rue du Faubourg Saint Antoine, F-75012 Paris, France

Amandine Baptiste
AP-HP, Hôpital Pitié-Salpêtrière, Département Biostatistique Santé Publique et Information Médicale, Centre de pharmacoépidémiologie (Céphépi), INSERM, CIC-P 1421, 75013 Paris, France

Dominique Bonnet-Zamponi
AP-HP, Hôpital Pitié-Salpêtrière, Centre de pharmacoépidémiologie (Céphépi), INSERM, UMR 1123, CIC-P 1421, 75013 Paris, France
Observatoire du Médicament des Dispositifs Médicaux et de l'Innovation Thérapeutique Ile de France, Paris, France

Florence Tubach
Sorbonne Université, Faculté de medicine Sorbonne Université, AP-HP, Hôpital Pitié-Salpêtrière, Département Biostatistique Santé Publique et Information Médicale, Centre de pharmacoépidémiologie (Céphépi), INSERM, UMR 1123, CIC-P 1421, 75013 Paris, France

Index